AF842487

Brain and Spine Surgery in the Elderly

Moncef Berhouma • Pierre Krolak-Salmon
Editors

Brain and Spine Surgery in the Elderly

Springer

Editors
Moncef Berhouma
Department of Neurosurgery,
University Hospital of Lyon
Lyon
France

Pierre Krolak-Salmon
Hôpital des Charpennes
Hospices civils de Lyon
Villeurbanne
France

ISBN 978-3-319-40231-4 ISBN 978-3-319-40232-1 (eBook)
DOI 10.1007/978-3-319-40232-1

Library of Congress Control Number: 2017932549

© Springer International Publishing Switzerland 2017
This work is subject to copyright. All rights are reserved by the Publisher, whether the whole or part of the material is concerned, specifically the rights of translation, reprinting, reuse of illustrations, recitation, broadcasting, reproduction on microfilms or in any other physical way, and transmission or information storage and retrieval, electronic adaptation, computer software, or by similar or dissimilar methodology now known or hereafter developed.
The use of general descriptive names, registered names, trademarks, service marks, etc. in this publication does not imply, even in the absence of a specific statement, that such names are exempt from the relevant protective laws and regulations and therefore free for general use.
The publisher, the authors and the editors are safe to assume that the advice and information in this book are believed to be true and accurate at the date of publication. Neither the publisher nor the authors or the editors give a warranty, express or implied, with respect to the material contained herein or for any errors or omissions that may have been made.

Printed on acid-free paper

This Springer imprint is published by Springer Nature
The registered company is Springer International Publishing AG
The registered company address is: Gewerbestrasse 11, 6330 Cham, Switzerland

Foreword

Geriatric Neurosurgery: A New Dimension of Modernity

The concept and reality of brain and spinal surgery in elderly individuals presents a new dimension in the ever-evolving subspecialty disciplines of neurosurgery.

Neurosurgery as an idea is both the oldest and newest of man's surgical endeavors. Dating back thousands of years, cranial trephinations were undertaken for what we believe were both medical and spiritual purposes. For centuries, epidural procedures were attempted with modicum of success. The nineteenth century provided the fundamental tools of antisepsis and anesthesia that allowed "giant steps" forward. These developments combined with accumulated comprehension of neuroanatomy and physiology allowed pioneers such as Harvey Cushing to establish what was the "modern" era of neurosurgery defining a true surgical specialty in the early part of the twentieth century.

Many of us have lived through the striking "reinvention" of neurosurgery that began in 1980 with the emergence of specialization, subspecialization, interdisciplinary cross federalization and the development of the departments of neurosurgery that now may be comprised of scores of individuals in larger institutions. All of this has been fueled by technical advances in supporting relevant fields of active and interdisciplinary cross-fertilization.

The concept and "modern" practice of neurosurgery has and is undergoing a striking metamorphosis as the field evolves in response to relevant areas of technical and medical sciences. The terms "molecular and cellular neurosurgery," "minimally invasive surgery," "nanoneurosurgery," "radiosurgery," "neuro-restoration," "virtual surgery," etc., are part of our vernacular.

I entered what was called "neurosurgery" as a resident at Yale in 1966. Nothing could have been farther from our minds than the idea of geriatric neurosurgery. What a difference five plus decades have made! Modern imaging, refined anesthesia, concepts of minimal invasion, and emerging molecular and nano methods offer new opportunities for approaching pathologies of the human nervous system. General medical care as well as environmental and social factors now present new challenges associated with an aging population. Viewpoint is striking! attending to these individuals from a neurological viewpoint is striking! Aside from the conventional general neurosurgical catalog, issues of mentation and neuropsychiatric disorders offer a particular challenge. What role the neurosurgeon will play is being defined. But whatever is it, the concept of geriatric neurosurgery is a current opportunity and represents significant social need. We have many tools to meet the challenge!

Moncef Berhouma and Pierre Krolak-Salmon have provided a well-designed, focused text dealing with elements of this critical issue. I suspect that this will be regarded as seminal work as we approach this somewhat new and important patient group. We have had "pediatric neurosurgery." Now dimensions of "geriatric neurosurgery" will be a focal point of our neurosurgical specialty as both ends of the human life term present their particular demanding needs.

New Haven, CT, USA Michael L.J. Apuzzo, MD

Preface

As the ratio of elderly population (>65 years old) is obviously rising in the majority of western countries, caregivers and particularly physicians are facing specific pathologies. This demographic trend mainly results from the association of decreasing fertility rates and increasing life expectancy. In geriatrics and in other medical specialties, a geriatric subspecialty has been developed during the last two decades (neurogeriatrics, oncogeriatrics, cardiogeriatrics, etc.) to answer specific questions as the management and the decision-making processes are not similar to young adult patients. Specifically in neurosurgery, the management of elderly patients raises several medical and ethical issues particularly in the fields of intracerebral hemorrhage and brain tumors. Thus the decision-making process should mandatorily include a multidisciplinary board discussion encompassing at least neurosurgeons, neurologists, geriatricians, and anesthesiologists.

After exposing the "raison d'être" for geriatric neurosurgery based mainly on demographic data, the physiological changes of the aging nervous system, and the neurological evaluation of the elderly, this volume gathers core chapters from world-renowned specialists in their respective fields. For each disease, good practices and rationale of treatment are detailed and debated. The ethical considerations specific to this age group are thoroughly examined for each neurosurgical disease. In fine, the reviews herein presented should assist the caregivers and particularly the general neurosurgeon in making appropriate choices keeping in mind primarily ratio profits on risks and the quality of life of elderly patients.

Lyon, France

Moncef Berhouma, MD, MSc, FEBNS
Pierre Krolak-Salmon, MD, PhD

About the Editor

Moncef Berhouma MD, MSc, FEBNS
Department of Neurosurgery B
Skull Base Surgery Program
Pierre Wertheimer University Hospital – Hospices Civils de Lyon – France

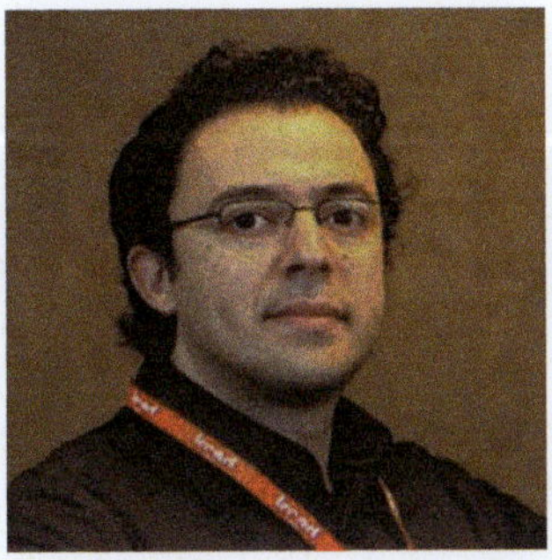

Moncef BERHOUMA is a consultant neurosurgeon at the University Hospital of Lyon. He is Associate Professor of Neurosurgery and surgical instructor at the European Association of Neurosurgical Societies (EANS). He is Master of Science in Philosophy of Neuroscience. He performed his research fellowship in the skull base surgery laboratory at the Ohio University in the USA in 2011. He is author of more than 50 scientific papers in peer-reviewed journals, more than 7 book chapters, and 2 books. His main interests are minimally invasive skull base surgery and geriatric neurosurgery.

Pierre Krolak-Salmon MD, PhD
Center of Memory, Ressources and Research of Lyon, France

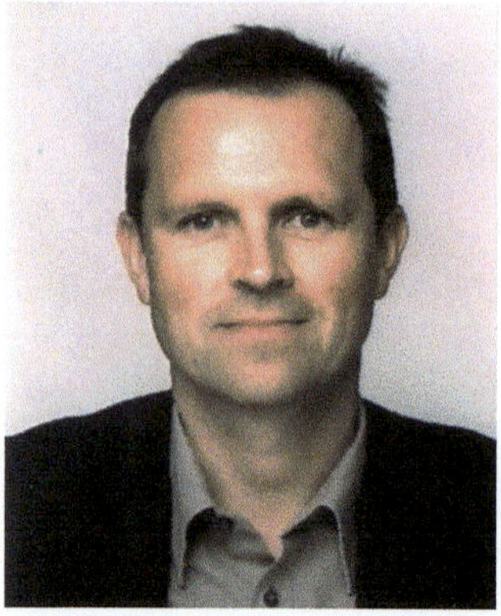

Pierre Krolak-Salmon is a neurologist and geriatrician at the University Hospital of Lyon (France), director of Clinical Research Memory Centre of Lyon and of the Clinical Research Centre "Elderly, Brain and Frailty", and head of the Social Cognition and Cognitive Disorders research group at Neuroscience Center of Lyon. Professor Krolak-Salmon attended medical school at the University of Lyon between 1987 and 1994; he completed his Neurosciences Master in 1999 and his PhD on brain dynamics of facial emotional expression recognition in 2004. During the course of his career, Professor Krolak-Salmon has also studied at the Wellcome Trust in London, UK, and Johns Hopkins Hospital in Baltimore, USA. Professor Krolak-Salmon currently has an active teaching role at the University Claude Bernard in Lyon, in the fields of geriatrics, neurology, neuroscience, and neuropsychology. His main areas of research interest include biomarkers (CSF and neuroimaging) and predictors of autonomy loss in dementia; social cognition and emotion recognition; and clinical neurology and geriatrics.

Acknowledgments

This collaborative work would not have been possible without the thorough efforts of our contributors, who are world-renowned experts in their respective fields. We would also like to thank the publishing team at Springer for their responsiveness and professionalism, particularly Ms Madona Samuel and Ms Nathalie Lhorset-Poulain. Finally, we would like to be grateful to our families for their constant support.

Moncef Berhouma
Pierre Krolak-Salmon

Contents

Part VII Miscellaneous

Contributors

Owoicho Adogwa Department of Neurosurgery, Rush University Medical Center, Chicago, IL, USA

Waleed A. Azab, MD Department of Neurosurgery, Ibn Sina Hospital, Kuwait city, Kuwait

Edward C. Benzel, MD Department of Neurosurgery, Center for Spine Health, Neurological Institute, Cleveland Clinic, Cleveland, OH, USA

Cleveland Clinic, Department of Neurological Surgery, Center for Spine Health, Cleveland, OH, USA

Moncef Berhouma, MD, MSc, FEBNS Department of Neurosurgery, University Hospital of Lyon – Hospices Civils de Lyon, Lyon, France

Desmond A. Brown, MD, PhD Department of Neurosurgery (DAB) and Division of Critical Care Neurology (EFMW), Mayo Clinic, Rochester, MN, USA

Michael Buchfelder, MD, PhD Department of Neurosurgery, Friedrich-Alexander-University Erlangen-Nürnberg, Erlangen, Germany

Chiara Caggiano, MD Division of Neurosurgery, Department of Neurosciences and Reproductive and Odontostomatological Sciences, Università degli Studi di Napoli Federico II, Naples, Italy

Paolo Cappabianca, MD Division of Neurosurgery, Department of Neurosciences and Reproductive and Odontostomatological Sciences, Università degli Studi di Napoli Federico II, Naples, Italy

Marina L. Castner, RN Department of Neurologic Surgery, College of Medicine, Mayo Clinic, Rochester, MN, USA

Luigi M. Cavallo, MD, PhD Division of Neurosurgery, Department of Neurosciences and Reproductive and Odontostomatological Sciences, Università degli Studi di Napoli Federico II, Naples, Italy

Jonathan Cohen University of Pittsburgh, Pittsburgh, PA, USA

Marialaura Del Basso De Caro, BS Department of Advanced Biomedical Sciences, Università degli Studi di Napoli Federico II, Naples, Italy

Rita De Micheli, MD Department of Oncology, Lausanne University Hospital, Lausanne, Switzerland

Colin L.W. Driscoll, MD Department of Neurologic Surgery, College of Medicine, Mayo Clinic, Rochester, MN, USA

Department of Otorhinolaryngology, College of Medicine, Mayo Clinic, Rochester, MN, USA

Francois Ducray NeuroOncology Department, Hôpital Neurologique Pierre Wertheimer, Hospices Civils de Lyon, Lyon, France

Roderic G. Eckenhoff, MD Department of Anesthesiology and Critical Care, University of Pennsylvania Perelman School of Medicine, Philadelphia, PA, USA

Ellie Edlmann Division of Neurosurgery, Department of Clinical Neurosciences, Addenbrooke's Hospital & University of Cambridge, Cambridge, UK

Per Enblad, MD, PhD Department of Neuroscience, Neurosurgery, Uppsala University Uppsala University Hospital, Uppsala, Sweden

Christian Ewald Department of Neurosurgery, University Hospital, Friedrich Schiller University, Jena, Germany

Michael G. Fehlings, MD, PhD, FRCSC, FACS Division of Neurosurgery, Department of Surgery, University of Toronto, Toronto, ON, Canada

Head Spinal Program, McEwen Centre for Regenerative Medicine, Toronto Western Hospital, University Health Network, Toronto, ON, Canada

Department of Surgery, Halbert Chair in Neural Repair and Regeneration, University of Toronto, Toronto, ON, Canada

Richard G. Fessler University of Chicago, Chicago, IL, USA

Ryan J. Filler Department of Neurosurgery, Center for Spine Health, Neurological Institute, Cleveland Clinic, Cleveland, OH, USA

Elizabeth M. Gabrielli, MD Department of Anesthesiology and Critical Care, University of Pennsylvania Perelman School of Medicine, Philadelphia, PA, USA

Cristina Izquierdo Gracia NeuroOncology Department, Hôpital Neurologique Pierre Wertheimer, Hospices Civils de Lyon, Lyon, France

Francesco Grandoni, MD Department of Oncology, Lausanne University Hospital, Lausanne, Switzerland

Elia Guadagno, MD Department of Advanced Biomedical Sciences, Università degli Studi di Napoli Federico II, Naples, Italy

Laureen D. Hachem Faculty of Medicine, University of Toronto, Toronto, ON, Canada

Mark G. Hamilton, MD, CM FRCSC, FAANS Division of Neurosurgery, Department of Clinical Neuroscience, University of Calgary, Calgary, AB, Canada

Adult Hydrocephalus Program, Department of Clinical Neuroscience, University of Calgary, Calgary, AB, Canada

Rodrigo Hasbun, MD, MPH University of Texas Health Sciences Center, Houston, TX, USA

Andreas F. Hottinger, MD, PhD Departments of Clinical Neurosciences & Oncology, Lausanne University Hospital, Lausanne, Switzerland

Peter J. Hutchinson Division of Neurosurgery, Department of Clinical Neurosciences, Addenbrooke's Hospital & University of Cambridge, Cambridge, UK

Albert M. Isaacs, BSc, MD Division of Neurosurgery, Department of Clinical Neuroscience, University of Calgary, Calgary, AB, Canada

Rajiv R. Iyer, MD Department of Neurosurgery, The Johns Hopkins University School of Medicine, Johns Hopkins All Children's Hospital, Baltimore, MD, USA

Timothée Jacquesson, MD, MSc Department of Neurosurgery, University Hospital of Lyon – Hospices Civils de Lyon, Lyon, France

George I. Jallo, MD Institute for Brain Protections Sciences, Johns Hopkins All Children's Hospital, St. Petersburg, FL, USA

Emmanuel Jouanneau, MD, PhD Department of Neurosurgery, University Hospital of Lyon – Hospices Civils de Lyon, Lyon, France

Andrea Kleindienst, MD, PhD Department of Neurosurgery, Friedrich-Alexander-University Erlangen-Nürnberg, Erlangen, Germany

Department of Neurosurgery, Klinikum Amberg, Amberg, Germany

W. Andrew Kofke Department of Anesthesiology and Critical Care, Department of Neurosurgery, University of Pennsylvania, Philadelphia, PA, USA

Angelos G. Kolias Division of Neurosurgery, Department of Clinical Neurosciences, Addenbrooke's Hospital & University of Cambridge, Cambridge, UK

Pierre Krolak-Salmon Lyon Institute for Elderly – Lyon University Hospital, Clinical and Research Memory Centre of Lyon, Lyon, France

Hôpital des Charpennes, Villeurbanne, France

Michael J. Link, MD Department of Neurologic Surgery, College of Medicine, Mayo Clinic, Rochester, MN, USA

Department of Otorhinolaryngology, College of Medicine, Mayo Clinic, Rochester, MN, USA

Chirstianto B. Lumenta, MD, PhD Neurosurgical Department, Municipal Hospital Munich, Teaching Hospital of the Technical University Munich, Munich, Germany

Karol Migliorati, MD Division of Neurosurgery, Department of Neurosciences and Reproductive and Odontostomatological Sciences, Università degli Studi di Napoli Federico II, Naples, Italy

Bianca Moura, MD Department of Oncology, Lausanne University Hospital, Lausanne, Switzerland

Hossein Mousavi University of Pittsburgh, Pittsburgh, PA, USA

Hideki Nagashima, MD, DMSc Department of Orthopedic Surgery, Faculty of Medicine, Tottori University, Yonago, Tottori, Japan

Chochlidakis Nikos, MD Neurosurgical Department, Municipal Hospital Munich, Teaching Hospital of the Technical University Munich, Munich, Germany

Louis G. Pol College of Business Administration, University of Nebraska Omaha, Omaha, NE, USA

Timothy T. Roberts Department of Neurosurgery, Center for Spine Health, Neurological Institute, Cleveland Clinic, Cleveland, OH, USA

Verena Röckelein Department of Neurosurgery, Friedrich-Alexander-University Erlangen-Nürnberg, Erlangen, Germany

Mats Ryttlefors, MD, PhD Department of Neuroscience, Neurosurgery, Uppsala University Uppsala University Hospital, Uppsala, Sweden

David B. Schul, MD Neurosurgical Department, Municipal Hospital Munich, Teaching Hospital of the Technical University Munich, Munich, Germany

Raymond F. Sekula Jr. University of Pittsburgh, Pittsburgh, PA, USA

Domenico Solari, MD, PhD Division of Neurosurgery, Department of Neurosciences and Reproductive and Odontostomatological Sciences, Università degli Studi di Napoli Federico II, Naples, Italy

Philip Y. Sun, MS Mayo Medical School, College of Medicine, Mayo Clinic, Rochester, MN, USA

Allan R. Tunkel, MD, PhD Warren Alpert Medical School of Brown University, Providence, RI, USA

Kathryn M. Van Abel, MD Department of Otorhinolaryngology, College of Medicine, Mayo Clinic, Rochester, MN, USA

Albrecht Waschke Department of Neurosurgery, University Hospital, Friedrich Schiller University, Jena, Germany

Eelco F.M. Wijdicks, MD, PhD Department of Neurosurgery (DAB) and Division of Critical Care Neurology (EFMW), Mayo Clinic, Rochester, MN, USA

Michael A. Williams, MD, FAAN Adult and Transitional Hydrocephalus and CSF Disorders, University of Washington School of Medicine, Seattle, WA, USA

Christopher D. Witiw, MD Division of Neurosurgery, Department of Surgery, University of Toronto, Toronto, ON, Canada

David A. Wyler, MD Jefferson Hospital of Neuroscience, Thomas Jefferson University, Philadelphia, PA, USA

Part I

Generalities

Rapid Growth in the Elderly Population of the World

1

Louis G. Pol

1.1 Introduction

Before information about and a discussion of the elderly segment of the global population is presented, it is important to consider what is meant by the terms elderly, old age, aging, and the like. The term elderly has no precise meaning, and past and current researchers throughout the globe have viewed the elderly population many different ways. Aging as a process has both biological and social components and must be seen from the perspectives of upward shifts in life expectancy, the growth of the older population, as well as how societies view old age.

From a biological perspective, for a number of years, demographers and others have been interested in both life expectancy at various ages and lifespan, the hypothetical length of life that would be realized if disease was eliminated. Life expectancy calculations rely on death rates specific to various ages, and often there is interest in examining death rates by cause of death or in calculating life expectancy if death due to one or more causes was eliminated (e.g., cancer). During the twentieth century, researchers from many scientific and social science fields focused on understanding why life expectancy was increasing as well as identifying the implications of increasing life expectancy on population size, population composition, and the changing social structure of populations. The cause-of-death transition during the nineteenth and twentieth centuries was comprised of falling death rates due to infectious and parasitic diseases along with increased death rates due to cancer and heart-related causes. These studies continue today, particularly as the age structures of the world and individual nations show that relatively rapid aging is ubiquitous.

The author offers a sincere thanks to Jackie Lynch and Kevin Mitchell for their assistance in the preparation of this chapter.

L.G. Pol (✉)
College of Business Administration, University of Nebraska Omaha, Omaha, NE, USA
e-mail: lpol@unomaha.edu

© Springer International Publishing Switzerland 2017

M. Berhouma, P. Krolak-Salmon (eds.), *Brain and Spine Surgery in the Elderly*,
DOI 10.1007/978-3-319-40232-1_1

From a social perspective, older age is seen in relative terms as individuals and groups compare themselves to others. There are appearance elements (e.g., does a person "look" old) as well as physiological limitation considerations (e.g., does a person have limitations with respect to walking or dressing). Product and service businesses have targeted the older population with respect to looking younger (e.g., getting a tummy tuck) and functioning better/younger (e.g., being prescribed a drug to address erectile dysfunction).

Since the beginning of the twentieth century, estimated life expectancy at birth for the world population has risen from 32 [7] to 72 years [10, 11], and today the average 50- or 60- or 70-year-old is much healthier at that age than her/his counterpart 100 or more years ago. If one looks at an even shorter time interval, for example, 1950 to present, the rise in life expectancy is from 47 to 72, an increase of 25 years [10, 11]. In either case, 116 years or 66 years, the rapid rise in life expectancy has resulted in a redefinition of elderly, middle age, and old age. Our languages are filled with pithy phrases such as "60 is the new 50" and "you are only as old as you feel," reflecting both the fact that we are living longer and that we have altered our ideas about what it means to be older.

This book of readings is about brain and spinal surgery in the elderly. The Free Dictionary and other publications that provide conceptual definitions of elderly use phrases like "being part of middle age," with single words such as "aged," "older," and "senior" often appearing [3]. Missing is a numeric-specific or operational definition. Even demographers are not consistent with respect to age, operationalizing differently terms such as "middle age," the "young-old," and the "old-old."

Much of the context of reporting on the aging of the USA and other country-specific populations has been set by the establishment of age 65 as the minimum age that one must achieve to receive social insurance. However, even that age minimum is shifting upward as the overall age structure of all nations change. The population age 65 and above is also observed with respect to its own age structure. That is, instead of simply reporting the absolute number of persons age 65 and above in a population or presenting a percentage of the total population that is age 65 and over, numeric and percentage data for age segments of the 65 and above population are provided (e.g., in five year intervals).

Later in the chapter, data with respect to age are used to describe the size and composition of the elderly population. For the purposes of this chapter, composition will focus on the age and sex structure of the total and the elderly populations. Also, the population age 60 or age 65 and above will most often be used as the operational definition for elderly. Introducing sex to the equation is important because, in general, females live longer than males. The population of the elderly is female dominated, and at the oldest ages, women outnumber men by a large margin. For example, in Eastern and Northern Europe at age 80 and above, there are two men for every five women [10, 11]. Both age and sex combined have implications regarding the need for and nature of brain and spinal surgery.[1]

[1] A more detailed description of the population age 60, 65 and 85 and over is presented in other publications (e.g., United Nations, 2015). The addition of other variables such as income, educational and immigrant status is important in many contexts.

It should be noted that the choice of age 65 and above as one operational definition of elderly has a long history. Germany was the first Western nation to adopt an old-age social insurance program. At its inception in 1881, the standard retirement age in Germany was set at 70. However, in 1916, the minimum was lowered to age 65 [8]. As the USA began to plan its social security program in the 1930s, President Franklin Roosevelt looked to Germany's program, borrowing the age 65 as the standard retirement age [9]. Other nations followed the lead of Germany and established their own retirement ages, very often age 65. Those nations currently utilizing a retirement age of 65 include Australia, Belgium, Canada, Denmark, and France. Lower retirement ages can be found in China (60), India (60), Japan (60), Turkey (45), and Vietnam (60) [4, 5]. In some nations, the retirement age for men is older than for women. Moreover, many nations are now in the process of increasing the minimum retirement age to reflect the aging population, once again supporting the claim that societies are redefining old age [1, 6].

1.2 Changes in the Age Structure

While increases in life expectancy tell us a great deal about the aging of the population of a region or a nation, understanding age structure involves the addition of two other factors: fertility and migration. With respect to the world population, only fertility need be added to the equation. The difference between fertility (births and birth rates) and mortality (deaths and death rates) over the long term determines the size and age structure of the population and sets the initial parameters for future demographic change. In simple equation form:

$$P_{t+1} = P_t + B_{t-t+1} - D_{t-t+1}$$

where:

$P_{(t+1)}$ is the population at some point in the future.
P_t is the population now.
$B_{(t-t+1)}$ is the number of births between now and some point in the future.
$D_{(t-t+1)}$ is the number of deaths between now and some point in the future.
For example, the world population in 2020 will begin with the population in 2016, adding the births that take place between 2016 and 2020 and subtracting the deaths that occur during that interval.

Overall, the size and composition of the world's population is subject to demographic change only through the addition (births) and subtractions (deaths). However, death can occur at any age, and to the extent that death rates fall, particularly at the younger ages, life expectancy rises.

For most of world history, birth and death rates both have been high leading to populations that exhibited slow growth. During periods of famine and

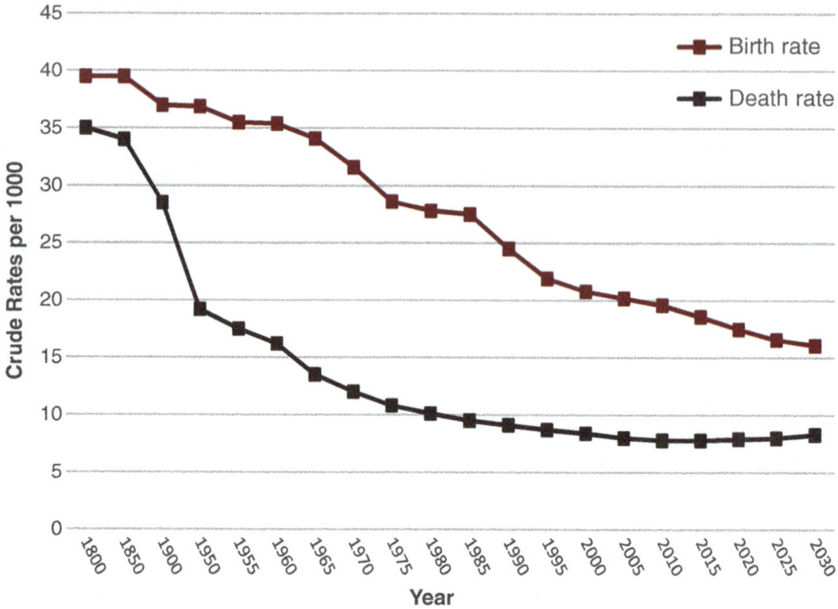

Fig. 1.1 Global birth and death rates: 1800–2030 (Source: United Nations [10])

outbreaks of disease, population size fell as death rates exceeded birth rates. For most of human history, high death rates resulted in life expectancy that was less than 40 years at birth [2]. Short-term upward fluctuations in birth rates led to limited population growth. Large increases in mortality (e.g., outbreak of the black plague during the fourteenth century) were responsible for significant population losses.

Falling death rates seen first in developed nations and then found in developing nations spurred rapid population growth beginning in the nineteenth century. The high birth rate/high death rate scenario gave way to a demographic transition where high fertility rates were paired with falling death rates [10, 11]. Over time, birth rates worldwide fell as well, although birth rates still exceed death rates. Therefore, the population of the world continues to grow, albeit less rapidly than in the twentieth century. Slowing growth in conjunction with rising life expectancy have resulted in population aging, giving way to a rapid rise in the elderly population.

Figure 1.1 shows the pattern of birth and death rates for the world beginning in 1800, when both rates were high, a birth rate of 40 births per 1,000 persons and a death rate of 35 deaths per 1,000 persons. Note that as death rates fell, particularly in the first five decades of the twentieth century, the gap between birth and death rates created a demographic environment that spurred rapid population growth. The birth rate/death rate difference of five (40 minus 35) found in 1800, grew to 20 by 1965. As the twentieth century progressed, falling fertility rates (death rates continued to fall but not as quickly) resulting in slower population growth. By 2030, the birth rate/death rate difference is forecast to be eight, only marginally higher than that seen in 1800.

The populations of some nations, and therefore regions, have aged even more rapidly than others because in addition to falling mortality rates there have been significant and rapid decreases in fertility rates. Today, most developed nations have below replacement fertility, which translates, over time, into population loss.[2] A combination of high life expectancy and low fertility also results in populations that age quickly, as expressed by rising median age and an increase in the percentage of the population at certain ages and above (e.g., 60, 65, or 75).

Population pyramids are used to illustrate the changing age and sex structure of populations over time. A population pyramid is a stacked bar graph with women represented from the center point to the right on the graph and men shown from the center to the left. Each bar represents the number or percentage of persons in a given age range (e.g., 5–9). Figure 1.2 presents world population pyramids for 1950, 2000, and 2030. In 1950, the population of the world was considerably younger than today as the result of higher birth rates and falling death rates. In addition, as noted earlier, the population was growing at a greater pace when compared to today. In 1950, the highest concentration of persons was in the youngest ages; thus, the base of the graph is large when compared to the rest of the pyramid-shaped figure. By 2000, birth and death rates had fallen and were relatively low, life expectancy had risen, and there was a marked increase of persons above age 30. The age distribution shown in this graph reflects an aging population and the pyramid-shaped picture has given way to one where the population for several age/sex groupings is similar. In the last image, 2030, birth rates have fallen further as noted earlier, life expectancy has risen, and the age structure observed has many age groupings of similar size, when compared to the figures from 1950 and 2000. This graph takes on a bullet shape, with a significant female-dominated anvil shape at the top representing the large population of persons age 80 and over.

Migration is the other variable in the equation because at the sub-global level (e.g., country) adding or subtracting net migrants is the third way to alter the size and the composition of a population. Introducing a large number of in-migrants or out-migrants over a short period of time can rapidly alter the size and age structure of a nation or a region. Moreover, the introduction of migration may exacerbate or ameliorate the aging process. Like fertility, migration may add to the size of a population, although at ages other than zero. Like mortality, migration may reduce a population, but again at selected ages. In nations such as Romania and Moldova, higher life expectancy, low fertility, and selective out-migration have produced populations that are declining in size and aging quickly. In the USA, net in-migration

[2] Replacement fertility is defined as the birth rate required to replace one woman and one partner. In developed nations, that rate is approximately 2.1 children over a woman's childbearing years (total fertility rate, TFR). The developed world has a TFR below 2.0, with a number of nations at or below 1.7.

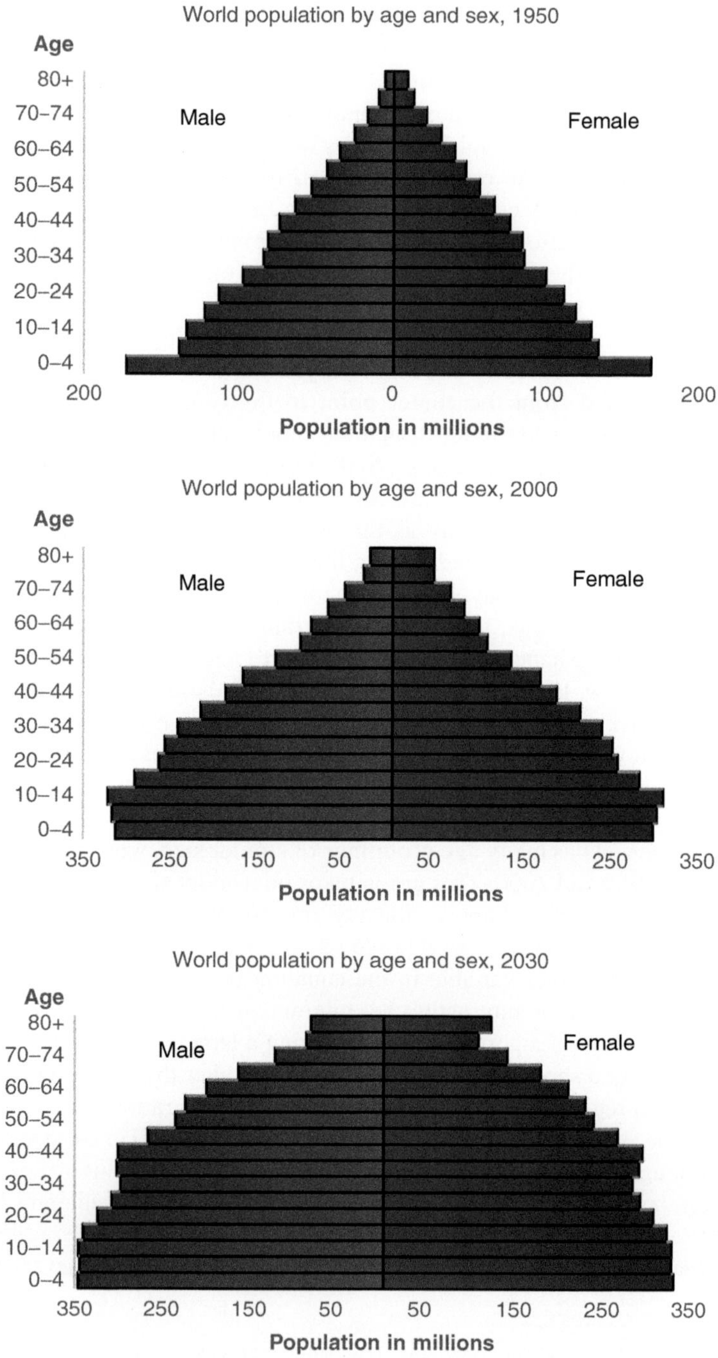

Fig. 1.2 Population pyramids for the world: 1950, 2000, and 2030 (Source: United Nations [10])

has offset below replacement fertility and has driven continued population growth. Migration from nation to nation tends to be dominated by younger populations; thus, the aging process speeds up in the country of origin when there is significant out-migration. Conversely, younger in-migrants and their offspring prevent a population from aging as fast as it might even though there has been a significant rise in life expectancy and low fertility.

Country- and region-specific population change can be expressed by the following equation:

$$P_{t+1} = P_t + B_{t-t+1} - D_{t-t+1} \pm M_{t-t+1}$$

where:

$P_{(t+1)}$ is the population at some point in the future.
P_t is the population now.
$B_{(t-t+1)}$ is the number of births between now and some point in the future.
$D_{(t-t+1)}$ is the number of deaths between now and some point in the future.
$\pm M_{(t-t+1)}$ is the number of net migrants between now and some point in the future.
So: The population of France in 2020, will begin with the population in 2016, adding the births that take place between 2016 and 2020, subtracting the number of deaths that occur between 2016 and 2020, and adding or subtracting the number of net migrants between 2016 and 2020.

Overall, it should be noted that regional and nation-specific populations are shaped and reshaped by the interaction of fertility, mortality, and migration. Fertility adds to the population, but only at age 0. Mortality occurs at all ages, and once again, falling mortality rates result in an increase in life expectancy. Migration may act in ways similar to fertility or mortality, except that additions to a population through migration can occur at any age.

The effect of migration on the population has additional levels of complexity. First, as noted previously, there can be a net migration effect addition or subtraction of persons to a population given that net migration is the point of focus. Second, while migration tends to be concentrated in the younger population, persons under age 40, it can involve the population at any age. Third, while the central focus in assessing population change is on net migration, it is possible that the population of in-migrants will be dissimilar to the population of out-migrants. In a situation where net migration is zero, the effect of in and out movement may still change a population. Last, migration may have a multiple dimension effect on a population. That is, migrants often arrive as part of families that also generate a number of births over time. In some regions and nations, the arrival of migrants brings about a younger population that is partly driven by an increase in the birth rate.

The remainder of the chapter is relatively straightforward. The population of the world is described with respect to its elderly population. Specific emphasis is placed on both numeric increases and proportional rises. Data are also provided for regions of the world.

1.3 Trends in Aging

Summary data describing the growth and the aging of the world population since 1950 are provided in Table 1.1. Using short-term population projections to the year 2025, the population is forecast to grow by over 5.4 billion persons over the 75-year interval covered in the table (a 215 percent increase). At the same time, the world's elderly population is projected to grow from 5.2 to 10.4 percent of the total population by 2025. At the world level, there will be 885 million elderly persons in 2025, a 675 percent increase from 1950. In addition, the population age 80 and over is forecast to grow even faster, from 0.5 to 1.9 percent of the population. Worldwide, there will be 151 million persons worldwide age 80 and above in 2025.

Table 1.1 contains other indicators of aging. The old-age dependency ratio, the ratio of persons age 65 and over divided by the population age 15–64 (working age population), increases from 8.6 to 15.9 in the 75-year interval, as falling birth rates yield fewer persons of working age over time. This ratio is frequently used to assess the solvency of social insurance/social security and health insurance programs in individual nations. Rapidly growing old-age dependency ratios raise concerns among policy makers, and drive politicians to pass legislation that increases the minimum age required before persons are eligible to begin receiving payments from those programs. In the USA, for example, the old-age dependency ratio is currently 22.8 [10, 11], or nearly 23 persons age 65 and above per 100 persons who are working age. The old-age dependency ratio varies considerably across countries with Finland and Sweden at 31, and Angola and Saudi Arabia at 5 and 4, respectively. Table 1.1 also shows the sex ratio, number of males per 100 females, for two age groups: 65 and over and 80 and over. These ratios do not change markedly over the 75-year period. They do reflect, as noted earlier, that life expectancy for men is lower than for women. At age 80 and over, there are fewer than 58 men for every 100 women.

Finally, the table presents figures for life expectancy[3] at three different ages: at birth, age 65 and above, and age 80 and above. Life expectancy at birth increases by nearly

Table 1.1 World population aging: 1950–2025

	1950	1975	2000	2025
Total population (in billions)	2,519	4,065	6,057	7,937
Percent 65+	5.2	5.7	6.9	10.4
Percent 80+	0.5	0.8	1.1	1.9
Old-age dependency ratio	8.6	9.9	10.9	15.9
Sex ratio 65+	75.5	73.7	76.2	79.9
Sex ratio 80+	61.4	58.1	53.1	57.7
Life expectancy				
Birth	46.5	59.8	66.0	72.4
65	11.3	13.7	15.3	17.2
80	5.3	6.3	7.2	8.2

Source: United Nations [12]

[3] Life expectancy at any age is the total number of years on average that a cohort of persons can expect to live given the assumption that current death rates remain constant.

Table 1.2 World population aging by region: 2015–2030 (numbers in thousands)

	Population age 60 and over		Percent of population age 60 and over	
	2015	2030	2015	2030
World	900,906	1,402,405	12.3	16.5
Africa	64,447	105,387	5.4	6.3
Eastern Africa	18,868	30,818	4.8	5.3
Middle Africa	6,901	11,267	4.5	4.9
North Africa	17,992	30,883	8.0	10.9
Southern Africa	4,680	6,958	7.5	9.9
Western Africa	16,006	25,462	4.5	4.9
Asia	507,954	844,487	11.6	17.2
Eastern Asia	267,797	435,155	16.7	26.4
South-Central Asia	159,803	265,554	8.4	11.9
Southern Asia	153,490	256,153	8.4	11.9
South-Eastern Asia	59,008	146,415	9.3	14.7
Western Asia	20,346	37,363	7.9	11.6
Europe	176,513	217,220	23.9	29.6
Eastern Europe	63,091	71,662	21.5	25.7
Northern Europe	23,968	30,820	23.4	28.0
Southern Europe	39,914	50,712	26.2	33.9
Western Europe	49,540	64,026	26.0	32.7
Latin America and the Caribbean	70,922	120,959	11.2	16.8
Caribbean	5,745	8,946	13.3	19.2
Central America	16,144	28,786	9.3	14.2
South America	49,033	83,227	11.7	17.7
Northern America	74,589	104,799	20.8	26.4
Oceana	6,481	9,553	16.5	20.2
Australia/New Zealand	5,808	8,391	20.4	25.0
Melanesia	555	950	5.8	7.7
Micronesia	51	95	9.7	15.6
Polynesia	67	117	9.8	15.6

Source: United Nations [11]

26 years between 1950 and 2025, a rise of over 55 percent. This increase alone provides considerable underlying explanation with respect to the growth in the elderly population. Focusing on the age groups 65 and over and 80 and over, there is a significant rise in life expectancy between 1950 and 2025. Life expectancy at age 65 and above is projected to rise nearly 6 years over the interval. At age 80 and above, the increase is nearly 3 years. The average person age 65 in 2025 can expect to live to over 82 years of age, and the average person age 80, to nearly 89. Moreover, the data for developed nations show even longer life expectancy at birth and at age 65 and 80. Thus, the aging of developed nations is much more pronounced than that seen for the rest of the world.

Table 1.2 shows the growth in the older population, operationalized as age 60 years and older, for the world and its regions, specific to the years 2015 and 2030. As can be seen in the first row of the table, a substantial increase in the population is forecast in the 15-year interval, an increase of nearly 502 million persons (56percent growth). The percentage of persons age 60 and over will rise from 12.3 to 16.5. When the data are subdivided by regions and subregions of the world, a significant diversity in the pattern of aging emerges. Africa (6.3percent in 2030) and its subregions have the lowest proportion population age 60 and over. More specifically, countries such as Burundi (4.9percent), Malawi (4.6percent), Zimbabwe (4.6percent), and Zambia (4.1percent) have the youngest populations in 2030. Europe has the oldest population (29.6percent of the population is age 60 or over in 2030), with Southern Europe (33.9percent) and Western Europe (32.7percent) showing the oldest subregional figures. Italy (36.6percent), Germany (36.1percent), and Portugal (34.7percent) all have more than one-third of their populations that are age 60 and over.

In examining large population nations, additional variations are observed. In 2030, the population age 60 and above in China is forecast to be over 358 million persons, or 25.3percent of the total population. A significant aging of the population will take place between 2015 and 2030 as the percent of population age 60 and above rises from 15.2 to 25.3. For India, the number of persons age 60 years and over is forecast to be nearly 191 million in 2030, with an increase in proportional representation from 8.9percent in 2015 to 12.5percent in 2030. Data for the USA show nearly 93 million persons age 60 and over in 2030, and a rise in percentage from 20.7 to 26.1. In Brazil, the total is nearly 43 million in 2030, an increase from 11.7 to 18.8percent [10, 11].

Overall, there are large variations in the proportion of elderly across the globe, as well as the pace at which regions, subregions, and nations are aging. While the largest "markets" for brain and spinal surgeries in the elderly are in the developed regions and nations of the world, major opportunities are found in nations such as India and Brazil. In addition, the most rapidly developing market with respect to current and future size is in China.

Table 1.3 presents data on life expectancy and healthy life expectancy for 2000 and 2012, cross-classified by region. Health-adjusted life expectancy (HALE), a measure of healthy life expectancy, refers to the average number of expected years of life at full health from birth that members of a cohort of persons can expect to live accounting for rates of comorbidity that lead to disability [13]. That is, HALE

Table 1.3 World life expectancy and HALE at birth: 2000 and 2012

	Life expectancy at birth		HALE at birth	
	2000	2012	2000	2012
World	66.2	70.3	58.0	61.7
High-income countries	76.0	78.9	67.3	69.8
Low- and median-income Countries	59.8	64.9	57.7	61.4
Africa region	50.2	57.7	43.1	49.6
Region of the Americas	73.9	76.4	64.9	67.1
Eastern Mediterranean Region	64.9	67.8	55.4	58.3
European Region	72.4	76.1	63.9	66.9
South East Asia Region	62.9	67.5	54.2	58.5
Western Pacific Region	72.3	75.9	64.8	66.1

Source: World Health Organization [14]

measures the average number of years from birth or another age that a cohort can expect to live without a disability of some type. Healthy life expectancy is an important concept because it indicates at what age, on average, persons can begin to experience more serious health challenges that effect day-to-day living.

Table 1.3 shows a large difference in life expectancy and HALE over time and region, between eight and more than nine years depending upon the region. In Europe, for example, there is a difference of 9.2 years between life expectancy and HALE in 2012. In Africa, the difference is smaller, 8.1 years. Moreover, both life expectancy and HALE for the world rose rapidly over the 12 years covered in the table, 4.1 years for life expectancy, and 3.7 years for healthy life expectancy. Table 1.3 also shows that there are large life expectancy and healthy life expectancy differences across regions of the world. In 2012, the longest life expectancy was found in Europe (76.1 years) and the lowest was experienced in Africa (57.7 years), an 18.4-year differential. For HALE, Europe, again, was highest in 2012, 66.9 years. Africa showed the lowest figure, 49.6 years, a difference of 17 years between the two regions. Table 1.3 also shows that over a relatively short period of time, there was a narrowing of the difference in HALE when comparing high income with low- and medium-income countries, from 9.6 years in 2000 to 8.4 years in 2012.

Table 1.4 offers 2013 life expectancy and HALE figures for the world and selected countries. The highest life expectancy nations, Singapore, Japan, and

Table 1.4 Life expectancy and HALE at birth for the world and selected nations: 2013

	Life expectancy at birth	HALE at birth
World	70	62.0
Singapore	83	76.3
Japan	84	75.0
Cyprus	82	74.4
Spain	83	73.2
South Korea	82	72.7
China	75	68.0
Kuwait	78	67.9
Croatia	78	67.8
Uruguay	77	67.7
Estonia	77	67.0
Ukraine	71	62.9
North Korea	70	62.6
Russian Federation	69	60.5
Yemen	64	54.7
Uganda	59	50.3
Afghanistan	61	50.0
Burundi	56	48.0
Central African Republic	51	43.7
Sierra Leone	46	39.4

Source: World Health Organization [15]

Spain, are also among the highest in regard to HALE, although not in the same order. Those nations with the lowest life expectancy and HALE are in Africa, although Afghanistan and Yemen are added to this list. The difference between the nations with the highest/lowest life expectancies and HALE is very large, 38 years between Jordan and Sierra Leone with respect to life expectancy and nearly 37 years for HALE when comparing Singapore with Sierra Leone.

Conclusion

The data presented show that the elderly population of the world is large, over 900 million persons age 65 and over in 2015, and is forecasted to grow rapidly in the foreseeable future. Significant differences in demographic conditions specific to countries and regions of the world have resulted in wide variations in the number of elderly persons, with the highest concentration found in Western Europe. Nevertheless, the elderly population in all countries and regions is growing faster than the remaining age segments, a reality that is not likely to change. Improved health conditions and advances in medicine will likely lead to further reductions in death rates and higher life expectancies. The rise in life expectancy will increase the pace of worldwide aging. The years of healthy life expectancy are also likely to grow, especially in the developing world. The major unknown on the mortality side of the population equation is the effect of epidemics and pandemics on death rates. While major outbreaks of Ebola or Zika may markedly influence death rates in some nations, they are less likely to have an impact on the death rates of the world. In recent years, each time one of these outbreaks occurs, worldwide response has kept the disease from having a widespread and sustained effect.

Fertility rates worldwide will continue to fall, and the below replacement reality that is found today in many nations of the world will be evident in other countries in the future. Historically, pro-natalist policies, those designed to foster increased fertility rates, have failed because irrespective of program offered, once a lower fertility expectation norm is achieved, women do not respond positively to financial and support inducements designed to encourage having additional children. China is now serving as the next "laboratory" for pro-natalist policy as the "one-child" policy has been altered.

Immigration will continue to have the greatest impact on the pace of aging for selected nations and regions. Countries with more restrictive migration policies, and cultural norms that reflect the lack of acceptance of migrants, will age much more rapidly than those with policies and cultures that encourage in-migration. Moreover, if there is a more global anti-immigration stance taken by developed nations, the pace of the elderly population growth differential between developed and developing nations will quicken.

Growth in the number of brain and spinal surgeries in the elderly is driven by both the improvement in technology/surgical skills and the number of persons who need/want such surgeries. The remainder of this book addresses the issue of improvements. With respect to need/want, the case is clear. The current size and rapid growth of the elderly population of the world, regions, and nations, will drive the demand for current and future treatment modalities. The rapid growth of the healthy older segments of the elderly population is likely to expand demand for surgeries, encouraging the development of technology and surgical skills targeted to the oldest members of society.

References

1. Fanti L (2014) Raising the mandatory retirement age and its effect on long-run income and pay-as-you-go (PAYG) pensions. Metroeconomica 65:619–645
2. Galor O, Moav O (2004) Natural selection and evolution of life expectancy. Brown University, Working Papers. http://www.brown.edu.leo.lib.unomaha.edu/Departments/Economics/Papers/2004/2004-14_paper.pdf. Accessed 1 Apr 2016
3. Merriam-Webster's Collegiate Dictionary (2003) 11th ed. Merriam-Webster, Springfield. http://www.merriam-webster.com/. Accessed 30 Mar 2016
4. OECD (2013) Pensions at a glance: Asia/Pacific 2013. OECD Publishing. http://dx.doi.org/10.1787/pension_asia-2013-en. Accessed 30 Mar 2016
5. OECD (2014) Average effective age of retirement versus the normal age in 2014 in OECD countries. http://www.oecd.org/els/emp/ageingandemploymentpolicies-statisticsonaverageeffectiveageofretirement.htm. Accessed 30 Mar 2016
6. Pestieau P (2003) Raising the age of retirement to ensure a better retirement. Geneva Pap Risk Insur 28:686–695
7. Riley JC (2005) Estimates of regional and global life expectancy, 1800–2001. Popul Dev Rev 31:537–543
8. Social Security Administration (2015) Age 65 retirement. https://www.ssa.gov/history/age65.html. Accessed 30 Mar 2016
9. U.S. Congress. Senate. *Social Security Act*. 74th Cong., 1st sess., 1935. http://www.legisworks.org/congress/74/publaw-271.pdf. Accessed 1 Apr 2016
10. United Nations (2015) Population division: world population prospects, the 2015 revision. http://esa.un.org/unpd/wpp/. Accessed 30 Mar 2016
11. United Nations (2015) World population ageing. Department of Economic and Social Affairs, Population Division. New York. http://www.un.org/esa/population/publications/worldageing19502050/
12. United Nations (2016) World population ageing: 1950–2050. Department of Economic and Social Affairs, Population Division. New York. www.un.org/esa/population/publications/worldageing1950/2050
13. World Health Organization (2014) WHO methods for life expectancy and health life expectancy. Global Health Technical Paper WHO/HIS/HIS/GHE/2014.5. Department of Health Statistics and Information Systems. WHO, Geneva
14. World Health Organization (2014) WHO methods for life expectancy and healthy life expectancy. Department of Health Statistics and Information Systems, WHO, Geneva, Table 6.1
15. World Health Organization (2015) Global health observatory, life expectancy-data by country. World Health Organization, Geneva

A Brief Physiology of the Aging

2

Moncef Berhouma

2.1 Introduction

The aging process of the brain encompasses specific changes including an overall decline in the brain weight and volume as well as an enlargement of cerebro-spinal fluid (CSF) spaces and ventricles. These changes appear to result from a neuronal cell and synapses loss. In the meantime some characteristic features of Alzheimer's disease are found in normal aging brains in a lesser amount, such as senile plaques and neurofibrillary tangles. Furthermore, spinal changes related to aging are difficult to differentiate from the so-called degenerative spinal alterations. Finally, several systemic changes occur with aging altering the reserve capacity of the elderly, i.e. the difficulty to maintain homeostasis during stressing situations, that may lead to systemic failure (Table 2.1). All these aging-related bodily features have to be considered during the management of neurosurgical elderly patients.

2.2 The Aging Brain

For the sake of clarity, the brain changes with aging can be categorized into structural both macroscopic and microscopic as well as functional alterations.

2.2.1 Structural Changes

The microscopic and macroscopic changes occurring in the aging brain are still debated. Their occurrence with a higher intensity in pathological conditions such as

M. Berhouma, MD, MSc, FEBNS
Department of Neurosurgery, University Hospital of Lyon – Hospices Civils de Lyon, Lyon, France
e-mail: berhouma.moncef@gmail.com

© Springer International Publishing Switzerland 2017

M. Berhouma, P. Krolak-Salmon (eds.), *Brain and Spine Surgery in the Elderly*,
DOI 10.1007/978-3-319-40232-1_2

dementia raises the question of a continuum between the normal aging brain and the pathological aging brain. The recent advances in noninvasive brain imaging answered some questions in this debate. Globally, the weight and volume of the brain decrease with age. It appears that the brain's weight diminishes of about 0.1 % per year between 20 and 60 years and faster thereafter [1–3], but these figures are extremely variable between studies and should therefore be interpreted carefully. The brain's volume decreases uniformly for the white matter but with some disparities for the gray matter [4]: The frontal, parietal, and hippocampus cortex are usually more affected than occipital and temporal lobes. A direct consequence is a passive enlargement of subarachnoid spaces and ventricles. The difficult differentiation between neuronal loss and neuronal shrinkage has led to disparate studies. Nevertheless, there is a global consensus that a certain amount of neurons are lost with aging particularly in the cerebral cortex, hippocampus, and amygdala. Specific regions appear to dodge this phenomenon including the nucleus basalis, contrary to what is observed during Alzheimer's disease [5].

Furthermore, several cellular changes are observed during the process of brain aging, and almost all of them are also present more intensely in Alzheimer's disease:

- Accumulation of lipofuscin in some neurons, a pigment composed of peroxidized protein and lipids that may result from the inability of aging cells to wash out the products of cell metabolism [6].
- Neurofibrillary tangles: These are composed of paired helical filaments resulting in the loss of the normal cytoskeleton of microtubules and neurofilaments, leading to neuronal loss. Along with senile plaques, neurofibrillary tangles represent the histopathological markers of Alzheimer's disease. Contrary to this latter, in the normal aging brain, the number of neurofibrillary tangles remains low and limited to the hippocampus, amygdala, and entorhinal cortex [7].
- Senile plaques: Also known as neuritic plaques, they are areas of gray matter comprising a core of proteins mainly amyloid β-peptide surrounded by swollen neurites [8].
- Granulovacuolar degeneration: These empty vacuoles are particularly seen in hippocampal pyramidal cells.
- Hirano bodies are rod-shaped structures also found in hippocampal pyramidal cells [9] probably composed by cytoskeletal proteins.
- Cerebral amyloid angiopathy, i.e., extracellular deposition of amyloid β-peptide in the walls of brain vessels.

2.2.2 Functional Changes

Several functional changes may be observed during the aging of the nervous system:

- Balance disturbances that can result in repeated falls in the elderly. They may be secondary to anomalies impacting cerebellar functions, vestibulocochlear integrity (degeneration of the otoconia), hearing and vision capacities, as well as muscular strength. Proprioception may also be disturbed secondary to muscle spindle and mechanoreceptor alterations.

- Cognitive anomalies are frequently reported but difficult to assess and to connect to pure aging of the brain. This aspect is detailed in Chap. 3. One of the most obvious features of brain aging is an impairment of selective attention and of the capacity to concentrate on complex tasks while attention is globally preserved.
- Vision impairment (accommodation weakening, glare tolerance, color discrimination, and attentional visual field) and hearing anomalies (presbycusis) are common features of the aging of the sensorial system.
- Muscle strength anomalies range from slight muscle mass decline to degenerative loss of skeletal muscle mass (sarcopenia).

2.3 The Aging Spine

Aging of the spine is very difficult to differentiate from common degenerative changes [10]. This aging process involves the vertebral bodies as well as the three-joint complex (intervertebral disc and the two posterior facet joints) and the spinal muscles (flexor and extensor groups). In addition to predetermined genetic cell degeneration, the spinal aging process mainly results from the exposure of tissues to physical stress particularly in case of demanding professional occupations. According to Yong-Hing and Kirkaldy-Willis [11], the process of spinal aging evolves in three stages: The first stage comprises minor chemical, physiological, and biomechanical modifications of the three-joint complex. The second stage results from hypermobility and instability, while the last stage is due to major changes in the biochemical profile of the disc as well as profuse osteophyte formation leading to vertebral stiffness.

Classically, the degeneration of the intervertebral disc is considered as the trigger phase of the aging process [12, 13]. The normal function of a disc rests on the metabolism of extracellular matrix and is certainly genetically predetermined at least in part. Therefore, the very early modifications comprise a decrease in aggrecan (a major proteoglycan in the articular cartilage), a loss of water leading to destructuring the matrix and ensuing a diminishing of the disc height. Simultaneously, the activity of proteases increases. The aging process includes a decrease in the permeability of the endplate that is the main source of nutrition of the intervertebral disc. This latter then suffers a tissue breakdown initiating in the nucleus, which is thought to begin as early as the second decade of life [13]. This breakdown leads to concentric fissuring and radial tears of the disc as well as the vanishing of the anatomical limits between the annulus and the nucleus during the third and fourth decades [14]. Aging of the intervertebral disc is also characterized by marked modifications of discal vascularization and innervation. While the normal healthy intervertebral disc is avascular except a bare vascularization in the periphery of the annulus, angiogenic factors intervene in the aging disc to facilitate the intrusion of factors modifying the extracellular matrix including cytokines and metalloproteinases [15–19].

The two facet joints play a crucial role in the stabilization of flexion/extension motion of the vertebral segment and help the intervertebral disc to support the load efforts. The degeneration of the facet joints results from the aging of the disc itself, i.e., from the height loss and the secondary instability [20]. This facet degeneration encompasses cartilage degradation, erosions and osteophytes, and articular hypertrophy as well with the risk of compressing neural structures. Degenerative instability leading to spondylolisthesis and scoliosis results also from the facet degeneration.

Aging of the ligaments includes biochemical and structural modifications particularly a decrease in tensile properties and hypertrophic degeneration [21–23]. These modifications of the ligaments are often associated to trunk and pelvic muscle alterations. These latter are of paramount importance in the stabilization of the spine and in locomotion. Lipomatous degeneration and muscle atrophy are well-known features of the aging spine. A massive fat degeneration of erectile muscles can result in the characteristic kyphotic lumbar attitude in the elderly suffering camptocormia [24].

Lastly, the bone changes are numerous in the aging spine. These include sclerosis and osteophytes of the endplates and compromise of the vascular supply to the intervertebral disc [11, 25]. The bone density decrease is also a paramount parameter that should be kept in mind when thinking of postoperative bone healing in the elderly.

Table 2.1 Features of the aging human body

Aging organ	Pathogenesis	Consequences
Brain	Neuronal loss	Brain weight and volume reduction
	Synapses decline	Enlargement of CSF spaces and ventricles
	Neuronal accumulation of lipofuscin	Balance disturbance
	Neurofibrillary tangles	Sensory anomalies
	Granulovacuolar degeneration	Cognitive decline
	Hirano bodies	Motor strength weakness
	Cerebral amyloid angiopathy	
Spine	Decrease in aggrecan	Disc degeneration
	Hypovascularization	Articular degeneration
	Protease activity increase	Camptocormia
	Articular facet instability	Sagittal imbalance
	Muscle atrophy	
Pulmonary system	Decreased respiratory muscle strength and altered elastic recoil	Susceptibility to pneumonia
	Impairment of ciliary activity	
	Alteration of inflammatory response	Diminution of vital capacity
	Modifications of thoracic and parenchymal compliance	

Table 2.1 (continued)

Aging organ	Pathogenesis	Consequences
Cardiovascular system	Degenerative fibrosis of pacemaking and conducting fibers	Dysautonomic anomalies (heart rate and cardiac output)
	Slowed isovolumic contraction	Increased rate of 1st degree atrioventricular and fascicular blocks
	Increased ventricular stiffness	
		Atrial fibrillation
	Vascular stiffening and reduction of arterial compliance	Impairment of cardiac output
		Systolic hypertension and ventricular hypertrophy
Renal system	Decreased thirst sensation	Dehydration
	Age-related decline in renal function (decrease in glomerular filtration and loss of cortical nephrons)	Dys-osmolar states
	Impairment of antidiuretic hormone (ADH) response	Majored toxicity for renal-excreted medications
	Alteration of sensitivity of baro- and osmoreceptors	

References

1. Dekaban AS (1978) Changes in brain weights during the span of human life: relation of brain weights to body heights and body weights. Ann Neurol 4:345–356
2. Skullerud K (1985) Variations in the size of the human brain. Influence of age, sex, body length, body mass index, alcoholism, Alzheimer changes, and cerebral atherosclerosis. Acta Neurol Scand Suppl 102:1–94
3. Ho KC, Roessmann U, Straumfjord JV, Monroe G (1980) Analysis of brain weight. II. Adult brain weight in relation to body height, weight, and surface area. Arch Pathol Lab Med 104:640–645
4. Pfefferbaum A et al (1994) A quantitative magnetic resonance imaging study of changes in brain morphology from infancy to late adulthood. Arch Neurol 51:874–887
5. Chui HC, Bondareff W, Zarow C, Slager U (1984) Stability of neuronal number in the human nucleus basalis of Meynert with age. Neurobiol Aging 5:83–88
6. Goyal VK (1982) Lipofuscin pigment accumulation in human brain during aging. Exp Gerontol 17:481–487
7. Mathis CA, Wang Y, Klunk WE (2004) Imaging beta-amyloid plaques and neurofibrillary tangles in the aging human brain. Curr Pharm Des 10:1469–1492
8. Cullen KM, Kócsi Z, Stone J (2006) Microvascular pathology in the aging human brain: evidence that senile plaques are sites of microhaemorrhages. Neurobiol Aging 27:1786–1796
9. Foncin JF (1981) Classical and ultrastructural neuropathology of aging processes in the human: a critical review (author's transl). Rev Electroencephalogr Neurophysiol Clin 10:215–227
10. Herkowitz HN, Spine IS; for S. of the L (2004) The lumbar spine. Lippincott Williams & Wilkins, Philadelphia

11. Yong-Hing K, Kirkaldy-Willis WH (1983) The pathophysiology of degenerative disease of the lumbar spine. Orthop Clin North Am 14:491–504
12. Bibby SR, Jones DA, Lee RB, Yu J, Urban JPG, null (2001) The pathophysiology of the intervertebral disc. Joint Bone Spine 68:537–542
13. Boos N et al (2002) Classification of age-related changes in lumbar intervertebral discs: 2002 Volvo Award in basic science. Spine 27:2631–2644
14. Hughes SPF, Freemont AJ, Hukins DWL, McGregor AH, Roberts S (2012) The pathogenesis of degeneration of the intervertebral disc and emerging therapies in the management of back pain. J Bone Joint Surg Br 94:1298–1304
15. Feng C et al (2016) Disc cell senescence in intervertebral disc degeneration: causes and molecular pathways. Cell Cycle 1–11. doi:10.1080/15384101.2016.1152433
16. Deng B et al (2015) Expression profiles of MMP-1 and TIMP-1 in lumbar intervertebral disc degeneration. Genet Mol Res 14:19080–19086
17. Li Y et al (2016) The imbalance between TIMP3 and matrix-degrading enzymes plays an important role in intervertebral disc degeneration. Biochem Biophys Res Commun 469:507–514
18. Liu H et al (2015) LIM mineralization protein-1 suppresses TNF-α induced intervertebral disc degeneration by maintaining nucleus pulposus extracellular matrix production and inhibiting matrix metalloproteinases expression. J Orthop Res 33:294–303
19. Le Maitre CL, Freemont AJ, Hoyland JA (2005) The role of interleukin-1 in the pathogenesis of human intervertebral disc degeneration. Arthritis Res Ther 7:R732–745
20. Cohen SP, Raja SN (2007) Pathogenesis, diagnosis, and treatment of lumbar zygapophysial (facet) joint pain. Anesthesiology 106:591–614
21. Panjabi MM, Goel VK, Takata K (1982) Physiologic strains in the lumbar spinal ligaments. An in vitro biomechanical study 1981 Volvo Award in Biomechanics. Spine 7:192–203
22. Iorio JA, Jakoi AM, Singla A (2016) Biomechanics of degenerative spinal disorders. Asian Spine J 10:377–384
23. Behrsin JF, Briggs CA (1988) Ligaments of the lumbar spine: a review. Surg Radiol Anat 10:211–219
24. Lenoir T, Guedj N, Boulu P, Guigui P, Benoist M (2010) Camptocormia: the bent spine syndrome, an update. Eur Spine J 19:1229–1237
25. Farfan HF (1980) The pathological anatomy of degenerative spondylolisthesis. A cadaver study. Spine 5:412–418

3 Neurological Assessment and Neurocognitive Evaluation of the Elderly

Pierre Krolak-Salmon

A formal neurological examination is necessary within the perisurgical period and in case of geriatric syndrome like repeated falls, cognitive complaint, atypical pain, or mood disorder. The neurological examination should be structured and hierarchized as a function of complaints and symptoms. Asymmetry of findings represents a good predictive value of neurological abnormalities, as opposed to mild symmetrical signs like distal lower limb hypoesthesia or reflex abolition. After an interview of the patient and possibly of a caregiver, an organized and thorough examination will determine whether neurological dysfunction exists. Antecedents and comorbidities should be formally collected, as well as full drug prescription. Any medical history should be deeply explored. Simply observing the patient during the course of the usual history and physical behaviors like watching the patient walk and get up and down from the exam table is the first step of examination. Then, as in adult, a formal examination will help to identify which components of the neurological system are affected (e.g., motor, sensory, cranial nerves, or possibly several systems simultaneously) and to determine the precise location of the problem, e.g., peripheral versus central nervous system.

P. Krolak-Salmon
Lyon Institute for Elderly – Lyon University Hospital, Clinical and Research Memory Centre of Lyon, Lyon, France

Hôpital des Charpennes, 27 rue Gabriel Péri, 69100 Villeurbanne, France
e-mail: pierre.krolak-salmon@chu-lyon.fr

© Springer International Publishing Switzerland 2017

M. Berhouma, P. Krolak-Salmon (eds.), *Brain and Spine Surgery in the Elderly*,
DOI 10.1007/978-3-319-40232-1_3

3.1 "Somatic" Neurological Examination

3.1.1 Gait and Coordination

Gait observation and examination are very informative. Multiple features may be examined, as speed, amplitude and regularity of steps, linearity, quality of the half-turn, and quality of standing up, especially feet together. The Romberg test (contrast of quality of standing eyes open versus eyes closed) will suggest sensorial disorders in particular sensory or vestibular impairments versus cerebellar syndrome.

Some global testing may quantify gait impairments and fall risks, in particular the "Timed Up and Go test" and monopodal standing, "walking, and talking" test.

Gait disorders and repeated falls imply a clinical research of cerebellar and vestibular syndrome, as well as sensory impairments. Romberg testing is essential, like in adult, as well as the star walking test. If this last test is difficult to perform, the Fukuda stepping test is really interesting. The patient stands up, closes both eyes and holds his arms outstretched directly in front of him, and starts stepping in place for 50–100 steps. His body may rotate to the side of the vestibular function impairment.

3.1.2 Muscle Strength, Tone, and Bulk

Muscle strength is important to systematically evaluate in the elderly. Four limb segments and right and left hemibodies should be compared to disclose any global or focal muscular deficit. Barré and Mingazzini testings are particularly profitable since old people should be able to perform them. Simply asking to rise from chair sitting or bed lying is very informative, for instance, to disclose any muscle syndrome. Formal muscular testing, group by group, is indicated by the complaint or handicap of the patient. Strength testing must take into account the age, sex, and fitness level of the patient. For example, a frail, elderly, bed-bound patient may have muscle weakness due to severe deconditioning and not to intrinsic neurological disease. Interpretation must also consider the expected strength of the muscle group being tested. The quadriceps group, for example, should be much more powerful then the biceps.

The classical 0–5 rating scale is applicable in the elderly for muscle strength:

0/5	No movement
1/5	Barest flicker of movement of the muscle, though not enough to move the structure to which it's attached
2/5	Voluntary movement which is not sufficient to overcome the force of gravity. For example, the patient would be able to slide their hand across a table but not lift it from the surface
3/5	Voluntary movement capable of overcoming gravity but not any applied resistance. For example, the patient could raise their hand off a table but not if any additional resistance were applied
4/5	Voluntary movement capable of overcoming "some" resistance
5/5	Normal strength

Muscular tonus should be normal, but very mild rigidity with subtle cogwheeling may be observed in the elderly without any real Parkinsonism. Spasticity has to be looked for, revealing often neurovascular disease or arthrosic myelopathy. Cubito-pronator and Achilles reflexes are often absent in the elderly, asymmetry being important to disclose. A Babinski sign is always pathologic. Cephalic extremity reflexes maintain a good semiological value in old age. Alternative movements are particularly efficient to disclose a Parkinsonian or cerebellar syndrome.

This assessment is somewhat subjective and quite dependent on the age, sex, and the activity or fitness level of the individual. A frail elderly person, for example, will have less muscle bulk than a 25-year-old body builder. With experience, you will get a sense of the normal range for given age groups, factoring in their particular activity levels and overall states of health.

Tremors are particularly frequent in the elderly, mostly resting tremor of the hand (the head and other body parts can also be affected) that diminishes when the patient voluntarily moves the affected limb, suggesting Parkinsonian syndrome, and benign essential tremor persisting throughout movement.

3.1.3 Sensory Function

Sensitivity should be examined like in adult, oriented by complaints and symptoms. The two main afferent pathways, i.e., spinothalamics and dorsal columns systems, should be tested.

Lower limb distal lemniscal abnormalities are common in the elderly, especially proprioception and vibratory sensation. Small-fiber impairment-related abnormalities are frequent, especially in case of diabetes or alcohol consumption.

3.1.4 Cranial Nerves

Cranial nerves should be explored in aged patients following classical procedures. Some specific issues should be mentioned.

Despite rareness of specific complaints, olfaction is often impaired in the elderly, for instance, in neurodegenerative diseases like Parkinson's disease or Alzheimer's disease or tumors of the skull base. Formal assessment of ability to smell would need a test tube filled with something that has a distinct, common odor to the open nostrils. The patient should be able to correctly identify the odor at approximately 10 cm. Standardized tests are now available.

Visual acuity is usually evaluated by an ophthalmologist or optometrist. Distinguishing fingers or hand movement in front of the patient's face, light detection, and pupil reflex are very useful. The Amsler grid is useful to detect macular degeneration or retina detachment. Holes in vision (referred to as visual field cuts) are caused by a disruption along any point in the path from the eyeball to the visual cortex of the brain. Visual fields assessment is performed for each eye separately, the examiner sitting in front of the patient, separated by approximately

8–12 in. The examiner closes one eye and the patient hides the one opposite. The examiner should move their hand out toward the periphery of his/her visual field on the side where the eyes are open. Since meaningful interpretation is predicated upon the examiner having normal fields, as they are using themselves for comparison, the fingers should be equidistant from both persons. The examiner should then move the wiggling finger toward them, along an imaginary line drawn between the two persons. The patient and examiner should detect the finger at more or less the same time.

Oculomotricity is usually full, despite some binocular elevation limitation after the late 70's. Formal oculomotricity examination is very useful in case of atypical Parkinsonism or repeated falls to help to disclose supranuclear palsy syndrome and any parietal, frontal, or brainstem syndrome.

Audition is often impaired, mostly by presbyacousia. A formal audiometry should be performed in case of clinical hypoacousia, since hearing aid may help several geriatric syndromes like gait disorders and falls, memory impairment and cognition, and depression. Identifying conductive versus sensorineural hearing deficits requires historical information as well as the results of Webber and Rinne testings.

3.2 Cognitive Assessment

3.2.1 Complaint

Any complaint should be sought and precisely explored before any neuropsychological testing. A memory complaint is different from a language complaint and a spatial disorientation. Behavioral changes must be explored with caregivers, because they may inaugurate some diseases like frontotemporal degeneration, Lewy body disease or vascular disease, as well as rare cases of frontal Alzheimer's disease.

The Cognitive Difficulties Scale (CDS, McNair and Kahn, 1984) and the following six questions [3] represent a good example of a tool exploring formally the cognitive complaint.

Compared to a few years ago:

- Does the patient have more trouble remembering things that have happened recently than he or she used to?
- Does he or she have more trouble recalling conversations a few days later?
- When speaking, does the patient have more difficulty in finding the right word or tend to use the wrong words more often?
- Is the patient less able to manage money and financial affairs (e.g., paying bills, budgeting)?
- Is the patient less able to manage his or her medication independently?
- Does the patient need more assistance with transport (either private or public)? (If the patient has difficulties due only to physical problems, e.g., bad leg, tick "no.")

(To get a total score, add the number of items answered "no," "don't know," or "N/A.")
Total score (out of 6).
If patient scores 0–3, cognitive impairment is indicated. Conduct standard investigations.

Before considering any extensive neuropsychological examination, simple tests may help to explore the main cognitive domains, i.e., episodic and semantic memory, verbal language, high-order visual function, praxies, executive function, and judgment.

A neuropsychological evaluation should be considered in cases presenting with a mild deficit (for instance, with a MMSE > 15–18) or to circumvent language disorders.

3.2.2 Tracking Tests

Several tests are available to explore global cognition, to provide a reference status and a follow-up, in particular the Mini-Mental State Examination [7] and the Montreal Cognitive Assessment [10]. The latter is particularly interesting in case of attention of executive dysfunction, like in subcortical and frontal lesions, Parkinson's disease, or vascular disease. Some functions like memory are better explored by specific tests like the MIS (Memory Impairment Screen) [4].

Verbal language should be explored first through interrogation of the patient. The physician should pay attention to verbal fluency and occurrence of verbal or phonemic paraphasia, should nominate several objects, and test verbal understanding and sentence repetition. Verbal fluencies may be formally explored through tests like the Isaac set test that needs also good executive function.

Besides cognition, it is crucial to quantify functional status and look for any autonomy loss, first by a good clinical history collection, second by formal testing, for instance, with the *Instrumental Activities of Daily Life* Scale [9]. Mood evaluation is also important through interrogation and if possible through a formal testing like the Geriatric Depression Scale [12].

3.2.3 Cognitive Function Declining with Aging

Attention is "the gate" to cognition. Attention is "multiple" and global, and selective, divided attention has to be considered. It is linked to vigilance and processing speed that may decline in aging [14]. Old-age people appear to be slower in cognitive processing and present some decline in selective and divided attention-related tasks. That may influence all specific cognitive function, especially memory and executive function.

Language is a frequent complaint in the elderly, particularly word-finding difficulties [1]. Access to lexicon may decline, what may be disclosed through naming and verbal fluency testing [5]. Semantic memory, vocabulary, orthography, verbal understanding, and reasoning are not classically sensitive to physiological aging [17, 18].

Visual recognition, praxies, and visuospatial processing are quite resistant to normal aging also. Visual perception may be slightly declining [2, 11], but visual function is often impaired in the elderly through ophthalmological disorders like cataract or macular degeneration.

Performance in *executive function* testing is particularly frail in normal aging, but speed processing influences deeply this kind of testing. Nevertheless, it is hypothesized in literature that executive function declines specifically during aging [19, 20]. Control, inhibition, planning, flexibility, and regulation processes may be particularly frail and may influence other cognitive domains like memory. Frontal cortex, especially orbitofrontal and anterior cingular cortex, may be involved in structural and metabolic changes during aging [6, 8, 13, 21].

Thus, two options have to be considered in normal aging: first, a global cognition decline mainly due to attention and speed-processing decline; second, some cognitive domains may be specifically weakened like executive, memory, and verbal language. Cognitive reserve may be important to consider in normal aging [15, 16]. Thus, cognitive reserve that is built thanks to genetic polymorphism, education, and social and professional interaction may help to resist to neurodegenerative diseases and to influence the duration of their asymptomatic period. Neural and cognitive reserve may be weakened by chronic diseases, especially neurovascular disease, cardiorespiratory or metabolic dysfunction, and also depression and anxiety.

References

1. Albert ML, Spiro A 3rd, Sayers KJ, Cohen JA, Brady CB, Goral M, Obler LK (2009) Effects of health status on word finding in aging. J Am Geriatr Soc 57:2300–2305
2. Benton AL, Eslinger PJ, Damasio AR (1981) Normative observations on neuropsychological test performances in old age. J Clin Neuropsychol 3:33–42
3. Brodaty H, Pond D, Kemp NM, Luscombe G, Harding L, Berman K, Huppert FA (2002) The GPCOG: a new screening test for dementia designed for general practice. J Am Geriatr Soc 50:530–534
4. Buschke H, Kuslansky G, Katz M, Stewart WF, Sliwinski MJ, Eckholdt HM, Lipton RB (1999) Screening for dementia with the memory impairment screen. Neurology 52:231–238
5. Coen RF, Maguire C, Swanwick GR, Kirby M, Burke T, Lawlor BA, Walsh JB, Coakley D (1996) Letter and category fluency in Alzheimer's disease: a prognostic indicator of progression? Dementia 7:246–250
6. Convit A, Wolf OT, de Leon MJ, Patalinjug M, Kandil E, Caraos C, Scherer A, Saint Louis LA, Cancro R (2001) Volumetric analysis of the pre-frontal regions: findings in aging and schizophrenia. Psychiatry Res 107:61–73
7. Folstein MF, Folstein SE, McHugh PR (1975) "Mini-mental state". A practical method for grading the cognitive state of patients for the clinician. J Psychiatr Res 12:189–198
8. Hedden T, Gabrieli JD (2004) Insights into the ageing mind: a view from cognitive neuroscience. Nat Rev Neurosci 5:87–96
9. Lawton MP, Brody EM (1969) Assessment of older people: self-maintaining and instrumental activities of daily living. Gerontologist 9:179–186

10. Nasreddine ZS, Phillips NA, Bedirian V, Charbonneau S, Whitehead V, Collin I, Cummings JL, Chertkow H (2005) The Montreal Cognitive Assessment, MoCA: a brief screening tool for mild cognitive impairment. J Am Geriatr Soc 53:695–699
11. Read DE (1988) Age-related changes in performance on a visual-closure task. J Clin Exp Neuropsychol 10:451–466
12. Reisberg B, Ferris SH, de Leon MJ, Crook T (1982) The Global Deterioration Scale for assessment of primary degenerative dementia. Am J Psychiatry 139:1136–1139
13. Resnick SM, Lamar M, Driscoll I (2007) Vulnerability of the orbitofrontal cortex to age-associated structural and functional brain changes. Ann N Y Acad Sci 1121:562–575
14. Salthouse TA (1996) The processing-speed theory of adult age differences in cognition. Psychol Rev 103:403–428
15. Stern Y (2012) Cognitive reserve in ageing and Alzheimer's disease. Lancet Neurol 11:1006–1012
16. Tucker AM, Stern Y (2011) Cognitive reserve in aging. Curr Alzheimer Res 8:354–360
17. Verhaeghen P (2003) Aging and vocabulary scores: a meta-analysis. Psychol Aging 18:332–339
18. Verhaeghen P, Steitz DW, Sliwinski MJ, Cerella J (2003) Aging and dual-task performance: a meta-analysis. Psychol Aging 18:443–460
19. West RL (1996) An application of prefrontal cortex function theory to cognitive aging. Psychol Bull 120:272–292
20. West R (2000) In defense of the frontal lobe hypothesis of cognitive aging. J Int Neuropsychol Soc 6:727–729; discussion 730
21. Willis MW, Ketter TA, Kimbrell TA, George MS, Herscovitch P, Danielson AL, Benson BE, Post RM (2002) Age, sex and laterality effects on cerebral glucose metabolism in healthy adults. Psychiatry Res 114:23–37

Part II

Neuroanesthesia and Critical Care

Neurosurgical Anesthesia for the Elderly: Is Age Really Just a Number?

4

David A. Wyler, Elizabeth M. Gabrielli, and W. Andrew Kofke

4.1 Introduction

Innovation in medicine has increased the survival and health of our population in recent years. The increasing age trend has grown the neurosurgical sector. Similarly, this expansion has led to the advent of many innovative procedures now available to seniors. From minimally invasive spine surgery to deep brain stimulation implant for Parkinson's disease, the innovation in neurosurgery has sparked new anesthetic techniques to best accommodate the growth in technology. For instance, awake craniotomy is now offered to elderly patients to determine which areas of the brain are responsible for abnormal functions and which ones are eloquent and must be avoided. The anesthetic technique should be tailored to best achieve these goals regardless of choice of anesthetic [1]. The fact is however that age alone is an independent risk factor for perioperative morbidity and mortality [2].

The geriatric patient with aging organ systems combined with neurologic disease presents unique challenges to the neuroanesthesiologist. It is important to discover through this chapter that the senescent brain does not age by itself independently. Rather multiple connections exist between each human system that influence the aging process in the brain and then consequently become further complicated with disease. Furthermore, not all patients age in equal form. Variability between aging patterns from patient to patient also makes it difficult to

D.A. Wyler, MD
Department of Anesthesiology & Critical Care, Neurosurgery, Jefferson Hospital of Neuroscience, Thomas Jefferson University, Philadelphia, PA, USA
e-mail: david.wyler@uphs.upenn.edu

W.A. Kofke (✉) • E.M. Gabrielli, MD
Department of Anesthesiology and Critical Care, Neurosurgery, University of Pennsylvania, 7 Dulles Building, 3400 Spruce St, Philadelphia, PA, USA
e-mail: William.Kofke@uphs.upenn.edu; elizabeth.mahannagabrielli@uphs.upenn.edu

© Springer International Publishing Switzerland 2017

M. Berhouma, P. Krolak-Salmon (eds.), *Brain and Spine Surgery in the Elderly*,
DOI 10.1007/978-3-319-40232-1_4

predict which organ systems to key in on while in the care of the perioperative physician. The aim of this chapter is to review the perioperative challenges of the elderly patient as they pertain to neurosurgical anesthesia. We will explore the perioperative experience for older adults and identify risk factors most relevant to the neurosurgical patient.

"Aging is a progressive and irreversible phenomenon characterized by degenerative changes in the structure and functional reserve of the organs and tissues" [3]. Obviously, in the modern era of medicine, polypharmacy coincides with advancing physiological age. Preoperatively, the neuroanesthesiologist is tasked with evaluating each of these organ systems and coinciding home medications paying special attention to their interactions with anesthetic drugs. In preparation for procedures targeting the brain and spinal cord, it is essential to establish baseline neurologic function and evaluate systems which are not only aged but more importantly physiologically dysfunctional.

4.2 Frailty

Recently, there has been considerable attention given to the concept of "frailty" in the elderly and its implications in the preoperative evaluation. Overwhelming evidence proves seniors have a higher risk for perioperative morbidity and mortality, and recent research demonstrates that "frailty" or lack of physiological reserve accounts for this phenomenon rather than chronological age alone [4, 5]. The old adage holds true: "age is just a number." One landmark study by Makary et al. demonstrated that frailty was associated with a significantly increased risk of postoperative complication (odds ratio [OR]=2.54) and institutionalization (OR=20.48) [5]. Historically, anesthesiologists and surgeons have visited their patients preoperatively to determine their patient's physical condition documenting physical exam phrases such as well nourished, well developed, or cachectic. Models such as the frailty phenotype and frailty index (fi) were created to help qualify the degree of frailty and replace the practice of "eyeballing" patients that we have done in years past [4, 5].

These assessment tools may help risk stratify elderly patients and serve as guides to clinicians in the patient selection/optimization process prior to surgery. Frailty phenotype meshes physical changes, namely, weight loss and sarcopenia (muscle atrophy) with performance measures such as endurance, slowness, gait, and handgrip [5, 6]. Alternatively, the fi represents a multidimensional risk state measured by the quantity of "deficits" an individual has accumulated. It incorporates dozens of dichotomized deficits including comorbidities, activities of daily living (ADL), and signs from the physical and neurological examination [5, 6]. Table 4.1 demonstrates an example of fi and demonstrates the inclusiveness of this comprehensive evaluation.

It is the opinion of this author that anesthesiologists can optimize seniors preoperatively and modify outcome. Certainly, in emergency surgery, where time lost

Table 4.1 Example of frailty index (fi) [5]

Deficits counted	Points (max denominator 55)
Cognition	Dementia = 1, mild cog. imp. = 0.5, delirium = 1, agitation = 1, delusions/hallucinations = 1
Emotional state	Anxiety = 1, recent bereavement = 1, depression = 1, fatigue = 1
Sleep	Poor or disrupted = 1, drowsiness = 1
Speech, hearing, vision	Impaired = 1 each
Hemiparesis	Weak arm = 1, weak leg = 1
Grip strength or proximal muscle strength (on non-hemiplegic side)	Weak = 1 each
Weight or weight change	Underweight = 1, obese = 1, slightly overweight = 0, loss = 1, gain = 1
Appetite	Poor = 1, fair = 0.5, normal = 0
Continence	Bowel or bladder incontinence = 1 each
Medical history (scoring 1 point each)	Hypertension, asthma/COPD, stroke/transient ischemic attack, angina/myocardial infarction, heart failure, diabetes, cancer/alcohol excess, pressure sores, hip fracture, osteoarthritis/osteoporosis, Parkinson's disease
No. of medications in 24 h	0–4 = 0, 5–9 = 1, 10–14 = 2, 15–19 = 3, 20–24 = 4, >25 = 5
Transfers or walking	Dependent = 1, assistance = 0.5
Movements (slow)	Yes = 1
Sitting balance	Impaired = 1
Falls in the last 6 months	Three or more = 1
Feeding, washing, and dressing (1 each)	Dependent = 1, assistance = 0.5
Manages own medications and finances	Dependent = 1, assistance = 0.5

may worsen neurologic injury, this would be a tall task. However, elective surgery should be preceded by a clinic visit [7, 8]. A visit to anesthesia clinic for preoperative evaluation could mean the start of an exercise program or physical therapy [1]. Perhaps, anemia can be worked up and nutritional deficiency addressed. Studies are under way that hypothesize that optimization based on frailty can benefit seniors.

4.3 Physiologic Reserve by Organ System

4.3.1 Central Nervous System Reserve

4.3.1.1 Cognitive Reserve

As "frailty" ensues, organ parenchyma atrophies. The brain is no exception. Loss of brain reserve can be considered in terms of cognitive or cerebrovascular reserve, and both relate to structural losses. Neurodegenerative conditions in the elderly cause destruction of neurons and synapses leading to cognitive dysfunction [3]. Structurally, this may be seen on neuroimaging as diffuse cortical atrophy, sulcal enlargement, and increased ventricular size. Alzheimer's disease (AD), the pathophysiology of which is highly complex, is best known to be associated with advanced age [9, 10]. In the late stages of AD, the above imaging findings are profound. These same structural changes are often present in patients older than 70 without cognitive impairment, albeit not to the extent as occurs in AD.

Extensive investigation looking at age-related loss of neuroplasticity has shown that decreased hippocampal regenerative capacity is key in senior's short-term memory loss and age-related cognitive decline [11]. Considerable research has also been conducted looking at anesthesia-related neurotoxicity and POCD. This will be covered at greater length in Chap. 3 "Neurotoxicity and the Elderly."

Medications taken by these elderly patients to treat their neurodegenerative disorders, movement disorders, and depression spark concern for the neuroanesthesiologist because many drug-drug interactions exist between them and anesthetic mediations. Centrally acting acetylcholine (ACh) inhibitors, the mainstay of AD therapy, may significantly interact with anesthetic drugs, namely, neuromuscular-blocking drugs (NMBDs) [10]. The duration of action of succinylcholine may be prolonged up to 50 min by inhibiting pseudocholinesterase with AD medications [10]. The half-life of non-depolarizing NMBDs such as vecuronium may decrease as a result of postsynaptic Ach receptor downregulation reducing receptor availability for the drug [10].

Parkinson's disease, also a disease primarily found in elderly, poses specific anesthetic challenges. Loss of dopamine-secreting cells in the substantia nigra leads to dysregulation in the basal ganglia and midbrain communications responsible for coordinating movement [12]. Not only does the Parkinson's phenotype present challenges during awake procedures, but issues arise such as autonomic instability, respiratory compromise, and cognitive impairment [12]. Resting tremor, rigidity, and bradykinesia of the respiratory muscles make emergence from anesthesia a challenge for the neuroanesthesiologist. The drugs used to combat Parkinson's disease also interact with anesthetic drugs. Bromocriptine and Sinemet, commonly used anti-Parkinson's medications, potentiate anesthetic-induced hypotension. Moreover, selegiline, a monoamine oxidase inhibitor B (MAOiB) frequently prescribed to patients in late-stage PD to help reduce Sinemet dose, should never be given with meperidine. In fact, caution should be taken with all opioids when a patient chronically takes selegiline. Meperidine in particular has been shown to cause hyperpyrexia, agitation, and rigidity in combination with selegiline [13]. All these medications for AD and PD should be continued at their regular suggested time during the perioperative period, and nasogastric route should be used during operative doses [9, 12, 13]. Because of long-term use of antiquated depression medications like MAOiAs and tricyclic antidepressants (TCAs), seniors at times present to the operating room taking medications with coexisting serious side effects. TCAs and MAOis are infamous for their numerous side effects. MAOis are known to cause hypertensive crisis by an interaction with ephedrine and other indirect-acting vasopressors. TCAs may lead to QRS prolongation, anticholinergic side effects, and hypotension under anesthesia due to catecholamine depletion. The elderly, given their numerous comorbid conditions, often have a long list of medications, and this polypharmacy brings higher risk for anesthetic interaction and medication error [14].

4.3.1.2 Cerebrovascular Reserve

As brain mass decreases with age, so does the brain's metabolism leading to a decrease in oxygen requirement and blood flow required to support brain function. Cerebral hemodynamics have been studied extensively in the elderly but still remain unclear [15–17]. We do know that a relationship exists between cerebral blood flow (CBF) and cerebral perfusion pressure (CPP). Figure 4.1 demonstrates an autoregulatory zone demonstrating cerebral vessel reactivity along the plateau phase. This plateau phase highlights varying degrees of vessel constriction and dilation (reactivity) in response to high- or low-pressure states, respectively. The plateau phase starts and ends with two inflection points termed the lower and upper limits of autoregulation. Outside of the autoregulatory zone, CPP and CBF have linear relationships and are termed nonreactive, perfusional, or outside the autoregulatory zone. Although highly debated, newer thought favors the notion that autoregulation and cerebrovascular reserve are not impaired when investigating age alone [18]. Elderly patients may have chronic hypertension which may shift the curve and corresponding lower inflection point to the right [16]. It is also logical to infer that known increases in sympathetic activity in the elderly shift the autoregulatory curve to the right [16]. A right shift in the autoregulatory curve may lead to ischemic stroke at borderline CPP values once thought to be safe.

Although chronological age alone seems unrelated to cerebral hemodynamics, elderly patients with carotid artery disease, peripheral vascular disease, advanced diabetes mellitus, or other comorbid conditions related to structurally abnormal cerebral vasculature have been found to lack the ability to vasodilate in focal

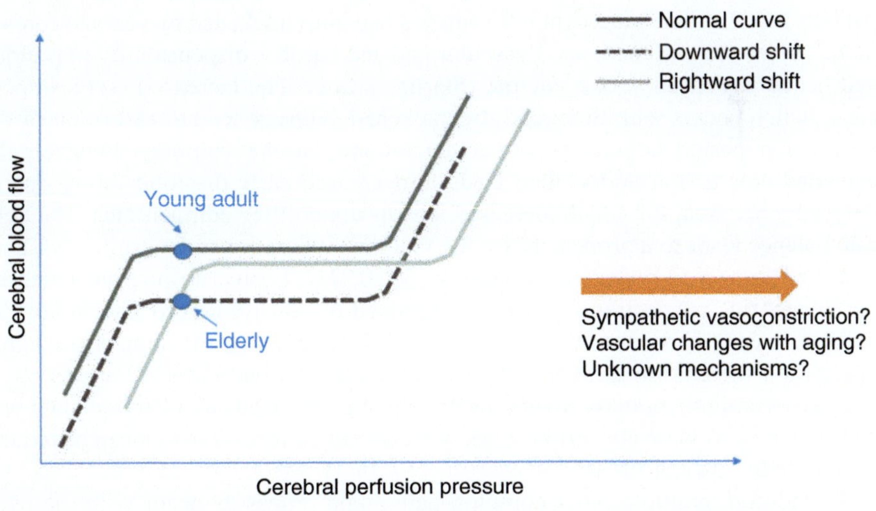

Fig. 4.1 Cerebral hemodynamics in the elderly [16]

regions susceptible to ischemia [15, 18, 19]. Thus, these patients have decreased cerebrovascular reserve and are at increased risk for perioperative stroke seen frequently in watershed areas of the brain [16, 17]. Patients with poor reserve fail to maximally dilate in susceptible regions in response to increased PCO2 from hypoventilation or an acetazolamide challenge. This "steal" phenomenon, where CBF actually decreases in areas of low reserve, has been demonstrated using transcranial Doppler (TCD) and stable xenon computed tomography (Xe/CT) [18]. This is hypothesized to be a mechanism of stroke in carotid artery stenting [18]. Alternatively, a patient with adequate reserve may not demonstrate stroke signs in response to the same emboli that break off from a proximal plaque or thrombus [18]. Evaluating cerebral reserve preoperatively using TCD, Xe/CT, or other perfusion scans may be a good way to stratify stroke risk preoperatively by evaluating a patient's cerebral reserve [17, 18].

4.3.2 Cardiovascular Reserve

Just as the aging process may affect cerebral hemodynamics by thickening the inner walls of cerebral arteries, the same changes occur in vessels all over the body as humans age. Arterial stiffening leads to chronic hypertension primarily isolated systolic hypertension and increased pulse pressure [3, 20, 21]. Reduced venous compliance exaggerates hypotension by dropping preload in hypovolemic states like blood loss, diuresis, and the insensible losses frequently seen in lengthy spine surgery. Concomitant anesthetic drugs exacerbate the above reduction of preload, and pooling of venous blood occurs primarily into the splanchnic venous circulation. Reduced preload accompanies the aged autonomic nervous system that lacks the neuron mass that their younger counterparts possess [22]. A reduced sympathetic response to stress underscores the reduced cardiovascular reserve seen in geriatric patients [21, 22]. The senescent left ventricle becomes thickened by years of forcing blood across the stiffened, aged vascular bed and has less dispensability to preload and hence a reduced stroke volume (Starling's law). The increased aortic impedance, which occurs with time, and the thickened ventricle lead to extension of the contraction period helping to offset the reduced stroke volume. However, the extended contraction period then leads to decreased early diastolic filling due to delayed relaxation, for which increased late diastolic filling compensates. The delicate balance leads to a propensity for the volume intolerance and diastolic dysfunction well known to occur in the elderly [3, 20, 21]. Lastly, despite an increased norepinephrine concentration, there is a reduced responsiveness to catecholamine, thus decreasing chronotropy and inotropy [20]. Essentially, the sum of the aging process on the cardiovascular system is a reduced cardiac output. Fortunately, a reduced overall organ mass favors lower demand. This leads to a very delicate balance of stroke volume and stroke work, which leads little reserve that can be readily overcome in times of stress.

In addition, multiple other common pathologic processes occur with the aged heart. A thickened left ventricle is also accompanied by increased left-sided filling pressure leading to a distended left atrium affecting the electrical conduction and frequently causing atrial fibrillation (AF). Since the elderly heart lacks the ability to fill efficiently during early diastole, it depends heavily on the atrial kick found in late diastole for optimal cardiac output [1, 21]. In the case of AF, the atrial kick is lost and often leads to acute pulmonary edema and florid cardiogenic shock in this vulnerable population. Moreover, thickening of the aortic valve commonly occurs in the elderly as well. Aortic stenosis can be viewed on a continuum from aortic sclerosis to severe aortic stenosis. Gradually, the valve area decreases creating a progressive pressure gradient to form between the left ventricle and the aorta. The result is reduced outflow to tissues such as the brain and coronary arteries. Vasodilation and reduced preload, as occur commonly during geriatric anesthesia, can be devastating with this valvular lesion. Since coronary blood flow and forward flow depend on maintaining diastolic blood pressure, maintaining vascular tone is essential. As such, phenylephrine, an alpha-1-agonist, is a good parenteral drug to optimize stroke volume and coronary perfusion during anesthesia-induced vasodilation [23]. Similarly, it avoids tachycardia with its intense alpha-1-vasoconstriction and reflex drop in the heart rate [23].

Since seniors, in general, are frequently prescribed antihypertensive and cardioprotective chronic medications, the neuroanesthesiologist must, in close consultation with cardiology and neurosurgery, decide cardiovascular perioperative best practice. Recent guidelines based on evidence-based medicine recommend the following: for higher-risk procedures such as craniotomy and multilevel spine procedures, pre-op evaluation should occur days prior. On the other hand, if the surgery is low risk like one-level diskectomy or percutaneous vertebroplasty, same-day management is appropriate [7, 24]. Currently, based on the POISE trials, the recommendations are to maintain current beta blockade on the day of surgery, but forego new prescriptions for the prevention of myocardial infarction on the day of surgery [25–27]. Angiotensin-converting enzyme inhibitors (ACE-I) and angiotensin receptor blockers (ARB) should be held on the day of surgery to prevent vasoplegic syndrome (VS) with anesthesia [28]. This is characterized by severe hypotension refractory to volume expansion and catecholamine therapy [28]. It is thought that since anesthesia blocks the sympathetic nervous system, vascular tone is then maintained by the vasopressinergic system and the renin-angiotensin system (RAS) [28, 29]. Since ACE-I and ARB block the RAS, these drugs are unique culprits of VS. Other antihypertensive meds can attribute to VS, but since they are less likely contributors, they often can be more safely maintained through the perioperative period. Aspirin and clopidogrel should be held for neurosurgery and held after the minimum 30 days have passed from bare-metal stent placement [25, 27]. Drug-eluting stents require 6 months of dual antiplatelet therapy (DAPT) to prevent stent re-thrombosis. Aspirin and a P2Y12 receptor blocker, most commonly clopidogrel, are prescribed. Other P2Y12 agents such as ticagrelor and prasugrel may be used, but improved safety has been found with clopidogrel [30, 31]. Elective surgery should therefore be postponed until these time periods have elapsed. However, in the emergency situation, this should be managed on case-by-case basis with multi-specialty involvement after a risk-benefit conversation [25, 27].

Anesthesiologists and surgeons frequently advocate that all elderly patients should be sent for EKG, echocardiography, and stress testing on the basis of advanced age alone. Actually, routine preoperative testing is not recommended by the ASA Practice Advisory for Preanesthesia Evaluation, even in older adults. Rather, they recommend anesthetic risk be assessed based on the severity of the patient's medical condition (s) and invasiveness of proposed procedure. Since the vast majority of neurosurgical procedures in the elderly are of intermediate to higher risk, most experts believe that even the fit elderly patients should undergo an EKG pre-op for the purpose of comparison. Stress testing, echo, and subsequent angiography should be reserved for patients with known or suspected cardiac disease, lower functional tolerance based on metabolic units (see Table 4.2), and

Table 4.2 Categories of functional tolerance based on (MET) metabolic units [32]

Light (<3 METs)	Moderate (3–6 METs)	Vigorous (>6 METs)
Walking	*Walking*	*Walking, jogging, and running*
Walking (slowly) = 2	Walking 3.0 mph = 3	Walking (very, very briskly, 4.5 mph) = 6.3
	Walking (very briskly, 4 mph) = 5	Walking/hiking (with moderate pace) = 7
		Hiking (steep grade with 10–40 lb pack) = 7.5–9
Household and occupation	*Household and occupation*	Jogging (5 mph) = 8
Sitting (at desk, typing, ate) = 1.5	Cleaning (heavy, washing windows, car) = 3	Jogging (6 mph) = 10
Standing (light work, making bed, dishes) = 2–2.5	Sweeping floors, vacuuming, mopping = 3–3.5	Running (7 mph) = 11.5
	Carpentry = 3.6	
Leisure time and sports	Carrying/stacking wood = 5.5	*Household and occupation*
	Mowing lawn (power mower) = 5.5	Shoveling sand, coal, etc. = 7
Boating (power) = 2.5		Carrying heavy loads = 7.5
Croquet = 2.5	*Leisure time and sports*	Heavy farming = 8
Darts = 2.5	Badminton (recreational = 4.5)	Shoveling, digging ditches = 8.5
Fishing (sitting) = 2.5	Basketball (shooting around) = 4.5	
Playing most musical instruments = 2–2.5	Bicycling on flat (light effort, 10–12 mph) = 6	*Leisure time and sports*
	Dancing (ballroom, slow) = 3	Basketball game = 8
	Dancing (ballroom, fast) = 4.5	Bicycling on flat (moderate, 12–14 mph) = 8
	Golf (walking, pulling clubs) = 4.3	Bicycling on flat (fast, 14–16 mph) = 10
	Sailing or windsurfing = 3	Cross-country skiing = 7

Recreated from Ainsworth et al. [32]

typical symptoms of angina or decompensated heart failure. Patients unable to exert four METs have increased cardiovascular risk and should undergo further evaluation.

4.3.3 Pulmonary Reserve

Just as aged cardiovascular systems work harmoniously at rest and falter under stress, respiratory resiliency also diminishes over time. Loss of respiratory reserve stems from anatomical changes that reduce mechanical advantage [1]. The emphysema-like change that occurs in the elderly lungs is characterized by the loss of alveolar architecture [33, 34]. Fractured alveolar membranes reduce lung elasticity and lung volumes rise. Figure 4.1 is a chest x-ray that characterizes the emphysema-like lungs demonstrating hyperinflation, flattened diaphragms, and increased lung volumes. Overall respiratory compliance does not change even though lung compliance increases [34]. Reduced chest wall compliance from the degenerative bony thorax offsets the increased lung compliance. Loss of alveoli reduces the surface area available for gas exchange increasing the physiological dead space. This in turn leads to intrapulmonary shunting reducing oxygen saturation at baseline and burdens seniors vulnerable to hypoxemia when threatened by any lesion that acutely worsens shunting and V/Q mismatch such as pneumonia, atelectasis, pulmonary embolus, pulmonary edema, or pulmonary contusion. The increased dead space also increases work of breathing during stress and initiates a vicious cycle of tachypnea, auto-PEEP, and pulmonary exhaustion that worsens the work of breathing. Auto-PEEP or extrinsic PEEP applied by the ventilator has an effect on ICP and brain volume if intrathoracic pressure is higher than ICP [35]. This would eliminate the "waterfall effect" (i.e., gradient required for venous drainage). However, in traumatic brain injury (TBI), where patients often have elevated ICP greater than PEEP, higher PEEP does not impede venous drainage or compromise CPP [36]. Paradoxically, in the elderly, PEEP can collapse alveolar capillaries, and less carbon dioxide can escape systemic circulation. Hypercarbia ensues and increases CBF and ICP [35]. The elderly respiratory system is thus at homeostasis, but when confronted with the stresses of an operation or illness, they often cannot adequately respond and hyperventilate appropriately to compensate.

Preoperative CXR was not found to improve morbidity and mortality although abnormalities were found more frequently in patients older than 70 [33] (Fig. 4.2).

4.3.4 Hepatic, Renal, and Nutritional Reserve

Predictably, as part of the aging process, reduced cardiac output in turn leads to lower flow to the kidneys and liver. Gradual reduction in organ perfusion gives rise to smaller and less functional kidneys and liver. Drop in glomerular filtration rate (GFR) is not always obvious because creatinine, our main tool besides urine output, also depends on muscle mass for secretion. Elderly patients with atrophied skeletal

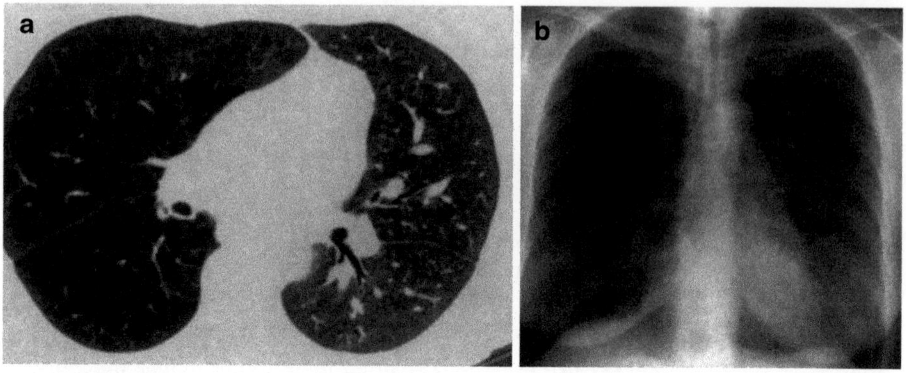

Fig. 4.2 (**a**) Emphysema-like changes demonstrate loss of alveolar architecture and low attenuation on CT scan of the right lung. (**b**) Hyperinflation and flattened diaphragm [37]

muscle secrete less, and so a high normal creatinine can be misleading and actually signify a low GFR in these patients. Reduced renal clearance causes many anesthetic drugs such as opioids and benzodiazepines to remain in the plasma and subsequently the brain longer [13]. Many anesthetic drugs are affected by an aged liver as well. While liver function tests are generally not affected by age, the amount of enzymes and plasma proteins produced by an atrophied liver are diminished. The result is less circulating plasma protein, less protein binding, and greater drug activity in the elderly [3, 13]. Furthermore, the aged adult's pharmacodynamics profile includes a reduced muscle mass, lower total body water, and greater fat content. This essentially means that water-soluble drugs like morphine have a lower volume of distribution (Vd) and more side effects. Fat-soluble anesthetic drugs like fentanyl, on the other hand, will store themselves in fat and have a higher Vd and hence a longer duration of action [14]. Likewise, reduced synthesis of liver enzymes (cytochrome P450 system) results in a decreased ability to degrade anesthetic drugs. In addition, the elderly neurosurgical patient may also be taking an antiseizure medication. Chronic therapy induces added cytochrome P450 enzymes in the liver accelerating the breakdown of non-depolarizing NMBD. Doses must be increased therefore to achieve the desired level of paralysis [38, 39]. The shrunken and functionally scaled-down capacity of the elderly organs underscores their diminished renal and hepatic reserve.

Elderly patients with and without neurologic disease frequently suffer from nutritional deficits as we discussed in the frailty section of this chapter. Low plasma albumin and prealbumin levels, proteins produced by the liver, have historically been used in ICUs to evaluate the nutritional status of patients. These measures may reflect nutritional status in the elderly; however, according to ASPEN guidelines, these acute phase reactants are not a substitute for history and physical indexes such as frailty. It is essential to also realize that nutritional status can affect many factors in neurosurgical anesthesia such as drug dosing and toxicity as well as retained intravascular volume and resuscitation.

4.3.5 Hematologic Issues

Hematologic issues and coagulopathies on all neurosurgical patients are of utmost importance. Outcomes in intracranial bleeding are influenced by hematoma size, growth, and location and the timing of evacuation, when indicated [40]. Common comorbid diseases in the elderly such as past MI, stroke, venous thromboembolism, and AF mandate that these patients take anticoagulation and antiplatelet medicine. In certain situations, the American Heart Association recommends continuing them into the perioperative period. This circumstance in conjunction with preexisting coagulopathies and perioperative transfusions combines to form a major concern for the neuroanesthesiologist. As such, perioperative strategies must be employed to best avoid serious intracranial bleeding. Table 4.2 lists the relevant antiplatelet and anticoagulants prescribed today along with their mechanism of action, indication, and current perioperative reversal strategy in elective and emergency surgery. We also include a post-op strategy to reinitiate therapy. Moreover, the bulk of the recommendations for reversal of antithrombotic that dictate practice patterns today are based off of expert opinion and studies with small populations (class C level I evidence). Nevertheless, the benefit of reducing hematoma expansion seems to be obvious to the neurosurgical community so the current guidelines recommend reversing or stopping the antithrombotic in the perioperative period. Moreover, in the case of intracerebral hemorrhage, a condition where hematoma formation expands and exerts mass effect and cellular injury, it is paramount that antithrombotic-induced coagulopathy be reversed as quickly as possible [41]. It is also worth mentioning that the American Heart Association guidelines for coagulation management in intracerebral hemorrhage provide no explicit instructions for perioperative care [42].

4.3.6 Musculoskeletal and Airway Changes

Derangements of the elderly musculoskeletal system are typified by degeneration of bone, collagen, and elastin fibers [1]. As tissues lose structure and flexibility, their reserve is compromised. As humans age, neuron mass declines, nerve denervation occurs, and skeletal muscle atrophies [3]. Preoperatively, the neuroanesthesiologist must recognize that changes in the musculoskeletal system translate to alterations of the airway that may lead to serious challenges. Elderly airway changes include loss of dentition and perioral atrophy, weakening the mask seal during bag mask ventilation [45]. Also due to osteoporosis and degenerative joint disease, a significant decrease in neck motion complicates the alignment of the axis known to improve laryngeal view in direct laryngoscopy [45]. Preparation to manage the elderly airway depends on the presence or suspicion of cervical fractures or instabilities. This requires that the necessary equipment to manage difficult airway be readily available. In the case of unstable spine, manual stabilization should be maintained throughout the airway securing process. The collar is usually removed and manual in-line stabilization is applied. If neurosurgical opinion is that a neurological exam should be maintained throughout the positioning process, then awake intubation should be performed. Fiber-optic intubation requires very little force and translation onto the cervical vertebra. Awake fiber-optic intubation is best performed with optimal airway preparation. This can be done by drying the airway with glycopyrrolate, an antimuscarinic agent, and then anesthetizing the airway. Airway anesthesia can be provided by topically nebulizing 4 % lidocaine or by injecting local anesthetic around the appropriate nerves that innervate the upper airway and the subglottic region. Videoscopic laryngoscopy is currently very popular in anesthetized patients with in-line stabilization because it translates less force onto the larynx than traditional laryngoscopy to obtain optimal view of cords [46, 47]. It should be known that studies demonstrating the force differences also showed that increased force did not correlate with increased cervical motion [46, 47]. It should be acknowledged that many various factors are at play when studying these techniques such as exclusion of difficult airway. In addition, there are other factors at play such as cooperation of the patient, skill of the anesthesia provider, and aspiration risk.

Besides making airway management challenging, degeneration of the spine also complicates traumatic spine injury. Elderly patients with spondylosis may present with central cord syndrome after hyperextension of the cervical spine. This syndrome is best known for classical signs of weakness and lack of sensation in the upper extremity with preserved lower extremity function.

4.3.7 Endocrine Reserve

The endocrine system is the "glue" that holds all the previous systems already discussed together. Its ability to regulate critical functions of other systems by interacting with the CNS, gastrointestinal, reproductive, and cardiovascular systems is remarkable. The aging process alters the precision and the tightly regulated function of the endocrine system, resulting in several malfunction-related disorders. Examples of age-related endocrine disorders, typified by age-related secretory wear down, are non-insulin-dependent DM, hypothyroidism, hypogonadism, hypopituitarism, and hypoadrenalism [48]. In addition, tumors of the elderly may lead to dysregulation and out-of-control secretion as occurs in hyperthyroidism and Cushing's disease. If left untreated, hyperthyroidism in the elderly could lead to rapid AF and imminent cardiovascular collapse. This is an example of how disruption of endocrine function if ignored can lead to physiological imbalance while younger adults may compensate. Frequently, patients take chronic steroids before and after neurosurgical procedures and may be at risk for adrenal insufficiency. More than twice as likely to occur in the elderly population, adrenal insufficiency should be addressed with intraoperative supplementation, and postoperative taper should be considered depending on the duration of administration [14, 49]. Data does not support stress dosing every patient, but consultation with an endocrinologist may be helpful to avoid perioperative complications. This is of particular importance in pituitary surgery. Elderly patients are frequently prescribed ACE inhibitors and angiotensin receptor blockers for BP control. Since these medications disrupt the renin-angiotensin-aldosterone system (RAAS), profound hypotension may occur under anesthesia in the elderly because of RAAS inhibition, diminished cardiac reserve, and sympathetic-blocking drugs [28].

4.3.8 Preoperative Anesthetic Planning

Once the preoperative evaluation is complete, the neuroanesthesiologist uses the information ascertained from patient history and physical combined with the positioning and invasiveness of the planned procedure to formulate the anesthetic plan. In certain neurosurgical situations, an awake procedure may be an option. However, in the elderly, the majority of procedures today are done with the patient under general anesthesia (GA). If the patient's airway, cognition, and physiological reserve are amenable, an awake procedure may be the best option. This requires in-depth discussion of the entire neurosurgical team along with discussion with the patient and family.

Decision at this time should be made regarding intravenous (IV) access, invasive monitoring, and patient positioning. Most neurosurgical procedures are deemed high on an estimation of bleeding risk; therefore, at least one and usually two large-bore IV lines are placed. Not only is the volume of blood loss considered high in spine surgery, but in the case of intracranial procedures, bleeding risk is high because bleeding in the brain leads to serious and sometimes irreversible complications. Similarly, because estimation of bleeding risk is high, it is customary to cross-match several units of different blood products for neurosurgical procedures. The bleeding risk in the elderly is higher than that of younger adults because elderly patients lose heat quickly, their renal and liver function is reduced, and medication prescribed for their comorbid conditions may still be lingering in their systemic circulation. Maintaining a reasonable temperature close to normothermia is important for hemostasis and avoidance of shivering in this patient population. Hypothermia interferes with coagulation by decreasing platelet and factor function. Shivering increases ICP and increases the metabolic rates of both the heart and the brain [50]. In the elderly population with reduced reserve of these organ systems, this could be disastrous.

A central venous line may be necessary and should be planned if the sitting position is required for posterior fossa surgery [51, 52]. The distal port should be placed at the SVC/right atrial junction so that if a large air embolus should occur, it could be aspirated out this port of the central line avoiding an air lock that could shut down forward flow. Monitoring for intradural procedures should include an arterial line to best manage the second-by-second hemodynamic changes and metabolic challenges of the surgery. In the setting of seated posterior fossa surgery, investigation using TEE to rule out patent foramen ovale (PFO) should be complete prior to seating the patient. Failure to rule out PFO could lead to paradoxical air embolus and ultimately stroke and MI [52]. In addition, since TEE has limitations, once PFO is ruled out, many neuroanesthesiologists prefer to monitor with precordial Doppler over TEE intraoperatively since TEE may cause tongue swelling with a flexed neck and may deactivate during the case if the critical temperature of the probe is reached. Precordial Doppler is very sensitive and picks up audible air well, but it cannot distinguish small amounts of air from large boluses that could lead to air lock [51, 52]. Above all, good communication with the surgeon as well as reviewing imaging data helps avoid wasteful moves in the operating room by positioning the patient in a way that facilitates the surgeon's trajectory to the pathology.

4.3.9 Anesthesia for Supratentorial Craniotomy

Frontal-temporal and pterional incisions are common craniotomy approaches to enter the brain for tumor excision and aneurysm clipping. General anesthesia for this traditional approach is done via an IV induction. The technique used should include a combination of a hypnotic to produce unconsciousness, an analgesic, and a muscle relaxant. Since propofol can lead to profound hypotension in the elderly, a cautious slow IV push should be given at a reduced dose. Etomidate may also be used to prevent hypotension in the elderly. For aneurysm surgery, the induction should be done very carefully not to increase transmural pressure in the aneurysm and rupture. The goal is to avoid rise in systolic blood pressure and strain on laryngoscopy or intubation. Different approaches have been offered to accomplish this goal: high-dose opioids, lidocaine, paralysis, and beta blockers. A combination of propofol, lidocaine, vecuronium, and fentanyl for induction works well. After administering high-dose fentanyl, a video laryngoscopy and laryngeal-tracheal lidocaine can be sprayed in the trachea prior to intubation. If during the video laryngoscopy there is a hemodynamic response, more fentanyl may be administered prior to reentering the mouth to intubate. Also sufentanil can be used at equianalgesic dose. In the elderly, it is important during any induction to prepare for fluctuations in blood pressure. A vasoconstrictor (phenylephrine) and a vasodilator (nicardipine) should be prepared in case significant fluctuations occur. In order to accurately monitor mean arterial pressure, the transducer should be placed at the tragus of the ear in the elderly. Since a hydrostatic gradient may exist between the aorta and the circle of Willis, it makes sense to maintain mean arterial pressure (MAP) of at least 65 at the tragus to ensure that the elderly brain is adequately profused. While positioning for these surgeries, the neuroanesthesiologist should verify that all bony prominences are well padded since peripheral nerves close to the surface of bones are susceptible to ischemic injury. During skull fixation, three fingerbreadths of space should also be confirmed to prevent ischemic over-flexion injury of cervical spinal cord.

4.3.10 Intraoperative Neuromonitoring (IONM)

In order to protect against cerebral injury intraoperatively, evoked potential (EP) and electroencephalogram (EEG) monitoring act as early warning systems. Ischemia from thrombus, temporary clip, or pressure from retractors during dissection should be detected with various neuromonitoring techniques. Focal slowing on EEG will alarm the team of surface ischemia but does not alarm against subcortical injury. Decreased somatosensory evoked potential (SSEP) amplitude or increased latency demonstrates interruption in signal transmission anywhere along the dorsal column-medial lemniscus (DCML) tract. The SSEP limitation is anatomical—it protects the sensory cortex, corresponding corona radiata, and internal capsule, but omits the more anterior motor tracts. Defending against injury to the motor tracts presents huge challenges for the neuroanesthesiologist. If the surgery necessitates motor evoked potential (MEP) monitoring, then muscle relaxant and volatile agents should not be prescribed. Otherwise, if muscle relaxation and volatiles are given, muscle action potentials will be technically difficult to assess. Although transcranial motor evoked potentials seldom lead to epileptiform activity, when direct cortical stimulation is utilized, then seizures both convulsive and nonconvulsive are risks to the patient. If MEPs are used, the neuroanesthesia community recommends a technique of total IV anesthesia (TIVA). If GA with TIVA is selected, a bispectral index (BIS) monitor may be helpful to maintain an adequate depth. TIVA is preferred over volatile anesthetics because volatile anesthetics impair neuromonitoring to a greater extent than propofol at the level of the synapses. In addition to propofol, TIVA may include an infusion with an opioid with predictable and stable context-sensitive half-times such as sufentanil or remifentanil. The dose of remifentanil must be adjusted for elderly patients over 65 years of age because EEG delta activity was comparable at 50 % dose when compared to healthy volunteers (25 years of age), and the package insert recommends reducing the dose in elderly patients by 50 % [53]. Depending on the size of the surgery, sometimes neuroanesthesiologists supplement analgesia and hypnosis with an adjunct such as ketamine or dexmedetomidine. BIS, a monitor which uses proprietary software to essentially process information from a single-lead EEG located on the surface of the frontal cortex, can be used to evaluate the depth of anesthesia. Its limitations are numerous, but it can be used to reduce the amount of medication used in the elderly. In addition, studies have shown that elderly have less POCD with its use [54]. TIVA for GA often begins with an induction dose of propofol followed by a maintenance dose for the remainder of the anesthetic. Fentanyl or sufentanil bolus during induction followed by an infusion of an opioid with predictable and stable context-sensitive half-time is customary. If an opioid infusion is not chosen, then fentanyl after 4 h of surgery if not closing may be administered. Remifentanil infusion may also be administered, but because of its ultrashort context-sensitive half-time, the neuroanesthesiologist may also need additional analgesic at the end of surgery to prevent hyperalgesia. Propofol, remifentanil, and sufentanil have the advantage of having a short context-sensitive half-time. Context-sensitive half-time is the time required for blood or plasma concentrations of a drug to decrease by 50 % after drug discontinuation. Remifentanil exemplifies short context-sensitive half-time regardless of dose used. It has obvious advantages in the older adults for its excellent intraoperative analgesia and complete independence of liver or renal metabolism. For larger incisions such as spine surgery, supplementation with intermediate-acting opioids helps avoid hyperalgesia in post-op period [55, 56].

4.3.11 Anesthesia for Transsphenoidal Surgery (TSS)

TSS, performed in a horizontal position with slight head-up tilt, is also frequently done on the elderly. Whatever anesthesia technique is employed, the strategy of the neuroanesthesiologist should be to maintain hemostasis for optimal endoscopic visualization. Some data supports TIVA over inhalational anesthesia at achieving better surgical conditions and rapidly controlling heart rate and blood pressure [57, 58]. The data is conflicting although since many studies do not report that TIVA is superior when clinically relevant doses are administered [57–59]. For years, deliberate hypotension has been the hallmark of reducing bleeding and improving visualization. This technique however presents challenges in the elderly because induced hypotension in a patient population with diminished cerebrovascular reserve may lead to ischemic stroke [59]. This is particularly important during resection of intradural lesions where perfusion to neural structures may be compromised [59]. Another challenge is with the use of high-dose opioids in the elderly to control the blood pressure. Ultrashort-acting opioids have advantage over high-dose longer-acting opioids since they allow for a smooth quick wake-up and an earlier neurological exam. The use of remifentanil may control BP and the surgical stimulation [59]. At the end of surgery, it is important for the neuroanesthesiologist to extubate with the patient awake since positive pressure ventilation by bag mask could lead to tension pneumocephalus with the breach in the sphenoid bone [60, 61]. If ventilation is required, using a laryngeal mask airway (LMA) should avoid mask ventilation and provide better sinus precaution (Fig. 4.3).

4.3.12 Awake Techniques and Local Anesthetics

Although GA frequently is performed for frontal-temporal craniotomy along with neurophysiological monitoring, the best way to avoid eloquent zones of the brain is frequent neurological exams in an awake patient. By stimulating with current the areas around the planned surgical target, the team will be able to differentiate centers of functional importance and avoid them. In addition, threshold testing is frequently done looking for epileptiform afterdischarges so a maximum current can be avoided during cortical mapping. In the case of epilepsy surgery, these centers can be removed. Successful awake procedures depend on careful patient selection. Frail patients with poor cognition and difficulty communicating will become confused during the procedure and are not good candidates. In addition, those patients with a history of difficult airway should not be operated awake because if the airway is lost as a consequence of seizure, air emboli, apnea, or hypotension, then hypoxia and hypercarbia could lead to a serious complication. Awake craniotomy is usually performed with a scalp block and sedation. The sedation technique frequently varies from a consistent monitored anesthesia care (MAC) to a technique where the patient status varies from asleep to awake then back asleep [63]. The former may include a combination of anxiolytic medicine and analgesics. Whatever the choice of sedative may be, the goal in the elderly is to avoid disinhibition and patient movement and maintain close to baseline

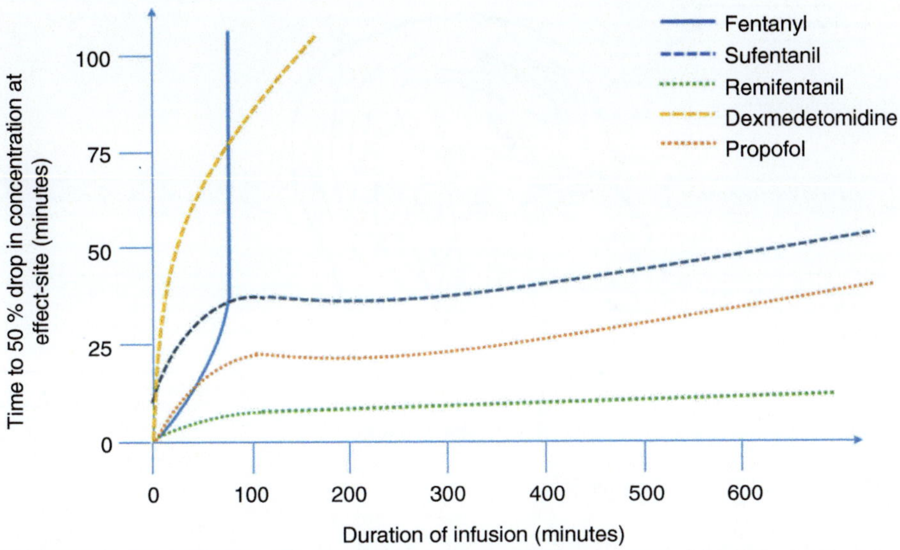

Fig. 4.3 Context-sensitive half-time of common TIVA infusions for neurosurgical procedures [62]

neurologic status so cortical mapping and functional neurosurgery can be conducted smoothly. A technique of combining dexmedetomidine and remifentanil may be employed for this purpose. Dexmedetomidine has the advantage of anxiolysis and analgesia without producing dreaded effects like hypoventilation and loss of airway. Its alpha-2-adrenergic agonist effect uniquely stimulates the locus coeruleus and allows for a very short context-sensitive half-time. A bolus is frequently followed by an infusion. Its main adverse effects are alterations in hemodynamics including bradycardia and during bolus dosing blood pressure variations, which may be biphasic—hypertension or hypotension. Asleep-awake-asleep techniques can be successfully done in a number of fashions. Initial asleep segment can be accomplished with augmenting the airway with nasal trumpets, LMA, and/or intubation [63]. The most effective techniques however are done with very little stimulation during removal of the artificial airway since the patient may be in skull traction. Moreover, the technique used should allow for quick offset so that cortical mapping can be accomplished in the awake state. Sivasankar et al. describe a technique making use of bilateral nasal trumpets connected to the anesthesia circuit [64]. This technique has the advantage that it is less stimulating to the airway so less coughing and straining occur, and therefore reduced dose propofol may be added to dexmedetomidine and remifentanil to achieve a deep plane of anesthesia that wears off quickly for cortical mapping. This technique may not secure the airway, but it does maintain relatively accurate end-tidal CO2 monitoring and ability to ventilate and rescue during apneic episodes.

Successful awake craniotomy relies on the effectiveness of the scalp block. The following nerves described in Fig. 4.4 should be blocked to provide adequate comfort during the procedure. These peripheral nerves are located close to the skin surface so by injecting around the head in a "sunglasses" pattern, starting above the orbit at the supraorbital nerve following around the ears and connecting the dots from the mastoid processes to the external occipital protuberance, this can be

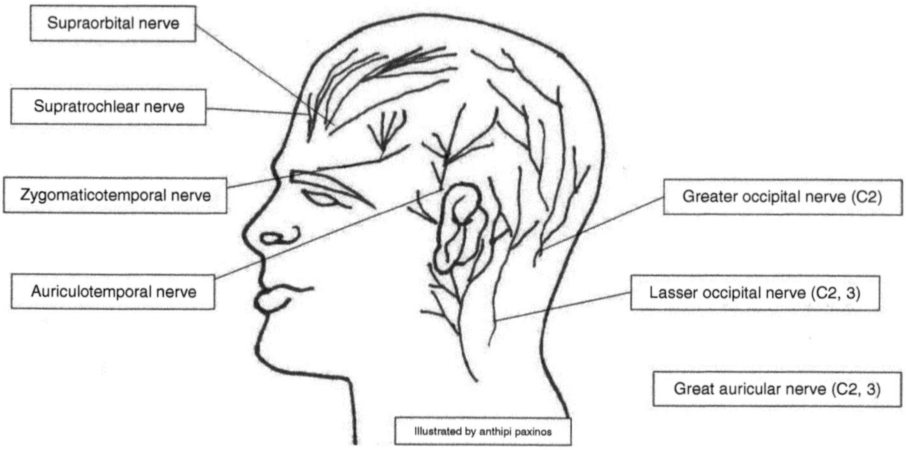

Fig. 4.4 Innervation of the scalp [65]

accomplished. Although all the nerves are superficial, the zygomaticotemporal has a branch deep to the temporalis muscle. It may be of benefit to block this nerve extensively on the surgical side to help with pain as the flap is raised [65]. Likewise, local anesthetic wheals may be raised at each pin sit prior to skull fixation [66]. Local anesthetic choice is made keeping in mind the length of the planned surgery. Table 4.3 describes the onset and duration of action of most clinically relevant local anesthetics and with added epinephrine. Longer-acting local anesthetics such as 0.5 % bupivacaine or 0.5 % ropivacaine supplementing with 1: 200,000 epinephrine are a good choice, keeping in mind that these surgeries are lengthy and the scalp is quite vascular. Lastly, in patients with prior craniotomies, and deeper dissections that lead to traction on the dura, it may be necessary to inject the dura with lidocaine or place lidocaine-soaked pledgets to block the afferent trigeminal nerve. Predictably, the effects of local anesthetics on older adults differ from their younger counterpart. The aged peripheral nervous system (PNS) is more sensitive to local anesthetics, and reduced hepatic-renal function leads to reduced metabolism. Since alpha-1-acid glycoprotein and albumin are produced by the liver and are responsible for binding local anesthetics, elderly with their reduced liver function therefore possess less local anesthetic binding capacity, and higher systemic levels occur. Moreover, the incidence of local anesthetic systemic toxicity (LAST) is higher in the elderly and includes both CNS and cardiovascular reactions. Seizures represent the late progression of CNS disturbance [67]. Anywhere from hypotension and dysrhythmia to complete cardiovascular collapse as in the case with bupivacaine can occur. Although acute seizure is usually terminated with a benzodiazepine such as lorazepam or midazolam, in the operative setting, a small dose of propofol will quickly and safely terminate a seizure [63, 68]. Intra-lipid therapy can also be used to treat LAST should it be refractory to other therapies. It works by engulfing the local anesthetic molecule and clearing it from systemic circulation [67] (Table 4.4).

Table 4.3 Antithrombotic agents and coinciding perioperative management strategies for neurosurgery and other surgeries with high bleeding risk [31, 40–44]

	Mechanism of action	Lab test	Reversal strategy elective surgery	Reversal strategy emergency surgery	Reinstitution strategy
Aspirin	Irreversibly blocks COX1/ thromboxane Inhibiting platelet function	Consider Thromboelastography® Platelet mapping™, ROTEM® platelet, or VerifyNow® aspirin	Hold 5–7 days Continue preoperatively for CEA	One unit (five pooled) Platelets	As early as possible: low bleeding risk within 24 h otherwise when bleeding risk passed
Plavix	Blocks adenosine phosphate (ADP) aggregation of platelet	Consider Thromboelastography® Platelet mapping™, ROTEM® platelet, or VerifyNow® PRU test	Hold 5–7 days	Two units (ten pooled) for 75 mg And 12 pooled for 150 mg	If usage required when bleeding risk has passed
Unfractionated heparin	Activates antithrombin	Partial thromboplastin time(PTT) Anti-X level ACT TEG with and without heparinase or ROTEM™ heptem	Hold 4–6 h Normalize PTT or ACT		24–48 h
Low molecular weight heparin (LMWH)	Primarily inhibits factor X	PTT? Anti-X level TEG with and without heparinase or ROTEM™ heptem	Hold at least 12 h	[a]Protamine Fresh frozen plasma (FFP)	24–48 h

(continued)

Table 4.3 (continued)

	Mechanism of action	Lab test	Reversal strategy elective surgery	Reversal strategy emergency surgery	Reinstitution strategy
Warfarin	Vitamin K antagonist (VKA)	Prothrombin time (PT) INR	• Hold 5 days prior • One day pre-op INR should be less than 1.5 if not give vitamin K 1–2.5 mg PO • [b]High risk for TE should be bridged with heparin or LMWH	• IV vitamin K • [c]Prothrombin complex concentrate (PCC) • FFP	24–48 h Use bridging agent for high-risk patients for thromboembolic events
Dabigatran	Direct thrombin inhibitor (DTI)	PTT TT ACT	GFR > 50 hold for 2 days + day of surgery prior GFR < 50 hold for 3 days + day of surgery [b]High risk for thromboembolic should be bridged with unfractioned heparin or LMWH	Idarucizumab (Praxbind) Activate charcoal if recent ingestion (<2 h) Hemodialysis	48–72 h [b]Consider bridging agent

Rivaroxaban, apixaban	Inhibits factor X	Anti-X level	GFR > 50 hold for 2 days + day of surgery prior GFR < 50 hold for 3 days + day of surgery [b]High risk for thromboembolic should be bridged with unfractioned heparin or LMWH	Activate charcoal if recent ingestion (<2 h) Antidote not available	48–72 h [b]Consider bridging agent

[a]Protamine reverses only 50 % of LMWH and may need repeat dosing.
[b]High-risk thromboembolism (TE) = AF with high CHADS score >5, recent DVT/PE (1 month), mechanical mitral valve, and late models of aortic mechanical valve, recent stent placed
[c]PCC has advantages over FFP—less volume and quicker administration—because it does not require thawing [42] and results to faster obtainment of INR of less than 1.3

Table 4.4 Pharmacokinetic effects of clinically relevant local anesthetics [69]

Anesthetic	Onset (min)	Duration of anesthesia (h)	Duration of analgesia (h)
3 % 2-chloroprocaine (+ HCO3)	10–15	1	2
3 % 2-chloroprocaine (HCO3+epinephrine)	10–15	1.5–2	2–3
1.5 % mepivacaine (+ HCO3)	10–20	2–3	3–5
1.5 % mepivacaine (+ HCO3 plus epinephrine)	10–20	2–5	3–8
2 % lidocaine (HCO3+epinephrine)	10–20	2–5	3–8
0.5 % ropivacaine	15–30	4–8	5–12
0.75 % ropivacaine	10–15	5–10	6–24
0.5 % bupivacaine or levobupivacaine (+ epinephrine)	15–30	5–15	6–30

4.3.13 Anesthesia for Skull Base Surgery

Skull base surgery and surgery of the posterior fossa are some of the most demanding cases for the neuroanesthesiologist. Positioning the patient, be it prone, lateral, park bench, or seated, generates unique challenges to the neurosurgical team as a whole. For starters, neuromonitoring, a pivotal means to protect neighboring structures, alters the anesthetic plan. Surgery of the posterior fossa may involve dissecting at an angular trajectory (retro-sigmoid) possibly compromising neighboring structures like the brainstem, cerebellum, and cranial nerves VII–X. Cranial nerve (CN) VII can be monitored with electromyogram (EMG) leads in the orbicularis oris and oculi. CN VIII is typically best protected with brainstem auditory evoked potentials. Bilateral SSEPs alarm the team of an interruption along the dorsal column-medial lemniscus pathway as it ascends before and after it crosses over at the cervical-medullary junction. Cranial nerve X may be monitored with EMG using an endotracheal tube with surface electrodes that stimulate the mucosa of the vocal cords [70]. The afferent and efferent signals are carried along the recurrent laryngeal nerve (RLN), a mixed nerve that is a branch of the vagus [70]. Otherwise, a more invasive technique of applying submucosal bipolar electrodes in the soft palate, cricothyroid muscle, trapezius, and tongue, respectively, for cranial nerves IX, X, XI, and XII, may be employed [70]. In the elderly patient, who may already have a compromised respiratory reserve, loss of CNs IX–X may lead to respiratory compromise and a need for post-op tracheostomy for airway protection.

Historically, the posterior fossa was best approached in the seating position. It had the advantage of accessing midline structures because anatomically the surgeon was faced onto the target. In addition, the airway was easily accessible, and gravity provided excellent cerebellar traction for pineal tumor surgery. Unfortunately, to a large extent, this position has become passé for its wide array of risks. Serious complications have occurred secondary to venous air embolism, paradoxical air embolism, tension pneumocephalus, quadriparesis from over-flexion of the cervical spinal cord, and macroglossia [51, 66]. Macroglossia in combination with the cranial nerve risks discussed above could lead to airway compromise. It is essential that in the seating position, the back should be firmly contacting the bed; otherwise, pressure forces will conduct to the pelvis and apply stress to this region [51]. A central venous line should be considered if the sitting position is required for posterior fossa surgery [51, 52]. The distal port should be placed at the SVC/right atrial junction so that if a large air embolus should occur, it could be aspirated out this port of the central line avoiding an air lock that could shut down forward flow. Monitoring for intradural procedures should include an arterial line to best manage the second-by-second hemodynamic changes and metabolic challenges of the surgery. In the setting of seated posterior fossa surgery, investigation using TEE to rule out patent foramen ovale (PFO) is advisable prior to seating the patient. Failure to rule out PFO could lead to paradoxical air embolus and ultimately stroke and MI [52]. In addition, since TEE has limitations, once PFO is ruled out, many neuroanesthesiologists prefer to monitor with precordial Doppler over TEE intraoperatively since TEE may cause tongue swelling with a flexed neck and may deactivate during the case if the critical temperature of the probe is reached. Precordial Doppler is very sensitive and picks up audible air well, but it cannot distinguish small amounts of air from large boluses that could lead to air lock [51, 52]. Above all, good communication between anesthetist and surgeon cuts lead time and promotes quick response to air embolus. Manuvers such as flooding the surgical field with saline, applying bone wax, and head down position can be instituted rapidly to prevent devastating outcomes.

Since historically the seating position presented safety concerns, the posterior fossa is currently more commonly approached with the patient horizontal. Prone, lateral, semi-lateral, and park bench are the typical horizontal approaches [66]. Prone surgery, to be discussed in the spinal surgery section, challenges the neuroanesthesiologist in many ways foremost by limiting access to the airway.

4.3.14 Anesthesia for Spine Surgery

Surgery of the lumbar and cervical spine is frequently performed on elderly patients. Degenerative changes in the elderly spine lead to conditions such as spondylosis, spinal stenosis, spondylolisthesis, degenerative scoliosis, and compression fractures [14]. Lengthy multiple-level spine surgeries in frail elderly patients are associated with multiple risks. In the setting of degenerative changes, older patients often require more aggressive surgeries imposing greater risk [14, 71]. Anesthesia for the more challenging cases will be tailored by the neurophysiological monitoring plan, whereas smaller spine cases usually do not necessitate monitoring. Multimodality monitoring for the spine may include SSEP, MEP, and EMG and may necessitate TIVA [14, 72]. Although SSEP monitoring protects the majority of the cord in the posterior approach, the vascular elements which supply anterior cord if dissected necessitate MEP for complete cord protection. Many neurosurgeons use EMG monitoring on the pedicle screws to make sure the screw is not "electrically close" to the nerve roots [72]. Visual evoked potentials to protect against intraoperative blindness have been studied but infrequently utilized clinically at this time due to many studies showing a lack of sensitivity and specificity [73, 74]. If neuromonitoring is necessary, TIVA with an opioid with a stable and predictable context-sensitive half-time is an excellent choice. Since postoperative pain following spine surgery is significant, the addition of a longer-acting opioid may provide superior analgesia. If propofol/remifentanil is chosen, a supplement with fentanyl or hydromorphone for postoperative pain is advisable to avoid hyperalgesia post-op [55, 56]. In addition, if the patient is opioid tolerant, one may supplement with dexmedetomidine or ketamine. Since opioids work by activating the mu receptor, a strategy to antagonize pain pathways using alternative pain receptors should be considered. Neuroanesthesiologists often utilize drugs like ketamine and dexmedetomidine which are NMDA receptor antagonists and alpha-2-agonists, respectively, for this purpose.

Perioperative visual loss is a rare but serious complication and includes both posterior ischemic optic neuropathy (ION) and central retinal artery occlusion (CRAO) as causes. The ASA practice advisory has stated large intraoperative blood loss and prolonged surgeries (greater than 6 h) as risk factors, and preoperative anemia, vascular disease, obesity, and tobacco use may be risk factors. They advise to avoid direct pressure to the eye to prevent CRAO, to monitor for acute blood loss anemia and hemoglobin to be maintained at minimum average of 9.4 g/dL, to monitor hemodynamics closely and caution when using deliberate hypotension, to use colloids along with crystalloids, to position the head in a neutral forward position even with or higher than the level of the heart, and to give consideration to stage complex procedures [75].

Consistent with other areas in neurosurgery, spinal surgery for the elderly is headed in a less invasive direction. Since larger surgeries on the spine lead to more complications and greater length of hospital stay in the elderly, this approach may enable seniors to benefit from future technology. Rosen et al. demonstrated benefit in a series of 50 patients with a mean age of 80 by showing in this series that minimally invasive lumbar decompression had no major complications or mortality [76]. As the geriatric population grows, innovation in decades to come will prove vital to improving the quality of seniors' lives as they age.

4.3.15 Anesthesia for Carotid Artery Surgery

Carotid endarterectomy, a surgery primarily performed for the elderly, can be done with GA or regional anesthesia. Induction is usually gentle, and a radial arterial line is placed in preparation for large swings in heart rate and blood pressure as the carotid sinus is mechanically manipulated. Neuromonitoring is accomplished with EEG and SSEP looking for signs of ischemia on the side being operated. As above in awake craniotomy, an awake carotid can also be done with a cooperative patient. An awake patient can act as an early warning system alarming the surgeon that shunting around the clamp will be necessary to avoid stroke. Regional anesthesia has traditionally been accomplished with deep and superficial cervical plexus blocks. Newer data supports benefit with superficial cervical plexus block alone, since the deep has been associated with complications like vertebral artery dissection and local anesthetic injection in the CSF or vertebral artery [77]. More opioid supplementation was needed however in the superficial cervical arm of the study. To supplement the superficial block, the surgeon can provide additional local anesthetic through the dissection and provide local anesthetic in areas stretched by the retractors.

4.3.16 Anesthesia for Decompressive Surgery

Intracranial bleeding and decompressive surgery occur more commonly in the elderly population. Falls, atrophy of the brain leading to more torsional force on bridging veins, and a greater predisposition for bleeding diathesis are some of the reasons for subdural hematomas to occur in older adults [78]. In addition, uncontrolled hypertension and amyloid angiopathy commonly occur in older adults and lead to intracerebral hemorrhage. Blood in the cranial vault expanding leads to mass effect, midline shift, and herniation syndromes [79, 80]. Evidence supports decompressive craniotomy when extradural blood is compressing the brain, when there is intracranial bleeding in the posterior fossa, and when malignant edema in middle cerebral artery (MCA) ischemic stroke is evolving [80, 81]. To provide optimal perioperative care for this vulnerable neurosurgical population, a multidisciplinary team of doctors and nurses including specialists in neurosurgery, neuroanesthesia, and neurology may improve outcome [82]. It has been shown that care in a neuro-ICU by a neuro-intensivist improves outcome. Surgeries in the prone position such as spine surgery and certain skull base surgery in older adults require respiratory monitoring and at times postoperative mechanical ventilation. In skull base surgery, two factors lead to respiratory compromise: vasogenic edema of the airway and cranial nerve injuries weakening laryngeal and pharyngeal protective reflexes. After a long spine surgery with massive blood loss, an ICU bed should be reserved for a frail patient for risk of airway edema, respiratory compromise, post-op hemorrhage, and thromboembolic events such as MI. A dedicated neuro-ICU is also best equipped to monitor neurologic complications as well. For instance, emergencies such as herniation, status epilepticus, and acute stroke should be monitored for after neurosurgery. Nurses in the neuro-ICU are well trained in the neurological exam and recognition of neurologic emergencies. In addition, continuous EEG is readily available and offered to rule out nonconvulsive status. Bedside CT scan may also be readily available and expertly read so that herniation can be managed swiftly. Neurosurgical presence in neuro-ICU makes delays unlikely. Having the expertise of a dedicated pharmacist in the neuro-ICU completes this multidisciplinary team who all work together to serve the neurosurgical elderly patient postoperatively.

The neuroanesthesiologist, in this emergency situation, must be prepared to apply temporary therapies as a bridge to reduce ICP until more surgical decompression is complete. Symptoms of elevated ICP include worsening of mental status and a fixed, midposition pupil down and out from compression of the midbrain which are also hallmarks of cranial nerve III compression due to uncal herniation. Imminent herniation often is accompanied by the Cushing reflex characterized by hypertension, bradycardia, and irregular breathing. Techniques at the neuroanesthesiologist disposal include minimally invasive techniques to improve brain venous drainage such as head-up position and clearing the external compressive elements around the neck [79, 80]. Pharmacologically, propofol can be given which decreases cerebral metabolic rate of oxygen (CMRO2) and CBF in turn reducing ICP. Care should be taken to avoid systemic hypotension which would decrease cerebral perfusion pressure. In the short term, hyperventilation can be used to rescue the patient. Hyperventilation greatly reduces ICP in the short term and works well to bridge to definitive decompression. While reducing PCO_2 effectively lowers CBF and ICP, the vasoconstrictive effect may have a deleterious effect on brain perfusion during aggressive hyperventilation past a PCO_2 of 30 mmHg [79, 80]. In the senescent brain with diminished reserve, this may not be well tolerated. Moreover, after several hours, the CSF bathing the medullary chemoreceptors re-equilibrates as CO2 diffuses. The result is CSF pH returns to pre-hyperventilation values, hence raising CBF and ICP. The next tool in our arsenal is hyperosmolar therapy. Although mannitol has historically been used to shrink the brain, the decision to use hypertonic saline versus mannitol should be based on the patient's volume status and risk for congestive heart failure. Mannitol, an osmotic diuretic, creates an osmotic gradient reducing brain volume [80, 83, 84]. The water that leaves the brain enters the plasma transiently and then exits the plasma via the kidney reducing overall water content and shrinking the intravascular compartment [83]. Mannitol may also improve cerebral perfusion by initially increasing plasma water content and altering blood cell rheology by decreasing blood viscosity [83]. Hypertonic saline (HTS) on the other hand enters the plasma and raises the solute concentration creating an osmotic gradient also drawing water from the brain, but HTS expands the intravascular compartment [84]. Increasing the volume could overwhelm the elderly heart which may not possess the compliance or systolic function to tolerate. It should be mentioned that sodium will increase with both therapies and mannitol will initially decrease the sodium until water escapes the systemic circulation. Any condition raising ICP such as ICH, subarachnoid hemorrhage (SAH) from traumatic brain injury (TBI) or aneurysm, or hydrocephalus may benefit from an external ventricular drain (EVD) placement and drainage [79, 80]. The Monro-Kellie hypothesis supports accelerating drainage of venous blood and CSF to make room for a swollen brain in a rigid box [79, 80, 83]. Other therapies include mild hypothermia and barbiturate coma [79, 80]. The neuroanesthesiologist should be comfortable with emergency neurologic treatment of elevated ICP.

4.3.17 Anesthesia in the Interventional Radiology Suite

Although brain bleeds are still commonly handled in the operating room, the twenty-first-century direction in interventional neuroscience is headed toward a noninvasive percutaneous path. As interventions such aneurysm coils, bleed embolization, and stent retrievals for ischemic stroke continue to develop, leaders in neuroanesthesiology must study and adapt new techniques to best serve the patients. Currently, the debate exists whether monitored anesthesia care (MAC) or GA best serves the patient. We assert that neuroanesthesia can never be done with a "one-size-fits-all" approach. There are few scenarios imaginable where this is more evident than in the elderly population. For example, a frail 90-year-old patient that has a good airway, is cognitively intact, and has a low National Institution of Health Stroke Scale (NIHSS) may benefit from the speed and hemodynamic stability of a MAC induction. On the other hand, a 65-year-old obese gentleman with severe sleep apnea and high NIHSS may move during the procedure with MAC requiring high-dose propofol to sedate him. Subsequently, without an airway supplemental device, he may suffer airway obstruction leading to hypoxemia, hypercarbia, and worst-case scenario loss of airway. This situation would have been much safer with GA and secure airway. While we do agree with the premise that "time is brain," we do not authorize offering the same anesthetic to every patient. Although small studies with strict exclusion criteria have shown benefit with MAC, this position is debatable. In fact, Sivasankar et al. showed GA to be highly variable and that techniques differ greatly in depth of anesthesia and airway management [85]. Nonetheless, more research should be dedicated to answer this question as the sector grows.

4.3.18 Postoperative Pain

Postoperative care of the elderly should include critical care and pain management ideally in a dedicated neuroscience intensive care unit (neuro-ICU). It is important to realize that frailty, diminished organ reserve, and neurologic diseases have a profound effect on how elderly patients perceive and communicate pain. A patent's baseline neurologic status or surgical events like perioperative stroke may prevent them from verbally communicating their pain. Therefore, in order to best serve the injured neurosurgical patient, neuro-ICU teams must have in place a means of assessing pain with a consistent scale [86]. A visual analog scale (VAS), numerical rating scale, faces pain scale, or other pain scales may be used for this purpose [87]. Asking elderly patients to describe pain in their own words may also be an effective means to assess post-op pain [86]. Caretakers in the neuro-ICU must also be aware that elderly patients have a higher threshold for pain, a fact that has been validated by level 1 evidence [87, 88]. It is a fact that neurophysiological differences do exist in the elderly such as reduced sensory fibers and cortical atrophy [3]. But perhaps seniors also complain less because they have different psychosocial influences and feel pain is part of the aging process [89]. Before treating acute postoperative pain, it is important to take into account several variables, namely, size and depth of the surgical incision, extent of patient frailty, and acute cognitive status. Reduction in hepatic, renal, and nervous system reserve makes cautious dosing of pain meds essential [86]. With this in mind, the use of pain medications with less toxicity and intermediate duration of action seems optimal. A reasonable approach, modified from the World Health Organization (WHO) ladder, would be to conceptualize a pain plan prior to administration [90]. The plan should start with low-potency medications with less addiction potential and increase potency and dose as needed [90]. The concept of "start low and go slow" pertains to post-op pain management of the elderly population [87]. Starting at the bottom of the ladder for mild pain, acetaminophen can be given up to 4 g in 24 h. However, nonsteroidal anti-inflammatory drugs (NSAIDS) can be highly toxic to elderly by injuring their kidneys or by inhibiting platelet function, thus worsening bleeding [14]. Although unadvised after neurosurgery, if used, NSAIDS should be given at a reduced dose given its highly protein-bound nature and likelihood to exist in high plasma concentration unbound in older adults [13]. For moderate pain, mild oral opioids like hydrocodone or low-dose oxycodone with acetaminophen can be attempted. In moderate-to-severe pain, low-dose fentanyl has the advantage of a higher duration of action in elderly because it is fat soluble, has higher Vd, and has longer time to clear given the reduced renal and hepatic function in elderly [3, 14]. However, water-soluble opioids such as morphine may be a bad choice because of immediate toxicity and the presence of morphine-6-glucuronide metabolite that is renally cleared. Similarly, longer-acting parenteral opioids should also be used with caution because they may have a less forgiving effect on the CNS. Of note, it may be challenging in the elderly brain-injured patient to tell the difference between pain, agitation, and hyperactive delirium. Pain after surgery in the elderly can easily be confused for delirium and therefore must be ruled out. If patients are on chronic opioids like methadone, it is important not to deny patients their chronic pain meds [14]. As stated, untreated pain can lead to delirium, unabated sympathetic outflow, and consequentially dysrhythmia, stroke, or MI. Medications such as AEDs, antidepressants, ketamine, or dexmedetomidine may also be used to supplement opioid analgesics. Gabapentin, a well-known AED, has been used for neuropathic pain. Its dose should be reduced in elderly because it is almost completely renally excreted. Antidepressants may also be effective to supplement opioids. Research linking pain and depression is a topic of ongoing research and a prevalent theme in elderly pain management. SSRIs are a safe choice, but TCAs should be avoided in seniors for their anticholinergic side effects.

References

1. Yang R, Wolfson M, Lewis MC (2011) Unique aspects of the elderly surgical population: an Anesthesiologist's perspective. Geriatr Orthop Surg Rehabil 2(2):56–64
2. Griffiths R et al (2014) Peri-operative care of the elderly 2014: Association of Anaesthetists of Great Britain and Ireland. Anaesthesia 69(Suppl 1):81–98
3. Sophie S (2007) Anaesthesia for the elderly patient. J Pak Med Assoc 57(4):196–201
4. Cesari M et al (2016) The geriatric management of frailty as paradigm of "The end of the disease era". Eur J Intern Med 31:11–4
5. Hubbard RE, Story DA (2014) Patient frailty: the elephant in the operating room. Anaesthesia 69:26–34
6. Axley MS, Schenning KJ (2015) Preoperative cognitive and frailty screening in the geriatric surgical patient: a narrative review. Clin Ther 37(12):2666–2675

7. Mantha S et al (2005) Usefulness of routine preoperative testing: a prospective single-observer study. J Clin Anesth 17(1):51–57
8. Roizen MF (1994) Preoperative evaluation of patients: a review. Ann Acad Med Singapore 23(6 Suppl):49–55
9. Inan G, Ozkose Satirlar Z (2015) Alzheimer disease and anesthesia. Turk J Med Sci 45(5):1026–1033
10. Kapoor MC (2011) Alzheimer's disease, anesthesia and the cholinergic system. J Anaesthesiol Clin Pharmacol 27(2):155–158
11. Jinno S (2015) Aging affects new cell production in the adult hippocampus: a quantitative anatomic review. J Chem Neuroanat. 76(Pt B):64–72
12. Nicholson G, Pereira AC, Hall GM (2002) Parkinson's disease and anaesthesia. Br J Anaesth 89(6):904–916
13. Burton DA, Nicholson G, Hall GM (2004) Anaesthesia in elderly patients with neurodegenerative disorders: special considerations. Drugs Aging 21(4):229–242
14. Brallier JW, Deiner S (2015) The elderly spine surgery patient: pre- and intraoperative management of drug theraph. Drugs Aging 32(8):601–609
15. Mariappan R et al (2015) Cerebrovascular reactivity to carbon dioxide under anesthesia: a qualitative systematic review. J Neurosurg Anesthesiol 27(2):123–135
16. Jorge M Serrador, William P Milberg, Lewis A Lipsitz (2005) Cerebral hemodynamics in the elderly. Springer/Humana Press Inc., Totowa, p. 75–83
17. Yonas H, Pindzola RR (2000) Clinical application of cerebrovascular reserve assessment as a strategy for stroke prevention. Keio J Med 49(Suppl 1):A4–A10
18. Chaer RA et al (2010) Cerebral reserve is decreased in elderly patients with carotid stenosis. J Vasc Surg 52(3):569–575
19. Goettel N et al (2016) Monitoring of cerebral blood flow autoregulation in adults undergoing sevoflurane anesthesia: a prospective cohort study of two age groups. J Clin Monit Comput 30(3):255–264
20. Murthy S et al (2015) Controversies in anaesthesia for noncardiac surgery in older adults. Br J Anaesth 115(Suppl 2):ii15–ii25
21. Priebe HJ (2000) The aged cardiovascular risk patient. Br J Anaesth 85(5):763–778
22. Ismail S, Azam SI, Khan FA (2002) Effect of age on haemodynamic response to tracheal intubation. A comparison of young, middle-aged and elderly patients. Anaesth Intensive Care 30(5):608–614
23. Thiele RH, Nemergut EC, Lynch C 3rd (2011) The clinical implications of isolated alpha(1) adrenergic stimulation. Anesth Analg 113(2):297–304
24. Apfelbaum JL et al (2012) Practice advisory for preanesthesia evaluation: an updated report by the American Society of Anesthesiologists Task Force on Preanesthesia Evaluation. Anesthesiology 116(3):522–538
25. Devereaux PJ, Sessler DI (2015) Cardiac complications in patients undergoing major noncardiac surgery. N Engl J Med 373(23):2258–2269
26. Halperin JL et al (2016) Further evolution of the ACC/AHA Clinical Practice Guideline Recommendation Classification System: a report of the American College of Cardiology/ American Heart Association Task Force on Clinical Practice Guidelines. J Am Coll Cardiol 67(13):1572–1574
27. Fleisher LA et al (2015) 2014 ACC/AHA guideline on perioperative cardiovascular evaluation and management of patients undergoing noncardiac surgery: executive summary: a report of the American College of Cardiology/American Heart Association Task Force on practice guidelines. Developed in collaboration with the American College of Surgeons, American Society of Anesthesiologists, American Society of Echocardiography, American Society of Nuclear Cardiology, Heart Rhythm Society, Society for Cardiovascular Angiography and Interventions, Society of Cardiovascular Anesthesiologists, and Society of Vascular Medicine Endorsed by the Society of Hospital Medicine. J Nucl Cardiol 22(1):162–215
28. Shear TG, Steven (2012) Vasoplegic syndrome and renin-angiotensin system antagonists, in Anesthesia Patient Safety Foundation Newsletter

29. Lange M et al (2008) Role of vasopressinergic V1 receptor agonists in the treatment of perioperative catecholamine-refractory arterial hypotension. Best Pract Res Clin Anaesthesiol 22(2):369–381
30. Levine GN et al (2016) ACC/AHA/SCAI focused update on primary percutaneous coronary intervention for patients with ST-elevation myocardial infarction: an update of the 2011 ACCF/AHA/SCAI guideline for percutaneous coronary intervention and the 2013 ACCF/AHA guideline for the management of ST-elevation myocardial infarction: a report of the American College of Cardiology/American Heart Association Task Force on Clinical Practice Guidelines and the Society for Cardiovascular Angiography and Interventions. Circulation 133(11):1135–1147
31. Kristensen SD et al (2014) 2014 ESC/ESA guidelines on non-cardiac surgery: cardiovascular assessment and management. Kardiol Pol 72(11):857–918
32. Ainsworth BE et al (2000) Compendium of physical activities: an update of activity codes and MET intensities. Med Sci Sports Exerc 32(9 Suppl):S498–S504
33. Joo HS et al (2005) The value of screening preoperative chest x-rays: a systematic review. Can J Anaesth 52(6):568–574
34. Sprung J, Gajic O, Warner DO (2006) Review article: age related alterations in respiratory function — anesthetic considerations. Can J Anesth 53(12):1244–1257
35. Metzger A et al (2015) Intrathoracic pressure regulation improves cerebral perfusion and cerebral blood flow in a porcine model of brain injury. Shock 44(Suppl 1):96–102
36. Huynh T et al (2002) Positive end-expiratory pressure alters intracranial and cerebral perfusion pressure in severe traumatic brain injury. J Trauma 53(3):488–492; discussion 492–3
37. Thurlbeck WM, Muller NL (1994) Emphysema: definition, imaging, and quantification. AJR Am J Roentgenol 163(5):1017–1025
38. Chowdhury L et al (2011) Chronic phenytoin therapy-induced vecuronium resistance. Indian J Pharmacol 43(2):214–215
39. Ornstein E et al (1987) The effect of phenytoin on the magnitude and duration of neuromuscular block following atracurium or vecuronium. Anesthesiology 67(2):191–196
40. Beshay JE et al (2010) Emergency reversal of anticoagulation and antiplatelet therapies in neurosurgical patients. J Neurosurg 112(2):307–318
41. Jauch EC, Pineda JA, Claude Hemphill J (2015) Emergency neurological life support: intracerebral hemorrhage. Neurocrit Care 23(Suppl 2):83–93
42. Hemphill JC 3rd et al (2015) Guidelines for the management of spontaneous intracerebral hemorrhage: a guideline for healthcare professionals from the American Heart Association/American Stroke Association. Stroke 46(7):2032–2060
43. Degos V et al (2013) Perioperative management of coagulation in nontraumatic intracerebral hemorrhage. Anesthesiology 119(1):218–227
44. Locatelli A, Musumeci G, Rossini R (2015) The POISE-2 aspirin trial. G Ital Cardiol (Rome) 16(5):261–264
45. Johnson KN et al (2015) Anatomic and physiopathologic changes affecting the airway of the elderly patient: implications for geriatric-focused airway management. Clin Interv Aging 10:1925–1934
46. Hindman BJ et al (2015) Intubation biomechanics: laryngoscope force and cervical spine motion during intubation in cadavers-cadavers versus patients, the effect of repeated intubations, and the effect of type II odontoid fracture on C1-C2 motion. Anesthesiology 123(5):1042–1058
47. Hindman BJ et al (2014) Intubation biomechanics: laryngoscope force and cervical spine motion during intubation with Macintosh and Airtraq laryngoscopes. Anesthesiology 121(2):260–271
48. Cai H et al (2012) Endocrine function in aging. Int J Endocrinol 2012:872478
49. Richards ML et al (1999) The rapid low-dose (1 microgram) cosyntropin test in the immediate postoperative period: results in elderly subjects after major abdominal surgery. Surgery 125(4):431–440
50. Tikuisis P, Bell DG, Jacobs I (1991) Shivering onset, metabolic response, and convective heat transfer during cold air exposure. J Appl Physiol (1985) 70(5):1996–2002

51. Porter JM, Pidgeon C, Cunningham AJ (1999) The sitting position in neurosurgery: a critical appraisal. Br J Anaesth 82(1):117–128
52. Pasternak JJ, Lanier WL (2013) Neuroanesthesiology update. J Neurosurg Anesthesiol 25(2):98–134
53. Ultiva (remifentanil hydrochloride) for Injection Prescribing Information, U.i.r.t.o.G.G. Limited, Editor.: www.ultiva.com. p. 10
54. Chan MT et al (2013) BIS-guided anesthesia decreases postoperative delirium and cognitive decline. J Neurosurg Anesthesiol 25(1):33–42
55. Angst MS, Clark JD (2006) Opioid-induced hyperalgesia: a qualitative systematic review. Anesthesiology 104(3):570–587
56. Zhang Y-L et al (2014) Effect of intraoperative high-dose remifentanil on postoperative pain: a prospective, double blind, randomized clinical trial. PLoS One 9(3):e91454
57. Beule AG et al (2007) Propofol versus sevoflurane: bleeding in endoscopic sinus surgery. Otolaryngol Head Neck Surg 136(1):45–50
58. Yoo HS et al (2010) Comparison of surgical condition in endoscopic sinus surgery using remifentanil combined with propofol, sevoflurane, or desflurane. Korean J Anesthesiol 59(6):377–382
59. Thongrong C et al (2013) Control of bleeding in endoscopic skull base surgery: current concepts to improve hemostasis. ISRN Surg 2013:191543
60. Kopelovich JC et al (2012) Pneumocephalus with BiPAP use after transsphenoidal surgery. J Clin Anesth 24(5):415–418
61. Zlotnik D et al (2014) Two cases of pneumocephalus following noninvasive continuous positive airway ventilation after transsphenoidal neurosurgery. Ann Fr Anesth Reanim 33(4):275–278
62. Miller R (2010) Miller anesthesia. Churchill Livingstone/Elsevier, Philadelphia
63. Skucas AP, Artru AA (2006) Anesthetic complications of awake craniotomies for epilepsy surgery. Anesth Analg 102(3):882–887
64. Sivasankar C et al (2016) Awake craniotomy: a new airway approach. Anesth Analg 122(2):509–511
65. Costello TG, Cormack JR (2004) Anaesthesia for awake craniotomy: a modern approach. J Clin Neurosci 11(1):16–19
66. Rozet I, Vavilala MS (2007) Risks and benefits of patient positioning during neurosurgical care. Anesthesiol Clin 25(3):631–653, x
67. Vasques F et al (2015) A review of local anesthetic systemic toxicity cases since publication of the American Society of regional anesthesia recommendations: to whom it may concern. Reg Anesth Pain Med 40(6):698–705
68. Heavner JE, Rosenberg P (1999) Propofol for lidocaine-induced seizures. Anesth Analg 88(5):1193
69. Gadsen J (2013) Local anesthetics: clinical pharmacology and rational selection. The New York Society of Regional Anesthesia. http://www.nysora.com/regional-anesthesia/foundations-of-ra/3492-local-anesthetics-clinical-pharmacology-andrational-selection.htlm
70. Holdefer RN et al (2013) Alternative sites for intraoperative monitoring of cranial nerves X and XII during intracranial surgeries. J Clin Neurophysiol 30(3):275–279
71. Cloyd JM, Acosta FL Jr, Ames CP (2008) Complications and outcomes of lumbar spine surgery in elderly people: a review of the literature. J Am Geriatr Soc 56(7):1318–1327
72. Stecker MM (2012) A review of intraoperative monitoring for spinal surgery. Surg Neurol Int 3(Suppl 3):S174–S187
73. Kodama K et al (2010) Standard and limitation of intraoperative monitoring of the visual evoked potential. Acta Neurochir (Wien) 152(4):643–648
74. Chung SB et al (2012) Intraoperative visual evoked potential has no association with postoperative visual outcomes in transsphenoidal surgery. Acta Neurochir (Wien) 154(8):1505–1510
75. American Society of Anesthesiologists Task Force on Perioperative Visual Loss (2012) Practice advisory for perioperative visual loss associated with spine surgery: an updated report

by the American Society of Anesthesiologists Task Force on Perioperative Visual Loss. Anesthesiology 116(2):274–285
76. Rosen DS et al (2007) Minimally invasive lumbar spinal decompression in the elderly: outcomes of 50 patients aged 75 years and older. Neurosurgery 60(3):503–509; discussion 509–10
77. Ivanec Z et al (2008) Superficial versus combined (deep and superficial) cervical plexus block for carotid endarterectomy. Acta Clin Croat 47(2):81–86
78. Ledic D et al (2014) Risk factors for subdural bleeding in elderly population. Coll Antropol 38(4):1195–1198
79. Lin AL, Avila EK (2015) Neurologic emergencies in the patients with cancer: diagnosis and management. J Intensive Care Med. 1–17 PMID 26704760
80. Stevens RD et al (2012) Emergency neurological life support: intracranial hypertension and herniation. Neurocrit Care 17(Suppl 1):S60–S65
81. Vahedi K et al (2007) Early decompressive surgery in malignant infarction of the middle cerebral artery: a pooled analysis of three randomised controlled trials. Lancet Neurol 6(3):215–222
82. Knopf L et al (2012) Impact of a neurointensivist on outcomes in critically ill stroke patients. Neurocrit Care 16(1):63–71
83. Davis M, Lucatorto M (1994) Mannitol revisited. J Neurosci Nurs 26(3):170–174
84. Knapp JM (2005) Hyperosmolar therapy in the treatment of severe head injury in children: mannitol and hypertonic saline. AACN Clin Issues 16(2):199–211
85. Sivasankar C et al (2015) Anesthetic variation and potential impact of anesthetics used during endovascular management of acute ischemic stroke. J Neurointerv Surg. 8:1101–1106
86. Calandese F et al (2010) Postoperative pain control in the elderly. BMC Geriatr 10(1):1–1
87. Falzone E, Hoffmann C, Keita H (2013) Postoperative analgesia in elderly patients. Drugs Aging 30(2):81–90
88. McCleane G (2007) Pharmacological pain management in the elderly patient. Clin Interv Aging 2(4):637–643
89. Gibson SJ, Helme RD (2001) Age-related differences in pain perception and report. Clin Geriatr Med 17(3):433–456, v-vi
90. Kumar N (2007) Report of a Delphi Study to determine the need for guidelines and to identify the number and topics of guidelines that should be developed by WHO, Geneva, p 9–13

Perioperative Neurotoxicity in the Elderly

5

Elizabeth M. Gabrielli and Roderic G. Eckenhoff

5.1 Introduction

Cognitive changes after anesthesia and surgery in elderly patients and the possible neurotoxicity of anesthetics has been postulated and debated for almost a century. As far back as 1955, a large retrospective review of almost 1,200 elderly patients undergoing surgery and anesthesia reported a 10 % incidence of "minor dementia" and a 1.5 % incidence of "extreme dementia" newly occurring after an operation [5]. As the elderly populations and the associated comorbidities continue to grow, the possibility of neurotoxicity of anesthesia and surgery has gained a significant amount of attention. Over the past decade we have seen a surge of manuscripts investigating the possibility of postoperative cognitive changes in people and the underlying mechanisms and pathophysiology in animals. As anesthesia almost always accompanies surgery, both the neurotoxicity of anesthesia and surgery are considered as a unit. This chapter will give an up-to-date review on terminology associated with perioperative neurotoxicity, preclinical and basic science studies, clinical studies, and future directions of research.

5.2 Terminology

An issue that has plagued this field is a lack of a consensus terminology and of diagnoses which are consistent with other fields of cognitive dysfunction. Broadly speaking, the perioperative neurotoxicity and subsequent cognitive change have been understood to be a decrement in cognitive function postoperatively as

E.M. Gabrielli, MD • R.G. Eckenhoff, MD (✉)
Department of Anesthesiology and Critical Care, University of Pennsylvania Perelman School of Medicine, Philadelphia, PA 19104, USA
e-mail: roderic.eckenhoff@uphs.upenn.edu

© Springer International Publishing Switzerland 2017

M. Berhouma, P. Krolak-Salmon (eds.), *Brain and Spine Surgery in the Elderly*,
DOI 10.1007/978-3-319-40232-1_5

compared to the preoperative state and occurring after full return of consciousness and after the anesthetic drugs have been eliminated. Studies to date, however, have used multiple different cognitive tests and criteria to classify patients as having a cognitive decline or not. And unfortunately, many studies have not considered other causes of cognitive change in the elderly population. Over the past few years, an expert working group, consisting of anesthesiologists, geriatricians, neurologists, and psychiatrists, has been convened in order to establish uniform nomenclature and diagnostic criteria which are in line with nomenclature and diagnostic criteria used in other fields of cognitive dysfunction, including the National Institute of Aging and the Alzheimer's Association, and in the DSM-V.

5.2.1 Postoperative Delirium

Delirium is an acute fluctuating condition, consisting of cognitive disruption and inattention as defined in the DSM-5. Currently the DSM-5 has specific categories of medication-induced, substance intoxication, substance withdrawal, delirium due to other medical conditions, and delirium due to medical etiologies but not postoperative delirium. This in spite of the fact that anesthesia and surgery are established risk factors for delirium with a high incidence in patients over the age of 65 years [29]. It has been proposed by Lis Evered that postoperative delirium (POD) should be defined as "delirium following a lucid interval after the conclusion of anesthesia and surgery and occurs in the hospital up to 1 week post procedure or until discharge."

5.2.2 Postoperative Cognitive Dysfunction

Postoperative cognitive dysfunction (POCD) is a syndrome in which an individual after anesthesia and surgery has an objective, measurable cognitive decline; it has rarely included a subjective complaint from the patient or caregiver. To date, criteria to establish this syndrome have not been made uniform. Early studies used only a decline from a baseline score, usually greater than one standard deviation, as criteria [50, 67]. A problem with this is it did not account for what could be a natural deterioration in cognition, independent of anesthesia and surgery, as there were no population controls. Some subsequent studies have included control groups, but there has been continued heterogeneity in how many cognitive tests have been used, how much of a decline is required, and in how many tests. Comparing the postoperative decline to an expected change which occurs in the control group is calculated as a reliable change index. One of the more strict definitions comes from the International Study of Postoperative Cognitive Dysfunction (ISPOCD) group. By their criteria, POCD is defined as a decline in greater than or equal to two standard deviations in two or more tests or a combined Z-score is less than two standard deviations. Published studies have also varied greatly with respect to how long after the surgery these tests have been performed. Assessments have been early (5–7 days), intermediate (60–90 days), or late (1–5 years), and all have been reported as "POCD."

As defined in DSM, neurocognitive disorders (NCD) are those in which there is objective evidence of cognitive decline and subjective complaints about cognition either from the individual, close informant, or clinician. Mild NCD is diagnosed when there is a decline of 1–2 standard deviations from an expected score based on the patient's age and education level. Major NCD is a decline of greater than two standard deviations. Both require the subjective complaint. It has been proposed that POCD should be considered a subtype of neurocognitive disorders (NCD) and classified as mild or major in a similar manner. If available, as in a research study, the decline would be compared against the individual's preoperative score. In order to make a clinical diagnosis, the subjective complaint would be required, but assessing this in early POCD might be difficult as changes may not yet be noticed by family members or the physical consequences of the surgery may camouflage the changes. Eliciting symptoms at 30 days and 90 days would be more feasible and could be incorporated into future studies to keep POCD aligned with the other forms of NCD. Which tests and how many tests are to be used are not defined in NCD and therefore should also not be specified in the clinical diagnosis of POCD. Whether or not specific tests should be promoted for research purposes is another area of future research and discussion.

By using unified nomenclature and criteria for diagnosis, which are aligned with the fields of neurology, psychiatry, and geriatrics, POD and POCD will not only be more readily recognized and diagnosed but also allow more robust treatment or prevention trials. Finally, consistent terminology should provide for more reliable meta-analyses when sufficient clinical studies are reported.

5.3 The Susceptible Elderly Brain

As the brain ages, both macroscopic and microscopic changes occur both as a normal process of aging and as age-related pathologic processes. Many such pathologic processes, as in many neurodegenerative disorders, also occur in people who do not exhibit cognitive deficits. These "subclinical" processes may provide an explanation of why the aged brain is more susceptible to stressful effects of anesthesia and surgery.

The aged brain has an exaggerated immune response to insults, which can then either directly produce injury or accelerate an ongoing process, both of which may adversely influence cognitive performance. For example, it has long been noticed that elderly patients who suffer an infection and immune challenge are at risk for delirium. These same patients then have a higher risk of acquiring Alzheimer's disease and dementia [21, 56]. The microglia play an important role in this phenomenon. Microglia, the primary innate immune cells of the central nervous system, have a complex role in both propagating an immune response to injury and inflammation and also in subduing inflammation and repairing injury and removing debris [56]. The balance between these opposing states and phenotypes is crucial to maintain homeostasis. In the aged brain, microglia have an increased expression of pro-inflammatory markers, leading to an exaggerated response to immune signaling from the periphery. For example, when activated in rodent models, aged brains produce both a greater amount and more sustained production of pro-inflammatory cytokines such as IL-1β, IL-6, and TNFα. Interleukin-1β may be especially important in cognitive changes occurring with immune challenges given its high concentration in the hippocampus. This pro-inflammatory state may also decrease the repair role of the microglia, including the removal of damaged synapses [56, 90].

While Alzheimer's disease is considered a pathologic process of aging, the hallmark pathology also occurs in people of normal cognitive ability and is perhaps a normal process of aging. These hallmarks include the amyloid-beta (Aβ) protein deposits and neurofibrillary tangles (NFTs) composed of the microtubule-associated protein, tau. While normally Aβ proteins are soluble, if they exceed a threshold, they will begin to aggregate and organize into large insoluble deposits called amyloid plaques [72]. These tend to be deposited extracellularly in a perivascular parenchyma and may be less of a source of neuronal dysfunction [72, 74]. Although still controversial, smaller aggregates appear to be the source of neuronal and synaptic damage [74]. The Aβ proteins can surpass the solubility threshold either via increased production or decreased clearance. Increased production can occur with increased activity of β-site-acting cleavage enzyme (BACE) or by mutations in the amyloid precursor protein (APP). Decreased clearance occurs in many states but notably in some ApoEε4 genotypes [74]. NFTs result when tau becomes phosphorylated and thereby dissociates from the microtubules. Neuronal dysfunction may then ensue either through microtubular instability or the loss of intracellular, organellar trafficking.

5.4 Preclinical Research

5.4.1 Anesthesia

Substantial evidence for post-anesthetic pathological and cognitive changes has been reported. In general, these changes are similar to those occurring in neurocognitive disorders such as Alzheimer's disease [4]. The earliest such work showed that even brief volatile anesthetic (halothane and isoflurane) exposure accelerated amyloid-beta aggregation and cellular cytotoxicity [20]. This was followed by several studies in both cell culture and mice that showed exposure to volatile anesthetics causes increased Aβ production, increased BACE, and increased cytotoxicity [19, 79, 91, 92]. Interestingly, desflurane may be less amyloidogenic unless combined with a hypoxic state [95]. Finally, tau hyperphosphorylation, via inhibition of protein phosphatase 2A activity, and detachment of tau from microtubules have also been shown to occur after anesthetic-induced hypothermia regardless of the anesthetic used [57, 58, 87]. Propofol, on the other hand, induced tau hyperphosphorylation even under normothermic conditions in mouse hippocampus and cortex [87]. Besides AD pathologic changes, calcium dysregulation has been implicated as a cause for anesthetic-induced apoptosis in multiple animal and cultured cell studies [86]. Further translational studies need to occur to test whether similar pathological processes happen in humans.

While the above studies have demonstrated widespread and in some cases pronounced effects of anesthetic exposure alone, subsequent effects on cognitive performance in normal wild-type animals have been much less convincing [84]. This may in part be due to varying rodent age, animal number, tests used, and when tested after anesthetic exposure. Nevertheless, some studies have reported that inhalational anesthesia produced durable but subtle impairment in spatial learning and memory [14–16, 41, 88, 93], while others found no effects of either inhalational or propofol anesthesia [9, 34]. In some studies, anesthetics actually improved cognition [60, 76]. Unfortunately, a valid animal model for postoperative delirium has yet to be developed. The conflicting results of many of these preclinical cognitive studies may have been predictable, since many were conducted in young wild-type animals and in the absence of surgery. In general, anything resembling POCD has not been reported in a similar human cohort.

Recognizing this, more recent studies have incorporated two features. First, surgery has been introduced to the animal model, and second, a preexisting vulnerability has been introduced. This vulnerability could be advanced age or the inclusion of disease-associated genes or combinations. And in general, these features, when combined with anesthesia, have produced more convincing and durable changes not only in pathology but also in cognitive performance.

5.4.2 Surgery

Anesthesia is rarely given without surgery, and surgery is a plausible contributor to POD and POCD because of its peripheral activation of innate immunity. Peripheral secretion of pro-inflammatory mediators interleukin-1β and tumor necrosis factor-α (TNFα), in particular, has been shown as causing elevations of CNS cytokines, microgliosis, and early memory impairments in a model of orthopedic surgery [13, 62, 79]. Both TNFα antibodies and knockout of IL-1 blocked the adverse effects of surgery on pathology and cognitive performance [13, 80]. It is important to note that these orthopedic surgery studies were conducted in young adult animals and that the cognitive deficits did not last beyond 7 days.

5.4.3 Age

In general, aged rodents have more significant pathology and durable cognitive impairments after anesthesia and surgery. For example, impairments in object recognition and increased microglial activation in the medial prefrontal cortex and dentate gyrus were noted up to 14 days after abdominal or cardiac surgery [26, 27, 33]. Markers of synaptic density and neuronal plasticity have also been shown to be decreased 1–3 days after surgery in the hippocampus in aged but not young rats after partial hepatectomy [33]. Another group found surgery-induced nociception reduced hippocampal learning and memory at 3–7 days but not 30 days in aged mice and not at all in young mice [96]. In addition, pathological markers of

Alzheimer's disease: microgliosis, astrogliosis, elevated β-APP, Aβ, and tau hyperphosphorylation in the hippocampus, have been shown to be induced after partial hepatectomy in comparison to sham surgery in aged mice [83].

5.4.4 Disease Genes

In addition to age, there exist specific genes associated with neurodegeneration that may also reflect a vulnerability to stresses like anesthesia and surgery. Most studied have been those associated with early-onset Alzheimer disease. In the Tg2576 mouse, the APP Swedish mutation causes amyloidosis and cognitive impairments at about 12 months of age. Exposure of these mice to volatile anesthetics alone resulted in accelerated amyloidosis but not changes in cognitive performance, in part because even the control animals were considerably compromised, and an incremental effect was difficult to detect [6]. Switching to a different triple-transgenic animal (3XTgAD) with the same and two other transgenes associated with Alzheimer's disease, this same group incorporated abdominal surgery and found that significant and essentially irreversible decrements in cognitive performance now occurred but only in those animals having surgery [77]. Only a transient cognitive effect occurred in the anesthesia-alone (desflurane) group. This strongly supports the "two-hit" notion, whereby a preexisting vulnerability is required for the added stress of anesthesia and surgery to have a significant, long-lasting effect on both CNS pathology and function.

5.5 Clinical Research

On a time scale of early to late postoperative CNS events, postoperative delirium is earliest and is a disturbing, reversible condition in which there is fluctuating attention, decreased cognitive function, and disorganized thinking [29]. POD is not only disturbing for the patient and family members but also incurs significant costs and is associated with increased early POCD, worse outcomes, and increased mortality [29, 63]. POD has been found to be the most common following cardiovascular, thoracic, and orthopedic procedures with incidences ranging from 10 to 50 %. Only one retrospective study has specifically examined neurosurgical patients, finding a delirium incidence of 21.4 % [53]. Significant predictors were prior dementia, diabetes, local anesthetic use, longer operative time, and severe postoperative pain. Many of these predictors are common features and comorbidities of the contemporary surgical patient.

There have been a plethora of studies examining POCD, and as previously discussed, this work has been plagued by a lack of uniformity on definition and diagnostic criteria. The majority of studies have been conducted in the cardiac population, and it was first thought that microemboli from the cardiopulmonary bypass were the culprit, a so-called pumphead. There have since been multiple studies showing no difference in the incidence of POCD between on and off bypass patients [2, 3]. Age, previous stroke, and major surgery have been found to be risk factors for early POCD [2, 52]. It is controversial whether early POCD predicts long-term decline, with some investigators showing that operative cardiac patients fare no worse than nonoperative controls matched for cardiac comorbidities [66]. Conflicting results have also been reported on whether general or regional anesthesia enhances risk [49, 52]. This may be due to the high doses of sedatives used during regional anesthesia in many of the studies. Similar to cardiac surgery, persistent POCD and risk of dementia after noncardiac surgery are controversial. The most recent meta-analysis of existing studies concluded that evidence is of insufficient quality to conclude whether anesthesia and surgery are associated with long-term (>6 months) cognitive decline or dementia diagnosis [65]. Since this review, a retrospective review from the Mayo Clinic found no association between surgery and dementia in the entire cohort, but when focusing on the elderly (>65) subgroup, a significant association was detected [73]. Similarly, a recent retrospective twin study (both identical and fraternal) showed a statistically significant association but concluded it was clinically nonsignificant [18]. Another study using a longitudinal prospective design also showed a significant association between surgery and incident dementia [64]. This last study also found that when the cohort was enriched for other risk factors, such as the apoEε4 allele, the association grew significantly. These observations are consistent with the "two-hit" idea mentioned above, in that enriching the study population for known neuropathology risk factors (age, apoEε4, prior cognitive impairment) enhances the risk of anesthesia and surgery of causing durable decline.

5.6 Biomarkers

5.6.1 Blood and CSF Biomarkers

Due to results of preclinical studies showing pathological changes similar to those found in AD after anesthesia and surgery, AD biomarkers have also been studied postoperatively. In a study of 11 patients undergoing nasal endoscopy for CSF leak, lumbar CSF total tau and phosphorylated tau (pTau) increased progressively for 48 h postoperatively, with no change in Aβ. The pro-inflammatory markers interleukin-6 and TNFα also increased at 24 h, as did the injury markers, S100β and total tau. Interestingly, the total tau/Aβ ratio approached values diagnostic of AD [75]. Patients undergoing cardiac surgery have also been shown to have increased CSF S100β and tau and decreased Aβ 6 months postoperatively [55]. Of note, CSF amyloid β levels are low in Alzheimer's disease, probably because of sequestration in the brain as plaque. A study on patients undergoing total hip replacement found a 24.6 % incidence of early POCD which was associated with significantly higher IL-1β, tau/Aβ, pTau/Aβ, and lower Aβ in the CSF 7 days after surgery [30]. Another recent study examining total hip replacement patients found POCD in 8.8 % of patients at 3 months, and a low preoperative CSF Aβ was found to be a significant predictor [22]. While these studies do point to a neuroinflammatory process associated with surgery and elements of neuronal injury, further studies are sorely needed to be able to solidify a relationship between the biomarkers and cognitive changes.

5.6.2 Neuroimaging Biomarkers

Neuroimaging biomarkers have long been examined in AD. In a prospective Alzheimer's disease cohort, significantly lower gray matter and hippocampal volumes were detected in subjects that had surgery an average of 6 months prior compared to nonoperative subjects [32]. Similarly, a prospective study found a statistically significant association between smaller hippocampal volume on MRI and early POCD in patients undergoing gastrointestinal surgery [11]. Preoperative hippocampal volume and leukoaraiosis, periventricular and perivascular white matter demyelination, and lacunar volume were examined in 40 total knee arthroplasty patients and compared to postoperative neurocognitive changes using comprehensive neuropsychological testing and the reliable change index. Greater preoperative leukoaraiosis and lacunar volumes were associated with worse postoperative executive function [59]. More studies examining neuroimaging biomarkers, using both structural and function MR, as well as PET for amyloid and tau, need to be performed to further elucidate the relationship between surgery and neuropathology [1]

5.6.3 Genetic Biomarkers

Few studies have examined genetic biomarkers and the association with POCD. One large prospective cohort study found a decreased risk of POCD in patients with C-reactive protein SNPs (*CRP* 1059G/C (odds ratio 0.37, 95% CI 0.16–0.78; $p=0.013$)) and the P-selectin SNPs (*SELP,* 1087G/A, OR 0.51, 95% CI 0.30–0.85; $p=0.011$) [45]. Apolipoprotein ε4 allele has also been studied with conflicting results of carrying a higher risk for POCD and POD [8, 37, 46, 64, 70]. Further work and meta-analyses should be performed to clarify the genetic predispositions to the postoperative cognitive syndromes.

5.7 Mitigating the Risk of Postoperative Cognitive Dysfunction

5.7.1 Neuroprotection

Interestingly, anesthetics have also been used as neuroprotective agents. Ketamine, an NMDA receptor antagonist, has been studied due to its anti-inflammatory properties, because it increases cerebral blood flow or because it prevents excitotoxic injury [61, 98]. However, ketamine has achieved mixed results as a neuroprotective agent in cardiac, abdominal, and in ophthalmic surgery [28, 51, 61, 98]. When given as a small bolus during induction, there was a significant decrease in cognitive dysfunction 1 week after cardiac surgery, although not when given as a larger bolus and infusion [28, 51]. When ketamine was combined with lidocaine, there was a decrease in POCD after abdominal surgery [98]. In elderly patients having ophthalmic surgery, a ketamine infusion improved postoperative cognition as compared to a control group [61]. In addition to the above, lidocaine has been studied alone in multiple other randomized controlled trials with mixed results [7].

Propofol is popular for induction of anesthesia, as a component of total intravenous anesthesia (TIVA), and for procedural sedation. Along with its anesthetic properties, it has been found to have anti-inflammatory, antioxidant, and neuroprotective properties [81]. In preclinical studies, propofol was found to attenuate apoptosis, production of reactive oxygen species, Aβ peptides, and caspase-3 activation due to sevoflurane and isoflurane in human neuroglioma cells [81, 97]. However, propofol infusions have failed to show a difference in POCD in cardiac surgery [7]. Thiopental and xenon also failed to decrease the incidence of POCD [7].

Multiple other drugs have been studied as neuroprotective agents. Magnesium sulfate, widely studied as a neuroprotective agent, has shown mixed results. Minocycline, a second-generation tetracycline derivative that has anti-inflammatory properties, crosses the blood-brain barrier and prevents isoflurane- and sevoflurane-induced cognitive dysfunction in elderly rats [38, 82]. It has yet to be studied in the clinical setting.

5.7.2 Anesthetic Depth

Controlling the "depth" of anesthesia may be a promising way to mitigate the risk of postoperative delirium and postoperative cognitive dysfunction. The association between deep anesthesia and poor outcomes has been increasingly studied. In elderly patients if anesthetic doses are based upon population estimates, they are often given more anesthesia than needed. This leads not only to hemodynamic complications, hypotension, and decreased cardiac output but also can lead to periods of very deep anesthesia and even burst suppression EEG patterns [36]. The depth of anesthesia is measured clinically with processed EEG monitors such as the bispectral index (BIS) or burst suppression ratio (BSR). BIS values vary from 0 to 100. Values greater than 80 correlated to sedation doses, between 50 and 60 to light general anesthesia, and less than 40 to deep general anesthesia. BIS values less than 30 are often associated with burst suppression patterns. Most of the current literature are retrospective analyses of other studies [36]. Both absolute lower BIS values, prolonged period of times with low BIS values, and BIS less than 40 have all been associated with lower survival [35, 40, 48]. However, this has not been consistently shown in multiple patient populations [36]. Suppression ratio, the time spent in an isoelectric state in the previous minute, was associated with higher 6-month mortality in one study but not with higher 90-day mortality in another [85]. Controlling for confounding factors, however, has proven difficult in these studies due to the retrospective nature. The Balanced Anesthesia Study, an international randomized controlled trial of deep (BIS = 35) and light (BIS =50) volatile anesthesia, is planning to recruit 6500 patients and is hypothesizing a 20 % relative risk reduction for 1-year mortality in the light anesthesia group.

The evidence for an association between anesthetic depth and postoperative delirium has proven to be more compelling. A randomized controlled trial looking at deep (BIS = 50) vs light (BIS >80) sedation in hip fracture patients under spinal anesthesia has found a lower incidence of POD in the light sedation group [69]. A recent meta-analysis of this study and four other studies looking at anesthetic depth under general anesthesia and postoperative delirium found a significantly reduced risk (OR 0.56, 95 % confidence interval: 0.40–0.77) [44].

Anesthetic sensitivity, defined here as a low BIS with a low concentration of anesthetic, may be a marker of increased patient frailty. It is conceivable, then, that low BIS in the above studies is simply a surrogate for frailty which might independently be associated with poor outcomes, rather than the anesthetic or BIS per se. Both this double-low state and triple-low state (low BIS, low anesthetic, and low mean arterial pressure) have been associated with increased 30-day mortality [12, 31, 68]. A randomized controlled trial is now underway in which anesthesiologists are either alerted or not alerted to low values, using a 90-day mortality as the primary outcomes (ClinicalTrials.org NCT00998894). The Balanced Anesthesia Study will also employ secondary analyses to evaluate the effect of anesthetic sensitivity on outcomes [89]. Thus, it remains unclear whether low BIS produced by a relative anesthetic "overdose" is associated with poor cognitive outcomes or whether the low BIS itself simply reflects the presence of significant neuropathology, which would be expected to correlate with poor cognitive outcomes.

5.7.3 Choice of Anesthetic

Few prospective studies have compared the choice of general anesthetic used in human populations. A Chinese prospective, randomized, parallel-group study examined 180 patients with mild cognitive impairment (MCI) having lumbar spinal surgery [43]. The patients were randomized to receive sevoflurane, propofol, or epidural anesthesia with lidocaine. At 2 years postoperatively, the groups had a similar conversion rate to dementia, but the sevoflurane group had a greater progression to amnestic MCI. Elderly patients receiving sevoflurane versus propofol for rectal surgery had the same incidence of POCD, but the sevoflurane group had a significantly higher severity of POCD as compared to the propofol group [78]. Another prospective cohort study examined 76 elderly patients who received either TIVA or sevoflurane and found no difference in the incidence of POD [17]. A meta-analysis that examined five studies comparing sevoflurane to desflurane found no difference in POCD [10]. Subsequently, another randomized controlled trial compared 110 patients who received either sevoflurane or desflurane general anesthesia, guided by processed EEG, and again found no difference in incidence of POCD between the groups [47]. Dexmedetomidine has shown promise in preventing delirium in the ICU and has been shown to decrease the incidence of POD in elderly patients both with and without mild cognitive impairment preoperatively [24, 42]. Dexmedetomidine has not yet been studied for POCD.

The established role for inflammation in neurodegeneration, and probably also POCD, has stimulated studies on whether dexamethasone could mitigate POCD. Recently, in a preplanned substudy of the Dexamethasone for Cardiac Surgery trial, a multicenter, randomized, double-blind, placebo controlled trial, assessed the effect of intraoperative high-dose dexamethasone on the incidence of POCD at 1 and 12 months after cardiac surgery and found no statistical significant difference in POCD [54]. In a study of 1000 patients having microvascular decompression for facial spasm, the incidence of early POCD was examined. Patients were randomized to no dexamethasone and to 0.1 mg/kg or 0.2 mg/kg of dexamethasone. The higher dose of dexamethasone was associated with a significantly higher rate of POCD at 5 days after surgery, 31.4 %, compared to the no dexamethasone group, 22.3 %, and the lower dose dexamethasone group, 20.6 % [23]. Although dexamethasone may decrease the inflammatory response of surgery, in aged rodents dexamethasone and glucocorticoids have been shown to elevate amyloid precursor protein expression, reduce its degradation, and augment tau protein [25, 39, 71, 94], effects that may underlie the unexpected effects in the clinical studies above.

5.8 Summary

In summary, POD and POCD are real and serious complications of surgery affecting a sizeable fraction of operative patients, especially the elderly. Their causes are yet to be completely elucidated but neuroinflammation and neurodegenerative changes of the Alzheimer type have been implicated both in preclinical studies and biomarker studies. Whether or not these changes cause persistent POCD and permanent neurological sequela is still debated. Consensus on definitions and diagnosis is necessary to allow further translational and clinical studies to be compared to one another and for meta-analyses to occur. Studies on elderly neurosurgical patients are especially needed to determine the incidence, risk factors, and sequelae of both POD and POCD as these patients have largely been excluded from studies.

References

1. Abildstrom H, Christiansen M, Siersma VD, Rasmussen LS (2004) Apolipoprotein E genotype and cognitive dysfunction after noncardiac surgery. J Am Soc Anesthesiol 101(4):855–861
2. Arora SS, Gooch JL, García PS (2014) Postoperative cognitive dysfunction, Alzheimer's disease, and anesthesia. Int J Neurosci 124(4):236–242
3. Avidan MS, Evers AS (2016) The fallacy of persistent postoperative cognitive decline. J Am Soc Anesthesiol 124(2):255–258
4. Baranov D, Bickler PE, Crosby GJ, Culley DJ, Eckenhoff MF, Eckenhoff RG, Hogan KJ, Jevtovic-Todorovic V, Palotás A, Perouansky M (2009) Consensus statement: first international workshop on anesthetics and Alzheimer's disease. Anesth Analg 108(5):1627

5. Bedford P (1955) Adverse cerebral effects of anaesthesia on old people. Lancet 266(6884):259–264
6. Bianchi SL, Tran T, Liu C, Lin S, Li Y, Keller JM, Eckenhoff RG, Eckenhoff MF (2008) Brain and behavior changes in 12-month-old Tg2576 and nontransgenic mice exposed to anesthetics. Neurobiol Aging 29(7):1002–1010
7. Bilotta F, Gelb A, Stazi E, Titi L, Paoloni F, Rosa G (2013) Pharmacological perioperative brain neuroprotection: a qualitative review of randomized clinical trials. Br J Anaesth 110(Suppl 1):i113–i120, aet059
8. Bryson GL, Wyand A, Wozny D, Rees L, Taljaard M, Nathan H (2011) A prospective cohort study evaluating associations among delirium, postoperative cognitive dysfunction, and apolipoprotein E genotype following open aortic repair. Can J Anesth 58(3):246–255
9. Callaway JK, Jones NC, Royse AG, Royse CF (2012) Sevoflurane anesthesia does not impair acquisition learning or memory in the Morris water maze in young adult and aged rats. J Am Soc Anesthesiol 117(5):1091–1101
10. Chen G, Zhou Y, Shi Q, Zhou H (2015) Comparison of early recovery and cognitive function after desflurane and sevoflurane anaesthesia in elderly patients: a meta-analysis of randomized controlled trials. J Int Med Res 43(5):619–628
11. Chen MH, Liao Y, Rong PF, Hu R, Lin GX, Ouyang W (2013) Hippocampal volume reduction in elderly patients at risk for postoperative cognitive dysfunction. J Anesth 27(4):487–492
12. Cheng XQ, Wu H, Zuo YM, Mei B, Zhang L, Cai YZ, Zhao Q, Lu XF, Liu XS, Gu EW (2016). Perioperative risk factors and cumulative duration of "triple-low" state associated with worse 30-day mortality of cardiac valvular surgery. J Clin Monit Comput doi:10.1007/s10877-016-9856-2
13. Cibelli M, Fidalgo AR, Terrando N, Ma D, Monaco C, Feldmann M, Takata M, Lever IJ, Nanchahal J, Fanselow MS (2010) Role of interleukin-1β in postoperative cognitive dysfunction. Ann Neurol 68(3):360–368
14. Culley DJ, Baxter M, Yukhananov R, Crosby G (2003) The memory effects of general anesthesia persist for weeks in young and aged rats. Anesth Analg 96(4):1004–1009
15. Culley DJ, Baxter MG, Yukhananov R, Crosby G (2004) Long-term impairment of acquisition of a spatial memory task following isoflurane–nitrous oxide anesthesia in rats. J Am Soc Anesthesiol 100(2):309–314
16. Culley DJ, Raghavan SV, Waly M, Baxter MG, Yukhananov R, Deth RC, Crosby G (2007) Nitrous oxide decreases cortical methionine synthase transiently but produces lasting memory impairment in aged rats. J Am Soc Anesthesiol 107(1):83–88
17. Deiner S, Lin H-M, Bodansky D, Silverstein J, Sano M (2014) Do stress markers and anesthetic technique predict delirium in the elderly? Dement Geriatr Cogn Disord 38(5–6):366–374
18. Dokkedal U, Hansen TG, Rasmussen LS, Mengel-From J, Christensen K (2016) Cognitive functioning after surgery in middle-aged and elderly Danish twins. J Am Soc Anesthesiol 124(2):312–321
19. Dong Y, Zhang G, Zhang B, Moir RD, Xia W, Marcantonio ER, Culley DJ, Crosby G, Tanzi RE, Xie Z (2009) The common inhalational anesthetic sevoflurane induces apoptosis and increases β-amyloid protein levels. Arch Neurol 66(5):620–631
20. Eckenhoff RG, Johansson JS, Wei H, Carnini A, Kang B, Wei W, Pidikiti R, Keller JM, Eckenhoff MF (2004) Inhaled anesthetic enhancement of amyloid-β oligomerization and cytotoxicity. J Am Soc Anesthesiol 101(3):703–709
21. Ehlenbach WJ, Hough CL, Crane PK, Haneuse SJ, Carson SS, Curtis JR, Larson EB (2010) Association between acute care and critical illness hospitalization and cognitive function in older adults. JAMA 303(8):763–770
22. Evered L, Silbert B, Scott DA, Ames D, Maruff P, Blennow K (2016) Cerebrospinal fluid biomarker for alzheimer disease predicts postoperative cognitive dysfunction. J Am Soc Anesthesiol 124(2):353–361
23. Fang Q, Qian X, An J, Wen H, Cope DK, Williams JP (2014) Higher dose dexamethasone increases early postoperative cognitive dysfunction. J Neurosurg Anesthesiol 26(3):220–225

24. Friedman JI, Soleimani L, McGonigle DP, Egol C, Silverstein JH (2014) Pharmacological treatments of non-substance-withdrawal delirium: a systematic review of prospective trials. Am J Psychiatry 171(2):151–159
25. Green KN, Billings LM, Roozendaal B, McGaugh JL, LaFerla FM (2006) Glucocorticoids increase amyloid-β and tau pathology in a mouse model of Alzheimer's disease. J Neurosci 26(35):9047–9056
26. Hovens IB, van Leeuwen BL, Mariani MA, Kraneveld AD, Schoemaker RG (2016) Postoperative cognitive dysfunction and neuroinflammation; cardiac surgery and abdominal surgery are not the same. Brain Behav Immun 54:178–193
27. Hovens IB, van Leeuwen BL, Nyakas C, Heineman E, van der Zee EA, Schoemaker RG (2015) Postoperative cognitive dysfunction and microglial activation in associated brain regions in old rats. Neurobiol Learn Mem 118:74–79
28. Hudetz J, Iqbal Z, Gandhi S, Patterson K, Byrne A, Hudetz A, Pagel P, Warltier D (2009) Ketamine attenuates post-operative cognitive dysfunction after cardiac surgery. Acta Anaesthesiol Scand 53(7):864–872
29. Inouye SK, Westendorp RG, Saczynski JS (2014) Delirium in elderly people. Lancet 383(9920):911–922
30. Ji M-H, Yuan H-M, Zhang G-F, Li X-M, Dong L, Li W-Y, Zhou Z-Q, Yang J-J (2012) Changes in plasma and cerebrospinal fluid biomarkers in aged patients with early postoperative cognitive dysfunction following total hip-replacement surgery. J Anesth 27(2):236–242
31. Kertai MD, White WD, Gan TJ (2014) Cumulative duration of "triple low" state of low blood pressure, low bispectral index, and low minimum alveolar concentration of volatile anesthesia is not associated with increased mortality. J Am Soc Anesthesiol 121(1):18–28
32. Kline RP, Pirraglia E, Cheng H, De Santi S, Li Y, Haile M, de Leon MJ, Bekker A (2012) Surgery and brain atrophy in cognitively normal elderly subjects and subjects diagnosed with mild cognitive impairment. J Am Soc Anesthesiol 116(3):603–612
33. Le Y, Liu S, Peng M, Tan C, Liao Q, Duan K, Ouyang W, Tong J (2014) Aging differentially affects the loss of neuronal dendritic spine, neuroinflammation and memory impairment at rats after surgery. PLoS One 9(9):e106837
34. Lee IH, Culley DJ, Baxter MG, Xie Z, Tanzi RE, Crosby G (2008) Spatial memory is intact in aged rats after propofol anesthesia. Anesth Analg 107(4):1211–1215
35. Leslie K, Myles PS, Forbes A, Chan MT (2010) The effect of bispectral index monitoring on long-term survival in the B-aware trial. Anesth Analg 110(3):816–822
36. Leslie K, Short TG (2016) Anesthetic depth and long-term survival: an update. Can J Anesth 63(2):233–240
37. Leung JM, Sands LP, Wang Y, Poon A, Kwok P-y, Kane JP, Pullinger CR (2007) Apolipoprotein E e4 allele increases the risk of early postoperative delirium in older patients undergoing noncardiac surgery. J Am Soc Anesthesiol 107(3):406–411
38. Li S-Y, Xia L-X, Zhao Y-L, Yang L, Chen Y-L, Wang J-T, Luo A-L (2013) Minocycline mitigates isoflurane-induced cognitive impairment in aged rats. Brain Res 1496:84–93
39. Li W-Z, Li W-P, Huang D-K, Kan H-W, Wang X, Wu W-Y, Yin Y-Y, Yao Y-Y (2012) Dexamethasone and Aβ 25–35 accelerate learning and memory impairments due to elevate amyloid precursor protein expression and neuronal apoptosis in 12-month male rats. Behav Brain Res 227(1):142–149
40. Lindholm ML, Traff S, Granath F, Greenwald SD, Ekbom A, Lennmarken C, Sandin RH (2009) Mortality within 2 years after surgery in relation to low intraoperative bispectral index values and preexisting malignant disease. Anesth Analg 108(2):508–512
41. Liu X-S, Xue Q-s, Zeng Q-W, Li Q, Liu J, Feng X-M, Yu B-W (2010) Sevoflurane impairs memory consolidation in rats, possibly through inhibiting phosphorylation of glycogen synthase kinase-3β in the hippocampus. Neurobiol Learn Mem 94(4):461–467
42. Liu Y, Ma L, Gao M, Guo W, Ma Y (2015) Dexmedetomidine reduces postoperative delirium after joint replacement in elderly patients with mild cognitive impairment. Aging Clin Exp Res 28:729–736

43. Liu Y, Pan N, Ma Y, Zhang S, Guo W, Li H, Zhou J, Liu G, Gao M (2013) Inhaled sevoflurane may promote progression of amnestic mild cognitive impairment: a prospective, randomized parallel-group study. Am J Med Sci 345(5):355–360
44. Luk TTH, Jia B, Pang EYT, Lau VNM, Lam CKM, Chu MHM, Han R, Chan MTV (2014) Depth of anesthesia and postoperative delirium. Curr Anesthesiol Rep 5(1):1–9
45. Mathew JP, Podgoreanu MV, Grocott HP, White WD, Morris RW, Stafford-Smith M, Mackensen GB, Rinder CS, Blumenthal JA, Schwinn DA (2007) Genetic variants in P-selectin and C-reactive protein influence susceptibility to cognitive decline after cardiac surgery. J Am Coll Cardiol 49(19):1934–1942
46. McDonagh DL, Mathew JP, White WD, Phillips-Bute B, Laskowitz DT, Podgoreanu MV, Newman MF (2010) Cognitive function after major noncardiac surgery, apolipoprotein E4 genotype, and biomarkers of brain injury. J Am Soc Anesthesiol 112(4):852–859
47. Meineke M, Applegate RL, Rasmussen T, Anderson D, Azer S, Mehdizadeh A, Kim A, Allard M (2014) Cognitive dysfunction following desflurane versus sevoflurane general anesthesia in elderly patients: a randomized controlled trial. Med Gas Res 4(1):6
48. Monk TG, Saini V, Weldon BC, Sigl JC (2005) Anesthetic management and one-year mortality after noncardiac surgery. Anesth Analg 100(1):4–10
49. Moyce Z, Rodseth R, Biccard B (2014) The efficacy of peri-operative interventions to decrease postoperative delirium in non-cardiac surgery: a systematic review and meta-analysis. Anaesthesia 69(3):259–269
50. Murkin J, Martzke J, Buchan A, Bentley C, Wong C (1995) A randomized study of the influence of perfusion technique and pH management strategy in 316 patients undergoing coronary artery bypass surgery: II. neurologic and cognitive outcomes. J Thorac Cardiovasc Surg 110(2):349–362
51. Nagels W, Demeyere R, Van Hemelrijck J, Vandenbussche E, Gijbels K, Vandermeersch E (2004) Evaluation of the neuroprotective effects of S (+)-ketamine during open-heart surgery. Anesth Analg 98(6):1595–1603
52. Newman S, Stygall J, Hirani S, Shaefi S, Maze M (2007) Postoperative cognitive dysfunction after noncardiac surgery a systematic review. J Am Soc Anesthesiol 106(3):572–590
53. Oh Y-S, Kim D-W, Chun H-J, Yi H-J (2008) Incidence and risk factors of acute postoperative delirium in geriatric neurosurgical patients. J Korean Neurosurg Soc 43(3):143–148
54. Ottens TH, Dieleman JM, Sauër A-MC, Peelen LM, Nierich AP, De Groot WJ, Nathoe HM, Buijsrogge MP, Kalkman CJ, Van Dijk D (2015) Effects of dexamethasone on cognitive decline after cardiac surgery: a randomized clinical trial. Surv Anesthesiol 59(4):166–167
55. Palotás A, Reis HJ, Bogáts G, Babik B, Racsmány M, Engvau L, Kecskeméti É, Juhász A, Vieira LB, Teixeira AL (2010) Coronary artery bypass surgery provokes Alzheimer's disease-like changes in the cerebrospinal fluid. J Alzheimers Dis 21(4):1153–1164
56. Patterson SL (2015) Immune dysregulation and cognitive vulnerability in the aging brain: Interactions of microglia, IL-1β, BDNF and synaptic plasticity. Neuropharmacology 96:11–18
57. Planel E, Bretteville A, Liu L, Virag L, Du AL, Yu WH, Dickson DW, Whittington RA, Duff KE (2009) Acceleration and persistence of neurofibrillary pathology in a mouse model of tauopathy following anesthesia. FASEB J 23(8):2595–2604
58. Planel E, Krishnamurthy P, Miyasaka T, Liu L, Herman M, Kumar A, Bretteville A, Figueroa HY, Yu WH, Whittington RA (2008) Anesthesia-induced hyperphosphorylation detaches 3-repeat tau from microtubules without affecting their stability in vivo. J Neurosci 28(48):12798–12807
59. Price CC, Tanner JJ, Schmalfuss I, Garvan CW, Gearen P, Dickey D, Heilman K, McDonagh DL, Libon DJ, Leonard C (2014) A pilot study evaluating presurgery neuroanatomical biomarkers for postoperative cognitive decline after total knee arthroplasty in older adults. J Ame Soc Anesthesiol 120(3):601–613
60. Rammes G, Starker LK, Haseneder R, Berkmann J, Plack A, Zieglgänsberger W, Ohl F, Kochs EF, Blobner M (2009) Isoflurane anaesthesia reversibly improves cognitive function and long-term potentiation (LTP) via an up-regulation in NMDA receptor 2B subunit expression. Neuropharmacology 56(3):626–636

61. Rascón-Martínez DM, Fresán-Orellana A, Ocharán-Hernández ME, Genis-Zarate JH, Castellanos-Olivares A (2016) The effects of ketamine on cognitive function in elderly patients undergoing ophthalmic surgery: a pilot study. Anesth Analg 122:969–975
62. Rosczyk H, Sparkman N, Johnson R (2008) Neuroinflammation and cognitive function in aged mice following minor surgery. Exp Gerontol 43(9):840–846
63. Saczynski JS, Marcantonio ER, Quach L, Fong TG, Gross A, Inouye SK, Jones RN (2012) Cognitive trajectories after postoperative delirium. N Engl J Med 367(1):30–39
64. Schenning KJ, Murchison CF, Mattek NC, Silbert LC, Kaye JA, Quinn JF (2015) Surgery is associated with ventricular enlargement as well as cognitive and functional decline. Alzheimers Dement 12(5):590–597
65. Seitz DP, Shah PS, Herrmann N, Beyene J, Siddiqui N (2011) Exposure to general anesthesia and risk of Alzheimer's disease: a systematic review and meta-analysis. BMC Geriatr 11(1):83
66. Selnes OA, Grega MA, Borowicz LM, Royall RM, McKhann GM, Baumgartner WA (2003) Cognitive changes with coronary artery disease: a prospective study of coronary artery bypass graft patients and nonsurgical controls. Ann Thorac Surg 75(5):1377–1386
67. Selnes OA, Royall RM, Grega MA, Borowicz LM Jr, Quaskey S, McKhann GM (2001) Cognitive changes 5 years after coronary artery bypass grafting: is there evidence of late decline? Arch Neurol 58(4):598–604
68. Sessler DI, Sigl JC, Kelley SD, Chamoun NG, Manberg PJ, Saager L, Kurz A, Greenwald S (2012) Hospital stay and mortality are increased in patients having a "triple low" of low blood pressure, low bispectral index, and low minimum alveolar concentration of volatile anesthesia. J Ame Soc Anesthesiol 116(6):1195–1203
69. Sieber FE, Zakriya KJ, Gottschalk A, Blute M-R, Lee HB, Rosenberg PB, Mears SC (2010) Sedation depth during spinal anesthesia and the development of postoperative delirium in elderly patients undergoing hip fracture repair. Mayo Clin Proc 85(1):18–26, Elsevier
70. Silbert BS, Evered LA, Scott DA, Cowie TF (2008) The apolipoprotein E ϵ4 allele is not associated with cognitive dysfunction in cardiac surgery. Ann Thorac Surg 86(3): 841–847
71. Sotiropoulos I, Catania C, Riedemann T, Fry JP, Breen KC, Michaelidis TM, Almeida OF (2008) Glucocorticoids trigger Alzheimer disease-like pathobiochemistry in rat neuronal cells expressing human tau. J Neurochem 107(2):385–397
72. Soto C (2003) Unfolding the role of protein misfolding in neurodegenerative diseases. Nat Rev Neurosci 4(1):49–60
73. Sprung J, Jankowski CJ, Roberts RO, Weingarten TN, Aguilar AL, Runkle KJ, Tucker AK, McLaren KC, Schroeder DR, Hanson AC (2013) Anesthesia and incident dementia: a population-based, nested, case-control study. Mayo Clin Proc 88(6):552–561, Elsevier
74. Tang J, Eckenhoff MF, Eckenhoff RG (2010) Anesthesia and the old brain. Anesth Analg 110(2):421–426
75. Tang JX, Baranov D, Hammond M, Shaw LM, Eckenhoff MF, Eckenhoff RG (2011) Human Alzheimer and inflammation biomarkers after anesthesia and surgery. J Ame Soc Anesthesiol 115(4):727–732
76. Tang JX, Mardini F, Caltagarone BM, Garrity ST, Li RQ, Bianchi SL, Gomes O, Laferla FM, Eckenhoff RG, Eckenhoff MF (2011) Anesthesia in presymptomatic Alzheimer's disease: a study using the triple-transgenic mouse model. Alzheimers Dement 7(5):521–531, e521
77. Tang JX, Mardini F, Janik LS, Garrity ST, Li RQ, Bachlani G, Eckenhoff RG, Eckenhoff MF (2013) Modulation of murine Alzheimer pathogenesis and behavior by surgery. Ann Surg 257(3):439
78. Tang N, Ou C, Liu Y, Zuo Y, Bai Y (2014) Effect of inhalational anaesthetic on postoperative cognitive dysfunction following radical rectal resection in elderly patients with mild cognitive impairment. J Int Med Res 42(6):1252–1261, 0300060514549781
79. Terrando N, Brzezinski M, Degos V, Eriksson LI, Kramer JH, Leung JM, Miller BL, Seeley WW, Vacas S, Weiner MW (2011) Perioperative cognitive decline in the aging population. Mayo Clin Proc 86(9):885–893, Elsevier

80. Terrando N, Monaco C, Ma D, Foxwell BM, Feldmann M, Maze M (2010) Tumor necrosis factor-α triggers a cytokine cascade yielding postoperative cognitive decline. Proc Natl Acad Sci 107(47):20518–20522
81. Tian Y, Guo S, Guo Y, Jian L (2015) Anesthetic propofol attenuates apoptosis, Aβ accumulation, and inflammation induced by sevoflurane through NF-kB pathway in human neuroglioma cells. Cell Mol Neurobiol 35(6):891–898
82. Tian Y, Guo S, Wu X, Ma L, Zhao X (2015) Minocycline alleviates sevoflurane-induced cognitive impairment in aged rats. Cell Mol Neurobiol 35(4):585–594
83. Wan Y, Xu J, Meng F, Bao Y, Ge Y, Lobo N, Vizcaychipi MP, Zhang D, Gentleman SM, Maze M (2010) Cognitive decline following major surgery is associated with gliosis, β-amyloid accumulation, and τ phosphorylation in old mice. Crit Care Med 38(11):2190–2198
84. Wang D-S, Orser BA (2011) Inhibition of learning and memory by general anesthetics. Can J Anesth 58(2):167–177
85. Watson PL, Shintani AK, Tyson R, Pandharipande PP, Pun BT, Ely EW (2008) Presence of electroencephalogram burst suppression in sedated, critically ill patients is associated with increased mortality. Crit Care Med 36(12):3171
86. Wei H (2011) The role of calcium dysregulation in anesthetic-mediated neurotoxicity. Anesth Analg 113(5):972
87. Whittington RA, Virág L, Marcouiller F, Papon M-A, Khoury NBE, Julien C, Morin F, Emala CW, Planel E (2011) Propofol directly increases tau phosphorylation. PLoS One 6(1):e16648
88. Wiklund A, Granon S, Faure P, Sundman E, Changeux J-P, Eriksson LI (2009) Object memory in young and aged mice after sevoflurane anaesthesia. Neuroreport 20(16):1419–1423
89. Willingham M, Abdallah AB, Gradwohl S, Helsten D, Lin N, Villafranca A, Jacobsohn E, Avidan M, Kaiser H (2014) Association between intraoperative electroencephalographic suppression and postoperative mortality. Br J Anaesth 113(6):1001–1008, aeu105
90. Wong WT (2015) Microglial aging in the healthy CNS: phenotypes, drivers, and rejuvenation. Front Cell Neurosci 7:22
91. Xie Z, Culley DJ, Dong Y, Zhang G, Zhang B, Moir RD, Frosch MP, Crosby G, Tanzi RE (2008) The common inhalation anesthetic isoflurane induces caspase activation and increases amyloid β-protein level in vivo. Ann Neurol 64(6):618–627
92. Xie Z, Dong Y, Maeda U, Alfille P, Culley DJ, Crosby G, Tanzi RE (2006) The common inhalation anesthetic isoflurane induces apoptosis and increases amyloid β protein levels. J Ame Soc Anesthesiol 104(5):988–994
93. Xiong W-X, Zhou G-X, Wang B, Xue Z-G, Wang L, Sun H-C, Ge S-J (2013) Impaired spatial learning and memory after sevoflurane–nitrous oxide anesthesia in aged rats is associated with down-regulated cAMP/CREB signaling. PLoS One 8(11):e79408
94. Yao Y-Y, Liu D-M, Xu D-F, Li W-P (2007) Memory and learning impairment induced by dexamethasone in senescent but not young mice. Eur J Pharmacol 574(1):20–28
95. Zhang B, Dong Y, Zhang G, Moir RD, Xia W, Yue Y, Tian M, Culley DJ, Crosby G, Tanzi RE (2008) The inhalation anesthetic desflurane induces caspase activation and increases amyloid β-protein levels under hypoxic conditions. J Biol Chem 283(18):11866–11875
96. Zhang X, Xin X, Dong Y, Zhang Y, Yu B, Mao J, Xie Z (2013) Surgical incision-induced nociception causes cognitive impairment and reduction in synaptic NMDA receptor 2B in mice. J Neurosci 33(45):17737–17748
97. Zhang Y, Zhen Y, Dong Y, Xu Z, Yue Y, Golde TE, Tanzi RE, Moir RD, Xie Z (2011) Anesthetic propofol attenuates the isoflurane-induced caspase-3 activation and Aβ oligomerization. PLoS One 6(11):e27019
98. Zhu M, Li Y, Wan Z, Zhang D, Wang X (2015) Effects of small-dose lidocaine combined with ketamine on early postoperative cognitive function in elderly patients undergoing gastrointestinal tumor surgery. Nan Fang Yi Ke Da Xue Xue Bao 35(7):1076–1078

Central Nervous System Infections in the Elderly

6

Rodrigo Hasbun and Allan R. Tunkel

6.1 Introduction

According to the United Nations, the number of persons living longer is increasing, and, by 2050, it is estimated that 21.5 % of the population will be older adults [1]; elderly patients are at increased risk for immune senescence and immunocompromise, placing them at higher risk for infections [2, 3]. Common presentations of central nervous system (CNS) infections include meningitis, encephalitis, and focal neurologic syndromes (e.g., brain abscess, subdural empyema, and epidural abscess) and may be caused by a variety of infectious agents (viruses, bacteria, fungi, and parasites) [4]. For the purposes of this chapter, we will focus on community-acquired and healthcare-associated meningitis and viral encephalitis among the elderly, highlighting the epidemiology, etiology, clinical features, prognosis, and approach to diagnosis and management.

6.2 Community-Acquired Meningitis

Community-acquired meningitis can be caused by several infectious and noninfectious etiologies and can present as urgent treatable conditions [5]. The most common infectious causes are viruses, bacteria (including *Mycobacterium tuberculosis*), and fungi. Meningitis in elderly patients can represent a diagnostic challenge,

R. Hasbun, MD, MPH (✉)
UT Health McGovern Medical School,
6431 Fannin St. 2.112 MSB, Houston, TX 77030, USA
e-mail: Rodrigo.Hasbun@uth.tmc.edu

A.R. Tunkel, MD, PhD
Warren Alpert Medical School of Brown University,
222 Richmond Street, Room G-M143, Providence, RI 02912, USA
e-mail: Allan_tunkel@brown.edu

© Springer International Publishing Switzerland 2017

M. Berhouma, P. Krolak-Salmon (eds.), *Brain and Spine Surgery in the Elderly*,
DOI 10.1007/978-3-319-40232-1_6

prompting the workup for other potential causes of altered mental status, thus delaying appropriate diagnosis and therapy [6–8]. In a study of 619 adults with community-acquired meningitis, elderly patients had more comorbidities and presented sicker than younger patients; the elderly had more abnormal neurological exam findings, higher CSF protein, and abnormalities on cranial imaging [6]. An adverse clinical outcome was also seen more frequently in elderly patients (51.9 % vs. 7.4 %, $P<0.001$). Furthermore, elderly patients were more likely to present with bacterial meningitis and West Nile encephalitis than the younger patients who more commonly had viral or fungal meningitis. Additionally, in a study of 567 adults with meningitis and a negative cerebrospinal fluid (CSF) Gram stain, the three independent predictors for an adverse clinical outcome were age >60 years of age, a CSF glucose <45 mg/dl, and an abnormal neurological exam [7]. Another study of 159 adults with meningitis showed that patients above the age of 60 years were more likely to have bacterial meningitis but were less likely to present with the typical meningitis symptoms [8].

6.3 Bacterial Meningitis

6.3.1 Community-Acquired Bacterial Meningitis

The most common pathogens that cause community-acquired bacterial meningitis are *Streptococcus pneumoniae*, *Neisseria meningitidis*, *Haemophilus influenzae*, *Listeria monocytogenes*, and group B streptococcus [8–10]. Bacterial meningitis continues to be associated with significant morbidity and mortality. Overall estimates of case fatality rates for bacterial meningitis were reported to be approximately 25 %, with increasing age as a risk factor for mortality [8–10]. In a study of 493 episodes of bacterial meningitis in adults, risk factors associated with mortality included age 60 years or older, obtundation, and seizure. In another retrospective study of 269 adults, hypotension, altered mental status, and seizures were used to create a prognostic model [8, 9]. In the largest prospective study to date including 1412 episodes of acute bacterial meningitis in adults, an adverse clinical outcome was seen in 38 % [10]; predictors of unfavorable outcome were age greater than 70 years, absence of otitis or sinusitis, alcoholism, tachycardia, lower score on the Glasgow Coma Scale, cranial nerve palsy, CSF white blood cell count lower than 1000 cells per μL, a positive blood culture, and a high serum C-reactive protein concentration. Adjunctive dexamethasone was found to be protective against an adverse outcome.

Bacterial meningitis is also associated with significant neurological sequelae such as cognitive deficits, hearing loss, seizures, visual impairment, and/or focal motor deficits [10]. In a worldwide review of 18,183 survivors of bacterial meningitis, risk for major neurological sequelae was pathogen dependent with *Streptococcus pneumoniae*, *Haemophilus influenzae* type b, and *Neisseria meningitidis* reported to be associated with at least one major neurological sequelae in 24.7 %, 9.5 %, and 7.2 % of patients, respectively [11].

The most common bacterial cause of meningitis in those 65 years of age and older is *S. pneumoniae* (~70 % of cases) [12]; *Listeria monocytogenes, N. meningitidis, H. influenzae, Streptococcus agalactiae,* and aerobic Gram-negative bacilli are less common in this age group. The use of pneumococcal and meningococcal conjugate vaccines in the United States has decreased the incidence of *S. pneumoniae* from 0.8 per 100,000 people in 1997 to 0.3 per 100,000 people in 2010 and of *N. meningitidis* from 0.72 per 100,000 people in 1997 to 0.12 per 100,000 people in 2010 [13]. Overall case fatality rates among all those with bacterial meningitis in the United States have not changed significantly from 15.7 % in 1999 to 14.3 % in 2007 [12].

In the United States, *S. pneumoniae* continues to be the leading pathogen in community-acquired bacterial meningitis and the one associated with the highest mortality [12]; death in those over 60 years of age is more commonly due to systemic complications from bacterial meningitis [14]. From 1999 to 2007, the percentage of adult patients with invasive pneumococcal disease who had underlying medical conditions increased from 52 to 59 % among those aged 18–64 years and from 69 to 81 % among those 65 years of age and older [12]. According to recommendations from the Centers for Disease Control and Prevention (CDC), all adults 65 years of age or older should receive both the 23-valent pneumococcal polysaccharide vaccine and the 13-valent pneumococcal vaccine [15]. Adult patients with functional asplenia or anatomic splenectomy, cerebrospinal fluid leak, cochlear implants, or immunosuppressing conditions should also be vaccinated [15].

L. monocytogenes is estimated to cause 2–8 % of all cases of bacterial meningitis in the United States; with serotypes 1/2b and 4b account accounting for up to 80 % of all cases [16]. Recently, serotype sequence type 6 (ST6) was shown to be a predictor of increasingly unfavorable outcomes among adults with *Listeria* meningitis in which poor outcomes rose from 27 to 61 % over the 14-year study period [17]. Predisposing factors in those who develop *Listeria* meningitis include age over 60 years, chronic corticosteroid therapy, alcohol dependence, immunosuppression, and malignancy [17–19]. A review of 820 cases of CNS listeriosis demonstrated an overall mortality rate of 26 %; patients with seizures and age greater than 65 years of age were at even higher risk [18]. Another study of 1959 cases of listeriosis in France showed that age greater than 65 years, underlying disease, and focal listeriosis were independently associated with increased mortality [19].

Streptococcus agalactiae (or group B streptococcus), although a common cause of meningitis in neonates, is also seen more frequently in adults over 60 years of age and in those with diabetes, cardiac disease, cirrhosis, renal failure, prior stroke, malignancy, alcoholism, neurogenic bladder, or decubitus ulcers [20–22]. The mortality rate in a study of 52 cases was 34.4 %, with factors associated with death being advanced age and complications on admission [22].

6.3.2 Healthcare-Associated Meningitis and Ventriculitis

Healthcare-associated meningitis and ventriculitis are serious complications of invasive neurosurgical procedures (e.g., craniotomy, placement of internal or external ventricular catheters, intrathecal infusions, spinal anesthesia, or lumbar puncture) or may occur after penetrating head trauma with or without cerebrospinal fluid leak [8, 13, 23, 24]. The incidence of staphylococcal and Gram-negative bacillary meningitis in the United States has significantly decreased from 1997 to 2010 but remains more common than two of the classic community-acquired pathogens (*Neisseria meningitidis* and *H. influenzae*) [13]. Healthcare-associated meningitis is usually caused by Gram-negative rods, *Staphylococcus* species, or *Propionibacterium acnes* [8, 13, 23, 24]. Gram-negative bacillary meningitis (e.g., caused by *Klebsiella* sp., *Escherichia coli, Serratia marcescens, Pseudomonas aeruginosa, Salmonella* spp., and *Acinetobacter* spp.) has been described in older adults, immunosuppressed patients, and those with a breach in the meninges as a result of trauma or neurosurgical procedures [8, 13, 20]. *Staphylococcus aureus* meningitis is also found in the early post-neurosurgical period, after trauma, in those with cerebrospinal fluid (CSF) shunts, or in those with underlying diseases (e.g., diabetes mellitus, chronic kidney disease requiring hemodialysis, injection drug use, and malignancies) [8,13,20,]. *Staphylococcus epidermidis* and *Propionibacterium acnes* may be seen in those with infected CSF shunts [24]. There is very limited data evaluating prognostic factors in healthcare-associated meningitis. A study of 91 cases of nosocomial meningitis from Korea found that septic shock and failure to remove the external ventricular drain were the two factors associated with a poor prognosis [25].

6.4 Clinical Features

Adult patients with acute bacterial meningitis typically present with fever, headache, neck stiffness, nausea, and altered mental status [10]. However, older patients may present insidiously with lethargy or obtundation, no fever, and variable signs of meningeal inflammation [5, 26–29]. Older patients also present with less complaints of headaches, nausea, and neck stiffness [5]. Bacterial meningitis should be considered in every elderly patient who has an acute febrile encephalopathy [28]. In a recent 30-year study of 185 patients who were 65 years of age and older, the diagnosis of community-acquired bacterial meningitis was more difficult because of the absence of characteristic meningeal signs; these patients presented more commonly with coma, seizures, and hemiparesis [29].

6.5 Diagnosis

Lumbar puncture with analysis of CSF remains an essential procedure in the diagnosis of bacterial meningitis [16]. The typical CSF findings in patients with bacterial meningitis include a pleocytosis (>1000 WBCs/mm^3), elevated protein (>100 mg/dL), and hypoglycorrhachia (CSF glucose <45 mg/dl or a CSF/serum glucose ratio $\leq$0.4). Older patients are more likely to have bacterial meningitis and present with higher rates of hypoglycorrhachia, elevated CSF protein, elevated CSF pleocytosis, and peripheral blood leukocytosis (serum WBC count >12,000/mm^3)

[5, 30]. In patients with suspected bacterial meningitis, a CSF Gram stain and culture should always be performed. The CSF Gram stain has a sensitivity between 50 and 90 % in the diagnosis of bacterial meningitis, and the likelihood of a positive Gram stain depends on the concentration of organisms within CSF, the specific meningeal pathogen, and the prior administration of antibiotic therapy [31]. The specificity of the CSF Gram stain approaches 100 %. Cultures are positive in 80–90 % of patients with community-acquired bacterial meningitis. Older adults presenting with community-acquired meningitis have a higher rate of having positive CSF Gram stains, CSF bacterial cultures, and blood cultures [5].

In those patients presenting with meningitis and a negative CSF Gram stain, the diagnosis of bacterial meningitis or another urgent treatable etiology may be more difficult to establish upon presentation to the emergency room [6, 32]. Clinical models, CSF lactate concentration, and CSF procalcitonin have all been used to try to identify patients at risk for bacterial meningitis, and a bacterial broad-range PCR and an immunochromatographic test for *S. pneumoniae* antigen have been utilized to identify specific etiologies [31–39]. A clinical model was derived and validated in 974 patients that identified a subgroup of patients at zero risk of having an urgent treatable cause [32]. Two meta-analyses, one including 1,692 patients [33] and the other including 1,885 patients [34], concluded that the diagnostic accuracy of CSF lactate was better than that of CSF WBC count, glucose, and protein in the differentiation of bacterial from aseptic meningitis. Nucleic acid amplification tests, such as polymerase chain reaction (PCR), have been used in patients with bacterial meningitis caused by several meningeal pathogens [35]; broad-based PCR has a sensitivity of 100 %, specificity of 98.2 %, positive predictive value of 98.2 %, and negative predictive value of 100 % [36]. An immunochromatographic test is also available for detection of *S. pneumoniae* in CSF and was found to be 99–100 % sensitive and 99–100 % specific in the diagnosis of pyogenic pneumococcal meningitis [37, 38], although requires further study.

6.6 Management

Bacterial meningitis is a medical emergency and delay in initiating antibiotic therapy can result in increased mortality [39, 40]. If a screening head CT scan is indicated, antimicrobial therapy should be administered after obtaining blood cultures [4]. Empiric antibiotic therapy should be bactericidal and able to achieve adequate cerebrospinal fluid concentrations. The choice of the initial empiric antibiotics should be based on age, local epidemiological patterns of pneumococcal resistance, and the need to add parenteral amoxicillin or ampicillin for *L. monocytogenes* (see Table 6.1). Listeria should be suspected in immunosuppressed and in those older than 50 years. Once the pathogen has been identified and antimicrobial susceptibilities determined, the antibiotics must be modified for optimal targeted treatment (Table 6.2). Penicillin resistance among *S. pneumoniae* strains has been increasing worldwide and has changed the initial therapy of patients with bacterial meningitis in several parts of the world. The Infectious Diseases Society of America (IDSA)

Table 6.1 Empirical antibiotics and antivirals for presumed community-acquired meningitis, healthcare-associated meningitis, and viral encephalitis

Type of CNS infections	Most common pathogens	Empirical therapy
Community-acquired bacterial meningitis		
Age <1 month	*Streptococcus agalactiae*, *Escherichia coli*, *Listeria monocytogenes*	Amoxicillin/ampicillin + cefotaxime or amoxicillin/ampicillin plus an aminoglycoside
Age 1–23 months	*S. agalactiae*, *E. coli*, *Streptococcus pneumoniae*, *Neisseria meningitidis*	Vancomycin + a third-generation cephalosporin (either cefotaxime or ceftriaxone)[a, b]
Age 2–50 years	*S. pneumoniae*, *N. meningitides*	Vancomycin + a third-generation cephalosporin (either cefotaxime or ceftriaxone)[a, b]
Age >50 years	*S. pneumoniae*, *N. meningitidis*, *L. monocytogenes*, aerobic Gram-negative bacilli	Vancomycin + ampicillin + a third-generation cephalosporin (either cefotaxime or ceftriaxone)
Immunocompromised state[c]	*S. pneumoniae*, *N. meningitidis*, *L. monocytogenes*, *Staphylococcus aureus*, *Salmonella* species, aerobic Gram-negative bacilli (including *Pseudomonas aeruginosa*)	Vancomycin + ampicillin + either cefepime or meropenem
Healthcare-associated meningitis or ventriculitis	*Staphylococcus* sp., *Streptococcus* sp., aerobic Gram-negative bacilli (including *P. aeruginosa)*, *P. acnes*	Vancomycin + antipseudomonal beta-lactam (cefepime, ceftazidime, meropenem)
Viral encephalitis	*Herpes simplex virus*, *varicella-zoster virus*, *West Nile virus, etc.*	Intravenous acyclovir

[a]If meningitis caused by *L. monocytogenes* is also suspected, add amoxicillin/ampicillin
[b]A third-generation cephalosporin alone is appropriate in countries where the prevalence of cephalosporin-resistant pneumococcus is <1 %
[c]Human immunodeficiency virus infection, posttransplantation, or receiving immunosuppressive therapies

guidelines recommend to initiate vancomycin and a third-generation cephalosporin (cefotaxime or ceftriaxone), but in countries where the prevalence of cephalosporin-resistant pneumococcus is <1 %, ceftriaxone alone is appropriate [41, 42].

In adult patients with suspected acute pneumococcal meningitis, adjunctive dexamethasone should also be administered [41]. This recommendation is based on a prospective, randomized, double-blind trial in 301 adults with bacterial meningitis in which the proportion of patients who had an unfavorable outcome (15 % vs. 25 %; $p = 0.03$) and who died (7 % vs. 15 %; $p = 0.04$) was significantly reduced in those who received adjunctive dexamethasone [42]; the benefits were most significant in

Table 6.2 Antibiotics and antivirals for community-acquired meningitis, healthcare-associated meningitis, and viral encephalitis after identifying pathogen and in vitro susceptibility testing

Isolated organism	Recommended therapy	Alternative therapies
Streptococcus pneumoniae		
Penicillin MIC ≤0.06 μg/mL	Penicillin G or amoxicillin/ampicillin	Cefotaxime, ceftriaxone, chloramphenicol
Penicillin MIC ≥0.12 μg/mL		
Cefotaxime or ceftriaxone MIC <1.0 μg/mL	Cefotaxime or ceftriaxone	Cefepime, meropenem
Cefotaxime or ceftriaxone MIC ≥1.0 μg/mL	Vancomycin + either cefotaxime or ceftriaxone[a]	Vancomycin + moxifloxacin or levofloxacin
Neisseria meningitides		
Penicillin MIC <0.1 μg/mL	Penicillin G or amoxicillin/ampicillin	Cefotaxime, ceftriaxone, chloramphenicol
Penicillin MIC ≥0.1 μg/mL	Cefotaxime or ceftriaxone	Cefepime, chloramphenicol, fluoroquinolone, meropenem
Listeria monocytogenes	Amoxicillin/ampicillin or penicillin G[b]	Trimethoprim-sulfamethoxazole
Streptococcus agalactiae	Amoxicillin/ampicillin or penicillin G[b]	Cefotaxime, ceftriaxone, vancomycin
Haemophilus influenzae		
β-lactamase negative	Amoxicillin/ampicillin	Cefotaxime, ceftriaxone, cefepime, chloramphenicol, aztreonam, fluoroquinolone
β-lactamase positive	Cefotaxime or ceftriaxone	Cefepime, chloramphenicol, aztreonam, fluoroquinolone
β-lactamase-negative ampicillin-resistant (BLNAR)	Meropenem	Fluoroquinolone
Escherichia coli	Amoxicillin/ampicillin plus an aminoglycoside	Cefotaxime
Pseudomonas aeruginosa	Cefepime, meropenem, ciprofloxacin	
Staphylococcus aureus or coagulase-negative staphylococcus	Vancomycin if methicillin resistant, nafcillin if susceptible	Linezolid, ceftaroline, daptomycin
Herpes simplex virus or varicella-zoster virus	Intravenous acyclovir for 14–21 days	Intravenous foscarnet

In the absence of clinical data, recommendations for use of some agents are based on CSF penetration and efficacy in experimental animal models of bacterial meningitis

[a]Addition of rifampin may be considered if the organism is demonstrated to be susceptible, the expected clinical or bacteriological response is delayed, or the cefotaxime/ceftriaxone MIC of the pneumococcal isolate is >4.0 μg/mL

[b]Consider adding gentamicin

the subset of patients with pneumococcal meningitis. An epidemiological study from 1997 until 2010 in the United States showed a decrease in the mortality of pneumococcal meningitis after the implementation of the IDSA guidelines, but a direct correlation with dexamethasone use could not be determined from the study [13]. In a nationwide observational cohort study from the Netherlands, adjunctive dexamethasone was administered for 1234 (89 %) of 1384 assessed episodes and was associated with a decrease in unfavorable outcomes [10].

In adults presenting with healthcare-associated meningitis and ventriculitis, empiric antibiotic therapy should include vancomycin and antipseudomonal beta-lactam antibiotic such as cefepime, ceftazidime, or meropenem [23, 24] (see Table 6.1). In patients with beta-lactam allergy, ciprofloxacin or aztreonam may be used. Antibiotic therapy should be modified based on in vitro susceptibility results. Hardware removal (e.g., CSF shunts, deep brain stimulators, etc.) should be done to improve the success of therapy. Intrathecal administration of antibiotics should be considered in patients failing appropriate intravenous antibiotic therapy or in patients with meningitis caused by carbapenem-resistant Gram-negative rods [43].

6.7 Encephalitis

6.7.1 Epidemiology and Etiology

Encephalitis represents a significant burden on the healthcare system with approximately 20,000 patients and a cost of $2 billion per year in the United States [44]. A review of the nationwide inpatient sample database in the United States between 1998 and 2010 estimated an average annual age-adjusted rate of 6.9 hospitalizations per 100,000 population [44]; adults aged 65 years or older had a relative risk of hospitalization 2.2 times that of those with encephalitis in the general population. Older patients also have a prolonged hospitalization and poor outcomes, including death and significant neurological disability.

Differentiating between encephalopathy and encephalitis is important [45, 46]. *Encephalitis* is defined as inflammation of the brain parenchyma associated with neurologic dysfunction. To standardize the definition of encephalitis, an international consortium recently published criteria that include the presence of one major (altered consciousness for more than 24 h) and several minor criteria (fever, new-onset seizure, new-onset focal neurological findings, CSF pleocytosis, and either abnormal MRI or EEG) [46]. *Encephalopathy* refers to a clinical state of altered mental status with or without inflammation of brain tissue and can be caused by several metabolic or toxic conditions. A specific etiology for encephalitis is often difficult to identify; studies range from 37 to 70 % of unknown causes depending on the routine use of PCR and evaluation for autoimmune etiologies [45–50]. Specific pathogens may be considered based on epidemiologic history, season of the year, outdoor activities, mosquito or tick exposure, animal and water exposure, living quarters, occupation, vaccination status, sick contacts, and immune status of the patient. It is beyond the scope of this chapter to provide information on all causes of encephalitis, so we will concentrate our discussion on specific viral pathogens (herpes simplex virus, varicella-zoster virus, and *West Nile virus*) that may be seen in elderly patients.

6.7.1.1 Herpes Viruses

The Alphaherpesvirinae subgroup includes infection with *herpes simplex virus* (HSV types 1 and 2) and *varicella-zoster virus* (VZV) [51]. HSV is the most common etiology of sporadic encephalitis in the United States. HSV encephalitis is an urgent treatable condition requiring prompt identification and administration of intravenous acyclovir [52]. In a multicenter study of 501 cases of HSV meningoencephalitis, age, Glasgow coma scale, and delay in antiviral therapy were all independently associated with an adverse outcome [52]. HSV meningitis is characterized by a benign clinical course regardless of the receipt of antiviral therapy [51]. HSV-1 has a predilection for the temporal lobes of the brain, and patients present with fever, seizures, altered mental status, and focal neurologic deficits [53]. Bilateral temporal lobe findings or lesions in the insula or cingulate are less likely seen in HSV encephalitis than in other etiologies [53].

Varicella-zoster virus (VZV) is one of the most commonly identified causes of encephalitis in adults especially in those older than 80 years of age [54], most often associated with viral reactivation causing a CNS vasculopathy [51]. VZV can also be associated with meningitis, radiculopathy, and myelitis, and intravenous acyclovir should be used [54]. The absence of a vesicular rash should not defer clinicians in ordering a CSF VZV PCR or a serum to CSF anti-VZV IgG as several patients can have *zoster sine herpete* [51, 54, 55]. A study of 30 patients with VZV vasculopathies showed a higher sensitivity of the anti-VZV CSF IgG than a CSF VZV PCR [55]. As older individuals are more likely to have reactivation of herpes zoster, herpes zoster vaccine should be administered to all adult patients above the age of 60 years [55].

6.7.1.2 Arboviruses

Arboviral CNS infections in the United States are most commonly seen in the summer or fall and include *West Nile virus* (WNV), eastern equine encephalitis virus, St. Louis encephalitis virus, and La Crosse virus [56]. WNV is the most common cause of epidemic viral encephalitis in the United States, causing more than 41,000 cases of neuroinvasive disease and approximately 3 million infections since its arrival in 1999 [57]. As only one-third of patients with meningitis and encephalitis are tested for WNV, this is most certainly an underestimate of the current scope of disease [58]. WNV can cause meningitis, encephalitis, acute flaccid paralysis, neuropathy, and retinopathy [57, 59]. Older patients are more likely to present with encephalitis and retinopathy and were associated with a higher risk of death in seven studies [59, 60].

West Nile virus has a predilection to affect the thalamus and the basal ganglia, and clinically patients can present with tremors, parkinsonism, and myoclonus [61]. WNV is also the most common cause of acute flaccid paralysis and can lead to lower extremity weakness and hyporeflexia that can persist for several years [62].

The diagnosis is established by obtaining a WNV IgM in the CSF or serum as the WNV PCR on CSF is not sensitive [63]. Both WNV IgM and IgG antibodies can persist in the serum (and less commonly the CSF) for many months after acute infection and, therefore, may not be indicative of a current ongoing infection [57]. There are currently no available therapies for patients with WNV neuroinvasive disease and there are no vaccines (except in horses). The most important protection is to avoid mosquito bites in endemic areas in the summer and fall [61, 62].

6.8 Diagnosis

A thorough diagnostic evaluation is important in patients with encephalitis, and the approach should consider endemic pathogens, risk factors, immunosuppression, and season of presentation [45, 46]. Identifying the offending pathogen is important for epidemiological, therapeutic, and prognostic reasons. Underutilization of current diagnostic tests such as an HSV PCR and WNV serologies could contribute to the high rate of "idiopathic" etiologies seen in CNS infections [58]. The CSF analysis in patients with encephalitis typically reveals a lymphocytic pleocytosis, an elevated protein, and a normal glucose [31]. CSF viral cultures are of limited usefulness and are not recommended in patients with viral encephalitis because of low sensitivity [32, 46]. The diagnosis of HSV encephalitis rests upon detection of HSV DNA in CSF by polymerase chain reaction (PCR). CSF PCR has a sensitivity of 98 %, specificity of 94 %, positive predictive value of 95 %, and negative predictive value of 98 % in the diagnosis of HSV encephalitis [31]. However, early in the disease (within the first 72 h), this test can be falsely negative [31, 64]. Therefore, if HSV encephalitis is strongly suspected, a repeat HSV PCR should be performed on a second CSF specimen from later (within 3–7 days) in the disease course [64]. VZV PCR and IgM should also be performed on CSF in patients with encephalitis [45, 46].

Magnetic resonance imaging (MRI) of the brain, combined with electroencephalography (EEG) and lumbar puncture, is an essential component in the diagnostic approach to encephalitis [46, 53, 61]; diffusion-weighted imaging is superior to conventional MRI for detection of abnormalities, especially those caused by HSV and WNV. In patients with HSV encephalitis, MRI may reveal significant edema and hemorrhage in the temporal lobes. Patients with WNV encephalitis may manifest characteristic patterns of mixed intensity or hypodense lesions on T1-weighted images in the thalamus, basal ganglia, and midbrain. EEG findings rarely identify a specific pathogen in patients with encephalitis but can be helpful in identifying the degree of cerebral dysfunction and specific area of the brain involved and detecting subclinical seizure activity.

Conclusions

As the prevalence of older and relatively immunosuppressed patients in the world increases, the evaluation of CNS infections among the elderly cannot be overestimated. Community-acquired and healthcare-associated meningitis and encephalitis are the most common CNS infection syndromes in the elderly and have distinct clinical presentations that frequently require prompt diagnosis and urgent treatment to reduce morbidity and mortality. Improved diagnostics have utility in rapidly and accurately identifying the causative pathogen in certain patients with meningitis and encephalitis but are being underutilized in clinical practice.

References

1. United Nations, Department of Economic and Social Affairs, Population Division, World Population Ageing 2013, ST/ESA/SER.A/348. 2013
2. Kared H, Camous X, Larbi A (2014) T cells and their cytokines in persistent stimulation of the immune system. Curr Opin Immunol 29C:79–85
3. Miller R (1996) The aging immune system: primer and prospectus. Science 273(5701):70–74
4. Tunkel AR (2015) Approach to the patient with central nervous system infection. In: Bennett JE, Dolin R, Blaser MJ (eds) Principles and practice of infectious diseases, 8th edn. Elsevier Saunders, Philadelphia, pp 1091–1096
5. Wang A, Machicado J, Khoury N, Wootton S, Salazar L, Hasbun R (2014) Community-acquired meningitis in older adults: clinical features, etiology, and prognostic factors. J Am Geriatric Soc 62(11):2064–2070
6. Khoury NT, Hossain M, Wootton SH, Salazar L, Hasbun R (2012) Meningitis with a negative cerebrospinal fluid gram stain in adults: risk classification for an adverse clinical outcome. Mayo Clin Proc 87:1172–1179
7. Delerme S, Castro S, Viallon A, Boutoille D, Bendahou M et al (2009) Meningitis in elderly patients. Eur J Emerg Med 16(5):273–276
8. Durand ML, Calderwood SB, Weber DJ et al (1993) Acute bacterial meningitis in adults: a review of 493 episodes. N Engl J Med 328(1):21–28
9. Aronin SI, Peduzzi P, Quagliarello VJ (1998) Community-acquired bacterial meningitis: risk stratification for adverse clinical outcome and effect on antibiotic timing. Ann Intern Med 129(11):862–869
10. Bijlsma M, Brouwer MC, Kasanmoentalib ES, Kloek AT, Lucas MJ et al (2016) Community-acquired bacterial meningitis in adults in the Netherlands, 2006–14: a prospective cohort study. Lancet Infect Dis 16: 339–347. Hoogman M, van de Beek D, Weisfelt M et al (2007) Cognitive outcome in adults after bacterial meningitis. J Neurol Neurosurg Psychiatry 78:1092–1096
11. Edmond K, Clark A, Korczak VS et al (2010) Global and regional risk of disabling sequelae from bacterial meningitis: a systemic review and meta-analysis. Lancet Infect Dis 10:317–328
12. Thigpen MC, Whitney CG, Messonnier NE et al (2011) Bacterial meningitis in the United States, 1998–2007. N Engl J Med 364:2016–2025
13. Lopez Castelblanco R, Lee M, Hasbun R (2014) Epidemiology of Bacterial Meningitis in the United States from 1997–2010: trends after conjugate vaccination and adjunctive dexamethasone recommendations: a population observational based study. Lancet Infect Dis 14(9):813–819
14. Weisfelt M, de Gans J, van der Poll T, van de Beek D (2006) Pneumococcal meningitis is adults: new approaches to management and prevention. Lancet Neurol 5(2):123–129
15. Tomczyk S, Bennett NM, Stoecker C et al (2014) Use of 13-valent pneumococcal conjugate vaccine and 23-valent pneumococcal polysaccharide vaccine among adults aged ≥65 years: recommendations of the Advisory Committee on Immunization Practices (ACIP). MMWR Morb Mortal Wkly Rep 63:822–825
16. Tunkel AR, van de Beek D, Scheld WM (2015) Acute meningitis. In: Bennett JE, Dolin R, Blaser MJ (eds) Principles and practice of infectious diseases, 8th edn. Elsevier Saunders, Philadelphia, pp 1097–1137
17. Koopmans MM, Brouwer MC, Bijlsma MW et al (2013) *Listeria monocytogenes* sequence type 6 and increased rate of unfavorable outcome in meningitis: epidemiologic cohort study. Clin Infect Dis 57(2):247–253

18. Mylonakis E, Hohmann EL, Calderwood SB (1998) Central nervous system infection with *Listeria monocytogenes*: 33 years' experience at a general hospital and review of 776 episodes from the literature. Medicine (Baltimore) 77(5):313–336
19. Goulet V, Hebert M, Hedberg C (2012) Incidence of listeriosis and related mortality among groups at risk of acquiring listeriosis. Clin Infect Dis 54(5):652–660
20. Dunne DW, Quagliarello V (1993) Group B streptococcal meningitis in adults. Medicine (Baltimore) 72:1–10
21. Jackson LA, Hilsdon R, Farley MM et al (1995) Risk factors for group B streptococcal disease in adults. Ann Intern Med 123:415–420
22. Domingo P, Barquet N, Alvarez M et al (1997) Group B streptococcal meningitis in adults: report of twelve cases and review. Clin Infect Dis 25:1180–1187
23. van de Beek D, Drake JM, Tunkel AR (2010) Nosocomial bacterial meningitis. N Engl J Med 362:146–154
24. Bhimraj A, Drake JM, Tunkel AR (2015) Cerebrospinal fluid shunt and drain infections. In: Bennett JE, Dolin R, Blaser MJ (eds) Principles and practice of infectious diseases, 8th edn. Elsevier Saunders, Philadelphia, pp 1186–1193
25. Kim HI, Kim SW, Park GY, Kwon EG, Kim HH et al (2012) The causes and treatment outcomes of 91 patients with adult nosocomial meningitis. Korean J Intern Med 27:171–179
26. Gorse GJ, Thrupp LD, Nudleman KL et al (1989) Bacterial meningitis in the elderly. Arch Intern Med 149:1603–1606
27. Choi C (2001) Bacterial meningitis in aging adults. Clin Infect Dis 33:1380–1385
28. Sheybani F, Naderi H, Sajjadi S (2016) The optimal management of acute febrile encephalopathy in the aged patient: a systematic review. Interdiscip Perspect Infect Dis 2016:5273651
29. Cabellos C, Verdaguer R, Olmo M et al (2009) Community-acquired bacterial meningitis in elderly patients: experience over 30 years. Medicine (Baltimore) 88(2):115–119
30. Shrikanth V, Salazar L, Khoury N, Wootton S, Hasbun R (2015) Hypoglycorrhachia in adults with community-acquired meningitis: etiologies and prognostic significance. Int J Infect Dis 39:39–43
31. Hasbun R (2014) Cerebrospinal fluid in central nervous system infections. In: Scheld WM, Whitley RJ, Marra CM (eds) Infections of the central nervous system, 4th edn. Lippincott Williams and Wilkins, Philadelphia
32. Hasbun R, Bijlsma M, Brouwer MC, Khoury N, Hadi CM, Ende AV, Wootton SH, Salazar L, Hossain M, Beilke M, van de Beek D (2013) Risk score for identifying adults with CSF pleocytosis and negative CSF Gram stain at low risk for an urgent treatable cause. J Infect 67(2):102–110
33. Huy NT, Thao NT, Diep DT, Kikuchi M, Zamora J, Hirayama K (2010) Cerebrospinal fluid lactate concentration to distinguish bacterial from aseptic meningitis: a systemic review and meta-analysis. Crit Care 14(6):R240
34. Sakashima K, Hayashino Y, Kawaguchi T, Jackson JL, Fukuhara S (2011) Diagnostic accuracy of cerebrospinal fluid lactate for differentiating bacterial meningitis from aseptic meningitis: a meta-analysis. J Infect 62(4):255–262
35. Saravolatz LD, Manzor O, VanderVelde N, Pawlak J, Belian B (2003) Broad-range bacterial polymerase chain reaction for early detection of bacterial meningitis. Clin Infect Dis 36(1):40–45
36. Werno AM, Murdoch DR (2008) Medical microbiology: laboratory diagnosis of invasive pneumococcal disease. Clin Infect Dis 46(6):926–932
37. Saha SK, Darmstadt GL, Yamanaka N et al (2005) Rapid diagnosis of pneumococcal meningitis: implications for treatment and measuring disease burden. Pediatr Infect Dis J 24(12):1093–1098
38. Moisi JC, Saha SK, Falade AG et al (2009) Enhanced diagnosis of pneumococcal meningitis with use of the Binax NOW immunochromatographic test of *Streptococcus pneumoniae* antigen: a multisite study. Clin Infect Dis 48(Suppl 2):S49–S56
39. Proulx N, Frechette D, Toye B, Chan J, Kravick S (2005) Delays in the administration of antibiotics are associated with mortality from adult acute bacterial meningitis. Q J Med 98:291–298

40. Lepur D, Barsic B (2007) Community-acquired bacterial meningitis in adults: antibiotic timing in disease course and outcome. Infection 35:225–231
41. Tunkel AR, Hartman BJ, Kaplan SL et al (2004) Practice guidelines for the management of bacterial meningitis. Clin Infect Dis 39(9):1267–1284
42. de Gans J, van de Beek D (2002) Dexamethasone in adults with bacterial meningitis. N Engl J Med 347(20):1549–1556
43. Shofty B, Neuberger A, Naffaa ME, Binawi T, Babitch T et al (2016) Intrathecal or intraventricular therapy for post-neurosurgical Gram-negative meningitis: matched cohort study. Clin Microbiol Infect 22:66–70
44. Vora NM, Holman RC, Mehal JM, Steiner CA, Blanton J, Sejvar J (2014) Burden of encephalitis-associated hospitalizations in the United States, 1998–2010. Neurology 82(5):443–451
45. Tunkel AR, Glaser CA, Bloch KC et al (2008) The management of encephalitis: Clinical practice guidelines by the Infectious Diseases Society of America. Clin Infect Dis 47:303–327
46. Venkatesan A, Tunkel AR, Bloch KC et al (2013) Case definitions, diagnostic algorithms, and priorities in encephalitis: consensus statement of the International Encephalitis Consortium. Clin Infect Dis 57(8):1114–1128
47. Granerod J, Ambrose H, Davies N et al (2010) Causes of encephalitis and differences in their clinical presentations in England: a multicenter, population-based prospective study. Lancet Infect Dis 10:835–844
48. Glaser C, Gilliam S, Schnurr D et al (2003) In search of encephalitis etiologies: diagnostic challenges in the California Encephalitis Project, 1998–2000. Clin Inf Dis 36:731–742
49. Davison KL, Crowcroft NS, Ramsay ME, Brown DW, Andrews NJ (2003) Viral Encephalitis in England, 1989–1998: what did we miss? Emerg Infect Dis 9:234–240
50. Mailles A, Stahl JP (2009) Infectious Encephalitis in France in 2007: a national prospective study. Clin Infect Dis 49:1838–4756
51. Kaewpoowat Q, Salazar L, Aguilera E, Wootton SH, Hasbun R (2016) Herpes simplex and varicella zoster CNS infections: clinical presentations, treatment and outcomes. Infection 44:337–345
52. Erdem H, Cag Y, Ozturk-Engin D, Defres S, Kaya S et al (2015) Results of a multinational study suggest the need for rapid diagnosis and early antiviral treatment at the onset of herpetic meningoencephalitis. Antimicrob Agents Chemother 59(6):3084–3089
53. Chow FC, Glaser CA, Sheriff H, Xia D, Messenger S, Whitley R, Venkatesan A (2015) Use of clinical and neuroimaging characteristics to distinguish temporal lobe herpes simplex encephalitis from its mimics. Clin Infect Dis 60(9):1377–1383
54. Parisi SG, Basso M, Del Vecchio C, Andreis S, Franchin E et al (2016) Viral infections of the central nervous system in elderly patients: a retrospective study. Int J Infect Dis 44:8–10
55. Nagel MA, Cohrs RJ, Mahalingam R, Wellish MC, Forghani B et al (2008) The varicella zoster vasculopathies: clinical, CSF, imaging and neurological features. Neurology 70(11):853–860
56. Gagliardi AM, Andriolo BN, Torloni MR, Soares BG (2016) Vaccines for preventing herpes zoster in older adults. Cochrane Database Syst Rev (3):3
57. Garcia MN, Hasbun R, Murray K (2015) Persistence of West Nile virus infection. Microbes Infect 17(2):163–168
58. Nesher L, Hadi CM, Salazar L, Wootton SH, Garey KW, Lasco T, Luce AM, Hasbun R (2016) Epidemiology of meningitis with a negative CSF Gram stain: under-utilization of available diagnostic tests. Epidemiol Infect 144(1):189–197
59. Hasbun R, Garcia MN, Kellaway J, Baker L, Salazar L, Woods SP, Murray KO (2016) West Nile virus retinopathy and associations with long term neurological and neurocognitive sequelae. PLoS One 11(3):e0148898
60. Patel H, Sander B, Nelder MP (2015) Long-term sequelae of West Nile virus-related illness: a systematic review. Lancet Infect Dis 15:951–959
61. Beattie GC, Glaser CA, Sheriff H, Messenger S, Preas CP, Shahkarami M, Venkatesan A (2013) Encephalitis with thalamic and basal ganglia abnormalities: etiologies, neuroimaging, and potential role of respiratory viruses. Clin Infect Dis 56(6):825–832

62. Weatherhead JE, Miller VE, Garcia MN, Hasbun R, Salazar L, Dimachkie MM, Murray KO (2015) Long-term neurological outcomes in West Nile virus–infected patients: an observational study. Am J Trop Med Hyg 92:1006–1012
63. Kapoor H, Signs K, Somsel P, Downes FP, Clark PA, Massey JP (2004) Persistence of West Nile virus (WNV) IgM antibodies in cerebrospinal fluid from patients with CNS disease. J Clin Virol 31:289–291
64. Weil AA, Glaser CA, Amad Z, Forghani B (2002) Patients with suspected herpes simplex encephalitis: rethinking an initial negative polymerase chain reaction result. Clin Infect Dis 3:1162–1167

Part III

Intracranial Tumors

Intracranial Meningiomas in the Elderly

7

David B. Schul, Chochlidakis Nikos,
and Chirstianto B. Lumenta

7.1 Introduction

Meningioma represents the most frequent brain tumor in the elderly. The prevalence of the disease is difficult to define due to subclinical manifestation in large portion of the population [15]. Great amount of these tumors are discovered incidentally through cranial or spinal radiological exams due to other causes. Others are diagnosed only on autopsy. The increase in average lifespan and the more frequent and easy use of diagnostic neuroimaging have resulted in a larger quantity of lesions being detected in the aging population.

Due to its usually benign biological behavior, many of those tumors are being handled conservatively. In general meningiomas in elderly patients have been considered to have a more benign course than meningiomas in young patients. Annual growth rate seems to be higher in younger patients [43–45]. Kuratsu et al. [34] reported 49 % of asymptomatic meningiomas for patients older than 70 years. This is in contrast to 34 % under this age.

Furthermore, due to limited life expectancy as well as generally more significant concomitant diseases in the elderly, surgeons tend to be more conservative in the management of these patients. Dolecek et al., evaluating the Surveillance, Epidemiology and End Results (SEER) Program database for the year 2004–2011, could clearly demonstrate that patients older than 75 years were substantially less likely to receive any kind of treatment (surgery, surgery + radiotherapy, or radiotherapy alone).

D.B. Schul, MD (✉) • C. Nikos, MD • C.B. Lumenta, MD, PhD
Neurosurgical Department, Municipal Hospital Munich,
Teaching Hospital of the Technical University Munich,
Englschalkingerstrasse 77, 81925 Munich, Germany
e-mail: david.schul@klinikum-muenchen.de

© Springer International Publishing Switzerland 2017

M. Berhouma, P. Krolak-Salmon (eds.), *Brain and Spine Surgery in the Elderly*,
DOI 10.1007/978-3-319-40232-1_7

The enormous improvement of peri-, intra-, and postoperative management of neurosurgical patients in the last decades allows neurosurgeon to safely operate on many of those lesions. However, new technologies such as radiosurgery, gamma knife, and improvement of conventional beam radiation offer more therapeutic alternatives. Nevertheless, the diagnosis of meningioma in the elderly poses an ethical as well as medical decision difficulty on whether it should be treated and which treatment risk is acceptable.

The interest in defining better criteria for dealing with such patients is increasing. In the last 20 years, many authors have reported their treatment results. Most of them have tried to isolate different risk factors for adverse outcomes. Some of these authors suggested different grading scores in order to facilitate patients' selection [1, 9, 17, 18, 28, 36, 56]. Unfortunately their conclusions differ or even contradictory.

7.2 Epidemiology

According to the World Health Organization as published in its classification for nervous tumors [37], meningiomas account for about 24–30 % of all primary intracranial tumors in the USA. Its annual incidence rate is reported to be up to 13 per 100,000 habitants. The Central Brain Tumor Registry of the United States (CBTRUS) [47] collects data regarding malignant and nonmalignant brain tumors in the USA. It is the largest register providing statistical data on the population-based incidence of primary CNS tumors. In its last report on CNS tumors between 2008 and 2012, meningiomas were the most frequently reported histology with 36.4 % of all brain tumors. They were much more frequent in female and in American Africans. Meningiomas were also the most common nonmalignant brain and CNS tumor (53.4 %). The incidence of all brain and CNS tumors was highest among the age 85+ years, and from age 35 years, it was the most common histology diagnosed (Table 7.1). Meningiomas' incidence was increasing with age, and it dramatically increases after age 65 years. Age had a large effect on relative survival after diagnosis of malignant meningioma.

Yearly relative survival rates decrease with age. This decline is much more evident in the age group 75+ years. This might be the result of therapy, but it is probably due to average life expectancy in this group.

Reports from different world regions confirm the data reported in the USA [21, 22, 29, 59].

Table 7.1 Rates of average annual age-related incidence of meningioma among all primary CNS and brain tumors per 100,000 adjusted to age (CBTRUS) [47]

Age (years)	Rate
0–19	0.14
20–34	1.39
35–44	4.82
45–54	9.02
55–64	14.77
65–74	25.96
75–84	38.70
85+	51.31

7.3 Histology

Approximately 80–90 % of meningiomas are classified as benign (WHO grade I). Atypical meningiomas (WHO grade II) were reported to account for 5–15 % of meningiomas. Nevertheless, the current WHO classification from 2007 includes cerebral tumor invasion as one of the criteria for WHO grade II even in the absence of cellular atypia or anaplasia. Therefore, an increase in the diagnosis of grade II tumors has been reported [48, 54]. This diagnosis could newly account for up to 20–35 % [50, 62]. The remnant 0.8–2 % account for WHO grade III tumors.

Park et al. [48] tried to look at the influence of age on histological grading. In 1083 surgical cases of 1067 patients, they reported 91.8 %, 6.8 %, and 1.4 % WHO grades I, II, and III tumors, respectively. However, they evaluated patients treated between the years 1991 and 2006; hence, the portion of WHO grade II tumors might have been higher if they had used the 2007 WHO definition. Statistical analysis showed though higher incidence of the combined grades II/III meningiomas with respect to age. In patients older than 60 year, incidence of grades II/III combined was 11.9 % as compared to 6.9 % in younger patients. The relative distribution of histological subtypes within a WHO grade did not show any statistically significant difference related to age.

Other authors reported only statistically significant increase in incidence of grades I and II and decline of grade III tumors [24]. Yet, diagnostic confirmation through pathology was inversely correlated to age confirming the somehow more conservative therapy tendency in this age group.

Similar results were obtained in an epidemiological study using the CTBRUS data between the years 2004 and 2010 [33]. Likewise a linear growth of the incidence of all three grades was noticed with peak incidence in the age group 75–84 years followed by a drop-off in incidence in the >85 year group. This as well could be the result of a more conservative approach in extreme elderly patient, which would result in lack of pathological confirmation.

The pathophysiology of the apparent incidence increasing in grade II and eventually grade III meningiomas with age might be explained through the long period of time in which tumor progresses before it becomes clinically evident. This long period of time might be enough for tumor cells to gain atypias and anaplasias or for tumor to grow enough to invade brain parenchyma, which would pose a higher grade upon diagnosis.

7.4 Proposed Scores and Risk Factors for Adverse Outcome

Decision-making in this patient population is challenging both for caregiver and for patients and their relatives. Any offered treatment should follow a simple concept, namely, treatment's benefit far outweighs the risks of treatment or the risk of non-treatment. A simple numerical representation of risk prediction might be helpful for counseling patients and relatives, simplify therapy plan, and predict outcome. Incorporating a set of risk factors for adverse outcome seems to be more robust than depending on only one single factor.

Numerous publications tried to analyze different risk factors for adverse outcome in this patient's population [1, 2, 4–7, 14, 17–20, 23, 28, 31, 39–41, 46, 52, 55–57, 61]. Most of the studies consist in retrospective analysis of patient's outcome. Only three of them were prospective studies [9, 32, 49]. To date, no randomized study dealing with this issue was published. Published data in the literature regarding outcome of meningioma surgery in the aged population is controversial and inconsistent. A summary of papers published to date with the respective morbidity and mortality figures as well as identified risk factors for either morbidity or mortality is shown in Table 7.2.

Numerous single risk factors for adverse outcome (either morbidity or mortality) were proposed and are listed below:

1. Age
2. Sex (male/female)
3. Resection grade
4. Peritumoral edema
5. Tumor size
6. Tumor location (eloquence, vessels, skull base)
7. Preoperative neurological condition/deficit
8. Preoperative Karnofsky Performance Scale
9. Concomitant disease
10. ASA Score (American Society of Anesthesiologists Physical Status Classification System)
11. Diabetes mellitus
12. Hypertension
13. Pulmonary disease
14. Race
15. Smoking
16. Alcohol use
17. Disseminated cancer elsewhere
18. Histology
19. Emergency procedures
20. History of previous meningioma surgery
21. History of previous radiation

The most frequently identified single factors in the cited studies include age, sex (male/female), presence of peritumoral edema, tumor size and location, neurological condition and Karnofsky Performance score, as well as the presence of concomitant disease or higher ASA score.

It seems that general health condition (expressed as the presence of concomitant disease or higher ASA score) remains a constant risk factor in most of the studies. This probably correlates to advanced age too. The older the patient is, the higher is the risk to have more concomitant diseases. Schul et al. [57], analyzing single risk factors of two proposed grading scores, could show that when nonsignificant risk factors were stepwise omitted from further calculation, only the elements of ASA score and concomitant disease remained significant. Cohen-Inbar et al. [17, 18] proposing a novel scoring score based on analysis of different risk factors in 250

Table 7.2 Summary of published literature on meningioma surgery in the elderly

A. Description of patients' numbers, age cut-off, and reported morbidity/mortality

Author	Year	No. pat.	Age cutoff (years)	Morbidity (%)	Mortality 30 days (%)	Mortality 90 days (%)	Mortality 1 year (%)
Djindjian et al.[a] [23]	1998	30	70	NA	23	37	NA
Awad et al. [2]	1989	25	70	52	8	8	NA
Arienta et al. [1]	1990	34	70	44	12	20	NA
Cornu et al. [19]	1990	96	65	43	16	NA	NA
Maurice Williams and Kitchen[a] [40]	1992	46	65	30	9	NA	NA
Umansky et al.[a] [61]	1992	37	70	40.5	5.4	NA	NA
McGrail and Ojemann[a] [41]	1994	56	70	11.3	3.6	NA	NA
Nishizaki et al. [46]	1994	78	70	13	NA	NA	NA
Mastronardi et al. [39]	1995	17	80	11.8	29	29	NA
Black et al. [5]	1998	57	65	15.8	1.8	NA	NA
Buhl et al.[a] [7]	2000	66	70	57.6	7.6	12	16
Caroli et al. [9]	2005	90	70	NA	6.7	7.8	15.6
D'Andrea et al. [20]	2005	37	80	2.7	10.8	13.5	13.5
Bateman et al. [4]	2005	2304	70	52.2	4	NA	NA
Boviatsis et al. [6]	2006	108	65	17,8	6,5	NA	NA
Sacko et al. [56]	2007	74	80	9.4	0	1.4	9.5
Rogne et al. [55]	2009	79	70	NA	2.5	NA	6
Cohen-Inbar et al. [17]	2010	250	65	NA	NA	8.4	NA
Patil et al. [49]	2010	258	70	29.8	12	NA	NA
Cohen-Inbar et al. [18]	2011	120	65	NA	NA	5.8	8.3
Grossman et al. [28]	2011	5717	65	17.5	3.2	NA	NA
Schul et al. [57]	2012	164	65	21	3.6	6.7	6.7
Konglund et al. [31]	2013	51	80	[b]	3.9	7.8	15.7
Konglund et al. [32]	2013	54	60	31.5	5.6	7.4	9.2
Poon et al. [52]	2013	92	65	69.6	0	2.2	4.3
Chen et al. [14]	2015	86	65	37.2	1.2	1.2	NA

(continued)

Table 7.2 (continued)

B. Description of investigated risk factors

Author	Risk factor identified for adverse outcome (morbidity and/or mortality)																			
	Age	Sex	Resection grade	Edema	Size	Tumor location	Neurological condition	KPS	Concomitant disease	ASA	Diabetes mellitus	Hypertension	Pulmonary disease	Race	Smoking	Alcohol abuse	Histology	Cancer	Surgery duration	Other
Djindjian et al.[a] [23]	y	NA	NA	y	n	NA	NA	y	NA	n	NA	NA	NA	NA	NA	NA	NA	NA	NA	
Awad et al. [2]	y	NA	NA	NA	y	y	y	NA	NA	NA	NA	NA	NA	NA	NA	NA	NA	NA	NA	
Arienta et al. [1]	NA	NA	NA	y	y	y	NA	n	y	NA	y	NA	NA	NA	NA	NA	NA	NA	n	
Cornu et al. [19]	n	n	NA	n	n	y	y	y	y	y	NA	NA	NA	NA	NA	NA	NA	NA	NA	
Maurice Williams and Kitchen[a] [40]	NA	NA	NA	NA	NA	NA	NA	NA	NA	NA	NA	NA	NA	NA	NA	NA	NA	NA	NA	
Umansky et al.[a] [61]	NA	NA	NA	NA	NA	NA	NA	NA	NA	NA	NA	NA	NA	NA	NA	NA	NA	NA	n	
McGrail and Ojemann[a] [41]	NA	NA	NA	NA	NA	NA	NA	NA	NA	NA	NA	NA	NA	NA	NA	NA	NA	NA	NA	
Nishizaki et al. [46]	n	n	n	NA	NA	n	y	NA	NA	NA	NA	NA	NA	NA	NA	NA	NA	y	NA	
Mastronardi et al. [39]	NA	NA	NA	n	y	NA	NA	y	NA	y	NA	NA	NA	NA	NA	NA	NA	NA	NA	
Black et al. [5]	NA	NA	NA	NA	NA	NA	NA	NA	NA	NA	NA	NA	NA	NA	NA	NA	NA	NA	NA	

Buhl et al.[a] [7]	n	NA	NA	y	y	y	NA	NA	y	NA	NA	NA	NA	NA	NA	NA	NA	NA	y	
Caroli et al. [9]	n	y	NA	y	y	y	y	n	y	NA	NA	NA	NA	NA	NA	NA	NA	NA	NA	
D'Andrea et al. [20]	NA	NA	NA	y	y	n	NA	y	NA	y	NA	NA	NA	NA	NA	NA	NA	NA	NA	
Bateman et al. [4]	y	NA	NA	NA	NA	NA	NA	NA	y	NA	NA	NA	NA	NA	NA	NA	NA	NA	NA	
Boviatsis et al. [6]	y	NA	NA	NA	NA	NA	NA	NA	NA	NA	NA	NA	NA	NA	NA	NA	NA	NA	NA	
Sacko et al. [56]	NA	y	y	y	y	y	NA	n	NA	y	NA	NA	NA	NA	NA	NA	n	NA	NA	
Rogne et al. [55]	n	n	n	NA	NA	NA	NA	NA	^{c}	n	NA	NA	NA	NA	NA	NA	n	NA	NA	PreOP ECOG^{c}
Cohen-Inbar et al. [17]	y	y	n	y	NA	y	y	y	y	NA	NA	y	y	NA	NA	NA	NA	NA	NA	
Patil et al. [49]	y	NA	NA	NA	NA	y	NA	y^{d}	NA	NA	NA	NA	NA	NA	NA	NA	NA	y	NA	
Cohen-Inbar et al. [18]	NA	NA	NA	NA	NA	NA	NA	NA	NA	NA	NA	NA	NA	NA	NA	NA	NA	NA	NA	
Grossman et al. [28]	y	n	NA	NA	NA	NA	NA	NA	NA^{c}	NA	NA	NA	NA	y	NA	NA	y	NA	NA	CCS^{c}, Elective procedure
Schul et al. [57]	n	n	n	n	n	n	n	n	y	y	NA	NA	NA	NA	NA	NA	NA	NA	NA	
Konglund et al. [31]	NA	y	NA	y	y	y	NA	y	NA	n	NA	NA	NA	NA	NA	NA	NA	NA	NA	

(continued)

Table 7.2 (continued)

B. Description of investigated risk factors																			
	Risk factor identified for adverse outcome (morbidity and/or mortality)																		
Author	Age	Sex	Resection grade	Edema	Size	Tumor location	Neurological condition	KPS	Concomitant disease	ASA	Diabetes mellitus	Hypertension	Pulmonary disease	Race	Smoking	Alcohol abuse	Histology	Cancer	Surgery duration	Other
Konglund et al. [32]	y	NA	NA	NA	NA	NA	NA	NA	NA	NA	NA	NA	NA	NA	NA	NA	NA	NA	NA	
Poon et al. [52]	y	y	n	NA	NA	y	NA	NA	NA	NA	NA	NA	NA	NA	NA	NA	n	NA	NA	Elective procedure
Chen et al. [14]	n	n	n	n	n	n	y	n	n	n	NA	NA	NA	NA	NA	NA	NA	NA	NA	

Detailed figures on mortality from recent publication are presented in Table 7.8:

y yes, *n* no, *NA* not available

[a]No statistical tests were applied

[b]13.7 serious, 25.5 Infection, 15.7 neurological deficits

[c]CCG/ECOG are also an expression of concomitant disease

[d]Reported as functional dependency

elderly patients divided concomitant disease into three singular diseases, namely, diabetes mellitus, hypertension, and pulmonary disease. The consequence was that concomitant disease gained threefold strength in their score. Grossman et al. [28] performed a multi-institutional retrospective cohort analysis of the American Nationwide Inpatient Sample relating it to the Charlson Comorbidity Score (CCS) [10, 11, 13, 51]. They as well showed a strong correlation of outcome (mortality, postoperative morbidity, length of stay in the hospital, and consequently costs of treatment) with comorbidity.

Further risk factors that regard tumor characteristics as size, location, and edema might relate to neurological status and Karnofsky score. These factors are also frequently presented in different studies.

These results were confirmed in the retrospective report of a personal series of Sade and Lee, consisted in 300 analyzed patients. They also added previous surgery and history of radiation treatment to reported risk factors [36]. Poon et al. [53] reviewing 13 published studies between 2002 and 2012 reported that mortality was commonly associated with ASA score, peritumoral edema, and Karnofsky Performance score. Among the 11 factors they isolated, which were associated with mortality, five were related to preoperative status and comorbidities.

7.5 Scores

In light of different identified risk factors mentioned above, several authors proposed various scoring systems meant to provide prognostic value and help clinical decision-making and patient's counseling.

A summary of the proposed scores is shown in Tables 7.3, 7.4, 7.5, 7.6, and 7.7.

- *Clinical Radiological Grading System (CRGS)* [1, 9] Table 7.3
  This grading system was first introduced in 1990 in order to standardize surgical decision-making in elderly patients with intracranial meningiomas.

Table 7.3 Clinical–Radiological Grading System (CRGS) [1, 9]

	Score		
Factor	1	2	3
Size of lesion (cm)	6	4–6	<4
Neurological condition[a]	Unrecoverable	Progressive	No deficits
KPS score	≤50	60–80	90–100
Critical location[b]	Highly	Moderately	Not critical
Peritumoral edema[c]	Severe	Moderate	Absent
Concomitant disease(s)[d]	Decompensated	Compensated	Absent

[a]Unrecoverable deficits: deficits complete and stabilized (e.g., hemiplegia or amaurosis); progressive deficits: deficits incomplete or worsening (e.g., hemiparesis or impairment of visual acuity)
[b]A critical location is present if the tumor is attached to a primary vascular or nervous structure (such as the cranial base or an eloquent area)
[c]Peritumoral edema is classified as moderate (only peritumoral) and severe (with a shift of midline structures)
[d]Concomitant diseases were evaluated as being compensated (controlled by medical therapy) or decompensated (uncontrolled despite medical therapy)

Table 7.4 SKALE (sex, Karnofsky, ASA, location, edema) grading system

Factors	Score		
	0	2	4
*S*ex	M	F	–
*K*arnofsky score	≤50	60–70	≥80
*A*SA class	IV	III	I or II
*L*ocation	Critical Highly	Not critical Moderately	– Not critical
*E*dema	Severe	Moderate	No edema

In red: modified SKALE (mSKALE) [31, 56]

Table 7.5 The Geriatric Scoring System (GSS) [17, 18]

Admission parameter	1 point	2 points	3 points
Size	>5 cm	3–5 cm	<3 cm
Neurological deficit	Progressive	Stable severe	None, minor
Karnofsky Performance Scale	<50	60–80	90–100
Tumor location	Falcine, parasagittal Foramen magnum	Tentorial Posterior fossa jugular foramen	Convexity Intraventricular Sphenoid wing Tuberculum sellae cavernous sinus Optic nerve
Peritumoral edema	Severe	Mild	None
Diabetes mellitus	Not controlled	Medically controlled	None
Hypertension	Not controlled	Medically controlled	None
Pulmonary disease	Severe	Mild	None

It was based on a retrospective analysis of 46 patients (of whom 34 were surgically treated) with an age cutoff of 70 years. It incorporates six preoperative factors regarding patient's status and radiological tumor's characteristics, namely, size of lesion, neurological condition, KPS score, critical location, peritumoral edema, and the presence of concomitant disease. The resulting score 6–18 was found to reflect mortality at 3 months. The same group has validated their system in 2005 on a group of 90 patients, confirming that patients with a score > 10 were the best candidates for surgery.

Some critics were expressed regarding the composition of this grading system [56, 57]. Initially, the CRGS was developed based on a small database of 34

Table 7.6 Charlson Comorbidity Index/Score (CCS) [10, 13, 28]

Weight	Clinical condition
1	Myocardial infarction
	Congestive heart failure
	Peripheral vascular disease
	Dementia
	Uncomplicated diabetes mellitus
	Cerebrovascular disease
	Chronic lung disease
	Peptic ulcer disease
	Chronic liver disease
2	Hemiplegia
	Moderate or severe kidney disease
	Diabetes mellitus with complications
	Any malignancy (leukemia, lymphoma)
3	Moderate or severe liver disease
6	Metastatic tumor malignancy
	Acquired immune deficiency syndrome
Assigned weights for each condition the patient has. For example: congestive heart failure – 1 point; moderate kidney disease – 2 points. Total score – 3	

Weighting for age	
Age group (years)	Weight
0–49	0
50–59	1
60–69	2
70–79	3
80–89	4
90–99	5

Aged weight is added to clinical condition weight

patients. That put in question its statistical power. Furthermore, correlation between Karnofsky Performance Scale and mortality was not statistically significant. Nevertheless, the authors of CRGS choose to include it. In further validation work 15 years later [9], KPS remained statistically insignificant. The same work found a substantial correlation of outcome to sex. Still they were reluctant to add it into the scale arguing that it has been the first time such a correlation was described.

Schul et al. [57] confirmed the predictive ability of this scale for mortality and better clinical outcome expressed in the Glasgow Outcome Score. However, as for SKALE (see below), analysis of single components revealed a lack of significance for all components except of the presence of concomitant disease and the statistical strength of total score was similar to the single component "concomitant disease."

Table 7.7 CLASS Algorithmic Scale [36]

	Score				
Factors	−2	−1	0	+1	+2
Comorbidity	ASA 3	ASA 2	ASA 1		
Location	Complex	Moderate	Simple		
Age (years)	≥71	61–70	≤60		
Size (cm)			≤2	2.1–4	>4
Signs and symptoms			Asymptomatic	Mild symptoms Irreversible neurologic deficits	Severe symptoms Reversible neurologic deficits
Other		Prior radiotherapy and/or surgery		Radiographic progression	

- *Sex, Karnofsky, ASA, Location, Edema Score (SKALE)* [56] Table 7.4
  Sacko et al. introduced a new scoring system in 2007 based on a retrospective study of 74 patients 80 years and older. They tried to correlate mortality at 1-year following intracranial meningioma surgery. They could identify five risk factors: sex, preoperative Karnofsky Performance Scale, American Society of Anesthesiology Class, tumor location, and the presence of peritumoral edema. Resulting score could range from 0 to 16. A correlation was found between increased mortality at 1 year with score equal to or lower than 8. Konglund et al. [31] proposed a modification for this scale (mSKALE) based on their data of 51 patients. They could reproduce the results of Sacko et al. regarding total SKALE score and 1-year survival. Nevertheless, assessing single components they could not demonstrate the significance of ASA score and tumor location in the multivariate analysis (ASA score was significant in the univariate analysis). The original definition of tumor location had only two possibilities: critical and not critical which could obtain 0 or 2 points respectively. In the mSKALE location was adapted to the three variable systems as in CRGS, namely, location could be appointed to highly, moderately, and not critical with assigned scores of 0, 2, and 4, respectively.
  As Konglund et al. reported, the resulting mSKALE score was therefore skewed +2 points. A score of ≥8 could predict mortality at 1 year. Schul et al. [57] confirmed the utility of the SKALE score to predict mortality at 1 year. Yet, single component analysis showed significance only for ASA score with an odds ratio of 5.17 per point increase in ASA score. The authors concluded that both SKALE and CRGS might be simplified to one component without losing their predictive ability.
- *Geriatric Scoring System (GSS)* [17, 18] Table 7.5
  Cohen-Inbar et al. proposed the GSS in 2010 based on a study of 250 patients 65 years and older. The GSS includes the same parameters as the CRGS except for concomitant disease, which was substitute by three parameters, namely, the

presence of diabetes mellitus, hypertension, and pulmonary disease. Tumor size was defined slightly differently and tumor location was subdivided in more details. In this study, the authors found correlation between GSS score and survival at 3 months and 5 years. Higher GSS score was additionally significant for performance level at 5 years after surgery as well as time spent in intensive care unit and length of hospitalization. Konglund et al. could not confirm the data regarding survival in their study. Major critic for this scale was that concomitant disease was divided into three factors gaining threefold power. Furthermore, diabetes mellitus was not statistically investigated separately even though 70 % of the patients suffered from it.

- *Charlson Comorbidity Index/Score (CCS)* [10, 13, 28] Table 7.6
  The Charlson Comorbidity Index was originally designed to classify prognostic comorbidity in longitudinal studies in order to predict survival at 1 year. It has been used and validated in numerous studies, some of them in neurosurgical pathologies, in order to stratify patients according to comorbid conditions and overall survival [3, 10–12, 25, 26, 28, 35, 38, 42, 58].
  The CCS assigns a weight of 1, 2, 3, and 6 for different clinical conditions. It is calculated by summing the weights for each condition in patient's medical history. Regardless of whether the conditions are obtained in the contest of clinical care or outcome data, the CSS weight for each condition is identical. CSS scores can range from 0 to 15 and is adjusted for age.
  Grossman et al. [28] performed a multi-institutional retrospective cohort analysis of the American Nationwide Inpatient Sample relating it to the Charlson Comorbidity Index (CCS) [28]. They could confirm a strong correlation of outcome (mortality, postoperative morbidity, length of stay in the hospital, and consequently costs of treatment) with comorbidity.
  Konglund et al. [31] found that survival was improved by CCS ≤ 6, but it did not reach statistical significance ($p=0.068$). It might be the consequence of the small patient's number ($n=51$).
  Laor et al. [35] reporting on outcome in general surgery of elderly patients indicated that increased age was associated with a higher death rate after emergency surgery and with late deaths after elective surgery. A higher mean CCS was noted in early non-survivors after both elective and emergency surgery with a more significant effect of the preoperative CCS than chronological age for the prediction of late postoperative death.
  CCS seems to be effective prognostic tool in further neurosurgical pathologies as glioblastoma multiforme or traumatic spine injury [25, 42]. Although the CCS was not designed to predict perioperative mortality in surgical cohorts, it correlates with a greater risk than age for perioperative death in the elderly.
- *CLASS Algorithmic Scale* [36] Table 7.7
  This algorithm aimed to balance the risks and benefits of meningioma surgery. The purpose of this scale is to suggest physician about surgical treatment in incidental tumors. Unlike the previous scales, this system suggests a raw of risk factors (comorbidity defined by ASA score, tumor location, and patient age) and benefit factors (tumor size, neurologic signs). A score is assigned to each factor

as follows: risk factors are graded from −2 to 0, while benefit factors are graded from 0 to +2. A score of +1 was added to total score in the presence of radiographic progression and −1 for previous history of surgery and/or radiotherapy. Patients are then divided into CLASS I (total score of +1 or above), CLASS II (total score of 0 or −1), and CLASS III (total score of −2 or below).
The validity of this scale was tested by the authors showing that patients in CLASS group I should be offered surgery and those in CLASS group III should not be offered surgery. Patients in CLASS group II should be discussed with caution.
Major disadvantage of this scoring system is that location was only defined subjectively by the senior author and not based of defined criteria; therefore, it might not be transferred to other centers. Additionally, no other study had until now tested this scale; thus, its utility is questionable.

In summary, all systems have their utility and disadvantages when considering patients for surgery. It seems that patients' general conditions play a crucial role in defining prognosis. Tumors' characteristics as location, size, and peritumoral edema seem to have an important role as well. Patient's age seems to correlate with outcome although it is not an independent factor and usually older age is associated with different risk factors. Moreover, physicians might improve patient's likelihood for better outcome by improving the "dynamic" factors such as improving general condition or reduce edema. Unchangeable factors as age, sex, or tumor size contribute for risk assessment but are not disposed to changes.

These scoring systems do provide useful help for decision-making but should not be used as guidelines when treating these patients. Best approach is probably careful judgment of all different factors and an open discussion with patients and relatives.

7.6 Outcome

The most important aim of all studies is to improve future outcome by identifying risk factors and developing systems. This would allow improving patients' selection and advise other practitioners on the best way to choose. An imperative task would be to look at one's own outcomes and identify adverse as well as good results. The advances of medical technology make it hard to compare historical series. Furthermore, differences in study designs and size of patients' collectives contribute to a large difficulty in comparing these studies. Reported mortality and morbidity rates vary widely and are sometimes even contradictory. A summary of published rates is shown in Table 7.2.

- *Morbidity*
  The definition of morbidity and operative complication differs largely. Identifying postoperative morbidity is not an easy task. First of all, surgery of intracranial lesions runs the risk of neurological complication such as motor deficits, speech

deficits, neurocognitive impairment, etc. Some of these complications are only temporary and resolve within few days. Others take much longer and some are unfortunately permanent.
Reporting such results depend largely on subjective measures especially when most of the studies are retrospective.
Somewhat easier task is to report morphological complications as postoperative hemorrhage or CSF fistula. Such complications might be reported then as need or need-not surgery.
Further medical complications as pneumonia, urinary tract infections, cardiac decompensation, etc. are easy to register, but correlation with preoperative factors might be difficult to achieve.
Reported morbidity figures are therefore heterogeneously reported and range from 2.7 to 69.6 % (Table 7.2). Comparing this data is an almost impossible task. Poon et al. [53] summarized complications' relevant published data between the years 2002 and 2012. The overall incidence of complications was 20.1 % per patient (range 2.7–60.5 %). The percentage of complications being neurological in nature ranged from 42.5 to 100 %.
In different studies comparing young to elderly patients, the last had significantly higher complication rate [6, 49, 52]. Patil et al. reported that elderly were more likely to have one or more complications (29.8 % vs. 13.1 %, $p>0.0001$). Poon et al. [52] described similar results with 69.6 % complications rate among older patients vs. 51.1 % ($p=0.01$) among young patients.

- *Mortality*
  Since death is a definitive state, it can be assessed on a set time point (in hospital, 30 days, 3 months, or 1 year). Its documentation is a much easier task to achieve and report.
  Reported numbers vary between high figures in historical reports and much lower figures in recent ones. This might be explained due to better operative and perioperative technologies as well as stricter patient's selection in recent reports. Mortality rates at 30 days are reported to range between 29 and 0 % (Table 7.2). Further reports on 3, 6, and 12 months as well as 5-year mortality rates in addition to death cause are summarized in Table 7.8. One-year mortality rate range from 4.3 to 15.7 % seems to be similar to rates reported in the general population [8]. Five-year mortality rates are rarely reported. They seem to be elevated yet it might represent the expected span of life in aged people.
- *Quality of life*
  Important information concerning the utility of surgery in these patients is reported through several indicators for quality of life (as postoperative Karnofsky Performance Scale or the Glasgow Outcome Score). Other indicators such as hospital discharge information are important, not only to caregivers but also for politics and insurance companies when planning health resources.
  Schul et al. [57] reported an improvement of the median Karnofsky Performance Scale from 80 to 90 in the surviving patients suggesting benefit of surgery to most of the operated patients. These results were confirmed by other authors [9]. Rogne et al. reported an improvement of ECOG Performance score (Eastern

Table 7.8 Summary of mortality figures in the elderly in some of the reports from 2002 to 2013

	Mortality (%)					Cause of death (%)	
Author	In hospital	30 days	90 days	1 year	5 years	Surgery related	Non-surgery related
Poon et al. [52]	–	0	2.2	4.3	–	25	75
Chen et al. [14]	1.2	1.2	1.2	–	–	100	0
Konglund et al. [32]	–	5.6	7.4	9.2	–	74	26
Konglund et al. [31]	–	3.9	7.8	15.7	–	–	–
Schul et al. [57]	–	3.7	6.7	6.7	–	81.8	18.2
Grossman et al. [28]	3.2	–	–	–	–	–	–
Cohen-Inbar et al. [18]	–	–	5.8	8.3	88.3[a]	–	–
Patil et al. [49]	–	12	–	–	–	–	–
Cohen-Inbar et al. [17]	–	.	6.8	–	–	–	–
Rogne et al. [55]	–	2.5	–	6.3	26.6	–	–
Sacko et al. [56]	–	0	1.4	9.4	27	–	–
Boviatsis et al. [6]	6.5	–	–	–	–	–	–
D'Andrea et al. [20]	–	10.8	13.5	13.5	–	–	–
Caroli et al. [9]	–	6.7	7.8	15.6	–	25	75

Adapted from Poon et al. [53]

[a]No availability of the numbers of patient in whom 5-year survival data was available

Cooperative Oncology Group) following surgery [55]. In further study, Konglund et al. [32] found no significant overall change in the level of independence after surgery measured through KPS. Nevertheless, an improvement of the Mini Mental State Examination (MMSE) postoperatively was noticed. Further quality of life questionnaire analysis revealed better mean functional scores in physical and social aspects, yet poorer cognitive functioning (comparing to population-based data). Tucha et al. [60] in the only study published specifically on the effects of surgery on cognitive function in elderly patients with intracranial meningioma could not reveal any significant deterioration. They could find marked improvements in attentional and memory functions as well as in task processing speed.

- *Hospital recovery*

  Due to the prevalence of concomitant disease in aged patients, it is expectable that these patients would spend much longer time in hospital. Grossman et al. could confirm it by using the CCS. Each one-point increase in CCS was associated with significantly longer length of stay in hospital and consequently higher hospital charges [28]. Increasing in ASA score and the presence of concomitant disease were correlated to increasing length of stay [14]. A close correlation to length of stay in the ICU was also linked to preoperative condition as expressed in the preoperative Karnofsky Performance Scale [17]

  Comparing young to old patients revealed significantly longer hospital stay for elderly patients (17.4 ± 20.4 days vs. 9.1 ± 4.98 days). Furthermore, elderly patients were more prone to be discharged into a facility than young patients [52]. It might be safe to assume that the ability to rehabilitate aged patients into independent self-care, if needed, pose a big challenge and might be impossible task.

7.7 Radiotherapy

Despite the notable decrease in surgery related complications, surgery is often not feasible. Not operable tumors, patient to ill for a surgical intervention, incomplete resection or recurrence of tumor, and patient or surgeon's preference might require seeking alternative therapy option. To date, there is no available chemotherapeutic agent widely acceptable for the treatment of meningiomas.

At least to date, there are only two retrospective works dealing specifically with stereotactic radiotherapy in the elderly [27, 30]. Both report a similar radiologic local control rate and overall survival rates (Table 7.9).

Table 7.9 Summary of radiologic local control rates/progression-free survival and overall survival followed stereotactical radiotherapy

	Progression-free survival %				Overall survival %		
Author, year	1 year	3 years	5 years	10 years	1 year	3 years	5 years
Kaul et al., 2015 [30]	–	93.7	91.1	82	–	–	–
Fokas et al., 2014 [27]	98.3	98.3	94.7	–	95.8	92.0	79.0

Procedure-related complications were reported only as toxicity grades I and II in about 50 % of patients. These consisted in headaches, alopecia, fatigue, vertigo, cranial nerve deficits, memory impairment, pyramidal dysfunction, and hearing loss. No mortality was related directly to the procedure. Fokas et al. [27] reported 13.2 % mortality rate due to other causes not related to the procedure during the follow-up period (median 40 months).

Cohen-Inbar et al. [16] tried to test their proposed Geriatric Scoring System (GSS) Score onto meningioma patients treated radiosurgically. Despite this scoring system designed to evaluate risk in elderly patients, it was tested on all patients collectively (young and old). An age stratification and analysis has not been reported.

It seems that stereotactic-based radiotherapy is an effective and safe therapeutic modality for intracranial meningiomas in elderly patients. It is a valuable alternative treatment option and should be discussed interdisciplinary and with patients.

Conclusion

Recent works suggest acceptable outcomes following intracranial meningioma surgery and radiosurgery. Yet these results should be used with caution. To date, studies should be interpreted as at best level II (most of them are evidence level III).

Decision-making should be based on thorough discussion of all parameters discussed above. Further, treatment recommendation should be openly discussed with patient and his relatives, defining treatment's goals with careful evaluation of pro- and contraindications. Individual's preoperative status, comorbidities, and tumor characteristics should be taken into consideration.

Radiosurgery seems to be a valid alternative for the treatment of intracranial meningiomas in this patient's group. Multidisciplinary exhaustive discussion is strongly recommended.

References

1. Arienta C, Caroli M, Crotti F et al (1990) Treatment of intracranial meningiomas in patients over 70 years old. Acta Neurochir 107:47–55
2. Awad IA, Kalfas I, Hahn JF et al (1989) Intracranial meningiomas in the aged: surgical outcome in the era of computed tomography. Neurosurgery 24:557–560
3. Bar B, Hemphill JC 3rd (2011) Charlson comorbidity index adjustment in intracerebral hemorrhage. Stroke 42:2944–2946
4. Bateman BT, Pile-Spellman J, Gutin PH et al (2005) Meningioma resection in the elderly: nationwide inpatient sample, 1998–2002. Neurosurgery 57:866–872; discussion 866–872
5. Black P, Kathiresan S, Chung W (1998) Meningioma surgery in the elderly: a case–control study assessing morbidity and mortality. Acta Neurochir 140:1013–1016; discussion 1016–1017
6. Boviatsis EJ, Bouras TI, Kouyialis AT et al (2007) Impact of age on complications and outcome in meningioma surgery. Surg Neurol 68:407–411; discussion 411
7. Buhl R, Hasan A, Behnke A et al (2000) Results in the operative treatment of elderly patients with intracranial meningioma. Neurosurg Rev 23:25–29
8. Cahill KS, Claus EB (2011) Treatment and survival of patients with nonmalignant intracranial meningioma: results from the Surveillance, Epidemiology, and End Results Program of the National Cancer Institute. Clinical article. J Neurosurg 115:259–267

9. Caroli M, Locatelli M, Prada F et al (2005) Surgery for intracranial meningiomas in the elderly: a clinical-radiological grading system as a predictor of outcome. J Neurosurg 102:290–294
10. Charlson M, Szatrowski TP, Peterson J et al (1994) Validation of a combined comorbidity index. J Clin Epidemiol 47:1245–1251
11. Charlson M, Wells MT, Ullman R et al (2014) The Charlson comorbidity index can be used prospectively to identify patients who will incur high future costs. PLoS One 9:e112479
12. Charlson ME, Charlson RE, Peterson JC et al (2008) The Charlson comorbidity index is adapted to predict costs of chronic disease in primary care patients. J Clin Epidemiol 61:1234–1240
13. Charlson ME, Pompei P, Ales KL et al (1987) A new method of classifying prognostic comorbidity in longitudinal studies: development and validation. J Chronic Dis 40:373–383
14. Chen ZY, Zheng CH, Tang L et al (2015) Intracranial meningioma surgery in the elderly (over 65 years): prognostic factors and outcome. Acta Neurochir (Wien) 157:1549–1557; discussion 1557
15. Claus EB, Bondy ML, Schildkraut JM et al (2005) Epidemiology of intracranial meningioma. Neurosurgery 57:1088–1095; discussion 1088–1095
16. Cohen-Inbar O, Lee CC, Schlesinger D et al (2015) The Geriatric Scoring System (GSS) for risk stratification in meningioma patients as a predictor of outcome in patients treated with radiosurgery. World Neurosurg 87:431–438
17. Cohen-Inbar O, Soustiel JF, Zaaroor M (2010) Meningiomas in the elderly, the surgical benefit and a new scoring system. Acta Neurochir (Wien) 152:87–97; discussion 97
18. Cohen-Inbar O, Sviri GE, Soustiel JF et al (2011) The Geriatric Scoring System (GSS) in meningioma patients--validation. Acta Neurochir (Wien) 153:1501–1508; discussion 1508
19. Cornu P, Chatellier G, Dagreou F et al (1990) Intracranial meningiomas in elderly patients. Postoperative morbidity and mortality. Factors predictive of outcome. Acta Neurochir 102:98–102
20. D'andrea G, Roperto R, Caroli E et al (2005) Thirty-seven cases of intracranial meningiomas in the ninth decade of life: our experience and review of the literature. Neurosurgery 56:956–961; discussion 956–961
21. Das A, Chapman CA, Yap WM (2000) Histological subtypes of symptomatic central nervous system tumours in Singapore. J Neurol Neurosurg Psychiatry 68:372–374
22. Das A, Tang WY, Smith DR (2000) Meningiomas in Singapore: demographic and biological characteristics. J Neurooncol 47:153–160
23. Djindjian M, Caron JP, Athayde AA et al (1988) Intracranial meningiomas in the elderly (over 70 years old). A retrospective study of 30 surgical cases. Acta Neurochir 90:121–123
24. Dolecek TA, Dressler EV, Thakkar JP et al (2015) Epidemiology of meningiomas post-Public Law 107–206: The Benign Brain Tumor Cancer Registries Amendment Act. Cancer 121: 2400–2410
25. Ening G, Osterheld F, Capper D et al (2015) Charlson comorbidity index: an additional prognostic parameter for preoperative glioblastoma patient stratification. J Cancer Res Clin Oncol 141:1131–1137
26. Fiorentino A, Ricchetti F, Mazzola R et al (2015) Regarding Ening et al. Charlson comorbidity index: an additional prognostic parameter for preoperative glioblastoma patient stratification. J Cancer Res Clin Oncol 141:1139–1140
27. Fokas E, Henzel M, Surber G et al (2014) Stereotactic radiotherapy of benign meningioma in the elderly: clinical outcome and toxicity in 121 patients. Radiother Oncol J Eur Soc Ther Radiol Oncol 111:457–462
28. Grossman R, Mukherjee D, Chang DC et al (2011) Preoperative charlson comorbidity score predicts postoperative outcomes among older intracranial meningioma patients. World Neurosurg 75:279–285
29. Ibebuike K, Ouma J (2014) Demographic profile of patients diagnosed with intracranial meningiomas in two academic hospitals in Johannesburg, South Africa: a 12-month prospective study. Afr Health Sci 14:939–945

30. Kaul D, Budach V, Graaf L et al (2015) Outcome of elderly patients with meningioma after image-guided stereotactic radiotherapy: a study of 100 cases. Biomed Res Int 2015:868401
31. Konglund A, Rogne SG, Helseth E et al (2013) Meningioma surgery in the very old-validating prognostic scoring systems. Acta Neurochir (Wien) 155:2263–2271; discussion 2271
32. Konglund A, Rogne SG, Lund-Johansen M et al (2013) Outcome following surgery for intracranial meningiomas in the aging. Acta Neurol Scand 127:161–169
33. Kshettry VR, Ostrom QT, Kruchko C et al (2015) Descriptive epidemiology of World Health Organization grades II and III intracranial meningiomas in the United States. Neuro Oncol 17:1166–1173
34. Kuratsu J, Kochi M, Ushio Y (2000) Incidence and clinical features of asymptomatic meningiomas. J Neurosurg 92:766–770
35. Laor A, Tal S, Guller V et al (2016) The Charlson Comorbidity Index (CCI) as a mortality predictor after surgery in elderly patients. Am Surg 82:22–27
36. Lee JH (2008) Meningiomas: diagnosis, treatment, and outcome. Springer, London
37. Louis DN, Ohgaki H, Wiestler OD et al (2007) The 2007 WHO classification of tumours of the central nervous system. Acta Neuropathol 114:97–109
38. Luber MP, Hollenberg JP, Williams-Russo P et al (2000) Diagnosis, treatment, comorbidity, and resource utilization of depressed patients in a general medical practice. Int J Psychiatry Med 30:1–13
39. Mastronardi L, Ferrante L, Qasho R et al (1995) Intracranial meningiomas in the 9th decade of life: a retrospective study of 17 surgical cases. Neurosurgery 36:270–274
40. Maurice-Williams RS, Kitchen ND (1992) Intracranial tumours in the elderly: the effect of age on the outcome of first time surgery for meningiomas. Br J Neurosurg 6:131–137
41. Mcgrail KM, Ojemann RG (1994) The surgical management of benign intracranial meningiomas and acoustic neuromas in patients 70 years of age and older. Surg Neurol 42:2–7
42. Menendez ME, Ring D, Harris MB et al (2015) Predicting in-hospital mortality in elderly patients with cervical spine fractures: a comparison of the charlson and elixhauser comorbidity measures. Spine 40:809–815
43. Nakamura M, Roser F, Michel J et al (2003) The natural history of incidental meningiomas. Neurosurgery 53:62–70; discussion 70–61
44. Nakamura M, Roser F, Michel J et al (2005) Volumetric analysis of the growth rate of incompletely resected intracranial meningiomas. Zentralbl Neurochir 66:17–23
45. Niiro M, Yatsushiro K, Nakamura K et al (2000) Natural history of elderly patients with asymptomatic meningiomas. J Neurol Neurosurg Psychiatry 68:25–28
46. Nishizaki T, Kamiryo T, Fujisawa H et al (1994) Prognostic implications of meningiomas in the elderly (over 70 years old) in the era of magnetic resonance imaging. Acta Neurochir 126:59–62
47. Ostrom QT, Gittleman H, Fulop J et al (2015) CBTRUS Statistical Report: primary brain and central nervous system tumors diagnosed in the United States in 2008–2012. Neuro Oncol 17:iv1–iv62
48. Park JS, Sade B, Oya S et al (2014) The influence of age on the histological grading of meningiomas. Neurosurg Rev 37:425–429; discussion 429
49. Patil GC, Veeravagu A, Lad SP et al (2010) Craniotomy for resection of meningioma in the elderly: a multicenter prospective analysis from the National Surgical Quality Improvement Program. J Neurol Neurusurg Psychiatry 81(5):502–505
50. Pearson BE, Markert JM, Fisher WS et al (2008) Hitting a moving target: evolution of a treatment paradigm for atypical meningiomas amid changing diagnostic criteria. Neurosurg Focus 24:E3
51. Peterson JC, Paget SA, Lachs MS et al (2012) The risk of comorbidity. Ann Rheum Dis 71:635–637
52. Poon MT, Fung LH, Pu JK et al (2013) Outcome comparison between younger and older patients undergoing intracranial meningioma resections. J Neurooncol 114:219–227
53. Poon MT, Fung LH, Pu JK et al (2014) Outcome of elderly patients undergoing intracranial meningioma resection–a systematic review and meta-analysis. Br J Neurosurg 28:303–309

54. Rogers L, Gilbert M, Vogelbaum MA (2010) Intracranial meningiomas of atypical (WHO grade II) histology. J Neurooncol 99:393–405
55. Rogne SG, Konglund A, Meling TR et al (2009) Intracranial tumor surgery in patients >70 years of age: is clinical practice worthwhile or futile? Acta Neurol Scand 120:288–294
56. Sacko O, Sesay M, Roux F-E et al (2007) Intracranial meningioma surgery in the ninth decade of life. Neurosurgery 61:950–954; discussion 955
57. Schul DB, Wolf S, Krammer MJ et al (2012) Meningioma surgery in the elderly: outcome and validation of 2 proposed grading score systems. Neurosurgery 70:555–565
58. Suidan RS, Leitao MM Jr, Zivanovic O et al (2015) Predictive value of the Age-Adjusted Charlson Comorbidity Index on perioperative complications and survival in patients undergoing primary debulking surgery for advanced epithelial ovarian cancer. Gynecol Oncol 138:246–251
59. Tamimi AF, Tamimi I, Abdelaziz M et al (2015) Epidemiology of malignant and non-malignant primary brain tumors in Jordan. Neuroepidemiology 45:100–108
60. Tucha O, Smely C, Lange KW (2001) Effects of surgery on cognitive functioning of elderly patients with intracranial meningioma. Br J Neurosurg 15:184–188
61. Umansky F, Ashkenazi E, Gertel M et al (1992) Surgical outcome in an elderly population with intracranial meningioma. J Neurol Neurosurg Psychiatry 55:481–485
62. Willis J, Smith C, Ironside JW et al (2005) The accuracy of meningioma grading: a 10-year retrospective audit. Neuropathol Appl Neurobiol 31:141–149

Brain Gliomas in the Elderly

8

Cristina Izquierdo Gracia and Francois Ducray

8.1 Introduction

Adult's gliomas are a group of primary central nervous system (CNS) neoplasms arising from neuroglial cells. In the World Health Organization, they are classified according to their phenotype and to a histological grading system. The grade I corresponds to pilocytic astrocytoma. The grade II corresponds to low-grade diffuse astrocytoma, oligodendroglioma and oligoastrocytoma. High-grade gliomas comprise anaplastic astrocytoma, anaplastic oligodendroglioma (grade III) and glioblastoma multiforme (GBM), which is the most frequent and most aggressive subtype (grade IV) [38]. However, this broad grouping contains tumours that are clinically, histologically and molecularly heterogeneous.

Low-grade gliomas are more common in young adults, while anaplastic gliomas and GBM occur more frequently in older patients [48]. Due to the global increase in life expectancy, the incidence of gliomas in elderly patients, especially GBM, is increasing [36]. The cut-off to define elderly patients with gliomas varies across studies between 65 and 70 years old [54].

Due to their frequently very poor prognosis and the fear that they may not tolerate brain radiotherapy (RT) and chemotherapy, elderly patients with gliomas have long been undertreated. However, within the last decade, several clinical trials conducted in this specific population have resulted in significant progress. This chapter attempts to summarize the main clinical, diagnostic and treatment features of brain gliomas in the elderly population.

C.I. Gracia • F. Ducray (✉)
NeuroOncology Department, Hôpital Neurologique Pierre Wertheimer,
Hospices Civils de Lyon, Lyon, France
e-mail: cizquierdogracia1@gmail.com; francois.ducray@chu-lyon.fr

© Springer International Publishing Switzerland 2017

M. Berhouma, P. Krolak-Salmon (eds.), *Brain and Spine Surgery in the Elderly*,
DOI 10.1007/978-3-319-40232-1_8

8.2 High-Grade Gliomas

8.2.1 Glioblastoma Multiforme

8.2.1.1 Epidemiology

Glioblastoma multiforme (GBM) is the most frequent malignant primary brain tumour in adults (46 %). Patients older than 65 years old represent nearly 50 % of all patients [48]. The definition of elderly patients with GBM varies, but in general a cut-off of 65 or 70 years old is well accepted. The median overall survival (OS) of elderly patients with GBM ranges from 4 to 8.6 months [26]. The incidence of elderly patients with GBM is increasing. Hence, elderly people represent an important part of the total number of newly diagnosed GBM, and consequently these patients need to be considered when new treatment approaches are developed [17].

8.2.1.2 Clinical Features

In elderly patients, focal neurological deficits (55 %) and cognitive impairment (48.5 %) are the most common symptoms at diagnosis [84]. Elderly patients present less likely with headache or seizures when compared to young patients. Since the onset of symptoms frequently occurs over a few weeks, it is important to perform a rapid diagnosis in order to start treatment before the performance status is too deteriorated [17, 39].

8.2.1.3 Prognostic Factors

Different prognostic factors have been evaluated in elderly patients with GBM [4]. Even in this population, an older age is associated with a poorer outcome [13]. As in younger patients, the Karnofsky Performance Status (KPS), with a cut-off at 70, or ECOG PS ≤ 2 has been shown to be associated with a poorer outcome [2, 55, 84]. Other prognostic factors include gross total resection [68] and *MGMT* promoter methylation status [16, 25]. Mutation of isocitrate dehydrogenase 1 (IDH1) has been identified in around 10 % of adult patients with GBM, and its positive impact on clinical outcome has also been demonstrated [6, 81]. The IDH1 mutation is less frequently reported in the geriatric population (1–2 %) which may partly explain the worse prognosis of those patients [24, 79]. The lack of other favourable prognostic biomarkers in elderly patients such as G34R H3F3A mutation, a G-CIMP, or PRDX1 methylation may also contribute to the overall worse outcome [79].

8.2.1.4 Radiology

On brain magnetic resonance imaging (MRI), GBMs typically present as large masses located in the supratentorial area. A hypo- or isointense lesion on T1 sequences with a central heterogeneous signal related to necrosis is usually observed. Sometimes, intratumoural bleeding is also present. T1 sequences after contrast administration frequently show thick and irregular ringlike contrast enhancement. Noteworthy, approximately one third of patients can present with lack of contrast enhancement, especially in elderly patients [61]. On FLAIR sequences, the tumour generally appears as a hyperintense mass surrounded by vasogenic fingerlike oedema. Multimodal MRI including diffusion, perfusion and MRI spectroscopy can help better characterize the tumour. MR spectroscopy provides information about metabolic tissue composition. The most useful metabolites in the diagnosis of GBM are choline which is related with membrane turnover, creatine reflecting basal metabolism, **N**-acetyl-aspartate (NAA) related to neuronal structures and lipids or lactate, both reflecting necrosis. MRI spectroscopy typically shows lactate or lipid peaks with an increased choline/NAA ratio. Perfusion MRI typically shows an elevated rCBV suggestive of neo-angiogenesis with higher values in geriatric population when compared to younger population [27, 29]. The differential diagnosis in this setting includes a unique brain metastasis and a pyogenic abscess, toxoplasmosis in HIV patients and tuberculoma in patients living in regions where tuberculosis is endemic [47]. Primary CNS lymphoma is rarely necrotic. In addition to a complete clinical exam, elderly patients with a suspicion of GBM should undergo thoracic-abdominal CT scan. Diffusion MRI should be carefully reviewed to exclude a pyogenic abscess which is frequently present without fever and any biological sign of inflammation. HIV serology should be systematic.

8.2.1.5 Treatment

Surgery

Surgery or biopsy is first required to obtain a definitive diagnosis. Even though MRI is frequently suggestive of the diagnosis, histology remains mandatory to exclude differential diagnosis. In addition, tumour tissue is needed for molecular analysis since molecular profiling is playing an increasing role in treatment decisions.

In younger patients, maximal safe surgical resection of the GBM is recommended. This recommendation however does not rely on randomized studies but on retrospective analysis of several clinical trials showing that in younger adults, a maximum safe resection is associated with a better OS independently of other prognostic factors [1, 65].

The role of surgery in elderly GBM patients remains debated. A retrospective analysis on the management of GBM in Spain between 2008 and 2010 showed that patients older than 70 years old presented a higher incidence of complications after surgery compared to their younger counterparts (12.6 % vs 18.8 %) and were less likely to undergo resection [22]. Another analysis of the perioperative complications in elderly population found similar results with an increased incidence of hematomas in the cavity and pneumonia [2]. On the other hand, some retrospectives studies support that elderly patients should be treated with a surgery as they present a better outcome with no increase of surgery-related morbidity [12, 49]. Yet a retrospective study of 289 patients concluded that despite maximum tumour resection should be attempted, surgery may be less useful in patients older than 80 years with a KPS less than 80 % [34]. Advances in intraoperative techniques have helped to maximize tumour resection and minimize morbidity in gliomas' surgeries. Awake craniotomy and the use of 5-aminolevulinic allow to perform more complete resections and also reduce the risk of postoperative deficits [41, 68]. A retrospective analysis suggested a benefit on survival of awake craniotomy in elderly population without increasing postoperative morbidities [23]. However, the value of these techniques in the geriatric population remains to be studied.

One prospective randomized trial compared resection versus biopsy in 30 elderly patients (median age was 70 years old) with newly diagnosed high-grade gliomas [75]. In this study, surgery was associated with longer survival compared to biopsy (171 days versus 85 days, respectively) and was also related with an improvement of the quality of life. Nevertheless, this study was limited by its small sample size and the inclusion of both GBM and anaplastic astrocytomas. The ANOCEF group (the French specialized association of neuro-oncology) has undertaken a randomized phase III study comparing surgery versus biopsy in elderly patients with GBM.

Initial Treatment in Patients with Good Performance Status

Radiotherapy

In young patients (<70 years old) with good KPS, since 2005, the standard of care for newly diagnosed GBM is maximal safe surgical resection followed by concomitant and adjuvant temozolomide radiochemotherapy (TMZ-RT) [70]. In patients aged <70 years, compared to RT alone, TMZ-RT was associated with increased median survival (12.1 vs 14.6 months) and an increase of the rate of patients alive at 2 and 3 years (27.2 % and 16 %, respectively) without important toxicity [69].

In elderly GBM patients, even in those with good KPS, whether oncological treatment might be beneficial has long remained debated. Keime-Guibert et al. conducted the first randomized trial in this population. This trial compared, in 85 patients aged ≥70 years and with a KPS ≥70, RT only (50.4 Gy, 28 fractions) versus best supportive care. Thirty-nine patients received RT and 42 patients received supportive care. The study was closed prematurely because the preliminary analysis showed clearly an increase in the OS of patients included in the RT arm (29 weeks versus 17 weeks ($p = 0.002$). Importantly, RT was well tolerated and was not associated with a decrease of the performance status, the quality of life or the cognitive function [33]. While in Keime-Guibert et al. study patients received a RT regimen close to that administered in LGG patients, several studies aimed at determining the optimal RT regimen in elderly patients. In 2004, a randomized trial compared an accelerated RT regimen (40 Gy, 15 fractions during 3 weeks) to a standard irradiation schedule (60 Gy in 30 fractions) in patients aged 60 years or more and showed no differences regarding median OS (5.6 and 5.1 months, respectively) and the KPS at the end of the treatment. However, patients treated with the classical schedule required more frequently an increase in the corticosteroid dose (49 % versus 23 %) suggesting a worse tolerance of the conventional dose [56]. Recently, a phase III randomized trial randomized elderly or frail patients to receive an even more accelerated hypofractionated regimen (25 Gy in five daily fractions over 1 week) or the most commonly schedule of RT used in elderly population (40 Gy in 15 daily fractions over 3 weeks). No differences in OS or survival (PFS) were identified [57].

Temozolomide

Besides RT, several retrospective studies suggested that TMZ could be an effective treatment in elderly GBM patients [21, 35], and this hypothesis was tested in two randomized phase 3 trials. Wick et al. conducted a non-inferiority phase III trial (NOA-08 study) where they compared TMZ vs RT in patients aged over 65 years old with a KPS ≥60 with a high-grade glioma. The patients were randomly assigned to receive either a dose-intensified TMZ regimen (100 mg/m^2/day days 1–7 of 1 week on, 1 week off) or standard RT (60 Gy over 6 weeks in 1.8–2 Gy fractions). No significant difference was found in terms of OS (8.6 months for the TMZ arm and 9.6 months for the RT arm), and no difference was identified in both groups regarding quality of life [78].

The second study, the Nordic trial, was conducted by Malmström et al. They enrolled 342 patients aged 60 years or older with a diagnosed GBM. Patients were randomized to receive one of the following three treatment arms: (a) TMZ (200 mg/m^2 for 5 consecutive days every 28 days), (b) hypofractionated RT (34 Gy in 10 fractions) and (c) standard schedule of RT (60Gy/30fractions). In the whole population, OS was significantly better in patients treated with TMZ than with the standard RT regimen (8.3 versus 6 months, $p=0.01$). In patients aged ≥70 years, TMZ and accelerated RT were equivalent and were superior to the standard RT regimen (OS 8.4 versus 7.4 months) [40]. At 3 months, TMZ was associated with a better quality of life than RT. Yet no subsequent analysis of quality of life was performed, and therefore these results need to be taken with caution. An example of good response to treatment with TMZ in an elderly patient is shown in Fig. 8.1.

MGMT Promoter Methylation

Interestingly, a retrospective analysis of *MGMT* methylation was performed in these two phase III trials, the NOA-8 and the Nordic trial [40, 78]. *MGMT* methylation was analysed in 56 and 69 % of patients in the NOA-8 and in the Nordic trial, respectively. In the NOA-8 trial (patients ≥65 years), *MGMT*-methylated patients had a longer PFS when treated with TMZ as opposed to RT (8.4 vs 4.6 months, $p=0.01$), while *MGMT* unmethylated patients had a longer PFS when treated with RT than with TMZ (4.6 vs 3.3 months, $p=0.01$). A similar yet not significant trend was observed for OS. The Nordic trial (patients ≥ 60 years) showed a non-significant trend towards longer OS in *MGMT*-methylated patients when treated with TMZ rather than with RT (hazard ratio = 0.64, $p=0.07$), but *MGMT*-unmethylated patients did not fare better when treated with RT than with TMZ. PFS data were not available for this trial, as these data were deliberately not collected. These results, together with another retrospective study, suggest that *MGMT* methylation could guide treatment decision in elderly patients with glioblastoma [79]. However, the data are not yet robust enough to be translated into the clinic and need prospective validation. Until now, the use of *MGMT* methylation as a predictive factor has also been limited by the fact that the optimal technique to study *MGMT* methylation is still debated. In Quillien et al., the rate of *MGMT* methylated patients varied from

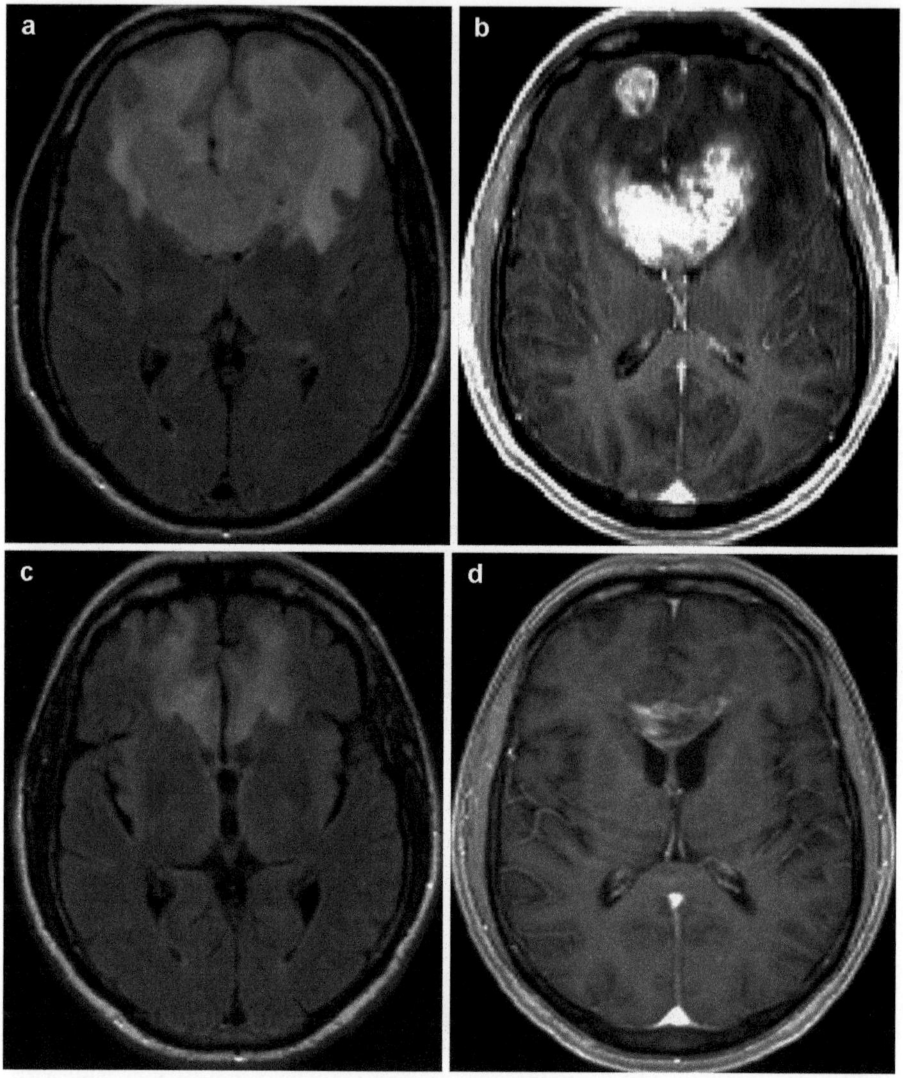

Fig. 8.1 (**a**, **b**) Magnetic resonance image (MRI) of an elderly male patient (71 years old) with newly diagnosed glioblastoma multiforme (GBM). Flair sequence shows a large and oedematous hyperintense lesion infiltrating both frontal lobes and corpus callosum (**a**). T1-weighted axial gadolinium-enhanced MRI showing two contrast enhancing lesions in the setting of a multicentric GBM (**b**). (**c**, **d**) Follow-up MRI from the same patient after six cycles of treatment with temozolomide. Flair sequence shows a marked reduction of the oedema (**c**). Dramatic improvement of the contrast enhancement lesions is observed after the administration of gadolinium (**d**). The patient presented a neurological improvement and the KPS increased from 50 to 70 %. The overall survival was 18 months

33 to 60 % depending on the method that was used [53]. Methylation-specific PCR has been used as a standard to study *MGMT* methylation, but this method is only qualitative and lacks automation. Therefore, alternative semi-quantitative and

quantitative techniques have been developed. However, these techniques do not study exactly the same regions of the *MGMT* promoter. Therefore, as the methylation pattern of the promoter can be heterogeneous, some patients are classified as methylated or as unmethylated depending on the technique used [53].

Radiotherapy and Temozolomide

Since temozolomide radiochemotherapy has improved the prognosis of younger patients with GBM, an important question until recently was whether this strategy may be beneficial in elderly patients and may not be too neurotoxic. Some non-randomized prospective studies had suggested the possible benefit of radiochemotherapy in elderly population [31, 44, 45]. This was also supported by a meta-analysis based on non-randomized studies comparing both therapeutic options (RT with TMZ versus RT alone) [82]. Finally the benefit of this strategy was recently proven by the results of the collaborative CCTG CE.6/EORTC 26062-22061/TROG 08.02/NCT00482677 trial which were presented at the 2016 ASCO meeting [50]. This trial compared RT alone (40 Gy in 15 fractions) vs RT/TMZ (40 Gy in 15 fractions associated with concomitant TMZ followed by up to 12 monthly TMZ cycles). Five hundred sixty-two patients were randomized, 281 on each arm; median age was 73 years, 77 % of patients had a KPS > 70 and 68 % had a resection. RT/TMZ significantly improved OS over RT alone (median 9.3 months vs 7.6 months, $p < 0.0001$) and significantly improved PFS (median 5.3 months vs 3.9 months, $p < 0.0001$). Preliminary *MGMT* analysis demonstrated a clear benefit of RT/TMZ vs RT alone in *MGMT* methylated patients (13.5 months vs 7.3 months, $p = 0.0001$) but also in *MGMT* unmethylated patients, however to a lesser extent (10 months vs 7.9 months, $p = 0.055$). Quality of life analyses showed no differences in functional domains of QLQC30 and BN20 but were worse in the RT/TMZ arm for nausea, vomiting and constipation. The authors concluded that the addition of concomitant and adjuvant TMZ to hypofractionated RT for elderly patients with GBM significantly improved OS and PFS in all patients and that it was well tolerated.

Initial Treatment in Patients with Poor KPS

The cut-off to define low KPS can vary in some reports but equal or less than 60 is well accepted. The optimal management of young patients with poor performance status is based mainly on retrospective studies and a subgroup analysis of prospective studies [14, 42]. A maximal safe resection is highly recommended when possible especially if it can improve the neurological status. Concerning the postsurgical treatment, it remains debated in the absence of prospective studies. Some patients may benefit from adding bevacizumab to TMZ radiochemotherapy [18].

In elderly patients with poor performance status, supportive care is frequently a reasonable option. However, in some patients, TMZ chemotherapy may be an alternative. The French ANOCEF group performed a phase II non-randomized trial in this population [19]. Seventy patients older than 70 years old with poor KPS and a newly diagnosed GBM received TMZ (150–200 mg/m^2/day, 5 days every 28 days). Median PFS and OS were 3.5 and 5.5 months, respectively, comparing favourably with historic controls only treated with supportive care. It is of note that 33 % of patients presented an improvement in their KPS by 10 or more points and that overall quality of life and cognition improved over time. In addition, *MGMT* promoter methylation was associated with longer survival even though only 44 % of patients could be analysed. Treatment was generally well tolerated with toxicity rates similar to those observed in young patients with good performance status [19]. More recently, the ANOCEF group conducted a prospective phase II non-randomized trial in the same population to evaluate the benefit of adding bevacizumab to TMZ. This study confirmed the benefit of TMZ, yet the addition of bevacizumab did not seem to confer additional benefit [20].

Recurrent Glioblastoma Multiforme

In young patients with glioblastoma, there is no standard of care at recurrence. Treatment options include re-surgery, re-challenge with TMZ, bevacizumab and nitrosoureas. Yet inclusion of patients in clinical trials is highly recommended.

Currently, there is no evidence for re-irradiation, and cognition toxicity is a limitation factor. Different studies showed controversies regarding the benefit of re-surgery in patients with poor performance status [43, 80]. However, a new tumour sample can be of utility in order to confirm the diagnosis, rule out a possible radionecrosis or perform molecular analysis.

Concerning chemotherapy, TMZ is one potential option at the recurrence in patients who present *MGMT* methylation [7, 83] and firstly presented a good response. However, the best schedule of TMZ at the recurrence is not well defined [76]. Nitrosoureas (carmustine, lomustine, fotemustine) have been a classical treatment in GBM recurrences, and several reports describe their benefit [8, 60] despite their haematological toxicity. Bevacizumab in monotherapy presents a clinical activity; however, its impact on survival is not clear. Furthermore, the combination with nitrosoureas improves the PFS despite their benefit on OS has not yet been confirmed [71]. In addition, many new target agents have emerged, but their efficacy remains to be confirmed [63].

In elderly patients with GBM, as in younger patients, there is no standard of care. All cases should be discussed on multi-disciplinary meetings, and the decisions should be based on the performance status. The main options are RT or preferably chemotherapy with TMZ or bevacizumab because of their relative safety side effect profile. Re-surgery or re-irradiation is not a feasible option in this fragile population. When performance status is not optimal, supportive care should be considered as a first option.

8.2.1.6 Conclusion

The management of elderly patients with GBM has evolved over the time, and several treatment options have emerged in the last few years. As an example, in Lyon, the median survival of elderly patients with GBM increased from 3 to 6 months between 2004 and 2008 [5]. However, the best therapy should be selected considering the functional status of the patient. Regarding the controversy of maximal safe resection versus biopsy, some retrospectives studies and one prospective study support that resection of the tumour should be done when feasible. The optimal treatment after surgery or biopsy in patients with good performance status is accelerated

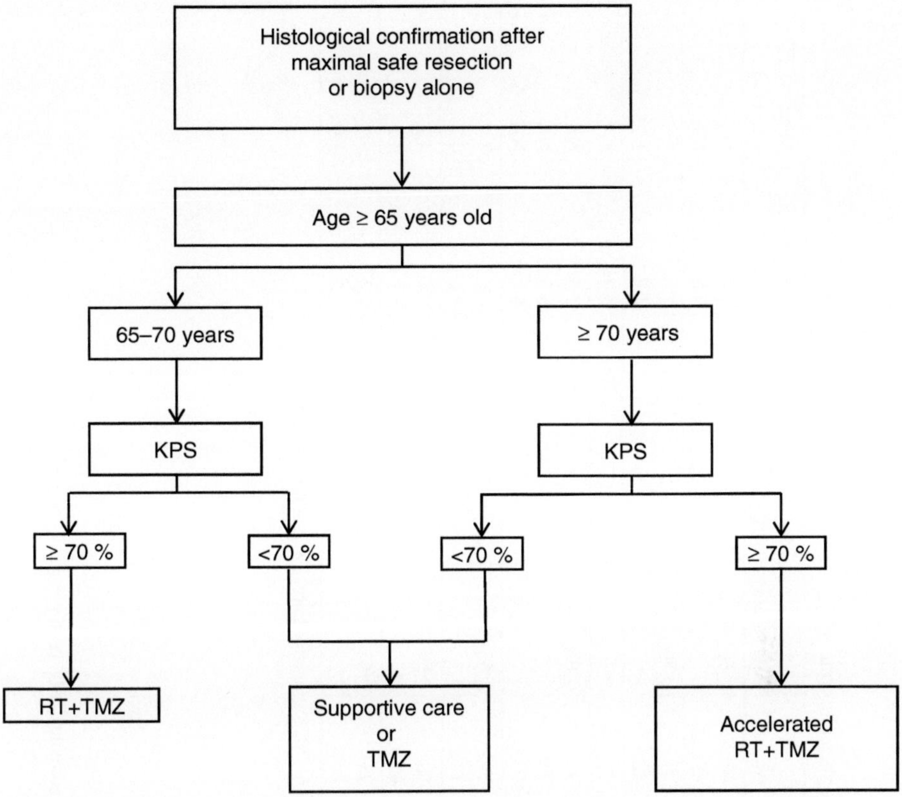

Fig. 8.2 Algorithm of treatment in newly diagnosed glioblastoma multiforme in elderly patients. *KPS* Karnofsky performance status, *RT* radiotherapy, *TMZ* temozolomide

RT/TMZ as recently shown in a large phase III trial. In some patients with poor performance status, TMZ may be an alternative to palliative care, especially in patients with a methylated *MGMT* promoter. However, the predictive impact of *MGMT* promoter methylation status in elderly patients still needs confirmation in prospective trials. An algorithm of treatment in these patients is proposed on Fig. 8.2. A summary of the main treatment studies in newly diagnosed GBM in the elderly population is also added (Table 8.1).

8.2.2 Anaplastic Gliomas

The exact incidence of anaplastic gliomas in elderly patients remains to be determined; however, they seem rare [48]. In young patients, anaplastic gliomas form a heterogeneous group of gliomas in terms of clinical, histological and molecular profiles. The survival times of patients range from a few years to more than 15 years [11]. This clinical heterogeneity reflects underlying molecular heterogeneity. From a

Table 8.1 Main studies of treatment in elderly patients with glioblastoma multiforme

Authors (Year)	Study design	Treatment	*N*	Age (years)	Median age (years)	KPS (%)	Median OS (months)	Median PFS (months)
Roa et al. [56]	Phase III	Standard RT[a] HypoRT[b]	47 48	≥60	72	≥50	5.1 5.6	NA NA
Keime-Guibert et al. [33]	Phase III	RT[c] SC	39 42	≥70	73	≥70	7.3 4.2	3.75 1.25
Gallego Perez-Larraya et al. [19]	Phase II	TMZ[d]	70	≥70	77	<70	6.25	4
Malmstrom et al. [40]	Phase III	HypoRT[e] TMZ[f] Standard RT[a]	98 93 100	≥65	70	≥60	7.5 8.3 6	NA NA NA
Wick et al. [78]	Phase III	TMZ[g] RT[a]	195 178	≥65	72	≥60	8.6 9.6	3.3 4.7
Roa et al. [57]	Phase III	HypoRT[b] Short-course RT[h]	50 48	≥50	NA	≥50	6.4 7.9	4.2 4.2
Perry et al. [50]	Phase III	HypoRT + TMZ[i] HypoRT[b]	281 281	≥65	73	≥70	9.3 7.6	5.3 3.9

RT radiotherapy, *NA* not available, *HypoRT* hypofractionated radiotherapy, *SC* supportive care, *TMZ* temozolomide

[a]60Gy/30fractions/6 weeks

[b]40Gy/15fractions/3weeks

[c]50Gy/28fractions/5–6weeks

[d]150–200 mg/m^2 per day for 5 days

[e]34Gy/10fractions/2weeks

[f]200mg/m^2per day for 5 days

[g]100mg/m^2 per day, for days 1–7 and 15–21

[h]26Gy/5fractions/1week

[i]40Gy/15fractions/weeks plus concomitant TMZ followed by monthly adjuvant TMZ until progression or 12 cycles

molecular point of view, three main subgroups can be distinguished based on two biomarkers, the 1p/19q co-deletion and the isocitrate dehydrogenase (IDH) mutation status. Gliomas with the 1p/19q co-deletion (which are virtually all IDH mutated) display the best prognosis [9]. The IDH-mutated gliomas, without 1p/19q co-deletion, have an intermediate prognosis. Finally, the non-1p/19q co-deleted and non-IDH-mutated gliomas have a poor prognosis. In younger patients, two randomized phase III studies have demonstrated that IDH-mutated patients (with or without 1p/19q co-deletion) benefit from adjuvant PCV chemotherapy in addition to RT which is not the case of patients without IDH mutation [10, 11, 74]. These patients have a prognosis close to that of GBM patients and are treated with TMZ radiochemotherapy.

In elderly patients, no prospective study has focused on anaplastic gliomas, and the rare retrospective studies in this population did not stratify patients according to the 1p/19q co-deletion and the IDH mutation [67]. IDH wild-type anaplastic gliomas in elderly patients should probably be treated like GBM patients. IDH-mutated anaplastic gliomas without 1p/19q co-deletion should probably receive RT plus adjuvant TMZ instead of PCV chemotherapy given (i) the potential toxicity of this regimen in patients over >70 years and (ii) the fact that TMZ may be equally effective as PCV even if this has not been formally demonstrated. In elderly patients with a 1p/19q co-deleted anaplastic glioma, chemotherapy only with TMZ may be

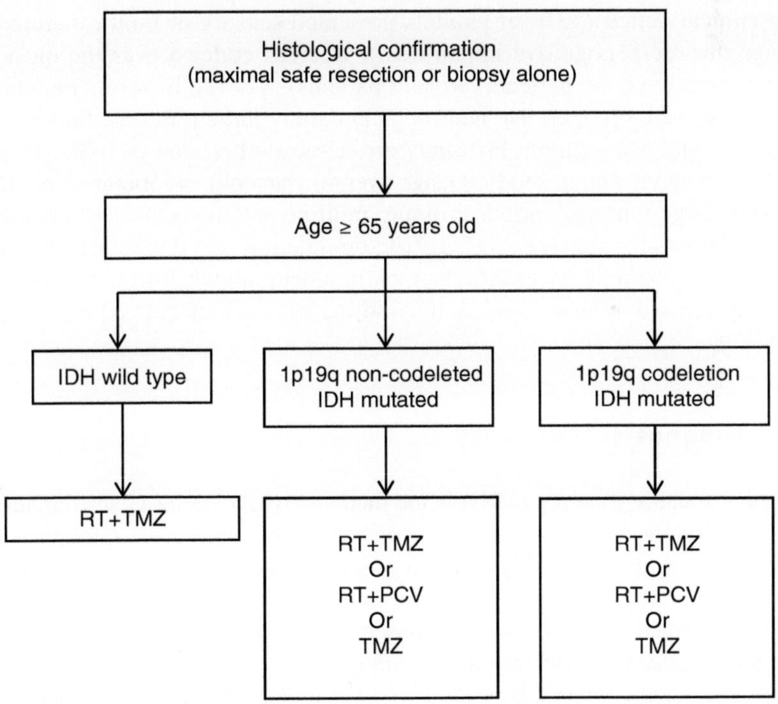

Fig. 8.3 Algorithm of treatment in newly diagnosed anaplastic gliomas in elderly patients. *IDH* isocitrate dehydrogenase, *RT* radiotherapy, *TMZ* temozolomide, *PCV* procarbazine, lomustine and vincristine

considered since these tumours are usually very chemosensitive [67]. A therapeutic algorithm is proposed on Fig. 8.3.

8.3 Low-Grade Gliomas

8.3.1 Epidemiology

LGG represent 15 % of all brain tumours in adults; the peak incidence occurs in people between 35 and 44 years old [51, 52]; nevertheless, nearly 8 % of LGG occur in patients of 60 years old [32]. However, this incidence may be underestimated because old patients are less likely to undergo surgery preventing histological confirmation of the diagnosis. The median OS in this population is shorter than in young population being around 3 years with a 5-year survival rate of 40 % [32, 52, 62].

8.3.2 Clinical Features and Prognostic Factors

Clinical manifestations in older population differ from their younger counterparts. A retrospective study identified that elderly patients presented more frequently with a clinical deficit (53 % of patients presented sensory or motor disturbances, language disorders, cognitive impairment), whereas epilepsy was the most common symptom in young patients (80 % of patients) [32, 51]. In young patients, age over 40 years old, preoperative neurological deficit, large tumours, tumour crossing midline and astrocytoma histology are associated related in LGG. In young patients with newly diagnosed LGG, age over 40 years old, preoperative neurological deficit, large tumour, tumour crossing midline and astrocytoma histology are pronostic factors for survival [51]. 1p/19q co-deletion and IDH mutation are also independent favourable prognostic factors. In older patients, astrocytic phenotype, increasing age and tumour crossing the midline were also negative prognostic factors [32].

8.3.3 Diagnosis

Magnetic resonance imaging (MRI) is the modality of choice for characterizing gliomas. These lesions are usually iso- or hypointense on T1 sequences and usually are confined to the white matter. T2 or FLAIR sequences show a hyperintensity lesion with a better delimitation of the lesion. They are commonly localized in supratentorial areas [52]. Contrast enhancement (CE) can be observed in up to 15 % of adults with LGG and is even more frequent in elderly population (44 %). However, it is mandatory to rule out an anaplastic glioma when CE is found. Furthermore, when a LGG is suspected in elderly population and despite the absence of CE, high-grade gliomas should be dismissed. Perfusion weighted imaging (PWI) may be an interesting tool in this setting [3, 37]. Conditions that may mimic an LGG in elderly patients are mostly stroke and pseudotumoural presentation of cerebral amyloid angiopathy-related inflammation. In most cases (85 %), this condition occurs in patients older than 60 years old presenting with cognitive impairment or focal deficits. The MRI demonstrates infiltrative white matter lesions with loco-regional mass effect, without contrast enhancement in most of cases and multiple microbleeds. Therefore, T2* sequences should be performed in elderly patients with a suspicion of LGG to rule out pseudotumoural presentation of cerebral amyloid angiopathy-related inflammation [58].

8.3.4 Treatment

8.3.4.1 Wait and See

Conservative management in young adults with LGG is characterized by a "wait and see" (WS) policy which consist in neuroimaging and clinical observation of those lesions that suggest LGG. Moreover, there is no evidence that early post-operative treatment is associated with improved survival [73]. Some authors suggest that for young patients with indolent LGG, the confirmation through stereotactic biopsy does not change the treatment; therefore, WS should be recommended [77]. When the lesion is surgically inaccessible or if the patients' symptoms are well controlled, WS could also be proposed. However, with this approach, there is a risk of tumour size increase.

In elderly patients, when an LGG lesion is suspected and the patient is practically asymptomatic, WS might be proposed as these tumours may have a very slow evolution.

8.3.4.2 Surgery

The surgery management of adults with LGG is controversial due to the lack of non-controlled studies. However, maximal safe resection is generally recommended in young patients.

Two recent large retrospectives studies in highly specialized centres support the benefit of early resection in the outcome of LGG and also highlight the minimal morbidity associated with surgery [30, 66]. There is evidence that awake craniotomy allows to perform more extensive safe resections [15, 59]. Noteworthy, histo-pathological diagnosis inconsistencies between surgery and biopsy have already been demonstrated, most especially in mixed gliomas with a low proliferation index [28, 46].

In elderly patients, there is no consensus on the optimal surgery management. Despite it is common to offer them biopsy or surgery without awake craniotomy, a recent report did not find significant differences in terms of perioperative mortality and morbidity when compared to young patients [23].

8.3.4.3 Radiotherapy

In adults, the role of adjuvant RT was investigated in the EORTC 22845 study, which compared early versus delayed RT. No differences between both groups in terms of OS were identified; however, PFS was higher in those patients firstly treated with RT at the expense of side effects [73]. Therefore, if the patient does not present risk factors, delay RT until progression is recommended.

In geriatric population, RT is one suitable treatment option. However, as neurotoxicity of RT increases with age, it would be recommendable to optimize the dose to minimize the incidence of side effects.

8.3.4.4 Chemo-Radiotherapy Treatment

In adult LGG patients, two randomized studies have addressed the question of the optimal treatment in patients who need another treatment than surgery: the RTOG 9802 and the EORTC 22033–26033 trials [64, 72]. Shaw et al. compared in the RTOG 9802 trial RT to RT with PCV. First results did not show any benefit on OS with the combined treatment despite an increase of PFS was identified. However, a further long-term follow-up concluded that patients with less than a gross total resection and older than 40 years presented a better outcome after treatment with PCV and RT [64, 72]. Nevertheless, information about the benefit on OS in LGG stratified by their molecular profile and histological type has not been yet provided. The EORTC 22033–26033 trial conducted by Baumert et al. was designed for patients with a bad prognostic profile in order to investigate the impact of temozolomide chemotherapy or RT on PFS and OS. No statistically significant difference between both treatments was observed for PFS, and OS was not reached. However, first molecular analyses showed that non-1p/19q co-deleted patients presented similar outcome when treated with RT or TMZ, while non-co-deleted patients presented better responses when treated with RT [72]. Survival analyses will require further maturation as well as more detailed molecular analyses. Based on the results of these two studies, RT plus PCV should be considered the standard of care for LGG who require postsurgical adjuvant treatment.

The best therapeutic option in elderly population with LGG who require another treatment than surgery is not defined. No prospective study has been performed. Based on the trials above commented, RT plus chemotherapy could be recommended for patients who conserve a good performance status. For those patients with lower KPS, especially if they present with a 1p/19q co-deleted glioma, TMZ chemotherapy could be a more interesting option because of its safety profile.

8.3.5 Conclusions

LGG in elderly patients are less frequent and present a worst outcome compared to younger patients. The clinical presentation and the radiological features also differ from the presentation in the young population. In patients with slowly progressive LGG who are asymptomatic or have been operated, WS and follow-up might be the best option. In symptomatic patients who require a treatment, it should be selected based on KPS and molecular profile. Figure 8.4 shows an algorithm of treatment in elderly population with LGG diagnosis.

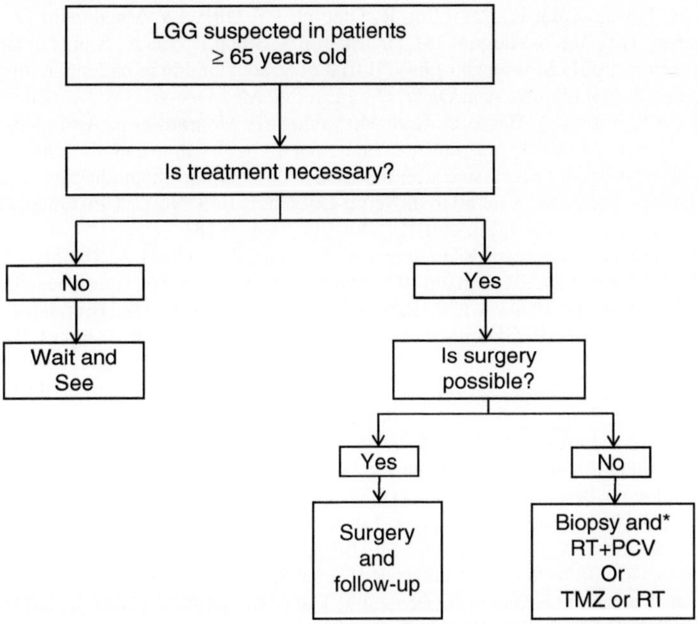

Fig. 8.4 Algorithm of treatment in newly diagnosed low-grade gliomas in elderly patients. *RT* radiotherapy, *TMZ* temozolomide, *PCV* Procarbazine, CCNU and Vincristine. *Patients should be treated acccording to their perfomance status and their molecular profile

Acknowledgement Cristina Izquierdo has been funded by La Fundación Alfonso Martín Escudero in the setting of a research grant.

References

1. Almeida JP, Chaichana KL, Rincon-Torroella J, Quinones-Hinojosa A (2015) The value of extent of resection of glioblastomas: clinical evidence and current approach. Curr Neurol Neurosci Rep 15(2):517. doi:10.1007/s11910-014-0517-x
2. Alvarez de Eulate-Beramendi S, Alvarez-Vega MA, Balbin M, Sanchez-Pitiot A, Vallina-Alvarez A, Martino-Gonzalez J (2016) Prognostic factors and survival study in high-grade glioma in the elderly. Br J Neurosurg 30(3):330–336. doi:10.3109/02688697.2016.1139049
3. Arvinda HR, Kesavadas C, Sarma PS, Thomas B, Radhakrishnan VV, Gupta AK, Kapilamoorthy TR, Nair S (2009) Glioma grading: sensitivity, specificity, positive and negative predictive values of diffusion and perfusion imaging. J Neurooncol 94(1):87–96. doi:10.1007/s11060-009-9807-6
4. Arvold ND, Reardon DA (2014) Treatment options and outcomes for glioblastoma in the elderly patient. Clin Interv Aging 9:357–367. doi:10.2147/CIA.S44259
5. Badaoui N, Meyronet D, Cartalat-Carel S, Guyotat J, Jouanneau E, d'Hombres A, Sunyach MP, Jouvet A, Louis-Tisserand G, Archinet A, Frappaz D, Bauchet L, Honnorat J, Ducray F (2014) Patterns of care and survival of glioblastoma patients: a comparative study between 2004 and 2008 in Lyon, France. Rev Neurol 170(3):222–227. doi:10.1016/j.neurol.2013.09.007
6. Balss J, Meyer J, Mueller W, Korshunov A, Hartmann C, von Deimling A (2008) Analysis of the IDH1 codon 132 mutation in brain tumors. Acta Neuropathol 116(6):597–602. doi:10.1007/s00401-008-0455-2

7. Brada M, Hoang-Xuan K, Rampling R, Dietrich PY, Dirix LY, Macdonald D, Heimans JJ, Zonnenberg BA, Bravo-Marques JM, Henriksson R, Stupp R, Yue N, Bruner J, Dugan M, Rao S, Zaknoen S (2001) Multicenter phase II trial of temozolomide in patients with glioblastoma multiforme at first relapse. Ann Oncol Off J Eur Soc Med Oncol/ESMO 12(2):259–266
8. Brandes AA, Tosoni A, Basso U, Reni M, Valduga F, Monfardini S, Amista P, Nicolardi L, Sotti G, Ermani M (2004) Second-line chemotherapy with irinotecan plus carmustine in glioblastoma recurrent or progressive after first-line temozolomide chemotherapy: a phase II study of the Gruppo Italiano Cooperativo di Neuro-Oncologia (GICNO). J Clin Oncol Off J Am Soc Clin Oncol 22(23):4779–4786. doi:10.1200/JCO.2004.06.181
9. Brat DJ, Verhaak RG, Aldape KD, Yung WK, Salama SR, Cooper LA, Rheinbay E, Miller CR, Vitucci M, Morozova O, Robertson AG, Noushmehr H, Laird PW, Cherniack AD, Akbani R, Huse JT, Ciriello G, Poisson LM, Barnholtz-Sloan JS, Berger MS, Brennan C, Colen RR, Colman H, Flanders AE, Giannini C, Grifford M, Iavarone A, Jain R, Joseph I, Kim J, Kasaian K, Mikkelsen T, Murray BA, O'Neill BP, Pachter L, Parsons DW, Sougnez C, Sulman EP, Vandenberg SR, Van Meir EG, von Deimling A, Zhang H, Crain D, Lau K, Mallery D, Morris S, Paulauskis J, Penny R, Shelton T, Sherman M, Yena P, Black A, Bowen J, Dicostanzo K, Gastier-Foster J, Leraas KM, Lichtenberg TM, Pierson CR, Ramirez NC, Taylor C, Weaver S, Wise L, Zmuda E, Davidsen T, Demchok JA, Eley G, Ferguson ML, Hutter CM, Mills Shaw KR, Ozenberger BA, Sheth M, Sofia HJ, Tarnuzzer R, Wang Z, Yang L, Zenklusen JC, Ayala B, Baboud J, Chudamani S, Jensen MA, Liu J, Pihl T, Raman R, Wan Y, Wu Y, Ally A, Auman JT, Balasundaram M, Balu S, Baylin SB, Beroukhim R, Bootwalla MS, Bowlby R, Bristow CA, Brooks D, Butterfield Y, Carlsen R, Carter S, Chin L, Chu A, Chuah E, Cibulskis K, Clarke A, Coetzee SG, Dhalla N, Fennell T, Fisher S, Gabriel S, Getz G, Gibbs R, Guin R, Hadjipanayis A, Hayes DN, Hinoue T, Hoadley K, Holt RA, Hoyle AP, Jefferys SR, Jones S, Jones CD, Kucherlapati R, Lai PH, Lander E, Lee S, Lichtenstein L, Ma Y, Maglinte DT, Mahadeshwar HS, Marra MA, Mayo M, Meng S, Meyerson ML, Mieczkowski PA, Moore RA, Mose LE, Mungall AJ, Pantazi A, Parfenov M, Park PJ, Parker JS, Perou CM, Protopopov A, Ren X, Roach J, Sabedot TS, Schein J, Schumacher SE, Seidman JG, Seth S, Shen H, Simons JV, Sipahimalani P, Soloway MG, Song X, Sun H, Tabak B, Tam A, Tan D, Tang J, Thiessen N, Triche T Jr, Van Den Berg DJ, Veluvolu U, Waring S, Weisenberger DJ, Wilkerson MD, Wong T, Wu J, Xi L, Xu AW, Zack TI, Zhang J, Aksoy BA, Arachchi H, Benz C, Bernard B, Carlin D, Cho J, DiCara D, Frazer S, Fuller GN, Gao J, Gehlenborg N, Haussler D, Heiman DI, Iype L, Jacobsen A, Ju Z, Katzman S, Kim H, Knijnenburg T, Kreisberg RB, Lawrence MS, Lee W, Leinonen K, Lin P, Ling S, Liu W, Liu Y, Lu Y, Mills G, Ng S, Noble MS, Paull E, Rao A, Reynolds S, Saksena G, Sanborn Z, Sander C, Schultz N, Senbabaoglu Y, Shen R, Shmulevich I, Sinha R, Stuart J, Sumer SO, Sun Y, Tasman N, Taylor BS, Voet D, Weinhold N, Weinstein JN, Yang D, Yoshihara K, Zheng S, Zhang W, Zou L, Abel T, Sadeghi S, Cohen ML, Eschbacher J, Hattab EM, Raghunathan A, Schniederjan MJ, Aziz D, Barnett G, Barrett W, Bigner DD, Boice L, Brewer C, Calatozzolo C, Campos B, Carlotti CG Jr, Chan TA, Cuppini L, Curley E, Cuzzubbo S, Devine K, DiMeco F, Duell R, Elder JB, Fehrenbach A, Finocchiaro G, Friedman W, Fulop J, Gardner J, Hermes B, Herold-Mende C, Jungk C, Kendler A, Lehman NL, Lipp E, Liu O, Mandt R, McGraw M, McLendon R, McPherson C, Neder L, Nguyen P, Noss A, Nunziata R, Ostrom QT, Palmer C, Perin A, Pollo B, Potapov A, Potapova O, Rathmell WK, Rotin D, Scarpace L, Schilero C, Senecal K, Shimmel K, Shurkhay V, Sifri S, Singh R, Sloan AE, Smolenski K, Staugaitis SM, Steele R, Thorne L, Tirapelli DP, Unterberg A, Vallurupalli M, Wang Y, Warnick R, Williams F, Wolinsky Y, Bell S, Rosenberg M, Stewart C, Huang F, Grimsby JL, Radenbaugh AJ (2015) Comprehensive, integrative genomic analysis of diffuse lower-grade gliomas. N Engl J Med 372(26):2481–2498. doi:10.1056/NEJMoa1402121
10. Cairncross G, Wang M, Shaw E, Jenkins R, Brachman D, Buckner J, Fink K, Souhami L, Laperriere N, Curran W, Mehta M (2013) Phase III trial of chemoradiotherapy for anaplastic oligodendroglioma: long-term results of RTOG 9402. J Clin Oncol Off J Am Soc Clin Oncol 31(3):337–343. doi:10.1200/JCO.2012.43.2674
11. Cairncross JG, Wang M, Jenkins RB, Shaw EG, Giannini C, Brachman DG, Buckner JC, Fink KL, Souhami L, Laperriere NJ, Huse JT, Mehta MP, Curran WJ Jr (2014) Benefit from

procarbazine, lomustine, and vincristine in oligodendroglial tumors is associated with mutation of IDH. J Clin Oncol Off J Am Soc Clin Oncol 32(8):783–790. doi:10.1200/JCO.2013.49.3726
12. Chaichana KL, Garzon-Muvdi T, Parker S, Weingart JD, Olivi A, Bennett R, Brem H, Quinones-Hinojosa A (2011) Supratentorial glioblastoma multiforme: the role of surgical resection versus biopsy among older patients. Ann Surg Oncol 18(1):239–245. doi:10.1245/s10434-010-1242-6
13. Chaichana KL, Halthore AN, Parker SL, Olivi A, Weingart JD, Brem H, Quinones-Hinojosa A (2011) Factors involved in maintaining prolonged functional independence following supratentorial glioblastoma resection. Clinical article. J Neurosurg 114(3):604–612. doi:10.3171/2010.4.JNS091340
14. Chaichana KL, Martinez-Gutierrez JC, De la Garza-Ramos R, Weingart JD, Olivi A, Gallia GL, Lim M, Brem H, Quinones-Hinojosa A (2013) Factors associated with survival for patients with glioblastoma with poor pre-operative functional status. J Clin Neurosci Off J Neurosurg Soc Australasia 20(6):818–823. doi:10.1016/j.jocn.2012.07.016
15. De Benedictis A, Moritz-Gasser S, Duffau H (2010) Awake mapping optimizes the extent of resection for low-grade gliomas in eloquent areas. Neurosurgery 66(6):1074–1084. doi:10.1227/01.NEU.0000369514.74284.78; discussion 1084
16. Esteller M, Toyota M, Sanchez-Cespedes M, Capella G, Peinado MA, Watkins DN, Issa JP, Sidransky D, Baylin SB, Herman JG (2000) Inactivation of the DNA repair gene O6-methylguanine-DNA methyltransferase by promoter hypermethylation is associated with G to A mutations in K-ras in colorectal tumorigenesis. Cancer Res 60(9):2368–2371
17. Gallego Perez-Larraya J, Delattre JY (2014) Management of elderly patients with gliomas. Oncologist 19(12):1258–1267. doi:10.1634/theoncologist.2014-0170
18. Gallego Perez-Larraya J, Ducray F (2014) Treating glioblastoma patients with poor performance status: where do we go from here? CNS Oncol 3(3):231–241. doi:10.2217/cns.14.20
19. Gallego Perez-Larraya J, Ducray F, Chinot O, Catry-Thomas I, Taillandier L, Guillamo JS, Campello C, Monjour A, Cartalat-Carel S, Barrie M, Huchet A, Beauchesne P, Matta M, Mokhtari K, Tanguy ML, Honnorat J, Delattre JY (2011) Temozolomide in elderly patients with newly diagnosed glioblastoma and poor performance status: an ANOCEF phase II trial. J Clin Oncol Off J Am Soc Clin Oncol 29(22):3050–3055. doi:10.1200/JCO.2011.34.8086
20. German Reyes-Botero JH, Chinot OL, Taillandier L, Catry-Thomas I, Barriere J, Guillamo JS, Fabbro M, Frappaz D, Amiel AB, Rhun EL, Campello C, Tennevet I, Ghiringhelli F, Tanguy M-L, Mokhtari K, Delattre J-Y, ANOCEF: Association des Neuro-Oncologues d'Expression Française; Service de Neurologie 2-Mazarin, Groupe Hospitalier Pitié-Salpêtrière, Paris, France; Hopital Pierre Wertheimer, Lyon, France; Centre Hospitalier Universitaire La Timone, Marseille, France; Centre Hospitalier Universitaire Nancy, Nancy, France; Hopital Saint-Andre CHU, Bordeaux, France; Centre Antoine Lacassagne, Nice, France; Centre Hospitalier Universitaire Caen, Caen, France; Centre Val d'Aurelle, Montpellier, France; Centre Léon Bérard, Lyon, France; Centre Hospitalier Universitaire Rangueil, Toulouse, France; Centre Oscar Lambret, Lille, France; Centre Hospitalier Universitaire Nimes, Nimes, France; Centre Henri Becquerel CLCC, Rouen, France; Georges-François Leclerc Cancer Center, Dijon, France; APHP-CHU Pitié-Salpêtrière, Paris, France; Hôpital Pitié-Salpêtrière, Paris, France; Pitie-Salpetriere Hospital-Pierre et Marie Curie Paris VI University, Paris, France (2013) Temozolomide plus bevacizumab in elderly patients with newly diagnosed glioblastoma and poor performance status: an Anocef phase II trial. J Clin Oncol 30:abstr 2020
21. Glantz M, Chamberlain M, Liu Q, Litofsky NS, Recht LD (2003) Temozolomide as an alternative to irradiation for elderly patients with newly diagnosed malignant gliomas. Cancer 97(9):2262–2266. doi:10.1002/cncr.11323
22. Graus F, Bruna J, Pardo J, Escudero D, Vilas D, Barcelo I, Brell M, Pascual C, Crespo JA, Erro E, Garcia-Romero JC, Estela J, Martino J, Garcia-Castano A, Mata E, Lema M, Gelabert M, Fuentes R, Perez P, Manzano A, Aguas J, Belenguer A, Simon A, Henriquez I, Murcia M, Vivanco R, Rojas-Marcos I, Munoz-Carmona D, Navas I, de Andres P, Mas G, Gil M, Verger E (2013) Patterns of care and outcome for patients with glioblastoma diagnosed during 2008–2010 in Spain. Neuro Oncol 15(6):797–805. doi:10.1093/neuonc/not013

23. Grossman R, Nossek E, Sitt R, Hayat D, Shahar T, Barzilai O, Gonen T, Korn A, Sela G, Ram Z (2013) Outcome of elderly patients undergoing awake-craniotomy for tumor resection. Ann Surg Oncol 20(5):1722–1728. doi:10.1245/s10434-012-2748-x
24. Hartmann C, Hentschel B, Wick W, Capper D, Felsberg J, Simon M, Westphal M, Schackert G, Meyermann R, Pietsch T, Reifenberger G, Weller M, Loeffler M, von Deimling A (2010) Patients with IDH1 wild type anaplastic astrocytomas exhibit worse prognosis than IDH1-mutated glioblastomas, and IDH1 mutation status accounts for the unfavorable prognostic effect of higher age: implications for classification of gliomas. Acta Neuropathol 120(6):707–718. doi:10.1007/s00401-010-0781-z
25. Hegi ME, Diserens AC, Gorlia T, Hamou MF, de Tribolet N, Weller M, Kros JM, Hainfellner JA, Mason W, Mariani L, Bromberg JE, Hau P, Mirimanoff RO, Cairncross JG, Janzer RC, Stupp R (2005) MGMT gene silencing and benefit from temozolomide in glioblastoma. N Engl J Med 352(10):997–1003. doi:10.1056/NEJMoa043331
26. Iwamoto FM, Reiner AS, Panageas KS, Elkin EB, Abrey LE (2008) Patterns of care in elderly glioblastoma patients. Ann Neurol 64(6):628–634. doi:10.1002/ana.21521
27. Jabehdar Maralani P, Melhem ER, Wang S, Herskovits EH, Voluck MR, Kim SJ, Learned KO, O'Rourke DM, Mohan S (2015) Association of dynamic susceptibility contrast enhanced MR Perfusion parameters with prognosis in elderly patients with glioblastomas. Eur Radiol 25(9):2738–2744. doi:10.1007/s00330-015-3640-4
28. Jackson RJ, Fuller GN, Abi-Said D, Lang FF, Gokaslan ZL, Shi WM, Wildrick DM, Sawaya R (2001) Limitations of stereotactic biopsy in the initial management of gliomas. Neuro Oncol 3(3):193–200
29. Jain R, Gutierrez J, Narang J, Scarpace L, Schultz LR, Lemke N, Patel SC, Mikkelsen T, Rock JP (2011) In vivo correlation of tumor blood volume and permeability with histologic and molecular angiogenic markers in gliomas. AJNR Am J Neuroradiol 32(2):388–394. doi:10.3174/ajnr.A2280
30. Jakola AS, Myrmel KS, Kloster R, Torp SH, Lindal S, Unsgard G, Solheim O (2012) Comparison of a strategy favoring early surgical resection vs a strategy favoring watchful waiting in low-grade gliomas. JAMA 308(18):1881–1888. doi:10.1001/jama.2012.12807
31. Jordan JT, Gerstner ER, Batchelor TT, Cahill DP, Plotkin SR (2016) Glioblastoma care in the elderly. Cancer 122(2):189–197. doi:10.1002/cncr.29742
32. Kaloshi G, Psimaras D, Mokhtari K, Dehais C, Houillier C, Marie Y, Laigle-Donadey F, Taillibert S, Guillevin R, Martin-Duverneuil N, Sanson M, Hoang-Xuan K, Delattre JY (2009) Supratentorial low-grade gliomas in older patients. Neurology 73(24):2093–2098. doi:10.1212/WNL.0b013e3181c6781e
33. Keime-Guibert F, Chinot O, Taillandier L, Cartalat-Carel S, Frenay M, Kantor G, Guillamo JS, Jadaud E, Colin P, Bondiau PY, Menei P, Loiseau H, Bernier V, Honnorat J, Barrie M, Mokhtari K, Mazeron JJ, Bissery A, Delattre JY (2007) Radiotherapy for glioblastoma in the elderly. N Engl J Med 356(15):1527–1535. doi:10.1056/NEJMoa065901
34. Konglund A, Helseth R, Lund-Johansen M, Helseth E, Meling TR (2013) Surgery for high-grade gliomas in the aging. Acta Neurol Scand 128(3):185–193. doi:10.1111/ane.12105
35. Laigle-Donadey F, Figarella-Branger D, Chinot O, Taillandier L, Cartalat-Carel S, Honnorat J, Kaloshi G, Delattre JY, Sanson M (2010) Up-front temozolomide in elderly patients with glioblastoma. J Neurooncol 99(1):89–94. doi:10.1007/s11060-009-0110-3
36. Laperriere N, Weller M, Stupp R, Perry JR, Brandes AA, Wick W, van den Bent MJ (2013) Optimal management of elderly patients with glioblastoma. Cancer Treat Rev 39(4):350–357. doi:10.1016/j.ctrv.2012.05.008
37. Law M, Yang S, Wang H, Babb JS, Johnson G, Cha S, Knopp EA, Zagzag D (2003) Glioma grading: sensitivity, specificity, and predictive values of perfusion MR imaging and proton MR spectroscopic imaging compared with conventional MR imaging. AJNR Am J Neuroradiol 24(10):1989–1998
38. Louis DN, Ohgaki H, Wiestler OD, Cavenee WK, Burger PC, Jouvet A, Scheithauer BW, Kleihues P (2007) The 2007 WHO classification of tumours of the central nervous system. Acta Neuropathol 114(2):97–109. doi:10.1007/s00401-007-0243-4

39. Lowry JK, Snyder JJ, Lowry PW (1998) Brain tumors in the elderly: recent trends in a Minnesota cohort study. Arch Neurol 55(7):922–928
40. Malmstrom A, Gronberg BH, Marosi C, Stupp R, Frappaz D, Schultz H, Abacioglu U, Tavelin B, Lhermitte B, Hegi ME, Rosell J, Henriksson R (2012) Temozolomide versus standard 6-week radiotherapy versus hypofractionated radiotherapy in patients older than 60 years with glioblastoma: the Nordic randomised, phase 3 trial. Lancet Oncol 13(9):916–926. doi:10.1016/S1470-2045(12)70265-6
41. Mandonnet E, De Witt HP, Poisson I, Whittle I, Bernat AL, Bresson D, Madadaki C, Bouazza S, Ursu R, Carpentier AF, George B, Froelich S (2015) Initial experience using awake surgery for glioma: oncological, functional, and employment outcomes in a consecutive series of 25 cases. Neurosurgery 76(4):382–389. doi:10.1227/NEU.0000000000000644; discussion 389
42. Marko NF, Weil RJ, Schroeder JL, Lang FF, Suki D, Sawaya RE (2014) Extent of resection of glioblastoma revisited: personalized survival modeling facilitates more accurate survival prediction and supports a maximum-safe-resection approach to surgery. J Clin Oncol Off J Am Soc Clin Oncol 32(8):774–782. doi:10.1200/JCO.2013.51.8886
43. McNamara MG, Lwin Z, Jiang H, Templeton AJ, Zadeh G, Bernstein M, Chung C, Millar BA, Laperriere N, Mason WP (2014) Factors impacting survival following second surgery in patients with glioblastoma in the temozolomide treatment era, incorporating neutrophil/lymphocyte ratio and time to first progression. J Neurooncol 117(1):147–152. doi:10.1007/s11060-014-1366-9
44. Minniti G, De Sanctis V, Muni R, Filippone F, Bozzao A, Valeriani M, Osti MF, De Paula U, Lanzetta G, Tombolini V, Maurizi Enrici R (2008) Radiotherapy plus concomitant and adjuvant temozolomide for glioblastoma in elderly patients. J Neurooncol 88(1):97–103. doi:10.1007/s11060-008-9538-0
45. Minniti G, Scaringi C, Lanzetta G, Terrenato I, Esposito V, Arcella A, Pace A, Giangaspero F, Bozzao A, Enrici RM (2015) Standard (60 Gy) or short-course (40 Gy) irradiation plus concomitant and adjuvant temozolomide for elderly patients with glioblastoma: a propensity-matched analysis. Int J Radiat Oncol Biol Phys 91(1):109–115. doi:10.1016/j.ijrobp.2014.09.013
46. Muragaki Y, Chernov M, Maruyama T, Ochiai T, Taira T, Kubo O, Nakamura R, Iseki H, Hori T, Takakura K (2008) Low-grade glioma on stereotactic biopsy: how often is the diagnosis accurate? Minim Invasive Neurosurg 51(5):275–279. doi:10.1055/s-0028-1082322
47. Omuro AM, Leite CC, Mokhtari K, Delattre JY (2006) Pitfalls in the diagnosis of brain tumours. Lancet Neurol 5(11):937–948. doi:10.1016/S1474-4422(06)70597-X
48. Ostrom QT, Gittleman H, Fulop J, Liu M, Blanda R, Kromer C, Wolinsky Y, Kruchko C, Barnholtz-Sloan JS (2015) CBTRUS Statistical Report: primary brain and central nervous system tumors diagnosed in the United States in 2008–2012. Neuro Oncol 17 Suppl 4:iv1–iv62. doi:10.1093/neuonc/nov189
49. Oszvald A, Guresir E, Setzer M, Vatter H, Senft C, Seifert V, Franz K (2012) Glioblastoma therapy in the elderly and the importance of the extent of resection regardless of age. J Neurosurg 116(2):357–364. doi:10.3171/2011.8.JNS102114
50. Perry JR, Laperriere N, O'Callaghan CJ, Brandes A, Menten J, Phillips C, Fay MF, Nishikawa R, Cairncross GJ, Roa W, Osoba D, Sahgal A, Hirte H, Wick W, Laigle-Donadey F, Franceschi E, Chinot O, Winch C, Ding K, Mason WP (2016) A phase III randomized controlled trial of short-course radiotherapy with or without concomitant and adjuvant temozolomide in elderly patients with glioblastoma. J Clin Oncol 34, 2016 (suppl; abstr LBA2)
51. Pignatti F, van den Bent M, Curran D, Debruyne C, Sylvester R, Therasse P, Afra D, Cornu P, Bolla M, Vecht C, Karim AB (2002) Prognostic factors for survival in adult patients with cerebral low-grade glioma. J Clin Oncol Off J Am Soc Clin Oncol 20(8):2076–2084
52. Pouratian N, Mut M, Jagannathan J, Lopes MB, Shaffrey ME, Schiff D (2008) Low-grade gliomas in older patients: a retrospective analysis of prognostic factors. J Neurooncol 90(3):341–350. doi:10.1007/s11060-008-9669-3
53. Quillien V, Lavenu A, Karayan-Tapon L, Carpentier C, Labussiere M, Lesimple T, Chinot O, Wager M, Honnorat J, Saikali S, Fina F, Sanson M, Figarella-Branger D (2012) Comparative

assessment of 5 methods (methylation-specific polymerase chain reaction, MethyLight, pyrosequencing, methylation-sensitive high-resolution melting, and immunohistochemistry) to analyze O6-methylguanine-DNA-methyltranferase in a series of 100 glioblastoma patients. Cancer 118(17):4201–4211. doi:10.1002/cncr.27392

54. Rampling R, Erridge S (2014) Management of central nervous system tumours in the elderly. Clin Oncol (R Coll Radiol) 26(7):431–437. doi:10.1016/j.clon.2014.03.009
55. Raysi Dehcordi S, De Paulis D, Marzi S, Ricci A, Cimini A, Cifone MG, Galzio RJ (2012) Survival prognostic factors in patients with glioblastoma: our experience. J Neurosurg Sci 56(3):239–245
56. Roa W, Brasher PM, Bauman G, Anthes M, Bruera E, Chan A, Fisher B, Fulton D, Gulavita S, Hao C, Husain S, Murtha A, Petruk K, Stewart D, Tai P, Urtasun R, Cairncross JG, Forsyth P (2004) Abbreviated course of radiation therapy in older patients with glioblastoma multiforme: a prospective randomized clinical trial. J Clin Oncol Off J Am Soc Clin Oncol 22(9):1583–1588. doi:10.1200/JCO.2004.06.082
57. Roa W, Kepka L, Kumar N, Sinaika V, Matiello J, Lomidze D, Hentati D, Guedes de Castro D, Dyttus-Cebulok K, Drodge S, Ghosh S, Jeremic B, Rosenblatt E, Fidarova E (2015) International Atomic Energy Agency randomized phase III study of radiation therapy in elderly and/or frail patients with newly diagnosed glioblastoma multiforme. J Clin Oncol Off J Am Soc Clin Oncol 33(35):4145–4150. doi:10.1200/JCO.2015.62.6606
58. Ronsin S, Deiana G, Geraldo AF, Durand-Dubief F, Thomas-Maisonneuve L, Formaglio M, Desestret V, Meyronet D, Nighoghossian N, Berthezene Y, Honnorat J, Ducray F (2016) Pseudotumoral presentation of cerebral amyloid angiopathy-related inflammation. Neurology. doi:10.1212/WNL.0000000000002444
59. Sacko O, Lauwers-Cances V, Brauge D, Sesay M, Brenner A, Roux FE (2011) Awake craniotomy vs surgery under general anesthesia for resection of supratentorial lesions. Neurosurgery 68(5):1192–1198. doi:10.1227/NEU.0b013e31820c02a3; discussion 1198–1199
60. Scoccianti S, Detti B, Sardaro A, Iannalfi A, Meattini I, Leonulli BG, Borghesi S, Martinelli F, Bordi L, Ammannati F, Biti G (2008) Second-line chemotherapy with fotemustine in temozolomide-pretreated patients with relapsing glioblastoma: a single institution experience. Anticancer Drugs 19(6):613–620. doi:10.1097/CAD.0b013e3283005075
61. Scott JN, Brasher PM, Sevick RJ, Rewcastle NB, Forsyth PA (2002) How often are nonenhancing supratentorial gliomas malignant? A population study. Neurology 59(6):947–949
62. Schomas DA, Laack NN, Brown PD (2009) Low-grade gliomas in older patients: long-term follow-up from Mayo Clinic. Cancer 115(17):3969–3978. doi:10.1002/cncr.24444
63. Seystahl K, Wick W, Weller M (2016) Therapeutic options in recurrent glioblastoma-An update. Crit Rev Oncol Hematol 99:389–408. doi:10.1016/j.critrevonc.2016.01.018
64. Shaw EG, Wang M, Coons SW, Brachman DG, Buckner JC, Stelzer KJ, Barger GR, Brown PD, Gilbert MR, Mehta MP (2012) Randomized trial of radiation therapy plus procarbazine, lomustine, and vincristine chemotherapy for supratentorial adult low-grade glioma: initial results of RTOG 9802. J Clin Oncol Off J Am Soc Clin Oncol 30(25):3065–3070. doi:10.1200/JCO.2011.35.8598
65. Simpson JR, Horton J, Scott C, Curran WJ, Rubin P, Fischbach J, Isaacson S, Rotman M, Asbell SO, Nelson JS et al (1993) Influence of location and extent of surgical resection on survival of patients with glioblastoma multiforme: results of three consecutive Radiation Therapy Oncology Group (RTOG) clinical trials. Int J Radiat Oncol Biol Phys 26(2):239–244
66. Smith JS, Chang EF, Lamborn KR, Chang SM, Prados MD, Cha S, Tihan T, Vandenberg S, McDermott MW, Berger MS (2008) Role of extent of resection in the long-term outcome of low-grade hemispheric gliomas. J Clin Oncol Off J Am Soc Clin Oncol 26(8):1338–1345. doi:10.1200/JCO.2007.13.9337
67. Strowd RE, Abuali I, Ye X, Lu Y, Grossman SA (2016) The role of temozolomide in the management of patients with newly diagnosed anaplastic astrocytoma: a comparison of survival in the era prior to and following the availability of temozolomide. J Neurooncol 127(1):165–171. doi:10.1007/s11060-015-2028-2

68. Stummer W, Pichlmeier U, Meinel T, Wiestler OD, Zanella F, Reulen HJ (2006) Fluorescence-guided surgery with 5-aminolevulinic acid for resection of malignant glioma: a randomised controlled multicentre phase III trial. Lancet Oncol 7(5):392–401. doi:10.1016/S1470-2045(06)70665-9
69. Stupp R, Hegi ME, Mason WP, van den Bent MJ, Taphoorn MJ, Janzer RC, Ludwin SK, Allgeier A, Fisher B, Belanger K, Hau P, Brandes AA, Gijtenbeek J, Marosi C, Vecht CJ, Mokhtari K, Wesseling P, Villa S, Eisenhauer E, Gorlia T, Weller M, Lacombe D, Cairncross JG, Mirimanoff RO (2009) Effects of radiotherapy with concomitant and adjuvant temozolomide versus radiotherapy alone on survival in glioblastoma in a randomised phase III study: 5-year analysis of the EORTC-NCIC trial. Lancet Oncol 10(5):459–466. doi:10.1016/S1470-2045(09)70025-7
70. Stupp R, Mason WP, van den Bent MJ, Weller M, Fisher B, Taphoorn MJ, Belanger K, Brandes AA, Marosi C, Bogdahn U, Curschmann J, Janzer RC, Ludwin SK, Gorlia T, Allgeier A, Lacombe D, Cairncross JG, Eisenhauer E, Mirimanoff RO (2005) Radiotherapy plus concomitant and adjuvant temozolomide for glioblastoma. N Engl J Med 352(10):987–996. doi:10.1056/NEJMoa043330
71. Taal W, Oosterkamp HM, Walenkamp AM, Dubbink HJ, Beerepoot LV, Hanse MC, Buter J, Honkoop AH, Boerman D, de Vos FY, Dinjens WN, Enting RH, Taphoorn MJ, van den Berkmortel FW, Jansen RL, Brandsma D, Bromberg JE, van Heuvel I, Vernhout RM, van der Holt B, van den Bent MJ (2014) Single-agent bevacizumab or lomustine versus a combination of bevacizumab plus lomustine in patients with recurrent glioblastoma (BELOB trial): a randomised controlled phase 2 trial. Lancet Oncol 15(9):943–953. doi:10.1016/S1470-2045(14)70314-6
72. van den Bent MJ (2015) Chemotherapy for low-grade glioma: when, for whom, which regimen? Curr Opin Neurol 28(6):633–938. doi:10.1097/WCO.0000000000000257
73. van den Bent MJ, Afra D, de Witte O, Ben Hassel M, Schraub S, Hoang-Xuan K, Malmstrom PO, Collette L, Pierart M, Mirimanoff R, Karim AB (2005) Long-term efficacy of early versus delayed radiotherapy for low-grade astrocytoma and oligodendroglioma in adults: the EORTC 22845 randomised trial. Lancet 366(9490):985–990. doi:10.1016/S0140-6736(05)67070-5
74. van den Bent MJ, Brandes AA, Taphoorn MJ, Kros JM, Kouwenhoven MC, Delattre JY, Bernsen HJ, Frenay M, Tijssen CC, Grisold W, Sipos L, Enting RH, French PJ, Dinjens WN, Vecht CJ, Allgeier A, Lacombe D, Gorlia T, Hoang-Xuan K (2013) Adjuvant procarbazine, lomustine, and vincristine chemotherapy in newly diagnosed anaplastic oligodendroglioma: long-term follow-up of EORTC brain tumor group study 26951. J Clin Oncol Off J Am Soc Clin Oncol 31(3):344–350. doi:10.1200/JCO.2012.43.2229
75. Vuorinen V, Hinkka S, Farkkila M, Jaaskelainen J (2003) Debulking or biopsy of malignant glioma in elderly people - a randomised study. Acta Neurochir 145(1):5–10. doi:10.1007/s00701-002-1030-6
76. Weller M, Tabatabai G, Kastner B, Felsberg J, Steinbach JP, Wick A, Schnell O, Hau P, Herrlinger U, Sabel MC, Wirsching HG, Ketter R, Bahr O, Platten M, Tonn JC, Schlegel U, Marosi C, Goldbrunner R, Stupp R, Homicsko K, Pichler J, Nikkhah G, Meixensberger J, Vajkoczy P, Kollias S, Husing J, Reifenberger G, Wick W (2015) MGMT promoter methylation is a strong prognostic biomarker for benefit from dose-intensified temozolomide rechallenge in progressive glioblastoma: the DIRECTOR trial. Clin Cancer Res Off J Am Assoc Cancer Res 21(9):2057–2064. doi:10.1158/1078-0432.CCR-14-2737
77. Wessels PH, Weber WE, Raven G, Ramaekers FC, Hopman AH, Twijnstra A (2003) Supratentorial grade II astrocytoma: biological features and clinical course. Lancet Neurol 2(7):395–403
78. Wick W, Platten M, Meisner C, Felsberg J, Tabatabai G, Simon M, Nikkhah G, Papsdorf K, Steinbach JP, Sabel M, Combs SE, Vesper J, Braun C, Meixensberger J, Ketter R, Mayer-Steinacker R, Reifenberger G, Weller M (2012) Temozolomide chemotherapy alone versus radiotherapy alone for malignant astrocytoma in the elderly: the NOA-08 randomised, phase 3 trial. Lancet Oncol 13(7):707–715. doi:10.1016/S1470-2045(12)70164-X
79. Wiestler B, Claus R, Hartlieb SA, Schliesser MG, Weiss EK, Hielscher T, Platten M, Dittmann LM, Meisner C, Felsberg J, Happold C, Simon M, Nikkhah G, Papsdorf K, Steinbach JP, Sabel

M, Grimm C, Weichenhan D, Tews B, Reifenberger G, Capper D, Muller W, Plass C, Weller M, Wick W (2013) Malignant astrocytomas of elderly patients lack favorable molecular markers: an analysis of the NOA-08 study collective. Neuro Oncol 15(8):1017–1026. doi:10.1093/neuonc/not043
80. Woernle CM, Peus D, Hofer S, Rushing EJ, Held U, Bozinov O, Krayenbuhl N, Weller M, Regli L (2015) Efficacy of surgery and further treatment of progressive glioblastoma. World Neurosurg 84(2):301–307. doi:10.1016/j.wneu.2015.03.018
81. Yan H, Parsons DW, Jin G, McLendon R, Rasheed BA, Yuan W, Kos I, Batinic-Haberle I, Jones S, Riggins GJ, Friedman H, Friedman A, Reardon D, Herndon J, Kinzler KW, Velculescu VE, Vogelstein B, Bigner DD (2009) IDH1 and IDH2 mutations in gliomas. N Engl J Med 360(8):765–773. doi:10.1056/NEJMoa0808710
82. Yin AA, Cai S, Dong Y, Zhang LH, Liu BL, Cheng JX, Zhang X (2014) A meta-analysis of temozolomide versus radiotherapy in elderly glioblastoma patients. J Neurooncol 116(2):315–324. doi:10.1007/s11060-013-1294-0
83. Yung WK, Albright RE, Olson J, Fredericks R, Fink K, Prados MD, Brada M, Spence A, Hohl RJ, Shapiro W, Glantz M, Greenberg H, Selker RG, Vick NA, Rampling R, Friedman H, Phillips P, Bruner J, Yue N, Osoba D, Zaknoen S, Levin VA (2000) A phase II study of temozolomide vs. procarbazine in patients with glioblastoma multiforme at first relapse. Br J Cancer 83(5):588–593. doi:10.1054/bjoc.2000.1316
84. Zouaoui S, Darlix A, Fabbro-Peray P, Mathieu-Daude H, Rigau V, Fabbro M, Bessaoud F, Taillandier L, Ducray F, Bauchet F, Wager M, Faillot T, Capelle L, Loiseau H, Kerr C, Menei P, Duffau H, Figarella-Branger D, Chinot O, Tretarre B, Bauchet L (2014) Oncological patterns of care and outcomes for 265 elderly patients with newly diagnosed glioblastoma in France. Neurosurg Rev 37(3):415–423. doi:10.1007/s10143-014-0528-8; discussion 423–414

Pituitary Adenomas

9

Paolo Cappabianca, Chiara Caggiano, Domenico Solari, Karol Migliorati, Waleed A. Azab, Elia Guadagno, Marialaura Del Basso De Caro, Emmanuel Jouanneau, and Luigi M. Cavallo

Abbreviations

ACTH	Adrenocorticotropin
ASA	American Society of Anesthesiologists
AVP	Arginine vasopressin
CAD	Coronary artery disease
CSF	Cerebrospinal fluid
DI	Diabetes insipidus
FSH	Follicle-stimulating hormone
GH	Growth hormone
GTR	Gross total removal
IHD	Ischemic heart disease
LH	Luteinizing hormone
NFPA	Non-functioning pituitary adenoma
PA	Pituitary adenoma

P. Cappabianca, MD (✉) • C. Caggiano, MD • D. Solari, MD, PhD
K. Migliorati, MD • L.M. Cavallo, MD, PhD
Division of Neurosurgery, Department of Neurosciences and Reproductive and Odontostomatological Sciences, Università degli Studi di Napoli Federico II, Via Pansini 5, 80131 Naples, Italy
e-mail: paolo.cappabianca@unina.it

W.A. Azab, MD
Department of Neurosurgery, Ibn Sina Hospital, Kuwait city, Kuwait

E. Guadagno, MD • M.D.B. De Caro, BS
Department of Advanced Biomedical Sciences, Università degli Studi di Napoli Federico II, Naples, Italy

E. Jouanneau, MD, PhD
Department of Neurosurgery, University Hospital of Lyon – Hospices Civils de Lyon, Lyon, France

© Springer International Publishing Switzerland 2017

M. Berhouma, P. Krolak-Salmon (eds.), *Brain and Spine Surgery in the Elderly*,
DOI 10.1007/978-3-319-40232-1_9

PRL	Prolactin
SIADH	Syndrome of inappropriate antidiuretic hormone
STR	Subtotal removal
TSH	Thyroid-stimulating hormone
VDF	Visual field deficit

9.1 Introduction

Pituitary adenomas (PA) are histological benign tumours of the adenohypophysis, representing the third most frequent intracranial neoplasia [1], with equal distribution in children, adults and elderly patients. These lesions can be identified as functioning or non-functioning adenomas according to the secretion of one or more pituitary hormones by the tumour mass. Diagnosis is easily ruled out in the cases of secreting lesions, upon the clinical features of hypersecretion that define a specific phenotypic syndrome, such as Cushing disease or acromegaly; conversely, in cases of non-functioning tumours, lesions are diagnosed when symptoms due to the mass effect, i.e. visual defects and/or oculomotor palsy, become evident. Finally, it should not be underestimated that a certain percentage of patients remain totally asymptomatic, receiving though accidental diagnosis.

The frequency of different subtypes of PA differs among age groups: the most common PAs in early childhood are ACTH-secreting; prolactinomas are the most encountered during the second, third and fourth decades of life, while after the age of 40 years, the most frequent are the non-functioning pituitary adenomas (NFPAs).

Nowadays, the average life can exceed 75 years in the developed countries and may increase in the future decades, with the threshold of elderly being considered 65 years. The incidence of PAs in this group of patients, i.e. the elderly, ranges between 7 and 9.9 % [12]: it is actually increasing, mostly due to the expanding number of elderly among population and to the increasing use of "secondary line" diagnostic tools, namely, the MRI for other neurological diseases, such as senile dementia, Alzheimer disease, cerebral transient ischemic attack, stroke, etc. [20]. As a matter of fact, non-functioning tumours represent the 70–80 % of all PAs in the elderly [2, 12, 17, 24, 26] and the main presenting symptoms are visual defects [12, 22, 31]. Otherwise, the most common functioning lesions in these patients are GH-secreting (14 %) and ACTH-secreting (4 %) [12].

9.2 Clinical Features

PAs in elderly are mainly represented by NFPAs, so that the most common symptoms observed at diagnosis are related to the mass effect: headache (29–43 %), visual field defects (VFD) and/or visual acuity loss (40–87 %) due to the compression of the optic chiasm and pathways and/or hypopituitarism (50–60 %) [20]. These clinical signs are often misdiagnosed, considering the presence of the different co-morbidities the elderly patients complain of.

In Table 9.1 the clinical features of elderly patients with PA as reported in literature are summarized. Other clinical presentations include pituitary intralesional

Table 9.1 The summary of the clinical feature series of elderly patients with PA in the last 20 years

Study	Visual symptoms	Endocrinological status	Others	Incidentally detected tumours	Time for diagnosis
Puchner (1995)	–	↑GH 100 %	NR	NR	NR
Benbow (1997) [2]	54.50 %	↑GH 11.3 % ↓TSH 33.3 % ↓ACTH 48.7 % ↑PRL 4.5 %	Neurological 20.45 % Apoplexy 2.2 %	15.90 %	NR
Turner (1999) [31]	39.3 %	Hypopituitarism 20.20 %	Hypernatraemia 9.5 %	9.50 %	NR
Fraioli (1999)	81.80 %	Hypopituitarism 90 %	III c.n. paralysis 9 %	NR	NR
Minniti (2005) [22]	66.6 %	↑PRL 100 %	Headache 33.3 % Cerebral ischaemia 11.1 %	NR	NR
Hong (2008) [14]	86.4 %	Hypopituitarism (35.9 %)	Headache 47.6 %	–	5.7years ±1.3 years
Sheehan (2008) [26]	58 %	↑GH 5 %	–	9 %	NR
Locatelli (2013) [21]	44 %	Hypopituitarism 44.1 % Single defect 30.2 % Multiple defect 13.9 %	–	–	–
Zhan (2015) [32]	84.2 %	–	Headache 75.9 %	NR	NR
Pereira (2014)	41.3 %	↑GH 3.8 % ↑ACTH 1.4 % ↓TSH 7.6 % ↓LH-FSH 1 % Hypopituitarism 3.8 %	Headache 5.8 % Apoplexy 3.8 %	22.5 %	NR
Gondim (2015) [12]	69 %	Hypopituitarism 38.2 %	Headache 29 % Apoplexy 10.9 %	–	–
Liu (2015) [20]	–	↑1 or more pituitary hormone 6.3 % ↓1 or more pituitary hormone 3.1 %	Mass effect 98.4 %	10.1 %	<5 years 64.5 % 5–10 years 21 % >10 years 14.5 %

haemorrhage/apoplexy (11–30 %) and/or ophthalmoplegia (3–10 %). Pituitary apoplexy occurs often in large adenomas and it results common in elderly as related to their co-morbidities, such as hypertension and coronary heart diseases, which are predisposing factors [20].

Visual deficit is the primary symptom in the majority of the published trials: different patterns of VFD have been described in patients with PA, in regard to the relationships between the tumour and the optic pathway. The most common VFD, also in the elderly patients with PA, is bitemporal hemianopia: the defect may be complete, involving the whole temporal field, or partial, usually affecting the superior quadrant. Anterior lesions, impinging pre-chiasmatic nerve, can cause central scotomas, while posterior lesions involving the optic tract can provide homonymous hemianopia. Despite several studies confirm that bitemporal hemianopia is the most prevalent VFD in elderly patients complaining of non-functioning tumours, it is quite common that this defect goes misdiagnosed [23]. Retinal degeneration, cataracts and amblyopia are common visual disturbances in the elderly: therefore, visual disturbances related to compression of optic pathways caused by the NFPA may be initially attributed to other age-related visual conditions and/or be unrecognized [6, 14].

Although clinical manifestations of hypopituitarism are not clearly evident, blood tests reveal in most cases pituitary function partial or complete hormonal failures. The majority of the studies show that most of the affected pituitary axes are the gonadic, with low LH/FSH levels in about 60 % of the cases, as well as the somatotrophic, with low IGF-1 levels in 50 % of the cases [7, 17]. On the other hand, the adrenocorticotrophic and thyrotrophic axes were deficient in about, respectively, 27 % and 23 % of the cases [7, 14, 31].

9.3 Preoperative Considerations

Preoperative evaluation must consider three main aspects:

- The type and size of PA
- The eventual patient co-morbidities
- The ASA (American Society of Anesthesiologists) score

As already mentioned, PAs in elderly are mostly NFPAs [14, 19, 20, 24, 31] generally large, but do not present more aggressive features as compared to those occurring in the younger patients [15, 20]: decrease of cell proliferation rate has been observed in adenomas, especially NFPA and GH-secreting tumours [15] of the elderly.

The main characteristics, i.e. tumour size, localization and type of adenomas, are summarized in Table 9.2.

The incidence of associated co-morbidities is highly variable (ranging from 17 to 90 %) with cardiovascular diseases being the most frequent, followed by respiratory diseases, diabetes mellitus and neurological disorders [21]. Most of these patients receive long-standing treatment with cardiological drugs, such as antihypertensive or

Table 9.2 Main tumour characteristics of PA in elderly patients

Study	Location	Size	Type
Fraioli (1999)	Intrasellar 9 % Intra-suprasellar 81,8 %	<1 cm 9 % >1 cm 91 %	NF 72,7 % PRL 9 % GH 9 % ACTH 9 %
Hong (2008) [14]	–	1–2 cm 6.8 % 2–3 cm 49.5 % 3–4 cm 35.9 % >4 cm 7.8 %	NF 72.8 % GH 9.7 % PRL 15.5 % ACTH 1.9 %
Locatelli (2010)	–	>1 cm 90.6 % >1 cm 9.4 %	NF 72 % GH 9.4 % ACTH18.6
Zhan (2015) [32]	Intrasellar 15.8 % Intra-suprasellar 40.5 % Parasellar 18.4 % Supra-parasellar 25.3 %	>1 cm 84.2 % <1 cm 15.8 %	NF 100 %
Gondim (2015) [12]	Knosp 2 5.4 % Knosp 3 9 % Knosp 4 14.5 %	–	NF 78.5 % GH 14.2 % PRL 2.8 % ACTH 4.2 %
Liu (2015) [20]	–	>1 cm 85.5 % >4 cm 14.5 %	NF 75.4 % GH 5.8 % ACTH 10.1 % Plurihormonal 5.8 % Apoplexy 2.9 %

antiarrhythmic agents, and a conspicuous number of patients in this group (59.4 %) complain of more than two co-morbidities: these factors can determine a longer preoperative hospitalization. Besides, endocrine and metabolic disorders, including significant changes in the hypothalamo-pituitary axis and pancreatic and thyroid malfunctioning, should be taken into account [18]; approximately 40 % of individuals between 65 and 74 years and ca. 50 % of individuals older than 80 years present impaired glucose tolerance or diabetes mellitus, often undiagnosed [16] (Table 9.3).

For these reasons, the preoperative clinical status of elderly patients with PA is commonly defined with ASA score of three or even four (Table 9.4), although there is no significant difference in terms of mortality (p 0.12) between young and elderly patients.

Owing that, surgery for the removal of a pituitary adenoma in an elderly can be indicated when patients present clear symptoms related to the adenoma, without severe co-morbidities that increase too much the overall risks of surgery.

It is preferable to choose a surgical approach as minimal invasive as possible, according to the localization and the inner features of the lesion. Nowadays, the endoscopic endonasal transsphenoidal approach represents a good option for the surgical treatment of pituitary adenomas in the elderly, because of its effectiveness in terms of tumoral removal, the excellent surgical outcomes in terms of visual outcome, its minimal invasiveness and the lower rates of morbidity and mortality related to the approach.

Table 9.3 Main co-morbidity in elderly patients with PA

Study	Co-morbidity
Hong (2008) [14]	Hypertension 33.9 %
	Cardiac disease 1.9 %
	Respiratory disease 23.3 %
	Hyperglycaemia 41.7 %
Sheehan (2008) [26]	Hypertension 26.9 %
	Cardiac disease 21.4 %
	Respiratory disease 8.3 %
	Coexisting malignancy 8.3 %
Locatelli (2013) [21]	Cardiac disease 86 %
	Respiratory disease 60.5 %
	Diabetes mellitus 18.6 %
	Neurological disease 11.6 %
Pereira (2014)	Hypertension 61.2 %
	Cardiac disease 10.7 %
	Hypercholesterolaemia 15.7 %
	Coexisting malignancy 13.7 %
	Diabetes mellitus 13 %
	Arthrosis 10.7 %

Table 9.4 Main complications after endoscopic endonasal transsphenoidal surgery

Authors	General complications	Specific complications
Turner (1999) [31]	Myocardial infarction 1.2 % Chest infection 1.2 % Small gastrointestinal bleed 1.2 % Meningitis 1.2 %	Transient DI 2.38 % Permanent DI 4.76 % Deterioration of visual function 5.9 %
Hong (2008) [14]	None	Transient DI 37.9 % CSF leak 4.9 % Deterioration of visual function 9.7 % Postoperative hypopituitarism 10.7 %
Sheehan (2008) [26]	None	DI 3.12 % Hypocortisolism 1.5 % Hypothyroidism 4.7 %
Grossman (2010) [13]	Death 3.75 % Pulmonary complications 3.50 % Stroke 2.52 %	Fluid or electrolyte abnormality 14.32 % CSF rhinorrhea 5.38 % DI 1.15 % Panhypopituitarism 0.5 %
Zhan (2015) [32]	None	DI 22.2 % CSF leak 3.8 % New hypopituitarism 9.5 % Meningitis 1.9 %
Liu (2015) [20]	Severe systemic complications (Clavien Classification ≥ IV) 4.3 %	DI 11.6 % CSF leak 1.4 % Panhypopituitarism 4.3 %
Gondim (2015) [12]	Refractory hypertension (7.2 %) Myocardial ischaemia (1.8 %)	CSF leaks (9 %), DI (3.6 %) Hypopituitarism 12.7 %

9.4 Surgical Technique and Outcome

Surgery yields the best outcomes when performed in dedicated centres, and it's targeted to achieve multiple goals, such as elimination of mass effect, restoration of normal pituitary function and/or visual acuity, prevention of tumour recurrence and normalization of excess of hormone secretion.

After general anaesthesia and orotracheal intubation, the patient is positioned supine with the head at 0° and rotated 10° to the surgeon. Disinfection with povidone-iodine into the nasal cavities and on the nasal skin is performed. Then eight cottonoids drenched of a solution with 2 ml of adrenaline 0.5 % and 5 ml of lidocaine are introduced into the nasal cavities and the draping is performed. In patients with history of ischemic heart disease (IHD) or coronary artery disease (CAD), we prefer to not use adrenaline in such solution for nasal decongestion. The technique consists in three parts: nasal, sphenoidal and sellar step [3, 4, 8, 28, 29].

- Nasal step
  We generally use a 0° angled lens, 4 mm in diameter endoscope, that is inserted in the right and then in the left nostril, between the nasal septum medially and the middle turbinate laterally. The cottons are then removed to promote the anti-bleeding effect, avoiding the nasal mucosa ischaemia, and the middle turbinate is carefully lateralized to increase the surgical corridor. Usually, in elderly patients the nasal mucosa and its vascular network appear hypotrophic, so that the nasal cavities are easily explored with the endoscope. Once the nasal choana is reached, the endoscope is pushed up for about 1.5–2 cm to identify the sphenoethmoid recess and the ostium of the sphenoid sinus.
- Sphenoidal step
  Once the mucosa is coagulated, the sphenoethmoid recess is opened and the posterior part of nasal septum is removed to expose the cavity of sphenoid sinus. The sphenoid mucosa is extensively removed to avoid postoperative sphenoid mucocele. After removal of eventual septa inside the sinus, several important anatomical landmarks are visible: at the centre the protuberance of the sellar floor, laterally the carotid protuberances, above the planum and below the clivus; above the carotid protuberance, there is the optic protuberance and between them the opto-carotid recess that corresponds to the anterior clinoid.
- Sellar step
  We generally perform this phase with four hands-two surgeons technique. The sellar opening is performed by microdrilling and can be extended up to the clivus below or the planum above, depending on the extension of the adenoma. The dural incision is performed in a cruciate fashioned at the midline. The adenoma is frequently soft and can be removed by suction and curetting, starting from the inferior and lateral parts, to retard the descent of the suprasellar cistern. After tumour removal, the osteodural defect is repaired depending to the opening entity and the presence of intraoperative CSF leak. In case of large macroadenomas, the bone exposure can involve the planum sphenoidale. In these cases the subarachnoid space is intentionally violated, and, because the surgery is performed through the basal cisterns, intraoperative CSF leakage occurs. However,

the goal of the reconstruction is a watertight closure of the skull base defect, to avoid postoperative CSF leak and infective complications.
It should be minded that in elderly patients, it is preferable to avoid opening of the suprasellar cistern, while accepting the risk of an incomplete tumour removal. This choice mostly relies on the fact that on one side the osteodural defect could be troublesome and take longer, but on the other the tumour growth is extremely slow.

9.5 Postoperative Management

All the patients, regardless the age, are generally mobilized on the same day of surgery.

The visual field deficits usually improve and/or are fully recovered, even if the defects were lasting for more than 6 months [20, 21]. Conversely, endocrine functions, above all in patients with preoperative hypopituitarism, do not change, maybe for a limited pituitary functional reserve in the elderly population [12, 20, 24].

The mean postoperative hospitalization stay is not different between elderly and young patients [12, 21].

Zhan et al. reported a total resection in 75.9 % of patients, subtotal resection in 22.8 % and a partial resection in 1.3 %, after pure endoscopic transsphenoidal surgery, with no significant difference compared to the younger group of control [32]. Also Gondim et al. in their series of elderly patients didn't find significant difference between the extent of resection obtained in elderly and young patients [12].

Postoperative fractionated radiotherapy is frequently administered to patients with residual or recurrent pituitary disease, but it is not recommended after surgery in elderly patients, considering the slow tumour growth rate, the low incidence of recurrences following total or subtotal resection and the shorter expectancy of life in this category of patients [30].

The use of adjuvant radiotherapy may be considered only in patients with large residual tumour that are unresponsive to medical treatment, although no consensus guidelines are available [22]. Chang et al. indeed recommend the use of adjuvant radiotherapy only in case of subtotal removal (STR), especially if the cavernous sinus is invaded, while not in case of gross total removal (GTR), due to the increased risk of death [5].

9.6 Complications

9.6.1 Medical Complications

Cardiopulmonary and vascular diseases, thromboembolic events, postoperative pneumonia, sepsis, stress ulcer bleeding, stroke and death represent the main dreaded postsurgical complications, when an elderly patient is submitted to a surgical procedure for the removal of a pituitary adenoma.

As previously reported, elderly patients have a higher rate of co-morbidities and are prone to develop systemic complications, so that incidence rates of complications are not claimed univocal.

Locatelli et al. reported the absence of major surgical complications, although about 70 % of patients had moderate or severe risk according to ASA class – this series accounts on 11 % of patients belonging to ASA score categories 4 and 5 [21].

Contrariwise, Gondim et al. reported a rate of systemic complications of 32.7 % in elderly group versus 10 % in younger patients, being this difference statistically significant ($p<0.05$). In this study, the higher rate of complications in elderly was referred to the postoperative high blood pressure peaks and subclinical pituitary apoplexy that occurs more frequently in elderly people; however, no significant mortality rate difference was observed between the two groups [12].

9.6.2 Approach-Related Complications

Potential complications of the endoscopic endonasal surgery include diabetes insipidus (DI) (11.6 %), postoperative hypopituitarism (22 %), cerebrospinal fluid (CSF) leak (5–16 %), meningitis (5.5 %), visual impairment (1.5 %), syndrome of inappropriate antidiuretic hormone (SIADH) secretion (8.5–25 %), haemorrhage (5 %), carotid artery injury (<1 %), ischemic stroke (2 %) and epistaxis (4.8 %) [12, 20] (Table 9.4).

Concerning endocrinological complications, postoperative DI results the most common: it can be transient, permanent or triphasic. Transient DI (30 % of patients) has its onset at 24–48 h post-op and it is usually resolved in 3–5 days. Permanent DI (10 % of cases) can be seen in patients in whom there is a direct damage to the pituitary stalk, hypothalamus and/or proximal infundibulum. The triphasic DI is extremely rare, with a first phase like transient DI and a second similar to SIADH, and finally it develops permanent DI. Untreated DI can cause or worsen hypernatraemia and serum hyperosmolality, potentially leading to dehydration, lethargy, irritability and, in the case of severe hypernatraemia, seizures [9, 25]. On the other side, as reported by Liu et al., there is no significant difference of postsurgical hypopituitarism rates between old and young patients [20].

Finally, notwithstanding recent advancements of the techniques and materials, CSF leak remains a frequent complication of this kind of surgery, also in elderly patients [11–13, 17]. It should be said though that intraoperative CSF fistula is the only significant predictive factor of postoperative leakage [10]: this complication is usually rare during removal manoeuvres of infradiaphragmatic lesions, whereas its risk raises when dealing with lesions that have breached the diaphragm. In these latter cases, an accurate reconstruction is mandatory of the osteodural defect [27].

Conclusion

Surgery in the elderly group is recommended for pituitary tumours causing neurological deficits – above all visual – and endocrinological syndrome, eventually resistant to pharmacological treatment. The endoscopic endonasal approach is the gold standard because of its safeness and efficacy. No mortality or major complications are observed, even in patients with elevated ASA scoring class; multiple co-morbidities, however, should be taken into account preoperatively, to achieve a long-term successful outcome and avoid threatening morbidities related to the surgery and to the approach itself. An adequate preoperative planning, careful surgical technique and rigorous postoperative care can reduce mortality and morbidity rates in this high-risk patient group.

References

1. Asa SL, Ezzat S (2002) The pathogenesis of pituitary tumours. Nat Rev Cancer 2(11):836–849. doi:10.1038/nrc926
2. Benbow SJ, Foy P, Jones B, Shaw D, MacFarlane IA (1997) Pituitary tumours presenting in the elderly: management and outcome. Clin Endocrinol (Oxf) 46(6):657–660
3. Cappabianca P, Cavallo LM, Colao A, Del Basso De Caro M, Esposito F, Cirillo S, Lombardi G, de Divitiis E (2002) Endoscopic endonasal transsphenoidal approach: outcome analysis of 100 consecutive procedures. Minim Invasive Neurosurg MIN 45(4):193–200. doi:10.1055/s-2002-36197
4. Cappabianca P, Cavallo LM, Solari D, Stagno V, Esposito F, de Angelis M (2014) Endoscopic endonasal surgery for pituitary adenomas. World Neurosurg 82(6 Suppl):S3–S11. doi:10.1016/j.wneu.2014.07.019
5. Chang EF, Zada G, Kim S, Lamborn KR, Quinones-Hinojosa A, Tyrrell JB, Wilson CB, Kunwar S (2008) Long-term recurrence and mortality after surgery and adjuvant radiotherapy for non-functional pituitary adenomas. J Neurosurg 108(4):736–745. doi:10.3171/JNS/2008/108/4/0736
6. Christensen K, Doblhammer G, Rau R, Vaupel JW (2009) Ageing populations: the challenges ahead. Lancet 374(9696):1196–1208. doi:10.1016/S0140-6736(09)61460-4
7. Del Monte P, Foppiani L, Ruelle A, Andrioli G, Bandelloni R, Quilici P, Prete C, Palummeri E, Marugo A, Bernasconi D (2007) Clinically non-functioning pituitary macroadenomas in the elderly. Aging Clin Exp Res 19(1):34–40
8. Di Maio S, Cavallo LM, Esposito F, Stagno V, Corriero OV, Cappabianca P (2011) Extended endoscopic endonasal approach for selected pituitary adenomas: early experience. J Neurosurg 114(2):345–353. doi:10.3171/2010.9.JNS10262
9. Dumont AS, Nemergut EC 2nd, Jane JA Jr, Laws ER Jr (2005) Postoperative care following pituitary surgery. J Intensive Care Med 20(3):127–140. doi:10.1177/0885066605275247
10. Duntze J, Litre CF, Graillon T, Maduri R, Pech-gourg G, Rakotozanany P, Gras R, Dufour H (2012) Cerebrospinal fluid rhinorrhea following endocopic trans-sphenoidal pituitary surgery: experience from 337 patients. Neurochirurgie 58(4):241–245. doi:10.1016/j.neuchi.2012.02.005
11. Ferrante L, Trillo G, Ramundo E, Celli P, Jaffrain-Rea ML, Salvati M, Esposito V, Roperto R, Osti MF, Minniti G (2002) Surgical treatment of pituitary tumors in the elderly: clinical outcome and long-term follow-up. J Neurooncol 60(2):185–191
12. Gondim JA, Almeida JP, de Albuquerque LA, Gomes E, Schops M, Mota JI (2015) Endoscopic endonasal transsphenoidal surgery in elderly patients with pituitary adenomas. J Neurosurg 123(1):31–38. doi:10.3171/2014.10.JNS14372
13. Grossman R, Mukherjee D, Chaichana KL, Salvatori R, Wand G, Brem H, Chang DC, Quinones-Hinojosa A (2010) Complications and death among elderly patients undergoing pituitary tumour surgery. Clin Endocrinol (Oxf) 73(3):361–368. doi:10.1111/j.1365-2265.2010.03813.x
14. Hong J, Ding X, Lu Y (2008) Clinical analysis of 103 elderly patients with pituitary adenomas: transsphenoidal surgery and follow-up. J Clin Neurosci Off J Neurosurg Soc Australasia 15(10):1091–1095. doi:10.1016/j.jocn.2007.11.003
15. Jaffrain-Rea ML, Di Stefano D, Minniti G, Esposito V, Bultrini A, Ferretti E, Santoro A, Faticanti Scucchi L, Gulino A, Cantore G (2002) A critical reappraisal of MIB-1 labelling index significance in a large series of pituitary tumours: secreting versus non-secreting adenomas. Endocr Relat Cancer 9(2):103–113

16. Kuchel GA, Minaker KL (1990) Dizziness in geriatric practice. J Am Geriatr Soc 38(8):957
17. Kurosaki M, Saeger W, Ludecke DK (2001) Pituitary tumors in the elderly. Pathol Res Pract 197(7):493–497. doi:10.1078/0344-0338-00117
18. Lamberts SW, van den Beld AW, van der Lely AJ (1997) The endocrinology of aging. Science 278(5337):419–424
19. Letournel F, Menei P, Guy G, Saint-Andre JP (2003) Transsphenoidal surgery in the elderly. J Am Geriatr Soc 51(5):729–730
20. Liu J, Li C, Xiao Q, Gan C, Chen X, Sun W, Li X, Xu Y, Chen J, Shu K, Lei T (2015) Comparison of pituitary adenomas in elderly and younger adults: clinical characteristics, surgical outcomes, and prognosis. J Am Geriatr Soc 63(9):1924–1930. doi:10.1111/jgs.13590
21. Locatelli M, Bertani G, Carrabba G, Rampini P, Zavanone M, Caroli M, Sala E, Ferrante E, Gaini SM, Spada A, Mantovani G, Lania A (2013) The trans-sphenoidal resection of pituitary adenomas in elderly patients and surgical risk. Pituitary 16(2):146–151. doi:10.1007/s11102-012-0390-z
22. Minniti G, Esposito V, Piccirilli M, Fratticci A, Santoro A, Jaffrain-Rea ML (2005) Diagnosis and management of pituitary tumours in the elderly: a review based on personal experience and evidence of literature. Eur J Endocrinol/Eur Fed Endocrine Soc 153(6):723–735. doi:10.1530/eje.1.02030
23. Ogra S, Nichols AD, Stylli S, Kaye AH, Savino PJ, Danesh-Meyer HV (2014) Visual acuity and pattern of visual field loss at presentation in pituitary adenoma. J Clin Neurosci Off J Neurosurg Soc Australasia 21(5):735–740. doi:10.1016/j.jocn.2014.01.005
24. Robenshtok E, Benbassat CA, Hirsch D, Tzvetov G, Cohen ZR, Iraqi HM, Gorshtein A, Toledano Y, Shimon I (2014) Clinical course and outcome of nonfunctioning pituitary adenomas in the elderly compared with younger age groups. Endocr Pract Off J Am Coll Endocrinol Am Assoc Clin Endocrinologists 20(2):159–164. doi:10.4158/EP13182.OR
25. Schreckinger M, Szerlip N, Mittal S (2013) Diabetes insipidus following resection of pituitary tumors. Clin Neurol Neurosurg 115(2):121–126. doi:10.1016/j.clineuro.2012.08.009
26. Sheehan JM, Douds GL, Hill K, Farace E (2008) Transsphenoidal surgery for pituitary adenoma in elderly patients. Acta Neurochir 150(6):571–574. doi:10.1007/s00701-008-1581-2; discussion 574
27. Shiley SG, Limonadi F, Delashaw JB, Barnwell SL, Andersen PE, Hwang PH, Wax MK (2003) Incidence, etiology, and management of cerebrospinal fluid leaks following trans-sphenoidal surgery. Laryngoscope 113(8):1283–1288. doi:10.1097/00005537-200308000-00003
28. Solari D, Cavallo LM, Cappabianca P (2014) Surgical approach to pituitary tumors. Handb Clin Neurol 124:291–301. doi:10.1016/B978-0-444-59602-4.00019-8
29. Solari D, Cavallo LM, De Angelis M, Villa A, Somma T, Esposito F, Del Basso De Caro M, Cappabianca P (2012) Advances in trans-sphenoidal pituitary surgery. Panminerva Med 54(4):271–276
30. Tanaka Y, Hongo K, Tada T, Sakai K, Kakizawa Y, Kobayashi S (2003) Growth pattern and rate in residual nonfunctioning pituitary adenomas: correlations among tumor volume doubling time, patient age, and MIB-1 index. J Neurosurg 98(2):359–365. doi:10.3171/jns.2003.98.2.0359
31. Turner HE, Adams CB, Wass JA (1999) Pituitary tumours in the elderly: a 20 year experience. Eur J Endocrinol/Eur Fed Endocrine Soc 140(5):383–389
32. Zhan R, Ma Z, Wang D, Li X (2015) Pure endoscopic endonasal transsphenoidal approach for nonfunctioning pituitary adenomas in the elderly: surgical outcomes and complications in 158 patients. World Neurosurg 84(6):1572–1578. doi:10.1016/j.wneu.2015.08.035

10 Vestibular Schwannoma Surgery in the Elderly

Philip Y. Sun, Marina L. Castner, Kathryn M. Van Abel, Colin L.W. Driscoll, and Michael J. Link

10.1 Introduction

Vestibular schwannoma (VS) is the most common cerebellopontine angle tumor encountered in neurosurgical and neuro-otological practice, with an incidence of 2,000–3,000 cases a year in the U.S [1]. A study in Denmark reports a diagnosis of VS in 17.4 per million inhabitants per year 1996–2001 [2]. Many small, minimally symptomatic tumors can be safely observed with serial imaging and audiologic

Funding The author(s) have received no financial support for the research, authorship, and/or publication of this chapter.

P.Y. Sun, MS
Mayo Medical School, Mayo Clinic, 200 1st St SW, Rochester, MN 55905, USA

M.L. Castner, RN
Department of Neurologic Surgery, College of Medicine, Mayo Clinic, 200 1st St SW, Rochester, MN 55905, USA

K.M. Van Abel, MD
Department of Otorhinolaryngology, College of Medicine, Mayo Clinic, 200 1st St SW, Rochester, MN 55905, USA

C.L.W. Driscoll, MD
Department of Neurologic Surgery, College of Medicine, Mayo Clinic, 200 1st St SW, Rochester, MN 55905, USA

Department of Otorhinolaryngology, College of Medicine, Mayo Clinic, 200 1st St SW, Rochester, MN 55905, USA

M.J. Link, MD (✉)
Department of Neurologic Surgery, College of Medicine, Mayo Clinic, 200 1st St SW, Rochester, MN 55905, USA

Department of Otorhinolaryngology, College of Medicine, Mayo Clinic, 200 1st St SW, Rochester, MN 55905, USA
e-mail: link.michael@mayo.edu

© Springer International Publishing Switzerland 2017

M. Berhouma, P. Krolak-Salmon (eds.), *Brain and Spine Surgery in the Elderly*,
DOI 10.1007/978-3-319-40232-1_10

follow-up, but when tumor growth is documented management options include radiation or microsurgical resection [7, 8]. Surgical resection is generally recommended for tumors with posterior fossa diameter >2.8 cm or when symptoms of mass effect (e.g., trigeminal neuralgia) predominate [3–6]. Post-op complications from either treatment modality can include hearing loss, facial numbness/tingling, and impaired balance function. Elderly patients (defined here as age > 65 years) may be more susceptible to certain complications due to overall diminished functional reserve, slower recovery, or possibility of more aggressive variants of VS.

A geriatric population, the fastest growing group in the U.S., may present with various comorbidities and potentially decreased tolerance for surgical intervention. Additionally, older patients may experience baseline hearing and balance functional decline simply due to age related degeneration of inner ear structures. The growth of this age group as well as the wide availability of advanced, non-invasive diagnostic imaging has led to increased discovery of VS in this population [2]. There are very few studies in the literature that have examined the outcome of VS surgery in older patients [9, 10]. We recently published our experience looking at the outcome of surgical resection of VS in patients greater than 70 years old [11].

Herein, we retrospectively describe our experience surgically managing VS patients > 65 years old over the past 16 years. We compare clinical presentation, tumor characteristics and outcomes to patients ≤ 65 years old operated during the same time period.

10.2 Methods

10.2.1 Patient Cohorts and Clinical Characteristics

After approval by the Institutional Review Board, we conducted a Health Insurance Portability and Accountability Act–compliant, retrospective review using the comprehensive electronic medical record system of patients who underwent microsurgical resection for VS from 9/1/1999 through 12/31/2015 at Mayo Clinic, Rochester, Minnesota. We identified patients over 65 years of age and reviewed patient demographics (i.e., age, sex, previous surgical history), operative characteristics (i.e., tumor size, approach), perioperative neurologic functions (i.e., hearing, facial nerve function), post-operative complications, and follow-up (i.e., recurrence). The control group consists of patients up to 65 years of age who also underwent microsurgical resection of sporadic VS at our institution.

10.2.2 Extent of Tumor Resection

Completeness of tumor resection was categorized into gross total resection (GTR) when the operating neurosurgeon and neuro-otologist independently agreed the entire tumor was removed and the 3-month follow-up MRI scan confirmed no residual tumor, near total resection (NTR) when a tumor remnant no greater than

5×5×2 mm was left in situ, usually for facial nerve function preservation. This small tumor remnant is likewise, not visible on a 3-month follow-up MRI scan. Subtotal tumor resection (STR) is defined as any tumor remnant larger than NTR. These remnants are always visible on the first follow-up MRI scan and can be subsequently targeted with stereotactic radiosurgery (SRS) or followed with serial imaging. Original tumor size and post-resection residual tumor sizes were the maximal axial dimension from the radiological or intraoperative measures, parallel to the petrous bone, excluding the portion within the internal auditory canal [11]. Recurrence was defined as progressive enlargement of an enhancing lesion following surgery or development of a new enhancing mass following GTR.

10.2.3 Hearing and Facial Nerve Functions

Facial nerve function was assessed using the House-Brackmann (HB) scale, postoperatively [12]. Hearing was reported according to the American Academy of Otolaryngology, Head and Neck Surgery guidelines [19].

10.2.4 Data Management and Statistical Methods

Study data were collected longitudinally from a prospectively maintained database and the Mayo medical record. Comparisons between the two groups were evaluated using two-sample t, Wilcoxon rank sum, chi-square, and Fisher exact tests. All tests were two-sided and p-values <0.05 were considered statistically significant. Data were analyzed using the Microsoft Excel and JMP 10.0 (SAS Institute Inc., Raleigh, NC) for descriptive statistics.

10.3 Results

10.3.1 Patient Demographics and Operative Characteristics (Table 10.1)

We identified a total of 550 patients with a diagnosis and microsurgical treatment for unilateral, sporadic vestibular schwannoma at our institution between 1999 and 2015. Four hundred eighty one patients (88 %) were up to the age of 65 years and 69 (12 %) patients were over 65 at the time of operation (mean ages 45.6 ± 11.9 and 71.9 ± 5.3, respectively). History of at least one non-curative prior surgery was reported in 32 (6.9 %) of the younger cohort and 12 (17.4 %) of the elderly cohort, respectively ($p=0.003$). Similarly, history of radiation surgery was more common in the elderly group (11.6 % vs. 4.2 %) ($p=0.009$). Predominately cystic tumors were more common in the elderly group (18.8 %) than the control (3.3 %) ($p<0.001$). The mean tumor size in the elderly group was 2.65 ± 0.98 cm (range 0.6, 4.5), significantly larger than that in the control, 2.29 ± 1.06 cm (range 0.5, 6.0) ($p=0.004$).

Table 10.1 Baseline demographic, surgical, and clinical features of 550 patients with vestibular schwannoma who underwent surgical resection from 1999 to 2015 at Mayo Clinic Rochester, Minnesota

	≤65 years (*n*=481)	>65 years (*n*=69)	*p* value
Sex, n (%)			
Male	230 (47.8)	37 (53.6)	0.37
Female	251 (52.2)	32 (46.4)	
Age, years, mean ± SD	45.6±11.9	71.9±5.3	NA
History of previous surgery, n (%)	32 (6.9)	12 (17.4)	0.003
History of radiation surgery, *n* (%)	20 (4.2)	8 (11.6)	0.009
Intra-canalicular tumor, n (%)	96 (20.0)	2 (2.9)	<0.001
Tumor size, cm, mean ± SD	2.29±1.06	2.65±0.98	0.004
Cystic appearance on the tumor, n (%)	16 (3.3)	13 (18.8)	<0.001
Approach, n (%)			
Middle fossa	37 (7.7)	0 (0)	0.028
Trans-labyrinthine	167 (34.7)	31 (45.0)	
Retrosigmoid	277 (57.6)	38 (55.0)	
Resection, n (%)			
Gross total resection (GTR)	356 (74.0)	22 (31.9)	<0.001
Subtotal resection (STR)	62 (12.9)	40 (58.0)	
Near-total resection (NTR)	63 (13.1)	7 (10.1)	

Patients in the older cohort were operated via a trans-labyrinthine route (45 %) when they presented with no useful hearing or had previously been operated via a retrosigmoid approach at a prior attempt to remove their tumor. The remaining 55 % were operated via a retrosigmoid approach and this route was chosen if they had useful hearing or had previously been operated via a translabryrinthine approach or had tumors greater than 3.5 cm in posterior fossa diameter. No patient in the elderly cohort underwent middle fossa surgery compared to 7.7 % of patients in the younger group. Additionally, 57.6 % of patients in the younger cohort underwent retrosigmoid resection and 34.7 % received a translabyrinthine operation. The extent of tumor resection in the elderly group was GTR (31.9 %), NTR (10.1 %) and STR (58.0 %), while those in the younger cohort were much more likely to receive GTR (74.0 %). The remaining patients in the younger group received either NTR (13.1 %) or STR (12.9 %).

10.3.2 Surgical and Perioperative Characteristics (Table 10.2)

Postoperative complications occurred in both groups and are summarized in Table 10.2. The mean follow-up in the older age group was 3.5 years (range 0.1–11.0 years) and 3.8 years (range 0.2–14.0 years) in the younger patients. In the elderly cohort, CSF leak occurred in 3 (4.4 %) patients, and in 55 (11.4 %) patients in the younger group (p=0.073). Post-op wound infection was reported in 1

Table 10.2 Post-op complications of 550 patients with vestibular schwannoma who underwent surgical resection from 1999 to 2015 at Mayo Clinic Rochester, Minnesota

	≤65 years (n=481)	>65 years (n=69)	p value
CSF leak, n (%)	55 (11.4)	3 (4.4)	0.073
Infection, n (%)	13 (2.7)	2 (2.9)	0.93
Hydrocephalus, n (%)	2 (0.4)	1 (1.5)	0.33
Subdural hematoma, n (%)	1 (0.2)	1 (1.5)	0.24
Posterior fossa hemorrhage, n (%)	1 (0.2)	1 (1.5)	0.24
Swallowing problems, n (%)	2 (0.4)	2 (2.9)	0.079
Pulmonary embolism, n (%)	2 (0.4)	0 (0)	1.0
DVT, n (%)	3 (0.6)	0 (0)	1.0

(1.5 %) elderly patient and 4 (0.8 %) younger patients (p=0.49). Swallowing problems were more common in the elderly patients. Two (2.9 %) patients had postoperative dysphagia with documented vocal fold weakness in the older group as did 2 (0.4 %) patients in the younger group (p=0.079). Fortunately, none of these lower cranial nerve palsies have been permanent, and no patient required a feeding tube. Hydrocephalus occurred postoperatively in 1 (1.5 %) of the elderly patients and 2 (0.4 %) in the younger group (p=0.33). Subdural hematoma, posterior fossa hemorrhage, pulmonary embolism, and deep venous thrombosis were rare in either group.

Two patients died in the elderly cohort in the 30 day postoperative period. An 82 year old, otherwise healthy man, presented with unilateral deafness, trigeminal neuropathy, severe imbalance with inability to ambulate independently and an MRI revealed a 4.5 cm polycystic unilateral VS (Fig. 10.1a). He underwent retrosigmoid STR of his tumor (Fig. 10.1b). His postoperative course was complicated by swallowing difficulties from which he was making a good recovery. He was discharged to a rehabilitation facility but developed C. difficile colitis and died on postoperative day #20 from sepsis. A 75 year old man presented with a 3.1 cm unilateral VS and unilateral hearing loss (Fig. 10.2a). He underwent translabyrinthine resection of his tumor without apparent complication. He was awakening slowly from anesthesia so he was taken directly from the operating room (OR) to the CT scanner where a non-contrast CT scan surprisingly revealed a large supratentorial hemispheric subdural hematoma (Fig. 10.2b). He was urgently taken back to the OR but he dilated his ipsilateral pupil en route. He underwent an emergent frontotemporoparietal craniotomy and evacuation of the subdural hematoma but never regained consciousness. The family elected to withdraw care and he died on postoperative day #12. One patient in the younger group suffered a fatal pulmonary embolus on postoperative day # 18. She was a 53 y/o woman who underwent translabyrinthine resection of a 2.1 cm VS. Her postoperative course was complicated by delayed CSF leak necessitating her return to our institution for wound re-exploration and packing of her Eustachian tube. She was recovering well and suddenly complained of chest pain and shortness of breath and lost consciousness. She could not be revived and autopsy confirmed large pulmonary embolus.

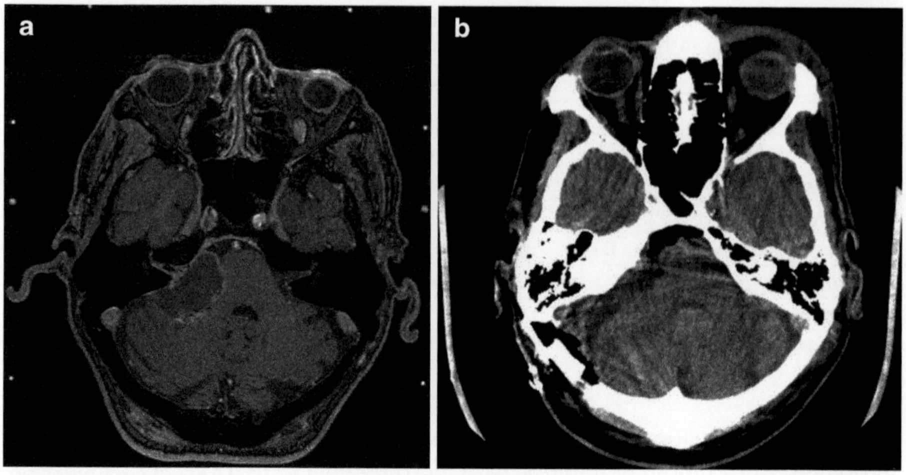

Fig. 10.1 (**a**) MRI on an 82 year old man who presented with unilateral deafness, trigeminal neuropathy, severe imbalance with inability to ambulate independently. Imaging revealed a 4.5 cm polycystic unilateral VS. (**b**) Post-op CT following retrosigmoid STR of his tumor. His postoperative course was complicated by swallowing difficulties from which he was making a good recovery. He was discharged to a rehabilitation facility but developed C. difficile colitis and died on postoperative day #20 from sepsis

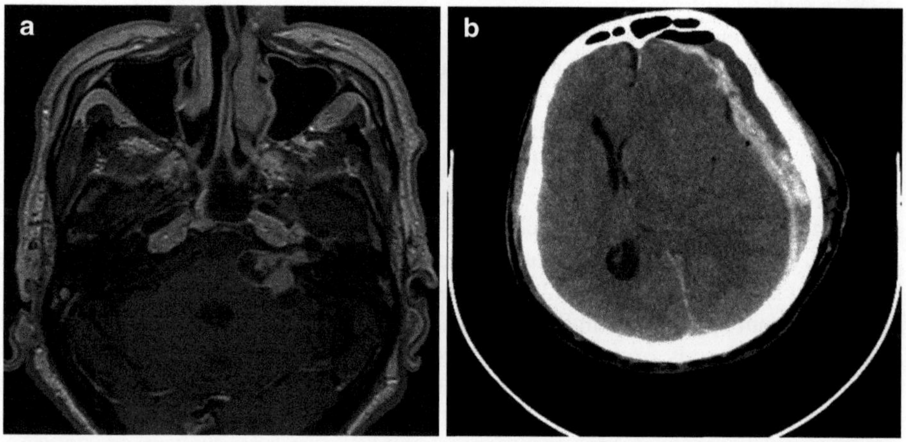

Fig. 10.2 (**a**) MRI on an 72 year old man who presented with unilateral hearing loss. Imaging revealed a 3.1 cm moderately cystic VS. (**b**) Post-op non-contrast CT following translabyrinthine resection on the patient shows an unexpected large supratentorial hemispheric subdural hematoma

10.3.3 Hearing and Facial Nerve Outcomes (Table 10.3)

At presentation, hearing function was significantly worse in the elderly group ($p<0.001$). Sixty three (91.3 %) elderly patients presented with Class D hearing, while only 42.5 % the younger cohort were Class D. Post-operatively, 417 (89.9 %) younger

Table 10.3 Perioperative information and prognosis of 550 patients with vestibular schwannoma who underwent surgical resection from 1999 to 2015 at Mayo Clinic Rochester, Minnesota

	≤65 years (n=481)	>65 years (n=69)	p value
Follow-up, months, mean ± SD	45.8±39.0	41.5±36.1	0.42
MRI showing remnant enhancement, n (%)	36 (7.5)	3 (4.4)	0.46
Pre-operative hearing score[a], n (%)			
A	187 (39.1)	1 (1.5)	<0.001
B	77 (16.1)	4 (5.8)	
C	11 (2.3)	1 (1.5)	
D	203 (42.5)	63 (91.3)	
Post-operative hearing score[a], n (%)			
A	36 (7.8)	0 (0)	0.007
B	10 (2.2)	0 (0)	
C	1 (0.2)	0 (0)	
D	417 (89.9)	66 (100)	
Post-operative facial nerve function[b], n (%)			
Grade I/II	393 (82.1)	50 (72.5)	0.035
Grade III/IV	70 (14.6)	11 (15.9)	
Grade V/VI	16 (3.3)	8 (11.6)	
Tumor recurrence, n (%)			
Recurrence	16 (3.3)	6 (8.7)	0.033
Recurrence tx with Gamma knife	16 (3.3)	5 (7.2)	
Recurrence with no intervention	0 (0.0)	1 (1.5)	

[a]AAO-HNS Hearing Class
[b]House-Brackmann scale

patients and all of 66 elderly patients with recorded post-op hearing exam were Class D. Facial nerve function at presentation and last follow-up were similar between the two age groups. At last follow-up, in both age groups, the majority of patients, 393 (82.1 %) younger patients and 50 (72.5 %) elderly patients, were HB grade 1 or 2. This was a statistically significant difference, however, including more patients with unacceptable facial nerve function (HB grade 5 or 6) in the elderly cohort (p=0.035). This may be explained by the older patients being operated for larger tumors and also having a higher likelihood of having undergone prior surgery. Most notably, 8.7 % of tumors progressed or recurred in the older cohort compared to only 3.3 % in the younger group after approximately 4 years of follow-up (p=0.033).

10.4 Discussion

Our review suggests that surgical treatment of VS yields a satisfactory outcome in carefully-selected elderly patients. Other studies have demonstrated that surgical resection of VS is effective in the management of tumor growth and symptoms with low perioperative risk in elderly patients [7, 8]. Piazza et al., from the University of

Parma operated 36 patients ≥ 65 years old, mostly via a translabyrinthine route. They achieved GTR in 94.4 %. While essentially 50 % had complete facial weakness at the time of discharge, only 6 % had complete (HB grade 6) facial palsy at 1 year follow-up. Complications occurred in 13.9 % of patients including one death due to pulmonary edema and renal infarction. One additional patient required urgent reoperation for a posterior fossa hematoma but subsequently made a good recovery. There was no tumor recurrence or growth of residual tumor at 5 year follow-up. Glasscock et al., from Nashville reported on 20 patients older than age 70 years in 1997 that had undergone surgery for VS. The mean tumor size was 2.8 cm. Once again, the majority were operated via the translabyrinthine route. Thirty percent of patients had their facial nerves anatomically sacrificed for tumor removal! Final facial nerve outcomes were not specified for the remaining patients. One patient (5 %) died and 3 (15 %) developed hydrocephalus. Half the patients had at least one complication. Compared to their experience treating more than 1300 tumors in non-elderly patients, in this group the mortality rate was only 0.5 % and 1 % of patients developed hydrocephalus. Roehm and Gantz from the University of Iowa operated 108 patients with a median age of 71 years (range, 65–92 years). At last follow-up 82.2 % had HB grade 1 or 2 facial nerve function. While there were 43 major complications (required return to the operating room or prolonged the hospital stay), they reported no mortality in their series. In a prior analysis at our institution by Van Abel et al., in which patients >70 years old were compared with tumor-size and sex-matched controls in a younger age group, the elderly group showed a higher likelihood of imbalance and coordination problems following surgery, but no notable impairment in facial nerve/hearing functionality as well as infection-related deaths compared to the younger age group [11]. A retrospective study by Ohgalai et al., reported lower chance of hearing preservation, but no difference in facial outcome, in patients older than 60 years of age, compared to younger than 40 years [10].

With very rare exception, we approach every VS operation with the goal of GTR. However, early in our experience with elderly patients in particular, we felt a NTR or more likely, STR to decompress the brainstem and cerebellum would be sufficient and would reduce the risk of facial weakness or any other cranial nerve morbidity, as well as potentially shortening the operative time and thus anesthetic risk. Considering the typical slow growth of VS, we reasoned that there would not be significant regrowth of any tumor remnant in the remaining life span of patients in the last few decades of life. However, we found a significant number of tumors will progress or recur, even in patients greater than 70 years old [11]. We think this may be due to a more aggressive tumor phenotype presenting at a large size in elderly patients, and therefore a more aggressive up front surgical strategy with GTR or SRS for any tumor remnant in the early postoperative period should be considered [11]. A recently published meta-analysis showed that STR followed by SRS 6 months postoperatively led to preservation of HB grades 1 or 2 in 142 of 151 adult patients, tumor growth control in 149 of 159 adult patients, and repeat therapy was required in 6 (3.7 %) patients [14]. This is a similar recurrence rate to our recurrence rate of 3.2 % in the younger age group, in which GTR was the preponderant treatment. This is consistent with our practice of supplementing STR or NTR with stereotactic radiosurgery in high-risk elderly group, which we hope can help reduce recurrence rate near the level of GTR. Due to the aggressiveness of recurrence following STR in elderly patients from our experience [11], we recommend an initial follow-up MRI scan at 3 months and 1 year post-STR, and then yearly for at least the next 5 years.

The most common complications following VS surgery in any age group are hearing loss and facial weakness. Baseline presbycusis can exacerbate or even mask the hearing loss caused by a unilateral VS. In elderly patients, great attention must be paid to the contralateral ear as ipsilateral hearing loss is highly likely with surgical resection of a VS. If there is significant contralateral hearing loss at presentation, even if the ipsilateral ear is functionally deaf (word recognition score < 50 %), we still often will try and preserve the cochlear nerve during resection of a VS in elderly patients. This potentially allows for cochlear implantation (CI) at a later date to rehabilitate the hearing. Also, we recommend elderly patients investigate all efforts to maximize contralateral hearing prior to undergoing surgery such as with the use of conventional hearing aids or even CI if they qualify as this will hopefully make their recovery from surgery easier.

Likewise, facial weakness may be especially difficult for elderly patients. This can manifest prominently if there is baseline visual impairment such as may occur with cataracts. In the rare patient who has a VS ipsilateral to their better seeing eye, if they develop complete facial weakness and difficulty protecting that cornea it may lead to significant visual difficulty. Combined with baseline age related balance dysfunction and a complete ipsilateral vestibulopathy from the tumor, further visual impairment can result in significant fall risk. Even if the eye is well protected by frequent application of drops or ointment these substances can cause blurring and loss of stereo vision and thus greater risk of falls. For all these reasons, postoperative vestibular rehabilitation and instruction with gait aids is a major component of the early postoperative recovery. Complete facial weakness can also result in impairment in the understandability of speech and difficulty with eating. Food may pocket in the weak side of the mouth and possibility exacerbate baseline age-related dysphagia. For all these reasons, every attempt to preserve facial nerve function should be made in elderly patients, balancing this against the knowledge that elderly patients that present with large symptomatic tumors thus requiring surgery, may be harboring a more aggressive tumor type and if GTR is not feasible due to risk of cranial nerve injury, then the tumor volume must be effectively reduced to allow safe and effective SRS.

For tumors less than 1.5 cm in posterior fossa diameter, almost regardless of age, we now favor an observational approach with follow-up MRI scan and audiogram every 6 months for the first year and then annually thereafter. At our center, most elderly patients choose to undergo SRS to treat an enlarging VS. To our knowledge, there is no evidence age affects outcome for patients treated with SRS for VS. Additionally, this treatment can be undertaken without interrupting oral anticoagulation, takes one day and is done on an out-patient basis. Therefore, our surgical series of patients >65 years of age who undergo surgical resection is very highly selected. These patients tend to have larger, more cystic (and anecdotally then less likely to respond to SRS) symptomatic tumors and are felt to be physiologically fit to undergo surgery in the posterior fossa. Anecdotally, we have found translabyrinthine surgery is better tolerated in the elderly population compared to retrosigmoid craniotomy as it relates to postoperative headache, fatigue and general well-being. While there is fairly good evidence even larger tumors can be treated safely with SRS, there is a higher risk of post-radiation hydrocephalus and we have found if the tumor fails SRS and requires resection, this is more difficult compared to non-radiated tumors [3]. Also, it may take on average 2–3 years following SRS before it is clear the tumor has failed radiation and requires resection and, of course, the patient will be 2–3 years older then at the time of surgical salvage. Also, as Roehm and Gantz have stressed, there is some risk the patient may become “lost to follow-up” and only return when the tumor is quite large and the risk of intervention is significantly higher [8]. Therefore, even in elderly patients, our bias is still to remove tumors with posterior fossa diameters >2.8 cm. While we attempt GTR, we understand the importance of maintaining good facial nerve function and will halt the resection if we feel we are putting the facial nerve at undo risk based on intraoperative facial nerve electrophysiologic testing [20]. However, we always perform a very extensive decompression of the posterior fossa component of the tumor and try to have any remnant less than a 1.5 cm^3 volume.

The current study has multiple strengths, including its focus on a large cohort of VS patients who underwent surgical resection to varying extents, allowing for a comprehensive review of demographics, imaging data, peri/intraoperative characteristics, complications, and follow-up, as well as effective comparison against younger age population to elucidate aging-specific differences that might yield insightful information on treating this growing population. This study is limited by retrospective data collection/analysis and significant selection bias as discussed above. With the variable clinical courses and treatments, our study shows that the elderly patients who underwent surgical resection mostly show a satisfactory outcome, but the recurrence rate tended to be high with the less aggressive approach. Therefore, consideration of adjuvant radiotherapy and close imaging follow-up is necessary in patients greater than 65 years old who undergo less than GTR.

References

1. Consensus Development Conference Statement December 11–13, 1991”. National Institutes of Health
2. Tos M, Stangerup SE, Cayé-Thomasen P, Tos T, Thomsen J (2004) What is the real incidence of vestibular schwannoma? Arch Otolaryngol Head Neck Surg 130:216–220
3. Milligan BD, Pollock BE, Foote RL et al (2012) Long-term tumor control and cranial nerve outcomes following gamma knife surgery for larger-volume vestibular schwannomas. J Neurosurg 116:598–604
4. Myrseth E, Møller P, Pedersen PH et al (2009) Vestibular schwannoma: surgery or gamma knife radiosurgery? A prospective, nonrandomized study. Neurosurgery 64:654–661
5. Anderson BM, Khuntia D, Bentzen SM et al (2014) Single institution experience treating 104 vestibular schwannomas with fractionated stereotactic radiation therapy or stereotactic radiosurgery. J Neurooncol 116:187–193

6. Choy W, Spasic M, Pezeshkian P et al (2013) Outcomes of stereotactic radiosurgery and stereotactic radiotherapy for the treatment of vestibular schwannoma. Neurosurgery 60:120–125
7. Piazza F, Frisina A, Gandolfi A, Quaranta N, Zini C (2003) Management of acoustic neuromas in the elderly: retrospective study. Ear Nose Throat J 82:374–378
8. Roehm PC, Gantz BJ (2007) Management of acoustic neuromas in patients 65 years or older. Otol Neurotol 28:708–714
9. Oghalai JS, Buxbaum JL, Pitts LH, Jackler RK (2003) The effect of age on acoustic neuroma surgery outcomes. Otol Neurotol 24:473–477
10. Nuseir A, Sequino G, De Donato G, Taibah A, Sanna M (2012) Surgical management of vestibular schwannoma in elderly patients. Eur Arch Otorhinolaryngol 269:17–23
11. Van Abel KM, Carlson ML, Driscoll CL, Neff BA, Link MJ (2014) Vestibular schwannoma surgery in the elderly: a matched cohort study. J Neurosurg 120(1):207–217
12. House JW, Brackmann DE (1985) Facial nerve grading system. Otolaryngol Head Neck Surg 93:146–147, 198
13. Glasscock ME III, Pappas DG Jr, Manolidis S, Von Doersten PG, Jackson CG, Storper IS (1997) Management of acoustic neuroma in the elderly population. Am J Otol 18:236–242
14. Brokinkel B, Sauerland C, Holling M, Ewelt C, Horstmann G, van Eck AT, Stummer W (2014) Gamma Knife radiosurgery following subtotal resection of vestibular schwannoma. J Clin Neurosci 21(12):2077–2082
15. Bloch O, Sughrue ME, Kaur R et al (2011) Factors associated with preservation of facial nerve function after surgical resection of vestibular schwannoma. J Neurooncol 102:281–286
16. Falcioni M, Fois P, Taibah A et al (2011) Facial nerve function after vestibular schwannoma surgery. J Neurosurg 115:820–826
17. Rinaldi V, Casale M, Bressi F et al (2012) Facial nerve outcome after vestibular schwannoma surgery: our experience. J Neurol Surg B Skull Base 73:21–27
18. Bloch DC, Oghalai JS, Jackler RK et al (2004) The fate of the tumor remnant after lessthan-complete acoustic neuroma resection. Otolaryngol Head Neck Surg 130:104–112
19. Monsell EM (1995) New and revised reporting guidelines from the Committee on Hearing and Equilibrium. American Academy of Otolaryngology-Head and Neck Surgery Foundation, Inc. Otolaryngol Head Neck Surg 113(3):176–178
20. Schmitt WR, Daube JR, Carlson ML, Mandrekar JN, Beatty CW, Neff BA, Driscoll CL, Link MJ (2013) Use of supramaximal stimulation to predict facial nerve outcomes following vestibular schwannoma microsurgery: results from a decade of experience. J Neurosurg 118(1):206–212

Management of Primary CNS Lymphoma in Elderly Patients

11

Andreas F. Hottinger, Bianca Moura, Francesco Grandoni, and Rita De Micheli

11.1 Definition of PCNSL and Epidemiology

Primary central nervous system lymphoma (PCNSL) describes a malignant extranodal non-Hodgkin's lymphoma (NHL) whose sole site of involvement is, by definition, the central nervous system. Most PCNSL cases present in the supratentorial space, most commonly in the frontal or temporo-parietal lobes, followed by the basal ganglia. Rarely, the disease may present in the cerebellum, brainstem or even the spinal cord. The disease may include the eyes and leptomeninges. PCNSL must be differentiated from systemic NHL with metastasis to the central nervous system.

It is commonly accepted that elderly patients should be defined as older than 60–65 years of age [1].

The peak age at diagnosis of PCNSL is 53–57 years in immunocompetent patients with a male/female ratio of 1.2–1.7:1 [2]. However, since 1990, the incidence has increased dramatically in those aged 60 and more [3]. The incidence of PCNSL is 28 per 10 million [4]. In immunocompromised patients, the typical age at presentation is younger with a mean age range between 31 and 35 years, consistent with the population that is most at risk of AIDS. Similarly, in this population the male/female ratio is 7.38:1 [2, 5].

A.F. Hottinger, MD, PhD (✉)
Departments of Clinical Neurosciences & Oncology, Lausanne University Hospital, Rue du Bugnon 46, 1011 Lausanne CHUV, Switzerland
e-mail: andreas.hottinger@chuv.com

B. Moura, MD • F. Grandoni, MD • R. De Micheli, MD
Department of Oncology, Lausanne University Hospital, Rue du Bugnon 46, 1011 Lausanne CHUV, Switzerland

© Springer International Publishing Switzerland 2017

M. Berhouma, P. Krolak-Salmon (eds.), *Brain and Spine Surgery in the Elderly*, DOI 10.1007/978-3-319-40232-1_11

11.2 Prognosis

Certain prognostic factors have a significant impact on the outcome of patients. Multiple prognostic scales have been developed, but in all, performance status and age have been consistently identified as treatment-independent prognostic factors [6, 7]. The fact that age plays a key role is critical as the median age of diagnosis for PCNSL in immunocompetent patients is around 65 years with most patients being between 45 and 70. Two scales are widely used as they have been validated in large multicentric populations of PCNSL patients. The IELSG prognostic index included five independent variables: age (>60), performance status (ECOG >1), serum LDH level (elevated), protein levels in the CSF (elevated) and involvement of deep structures [7]. This index shows a survival rate at 2 years of 80 % for patients with up to 1 abnormal factor, 48 % for up to 3 abnormal factors and 15 % for 4 or more abnormal prognostic factors. The Memorial Sloan Kettering prognostic index identified age and performance status as sole independent prognostic factors (Fig. 11.1) [8].

11.3 Predisposing Conditions

The only characteristics shared by immunocompetent patients with PCNSL are advanced age and a slight propensity for male gender. Next to AIDS, conditions that favour the development in immunocompromised patients include iatrogenic immunosuppression for transplantation or for autoimmune diseases (such as rheumatoid arthritis and rare congenital immunodeficiency syndromes such as severe combined immunodeficiency, Wiskott-Aldrich or ataxia-telangiectasia syndromes) [9]. The risk of PCNSL directly correlates with the degree of immune suppression as illustrated in AIDS patients, where the median CD4 count in patients with PCNSL is 30 cells/mm^3 [10].

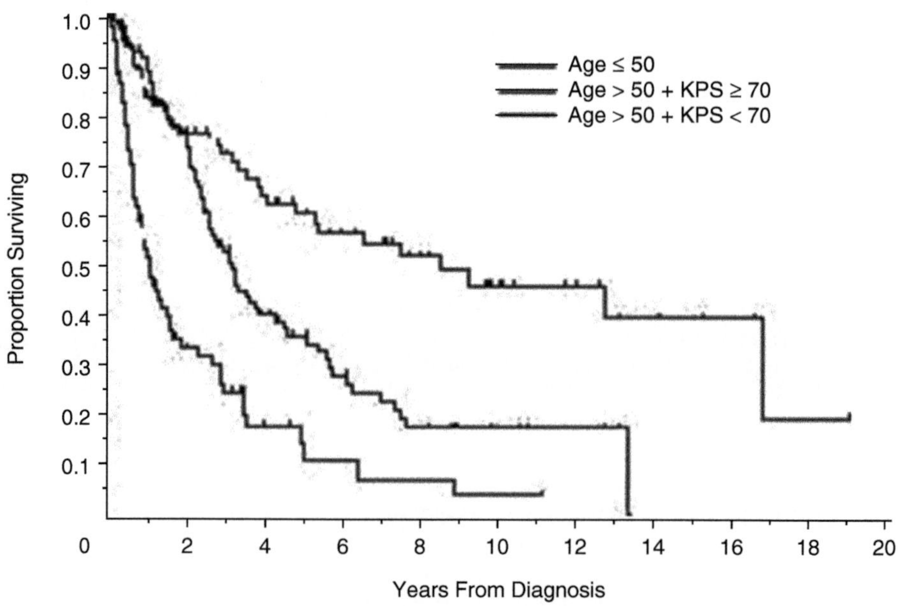

Fig. 11.1 The Memorial Sloan-Kettering Cancer Center (MSKCC) prognostic model

11.4 Clinical Features

11.4.1 Anatomic Distribution of the Lesions

The signs and symptoms of PCNSL reflect the neuroanatomic localization of the lesions. PCNSL can be separated into four distinct anatomic distributions: (1) intracranial mass lesions that can be solitary or multiple, often in contact with the ventricular surface; (2) leptomeningeal lesions; (3) ocular lymphoma that can present either without or with associated cerebral lesions; and (4) spinal cord lesions (extremely rare).

Intracranial PCNSL lesions appear as a solitary lesion in about 70 % of immunocompetent patients, whereas AIDS-associated PCNSL is as likely to present with either multiple or solitary lesions [5, 11]. Approximately 85 % of the lesions are found in supratentorial site, whereas only 15 % will be localized in an infratentorial location [11]. Of the lesions localized supratentorially, more than 60 % are periventricular and may involve the basal ganglia, thalamus or corpus callosum, which is especially suggestive of the presence of PCNSL [12]. When considering the distribution between cerebral lobes, the frontal (20 %) parietal (18 %) and temporal (15 %) lobes are more often involved than the occipital lobe (4 %) [11].

Primary leptomeningeal lymphoma is defined as PCNSL limited to the meninges, without presence of parenchymal cerebral or systemic disease. It is rare and represents only about 7 % of all immunocompetent PCNSL [13]. In contrast, involvement of the meninges by intracranial PCNSL is much more common and can be observed in up to 41 % of cases [14].

Primary intraocular lymphoma involves the vitreous, retina, choroid or the optic nerve. It is a rare malignancy, but the exact incidence is unknown. Of note, about 10–20 % of immunocompetent patients with intracerebral PCNSL are found to have ocular involvement of the disease at time of diagnosis [15].

With less than 1 % of presenting cases, the spinal cord is rarely involved in PCNSL. In multifocal PCNSL, dissemination to the spinal cord may result from direct invasion from the caudal brainstem or through dissemination through the CSF [16].

11.5 Presenting Signs and Symptoms

The average time from presentation of symptoms to diagnosis is 2–3 months [5]. The localization of the PCNSL will determine the clinical presentation in each patient. In a large series of 248 immunocompetent patients, 70 % of patients showed focal neurological deficits; 43 % showed neuropsychiatric symptoms including apathy, depression and confusion. These symptoms have been linked to infiltration and function disruption of the white fibre tracts that surround the periventricular regions and the corpus callosum. Signs and symptoms suggestive of intracranial hypertension (headache, nausea and vomiting) were seen in 33 % of patients. Merely 14 % of patients presented with seizures. This low number reflects the deep localization of

Table 11.1 Signs and symptoms of PCNSL at presentation

Signs or symptoms	Percentage
Focal neurological deficit	70 %
Neuropsychiatric symptoms Apathy Depression Confusion	43 %
Increased intracranial pressure Headache Nausea Vomiting	33 %
Seizures	14 %
Ocular symptoms Floaters Blurred vision Decrease in acuity Painful red eye	4 %
Cranial nerve palsies	5–31 %

Adapted from Bataille et al. [11]

the tumour, away from the cortical grey matter. Four percent of patients present with ocular symptoms (Table 11.1). In contrast to immunocompetent patients, immunocompromised patients are more likely to present with mental status changes and seizures [5].

Leptomeningeal involvement is asymptomatic in the majority of cases [14]. Cranial nerve palsies have been reported in 5–31 % of patients [9, 17].

In case of ocular lymphoma, both eyes will be affected in the majority of cases, and patients will complain of floaters and blurred vision. More rarely, patient will present with loss of visual acuity or painful red eyes. Up to 20 % of patients will be asymptomatic [15].

Symptoms and signs of intramedullary spinal tumours may include limb numbness or paraesthesia, weakness (often asymmetrical) and bowel or bladder dysfunction.

11.6 Diagnosis and Staging

The diagnosis of PCNSL will usually be established based on the clinical presentation of the patient and the radiological appearance. It cannot be stressed enough that the initiation of a steroid treatment might compromise the further work-up and should only be performed after careful consideration of the situation (e.g. given the presence of important neurological deficits). There is a common belief that any cerebral lesion that shows a partial or complete response following administration of steroids will be a PCNSL by definition. Recent studies over show that merely 50 % of these lesions will be PCNSL [18].

11.6.1 Neuroimaging

The appearance of PCNSL presents some characteristic features both on CT and MRI. A solitary lesion that infiltrates the corpus callosum and shows a very intense and homogeneous enhancement and little peritumoral oedema is highly suggestive of PCNSL. On CT, masses appear most commonly iso- or hyperdense and show homogeneous enhancement following contrast injection. On MRI, lesions are typically hypointense on T1 sequences and iso- or hyperintense on T2 weighted sequences (Fig. 11.2). They will show homogeneous contrast enhancement following gadolinium contrast injection [19]. Linear enhancement at the margins of a lesion tracking along the Virchow-Robin perivascular spaces has been described as highly specific for PCNSL. Evidence of calcifications, intratumoral haemorrhages or necrosis are rarely observed in untreated PCNSL lesions.

Moreover, these lesions often show a high hyperintensity on diffusion-weighted images, based on the relative restriction of water diffusion. This is however not exclusive to PCNSL and may also be observed in acute stroke, cerebral abscess and other high-grade tumours. On perfusion sequences, PCNSL lesions typically present a low rCBV, which might be attributed to the typical angiocentric growth pattern. This also explains the important leakage of contrast media into the interstitial space and the high and homogeneous contrast enhancement observed in these lesions [20]. MR spectroscopy often shows increased choline and decreased NAA along with the presence of lipid peaks. This pattern does not allow for a clear discrimination from glioblastoma or metastases but may help in differentiating PCNSL from other lesions [20].

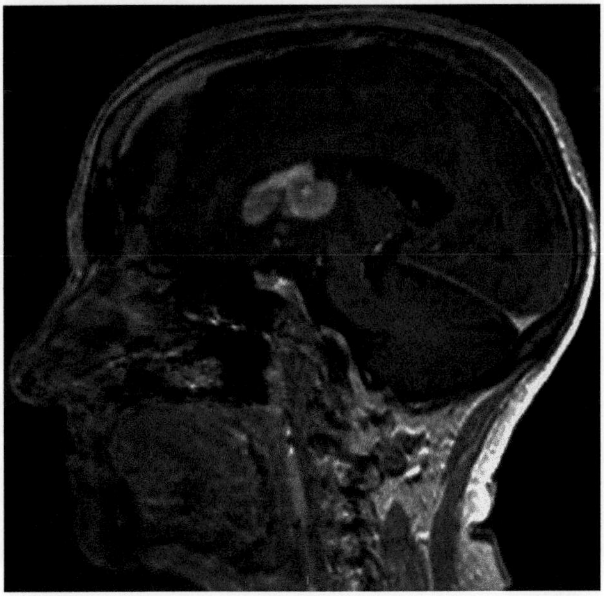

Fig. 11.2 Typical MRI T1 contrast-enhanced image of PCNSL

As spinal cord involvement is rare, enhanced MRI of the spine is not recommended routinely but should be reserved for patients where the clinical suspicion of PCNSL involvement is high [21].

11.6.2 Radiological Differential Diagnosis

In most instances the differential diagnosis will be established based on MRI findings. Many patients however present with atypical lesions that do not include all the hallmarks of PCNSL. The differential diagnosis of such a lesion on MRI includes glioma, metastatic brain tumour or focal demyelinating lesions. For immunocompromised patients, the differential diagnosis must further include toxoplasmosis cerebri, which has a similar incidence than PCNSL in AIDS patients.

11.7 Patient Work-Up

Once PCNSL is suspected, because of the clinical history of the patient and based on findings on the MRI, a definitive diagnosis must be established through other diagnostic modalities before initiation of treatment (Table 11.2). The work-up must be performed not only to establish the diagnosis of PCNSL but also to exclude the possibility of a systemic lymphoma, to tailor the optimal treatment and to ensure that the patient will not present exclusion criteria for the planned treatment. A spinal tap, if not contraindicated, and ophthalmologic evaluation in all patients are recommended, including those without ocular symptoms [1]. In the presence of a high clinical and radiological suspicion of PCNSL, identification of lymphoma cells in the vitreous fluid or the CSF might obviate the need for a stereotactic biopsy to confirm the diagnosis. In a prospective study of 96 immunocompetent patients with

Table 11.2 Diagnostic studies and work-up

Diagnostic studies	Evaluation
Radiological studies	Contrast-enhanced cranial CT Contrast-enhanced cranial MRI Body CT of the chest, abdomen and pelvis FDG-PET
Biopsy	Stereotactic brain biopsy Bone marrow biopsy
CSF lumbar puncture	Cell count, total protein Cytology, flow cytometry Search for clonal rearrangement EBV PCR (immunocompromised patients)
Blood	Lactate dehydrogenase (LDH) levels HIV serology Electrolytes Kidney and hepatic functions
Ocular evaluation	Slit-lamp examination

PCNSL, 15 % could be diagnosed by CSF cytology alone; in contrast 5 % were diagnosed by vitrectomy and 78 % by operative means [14].

The blood work-up should include determination of complete blood counts (CBC), serum lactate and dehydrogenase (LDH) levels, HIV testing and determination that electrolytes and kidney and liver functions are within normal limits.

At diagnosis, evidence of systemic lymphoma will be found in 2–3 % of "PCNSL" cases. This might however represent an underestimation of the true rate as many cases will not be included in PCNSL case series. Over the course of the disease, 7–10 % of cases will develop systemic involvement, usually late in the course of the disease [22, 23]. Systemic staging should include at least a physical examination, bone marrow biopsy, testicular ultrasonography and CT scan of the chest, abdomen and pelvis. Whole-body fluorodeoxyglucose PET might be an alternative to testicular sonography and the body CT [1].

11.7.1 Cerebrospinal Fluid

Analysis of cerebrospinal fluid (CSF) is an important part of the work-up. As a note of caution, as with any other patient presenting an intracerebral mass lesion, a lumbar puncture should however only be performed on PCNSL patients once the risk of herniation could be reasonably excluded. The CSF examination should include (1) basic studies including white blood cell count, protein and glucose levels (the glucose level will have to be compared to the serum glucose level); (2) cytology and/or (flow cytometry); and (3) determination of the presence of clonal immunoglobulin gene rearrangements or, in AIDS patients, PCR for Epstein-Barr virus DNA [24]. Most neuropathologists will rely on CSF cytology. In many immunocompetent patients, basic CSF parameters may be within normal limits or only slightly abnormal: in a study of 96 patients, a mild pleocytosis was present in only slightly more than half the patients (54 %), with a median WBC count of 8 cells/mm^3 (normal, $\leq$7 cells/mm^3). In the same study proteins were elevated in 67 % of patients, and low glucose was found in 10 % [14]. CSF cytology can be sufficient to establish the diagnosis in a significant percentage of cases: positive CSF cytology will be positive in 26–31 % of cases [5]. Serial samples of CSF might increase the probability of establishing the diagnosis through CSF cytology; this approach must however be balanced against the possibility to quickly perform a cerebral biopsy. Given the relatively low yield of cytology, the search for clonal rearrangements of the immunoglobulin heavy chains by PCR can establish monoclonality of a lymphocyte population in the CSF and thus confirm the diagnosis of PCNSL [25–27].

11.7.2 Neurosurgical Approach: Biopsy

Biopsy remains the standard procedure to obtain tissue that is adequate for pathologic diagnosis of PCNSL [1]. As administration of steroids may prevent to establish a histopathological diagnosis, its use should be avoided prior to the biopsy. In the case when, following administration of steroids, the neuropathologist is unable to establish a diagnosis due to remission or the presence of an aspecific inflammation, the patient should be carefully followed clinically and radiologically with serial MRIs and be rebiopsied once the lesion recurs [1].

The immunohistochemical markers should include pan-B-cell markers (CD19, CD20, PAX5) BCL6, MUM1/IRF4 and CD10). In difficult cases PCR analysis of immunoglobulin gene families might help to establish the diagnosis by demonstrating monoclonal rearrangement.

In immunocompromised patient, both the morbidity and mortality are higher compared to non-immunocompromised patients as these patients present both a higher risk of haemorrhages and of infections [28]. The diagnostic accuracy of a biopsy in AIDS patients ranges from 88 to 96 % [29]. In this patient population, the most common differential diagnosis includes toxoplasmosis. As all HIV-associated PCNSL are associated with EBV, PCR detection of EBV DNA in the CSF has become an established tool for the diagnosis and can obviate the need for a biopsy. It has a high sensitivity (83–100 %) and a high specificity (>90 %) [30–32].

11.7.3 Surgery Versus Biopsy?

Of note, traditionally, surgery has been deemed to have no role in the treatment of PCNSL. This view is based on small retrospective series, which suggest that there is no clear benefit of outcome for patients when compared with supportive care and to patients who underwent biopsy [33]. Similarly, patients who undergo maximal treatment with chemo- and radiotherapy have the same outcome regardless whether they had undergone prior resection or biopsy [11, 34]. This lack of efficacy of surgical resection might be attributed to a number of reasons, including the possibility that, due to its infiltrative nature, there is microscopic disease localized at distance from the visible site of disease [35]. Moreover, any potential benefit of a larger resection might be mitigated as PCNSL is highly sensitive to chemotherapy and radiation therapy. Given the usually deep localization of the disease, a neurosurgical approach is often also linked with a significant risk of postoperative morbidity. The recommendation to discourage neurosurgical resection is however not based on any randomized trial data. Interestingly a retrospective analysis of the German PCNSL study group-1 phase III trial evaluated the association between outcome and surgery. Interestingly, patients with subtotal or total resections had significantly longer progression-free survival and overall survival than did patients who received biopsies [36]. This was independent of age and of postoperative performance status. There is a possibility that this difference in outcome might have been influenced by the fact that the resected lesions were localized more frequently in more superficial localizations. It must also be noted that once adjusted for the number of lesions present, the outcome difference remained statistically significant for PFS but not for OS. Presently, an aggressive resection approach can therefore not be recommended as a standard approach. It might however be considered in patients with large lesions and symptoms of acute herniation to rapidly reduce intracranial pressure and potentially in unifocal and resectable lesions [1].

11.7.4 Ocular Evaluation

As part of the assessment of any PCNSL patient, an ocular evaluation including visualization of the fundus and a slit lamp should be performed. Typically, a cellular infiltration can be observed in the vitreous, and subretinal infiltrates may be seen. If indicated, vitrectomy may establish the diagnosis of PCNSL. It should be performed in the eye with the worst vision and most severe vitritis [1]. The specimen can also be analyzed by immunohistochemistry or flow cytometry to establish monoclonality.

11.8 Treatment

In general, PCNSL is an extremely radio- and chemosensitive tumour. Relapse is however common, and the ideal combination of chemotherapy and radiotherapy has not yet been established. Moreover, balancing the efficacy of treatment with the risk of serious, permanent long-term neurological deficits must be considered.

11.9 Steroids

Administration of steroids can delay or confound the diagnosis as steroids induce cytolysis of lymphoma cells, by way of cytoplasmic steroid receptors that are translocated to the nucleus [37]. This effect is independent from wild-type p53 activity but attenuated by the Bcl-2 proto-oncogene product [38]. Initial treatment of PCNSL with steroids may result in complete and partial remissions of 15 % and 25 %, respectively [39, 40]. This remission may outlast steroid administration, but the effect is usually temporary and recurrence is common. At that point the tumour is most often resistant to re-exposure to steroids. Because of this direct cytotoxic effect of steroids, they should, whenever possible, be avoided before biopsy to avoid false-negative results. Optimally, they should be withheld during the initial clinical evaluation, especially before CSF and ocular examination are performed. Steroids will have a rapid and important impact on peritumoral oedema and will decrease the mass effect induced by the PCNSL. If needed, they may therefore represent a key tool to improve neurological deficits in patients [39, 40]. To date, it remains however unclear whether steroids are an essential component of chemotherapy regimen against PCNSL, comparable to their use in systemic NHL. In summary, corticosteroids are useful to control increased intracranial pressure. The dose should be tapered off as quickly as possible to the lowest dose possible allowing to control neurological symptoms and can usually be tapered off once definitive treatment has been started.

The most common secondary complication of steroids include glucose intolerance, weight gain, myopathy, insomnia, adrenal insufficiency and increased rate of *Pneumocystis jiroveci* pneumonia. Steroids should be, whenever possible, avoided in immunocompromised patients because of the high risks of reactivated tuberculosis, *Pneumocystis jiroveci* infection and other life-threatening infections.

11.10 Radiation Therapy Alone

When used alone, whole brain radiation therapy targeting the whole brain and eyes achieves response rates of 60 %, but recurrences are usually rapid and median overall survival remains limited to 12–18 months and the 5-year survival rate is 4 % [41, 42]. This poor outcome might be attributed to several factors, including the microscopically diffuse and multifocal nature of PCNSL. A phase II radiation therapy oncology group (RTOG) trial delivered a total dose of 40 Gy with a 20 Gy boost to the contrast enhancing lesions. The results were disappointing with a median overall survival of 11.6 months and most recurrences occurring within the areas that had received the highest doses of RT [41]. These results strongly suggest that WBRT does not have any significant role in the management of PCNSL.

In various trials, the combination of high-dose methotrexate with WBRT has been suggested to result in better outcomes than WBRT alone with longer median overall survivals of 30–72 months and by increasing the percentage of long-term survivors (20–50 % of patients alive at 5 years) [43–50]. The optimum dose and fractionation schema have never been evaluated prospectively in PCNSL. Most protocols use a total dose of 40–45 Gy without a boost with 1.8–2 Gy delivered per fraction. A randomized phase III trial (G-PCNSL-SG1 trial) has evaluated RT following chemotherapy versus watch and wait. This non-inferiority trial randomized patient that had achieved a complete response following high-dose methotrexate chemotherapy to receive either consolidation RT (45 Gy in 30 fractions of 2 Gy) vs no further treatment. 318 patients were treated per protocol, and the overall survival was similar in both groups. In the protocol population, there was a slight but statistically non-significant outcome advantage in progression-free survival but not for OS for patients that had received WBRT [51]. The results of this trial have been hotly debated as the trial did not meet its primary endpoint and as there were a high number of patients that violated the protocol. Nevertheless, many experts estimate that these results contribute strongly to the accumulating retrospective evidence that suggest that omission of WBRT results in shorter progression-free survival but does not compromise overall survival [1].

11.11 Chemotherapy

Methotrexate-based regimens are the only that have demonstrated a significant advantage in outcome. Standard therapies for systemic NHL, such as cyclophosphamide-doxorubicin-vincristine-prednisone (CHOP), have not resulted in any sustained responses in PCNSL, probably linked to the poor CNS penetration of these agents due to the BBB [52–55]. Rapid infusion of high-dose MTX over 3 h greatly increases the drug level in the CSF [56]. As the efficacy of methotrexate can likewise depend on duration of exposure, MTX administration interval should range between 10 and 21 days [57]. High-dose administration of MTX however requires expertise for its administration, as attention to proper supportive care after administration must be scrupulous. All patients must have adequate creatinine clearance of ≥50 ml/min. The patient must be able to support important hydration and alkalinization of the urine and leucovorin rescue to reduce any morbidity associated with MTX. Leucovorin is a folate antagonist that is unable to cross the BBB, which will reverse the effect of MTX at the systemic level and will prevent hematologic and gastrointestinal toxicities. MTX is usually combined with a number of other agents that have demonstrated activity in PCNSL. In most protocols, a minimum of 4–6 injections are delivered, especially if no consolidation treatment (radiotherapy or intensive chemotherapy) is planned. Additional rounds of treatment might improve the complete remission rate in patients who achieve only a partial response [58]. Currently, most protocols combine high-dose MTX with various other agents to improve the response rate and duration of the remission. The best illustration comes from the IELSG phase II trial that compared high-dose MTX (3 g/m^2 every 21 days) alone versus high-dose MTX combined with cytarabine (2 g/m^2 twice per day on days 2 and 3 of every cycle). The patients receiving the combination treatment showed improved outcome in terms of response rate, percentage of complete remission and PFS [59].

The value of intrathecal chemotherapy as prophylaxis remains unclear. Intrathecal chemotherapy (intralumbar or preferably intraventricular through an Ommaya reservoir) can be proposed whenever meningeal involvement is documented [1].

11.12 Specific Considerations for the Treatment of Elderly Patients

For PCNSL patients, older age has been correlated with poorer outcome. The definition of older is however variable from study to study and may in some instances include patients as young as 50 years old. Moreover, older age (usually defined as >60 years) is associated with an increased risk of suffering from neurotoxic effects of treatments. The cut-off for elderly is therefore 60 years of age in most studies. A RTOG phase II trial demonstrated that WBRT alone in patients over 60 years of age resulted in a median overall survival of only 7.8 months [41]. Following MTX-based therapy of at least 1 g/m^2, median PFS and OS were between 6 and 16 months and 14–37 months respectively [50, 60–71]. Formal comparisons between the different high-dose methotrexate-based regimens have not been performed. However, a recent phase II study of elderly patients compared methotrexate, procarbazine, vincristine and cytarabine (MPV-A) and methotrexate-temozolomide. Side effects were similar in both arms, and there was a slight although not statistically significant better outcome in the MPV-A arm in regard to response rate, percentage of patients with complete responses, PFS and OS [64].

It must be noted that in most studies, administration of high-dose MTX up to doses of 3.5 g/m^2 was usually well tolerated by elderly patients [61, 62, 72, 73]. In the different trials, less than 10 % of elderly patients developed grade 3–4 nephrotoxic effects, and 7–10 % of patients needed to discontinue treatment related to adverse toxic events. It is however essential to adequately monitor renal function [74]. The risk of developing delayed leucoencephalopathy with neurocognitive deficits is also of great concern in elderly PCNSL patients [75, 76].

Because of this, it is recommended that patient with a KPS $\geq$ 70 be treated with high-dose MTX with deferral or omission of WBRT. In patients with a poor performance status and those older than 80 years, the treatment strategies must be weighted individually, based on co-morbidities and the poorer prognosis of any survival benefit as those patients have a worse prognosis and increased risk of treatment-related toxicities [1].

11.13 Rare Forms of PCNSL

11.13.1 Primary Leptomeningeal PCNSL

Primary leptomeningeal lymphoma is defined as PCNSL limited to the meninges, without presence of parenchymal cerebral or systemic disease. It is rare and represents only about 7 % of all immunocompetent PCNSL [13]. In contrast, involvement of the meninges by intracranial PCNSL is much more common and can be observed in up to 41 % of cases [14].

11.13.2 T-Cell Primary CNS Lymphoma

The clinical characteristics of T-cell PCNSL appear similar to the presentation of classical NHL PCNSL with similar median age of onset, performance status and location of lesions. There might be a male preponderance in T-cell lymphoma, and patients may present more commonly with B symptoms. Ocular involvement is uncommon [77]. The pathology is heterogeneous: one subtype shows CD30-positive anaplastic large cell lymphoma [78, 79]. Another subtype is a small cell variant [80, 81]. In most reported cases, the treatment consisted in combined modality therapy with systemic chemotherapy with either high-dose MTX alone or combined with other agents. The 2-year overall survival rate is around 37 % and the median disease-free interval 25 months [82].

11.13.3 Neurolymphomatosis

Neurolymphomatosis is a very rare syndrome, defined as a neuropathy of the peripheral nerves, nerve root, plexus or cranial nerve infiltration by NHL [83]. The clinical presentation mimics paraneoplastic or autoimmune neuropathies and may present as painful polyneuropathy or polyradiculopathy, cranial neuropathy or a painless neuropathy. In most cases, many months to years elapse between symptom presentation and diagnosis. In most cases, the diagnosis is made by biopsy of a mass lesion or through CSF analysis.

References

1. Hoang-Xuan K, Bessell E, Bromberg J et al (2015) Diagnosis and treatment of primary CNS lymphoma in immunocompetent patients: guidelines from the European Association for Neuro-Oncology. Lancet Oncol 16:e322–e332

2. Schabet M (1999) Epidemiology of primary CNS lymphoma. J Neurooncol 43:199–201
3. Kadan-Lottick NS, Skluzacek MC, Gurney JG (2002) Decreasing incidence rates of primary central nervous system lymphoma. Cancer 95:193–202
4. Cote TR, Manns A, Hardy CR et al (1996) Epidemiology of brain lymphoma among people with or without acquired immunodeficiency syndrome. AIDS/Cancer Study Group. J Natl Cancer Inst 88:675–679
5. Fine HA, Mayer RJ (1993) Primary central nervous system lymphoma. Ann Intern Med 119:1093–1104
6. Corry J, Smith JG, Wirth A et al (1998) Primary central nervous system lymphoma: age and performance status are more important than treatment modality. Int J Radiat Oncol Biol Phys 41:615–620
7. Ferreri AJ, Blay JY, Reni M et al (2003) Prognostic scoring system for primary CNS lymphomas: the International Extranodal Lymphoma Study Group experience. J Clin Oncol 21:266–272
8. Abrey LE, Ben-Porat L, Panageas KS et al (2006) Primary central nervous system lymphoma: the Memorial Sloan-Kettering Cancer Center prognostic model. J Clin Oncol 24:5711–5715
9. Herrlinger U, Schabet M, Bitzer M et al (1999) Primary central nervous system lymphoma: from clinical presentation to diagnosis. J Neurooncol 43:219–226
10. Besson C, Goubar A, Gabarre J et al (2001) Changes in AIDS-related lymphoma since the era of highly active antiretroviral therapy. Blood 98:2339–2344
11. Bataille B, Delwail V, Menet E et al (2000) Primary intracerebral malignant lymphoma: report of 248 cases. J Neurosurg 92:261–266
12. Camilleri-Broet S, Martin A, Moreau A et al (1998) Primary central nervous system lymphomas in 72 immunocompetent patients: pathologic findings and clinical correlations. Groupe Ouest Est d'etude des Leucenies et Autres Maladies du Sang (GOELAMS). Am J Clin Pathol 110:607–612
13. Lachance DH, O'Neill BP, Macdonald DR et al (1991) Primary leptomeningeal lymphoma: report of 9 cases, diagnosis with immunocytochemical analysis, and review of the literature. Neurology 41:95–100
14. Balmaceda C, Gaynor JJ, Sun M et al (1995) Leptomeningeal tumor in primary central nervous system lymphoma: recognition, significance, and implications. Ann Neurol 38:202–209
15. Grimm SA, McCannel CA, Omuro AM et al (2008) Primary CNS lymphoma with intraocular involvement: International PCNSL Collaborative Group Report. Neurology 71:1355–1360
16. Kawasaki K, Wakabayashi K, Koizumi T et al (2002) Spinal cord involvement of primary central nervous system lymphomas: histopathological examination of 14 autopsy cases. Neuropathology 22:13–18
17. Braus DF, Schwechheimer K, Muller-Hermelink HK et al (1992) Primary cerebral malignant non-Hodgkin's lymphomas: a retrospective clinical study. J Neurol 239:117–124
18. Shaw A, Iyer V, Rooney N et al (2014) Diagnosis of primary cerebral lymphomas: possible value of PCR testing in equivocal cases requiring rebiopsy. Br J Neurosurg 28:214–219
19. Mansour A, Qandeel M, Abdel-Razeq H, Abu Ali HA (2014) MR imaging features of intracranial primary CNS lymphoma in immune competent patients. Cancer Imaging 14:22
20. Haldorsen IS, Espeland A, Larsson EM (2011) Central nervous system lymphoma: characteristic findings on traditional and advanced imaging. AJNR Am J Neuroradiol 32:984–992
21. DeAngelis LM (1999) Primary central nervous system lymphoma. Curr Opin Neurol 12:687–691
22. Nasir S, DeAngelis LM (2000) Update on the management of primary CNS lymphoma. Oncology (Williston Park) 14:228–234; discussion 237–242, 244
23. Pasricha S, Gupta A, Gawande J et al (2011) Primary central nervous system lymphoma: a study of clinicopathological features and trend in western India. Indian J Cancer 48:199–203
24. Ivers LC, Kim AY, Sax PE (2004) Predictive value of polymerase chain reaction of cerebrospinal fluid for detection of Epstein-Barr virus to establish the diagnosis of HIV-related primary central nervous system lymphoma. Clin Infect Dis 38:1629–1632
25. Gleissner B, Siehl J, Korfel A et al (2002) CSF evaluation in primary CNS lymphoma patients by PCR of the CDR III IgH genes. Neurology 58:390–396

26. Galoin S, Daste G, Apoil PA et al (1997) Polymerase chain reaction on cerebrospinal fluid cells in the detection of leptomeningeal involvement by B-cell lymphoma and leukaemia: a novel strategy and its implications. Br J Haematol 99:122–130
27. Yanagisawa K, Tanuma J, Hagiwara S et al (2013) Epstein-Barr viral load in cerebrospinal fluid as a diagnostic marker of central nervous system involvement of AIDS-related lymphoma. Intern Med 52:955–959
28. Pell MF, Thomas DG, Whittle IR (1991) Stereotactic biopsy of cerebral lesions in patients with AIDS. Br J Neurosurg 5:585–589
29. Luzzati R, Ferrari S, Nicolato A et al (1996) Stereotactic brain biopsy in human immunodeficiency virus-infected patients. Arch Intern Med 156:565–568
30. Cinque P, Brytting M, Vago L et al (1993) Epstein-Barr virus DNA in cerebrospinal fluid from patients with AIDS-related primary lymphoma of the central nervous system. Lancet 342:398–401
31. De Luca A, Antinori A, Cingolani A et al (1995) Evaluation of cerebrospinal fluid EBV-DNA and IL-10 as markers for in vivo diagnosis of AIDS-related primary central nervous system lymphoma. Br J Haematol 90:844–849
32. Arribas JR, Clifford DB, Fichtenbaum CJ et al (1995) Detection of Epstein-Barr virus DNA in cerebrospinal fluid for diagnosis of AIDS-related central nervous system lymphoma. J Clin Microbiol 33:1580–1583
33. Henry JM, Heffner RRJ, Dillard SH et al (1974) Primary malignant lymphomas of the central nervous system. Cancer 34:1293–1302
34. Bellinzona M, Roser F, Ostertag H et al (2005) Surgical removal of primary central nervous system lymphomas (PCNSL) presenting as space occupying lesions: a series of 33 cases. Eur J Surg Oncol 31:100–105
35. Lai R, Rosenblum MK, DeAngelis LM (2002) Primary CNS lymphoma: a whole-brain disease? Neurology 59:1557–1562
36. Weller M, Martus P, Roth P et al (2012) Surgery for primary CNS lymphoma? Challenging a paradigm. Neuro Oncol 14:1481–1484
37. Roth P, Happold C, Weller M (2015) Corticosteroid use in neuro-oncology: an update. Neurooncol Pract 2:6–12
38. Weller M (1999) Glucocorticoid treatment of primary CNS lymphoma. J Neurooncol 43:237–239
39. Singh A, Strobos RJ, Singh BM et al (1982) Steroid-induced remissions in CNS lymphoma. Neurology 32:1267–1271
40. Todd FD, Miller CA, Yates AJ, Mervis LJ (1986) Steroid-induced remission in primary malignant lymphoma of the central nervous system. Surg Neurol 26:79–84
41. Nelson DF, Martz KL, Bonner H et al (1992) Non-Hodgkin's lymphoma of the brain: can high dose, large volume radiation therapy improve survival? Report on a prospective trial by the Radiation Therapy Oncology Group (RTOG): RTOG 8315. Int J Radiat Oncol Biol Phys 23:9–17
42. Ling SM, Roach M, Larson DA, Wara WM (1994) Radiotherapy of primary central nervous system lymphoma in patients with and without human immunodeficiency virus. Ten years of treatment experience at the University of California San Francisco. Cancer 73:2570–2582
43. DeAngelis LM, Yahalom J, Thaler HT, Kher U (1992) Combined modality therapy for primary CNS lymphoma. J Clin Oncol 10:635–643
44. Blay JY, Bouhour D, Carrie C et al (1995) The C5R protocol: a regimen of high-dose chemotherapy and radiotherapy in primary cerebral non-Hodgkin's lymphoma of patients with no known cause of immunosuppression. Blood 86:2922–2929
45. O'Brien P, Roos D, Pratt G et al (2000) Phase II multicenter study of brief single-agent methotrexate followed by irradiation in primary CNS lymphoma. J Clin Oncol 18:519–526
46. Omuro AM, DeAngelis LM, Yahalom J, Abrey LE (2005) Chemoradiotherapy for primary CNS lymphoma: an intent-to-treat analysis with complete follow-up. Neurology 64:69–74
47. Bessell EM, Graus F, Lopez-Guillermo A et al (2004) Primary non-Hodgkin's lymphoma of the CNS treated with CHOD/BVAM or BVAM chemotherapy before radiotherapy: long-term survival and prognostic factors. Int J Radiat Oncol Biol Phys 59:501–508

48. Poortmans PM, Kluin-Nelemans HC, Haaxma-Reiche H et al (2003) High-dose methotrexate-based chemotherapy followed by consolidating radiotherapy in non-AIDS-related primary central nervous system lymphoma: European Organization for Research and Treatment of Cancer Lymphoma Group Phase II Trial 20962. J Clin Oncol 21:4483–4488
49. Gavrilovic IT, Hormigo A, Yahalom J et al (2006) Long-term follow-up of high-dose methotrexate-based therapy with and without whole brain irradiation for newly diagnosed primary CNS lymphoma. J Clin Oncol 24:4570–4574
50. Ghesquieres H, Ferlay C, Sebban C et al (2010) Long-term follow-up of an age-adapted C5R protocol followed by radiotherapy in 99 newly diagnosed primary CNS lymphomas: a prospective multicentric phase II study of the Groupe d'Etude des Lymphomes de l'Adulte (GELA). Ann Oncol 21:842–850
51. Thiel E, Korfel A, Martus P et al (2010) High-dose methotrexate with or without whole brain radiotherapy for primary CNS lymphoma (G-PCNSL-SG-1): a phase 3, randomised, non-inferiority trial. Lancet Oncol 11:1036–1047
52. Lachance DH, Brizel DM, Gockerman JP et al (1994) Cyclophosphamide, doxorubicin, vincristine, and prednisone for primary central nervous system lymphoma: short-duration response and multifocal intracerebral recurrence preceding radiotherapy. Neurology 44:1721–1727
53. Schultz C, Scott C, Sherman W et al (1996) Preirradiation chemotherapy with cyclophosphamide, doxorubicin, vincristine, and dexamethasone for primary CNS lymphomas: initial report of radiation therapy oncology group protocol 88-06. J Clin Oncol 14:556–564
54. Shibamoto Y, Tsutsui K, Dodo Y et al (1990) Improved survival rate in primary intracranial lymphoma treated by high-dose radiation and systemic vincristine-doxorubicin-cyclophosphamide-prednisolone chemotherapy. Cancer 65:1907–1912
55. Stewart DJ, Russell N, Atack EA et al (1983) Cyclophosphamide, doxorubicin, vincristine, and dexamethasone in primary lymphoma of the brain: a case report. Cancer Treat Rep 67:287–291
56. Hiraga S, Arita N, Ohnishi T et al (1999) Rapid infusion of high-dose methotrexate resulting in enhanced penetration into cerebrospinal fluid and intensified tumor response in primary central nervous system lymphomas. J Neurosurg 91:221–230
57. Glass J, Gruber ML, Cher L, Hochberg FH (1994) Preirradiation methotrexate chemotherapy of primary central nervous system lymphoma: long-term outcome. J Neurosurg 81:188–195
58. Morris PG, Correa DD, Yahalom J et al (2013) Rituximab, methotrexate, procarbazine, and vincristine followed by consolidation reduced-dose whole-brain radiotherapy and cytarabine in newly diagnosed primary CNS lymphoma: final results and long-term outcome. J Clin Oncol 31:3971–3979
59. Ferreri AJ, Reni M, Foppoli M et al (2009) High-dose cytarabine plus high-dose methotrexate versus high-dose methotrexate alone in patients with primary CNS lymphoma: a randomised phase 2 trial. Lancet 374:1512–1520
60. Pels H, Schmidt-Wolf IG, Glasmacher A et al (2003) Primary central nervous system lymphoma: results of a pilot and phase II study of systemic and intraventricular chemotherapy with deferred radiotherapy. J Clin Oncol 21:4489–4495
61. Hoang-Xuan K, Taillandier L, Chinot O et al (2003) Chemotherapy alone as initial treatment for primary CNS lymphoma in patients older than 60 years: a multicenter phase II study (26952) of the European Organization for Research and Treatment of Cancer Brain Tumor Group. J Clin Oncol 21:2726–2731
62. Fritsch K, Kasenda B, Hader C et al (2011) Immunochemotherapy with rituximab, methotrexate, procarbazine, and lomustine for primary CNS lymphoma (PCNSL) in the elderly. Ann Oncol 22:2080–2085
63. Ney DE, Reiner AS, Panageas KS et al (2010) Characteristics and outcomes of elderly patients with primary central nervous system lymphoma: the Memorial Sloan-Kettering Cancer Center experience. Cancer 116:4605–4612
64. Omuro AM, Taillandier L, Chinot O et al (2007) Temozolomide and methotrexate for primary central nervous system lymphoma in the elderly. J Neurooncol 85:207–211
65. Roth P, Martus P, Kiewe P et al (2012) Outcome of elderly patients with primary CNS lymphoma in the G-PCNSL-SG-1 trial. Neurology 79:890–896

66. Illerhaus G, Muller F, Feuerhake F et al (2008) High-dose chemotherapy and autologous stem-cell transplantation without consolidating radiotherapy as first-line treatment for primary lymphoma of the central nervous system. Haematologica 93(1):147–148
67. Schuurmans M, Bromberg JE, Doorduijn J et al (2010) Primary central nervous system lymphoma in the elderly: a multicentre retrospective analysis. Br J Haematol 151:179–184
68. Taoka K, Okoshi Y, Sakamoto N et al (2010) A nonradiation-containing, intermediate-dose methotrexate regimen for elderly patients with primary central nervous system lymphoma. Int J Hematol 92:617–623
69. Zhu JJ, Gerstner ER, Engler DA et al (2009) High-dose methotrexate for elderly patients with primary CNS lymphoma. Neuro Oncol 11:211–215
70. Kurzwelly D, Glas M, Roth P et al (2010) Primary CNS lymphoma in the elderly: temozolomide therapy and MGMT status. J Neurooncol 97:389–392
71. Welch MR, Omuro A, Deangelis LM (2012) Outcomes of the oldest patients with primary CNS lymphoma treated at Memorial Sloan-Kettering Cancer Center. Neuro Oncol 14:1304–1311
72. Illerhaus G, Marks R, Muller F et al (2009) High-dose methotrexate combined with procarbazine and CCNU for primary CNS lymphoma in the elderly: results of a prospective pilot and phase II study. Ann Oncol 20:319–325
73. Jahnke K, Korfel A, Martus P et al (2005) High-dose methotrexate toxicity in elderly patients with primary central nervous system lymphoma. Ann Oncol 16:445–449
74. Bessell EM, Dickinson P, Dickinson S, Salmon J (2011) Increasing age at diagnosis and worsening renal function in patients with primary central nervous system lymphoma. J Neurooncol 104:191–193
75. Omuro A, Chinot O, Taillandier L et al (2015) Methotrexate and temozolomide versus methotrexate, procarbazine, vincristine, and cytarabine for primary CNS lymphoma in an elderly population: an intergroup ANOCEF-GOELAMS randomised phase 2 trial. Lancet Haematol 2:e251–e259
76. Correa DD, Shi W, Abrey LE et al (2012) Cognitive functions in primary CNS lymphoma after single or combined modality regimens. Neuro Oncol 14:101–108
77. Ferreri AJ, Blay JY, Reni M et al (2002) Relevance of intraocular involvement in the management of primary central nervous system lymphomas. Ann Oncol 13:531–538
78. Ponzoni M, Terreni MR, Ciceri F et al (2002) Primary brain CD30+ ALK1+ anaplastic large cell lymphoma ('ALKoma'): the first case with a combination of 'not common' variants. Ann Oncol 13:1827–1832
79. Shenkier TN, Blay JY, O'Neill BP et al (2005) Primary CNS lymphoma of T-cell origin: a descriptive analysis from the international primary CNS lymphoma collaborative group. J Clin Oncol 23:2233–2239
80. McCue MP, Sandrock AW, Lee JM et al (1993) Primary T-cell lymphoma of the brainstem. Neurology 43:377–381
81. Villegas E, Villa S, Lopez-Guillermo A et al (1997) Primary central nervous system lymphoma of T-cell origin: description of two cases and review of the literature. J Neurooncol 34:157–161
82. Ferreri AJ, Reni M, Pasini F et al (2002) A multicenter study of treatment of primary CNS lymphoma. Neurology 58:1513–1520
83. Baehring JM, Damek D, Martin EC et al (2003) Neurolymphomatosis. Neuro Oncol 5:104–115

Management of Brain Metastases: Distinctive Features in the Elderly

12

Moncef Berhouma

12.1 Generalities

Metastases represent the majority of brain tumors in the elderly. Up to 25% of elderly patients dying of cancer harbor one or more brain metastases at autopsy. Despite recent advances in chemotherapy, targeted treatments, and radiotherapy including radiosurgery, median survival remains poor usually ranging from 3 to 6 months in average as does the functional outcome. The most frequent sources of brain metastases in the elderly are the respiratory tract cancer, particularly small-cell cancer, and breast cancer. Melanoma is also a common provider of brain metastasis in the elderly, representing 10% of all brain metastases. Almost 40% of patients with melanoma have brain metastases at autopsy (Figs 12.1 – 12.6) [1, 2].

Obviously, the incidence of brain metastases in the elderly is increasing secondary to several factors. Firstly the widespread use of brain imaging either CT scan or MRI allows precocious diagnosis even in asymptomatic patients. Secondly, a longer survival of patients with cancer in general provides enough time to develop brain dissemination. Finally, the absence of chemotherapy drugs that penetrates efficiently the blood–brain barrier which still leaves the brain as a therapeutic sanctuary for chemotherapy [3].

In about 10% of elderly patients presenting with brain metastases, the primary neoplasm remains untraceable despite exhaustive explorations. The preferential location is the cortico–subcortical junction with a clear majority of supratentorial locations (90%) versus infratentorial ones (10%).

In contrast with younger patients whom usually present with intracranial hypertension signs and/or seizures, elderly patients with brain metastases commonly

M. Berhouma, MD, MSc, FEBNS
Department of Neurosurgery, University Hospital of Lyon – Hospices Civils de Lyon, Lyon, France
e-mail: berhouma.moncef@gmail.com

© Springer International Publishing Switzerland 2017

M. Berhouma, P. Krolak-Salmon (eds.), *Brain and Spine Surgery in the Elderly*,
DOI 10.1007/978-3-319-40232-1_12

suffer from more insidious symptoms such as cognitive changes and progressive focal deficits [4, 5]. In some cases, the clinical presentation can even be acute pseudovascular either secondary to intra-tumoral hemorrhage or to post-seizure motor deficit, leading to misdiagnoses of stroke. About one third of elderly patients with brain metastases will suffer from seizures during the course of their disease, particularly those harboring hemorrhagic metastases (melanoma, kidney, and thyroid).

12.2 Management in the Elderly

In the majority of cases, there is a relatively large amount of peri-tumoral edema that can be more threatening than the metastasis itself. The benefic role of corticosteroids has been clearly proven, reducing the signs of intracranial hypertension and usually improving neurological deficits. In the elderly, the use of high doses of corticosteroids should be closely monitored to prevent and timely detect specific complications such as diabetes mellitus, gastroduodenal ulcerations, and venous thrombosis. Roughly one third of elderly patients with brain metastases will have seizures during the course of their disease, reaching even 50% in hemorrhagic lesions or melanoma metastases, and therefore may require anticonvulsant therapy. This latter should not be systematic and prescribed only in cases of proven seizures because of the risk of interference with chemotherapy agents and may even cause complications (psychiatric morbidity, allergy, etc.). The doses should be rigorously adapted to the renal function.

12.3 Role of Neurosurgery

Neurosurgery can be useful in life-threatening solitary brain metastases (temporal lobe and cerebellar locations) or in hemorrhagic cases. Surgery can be helpful as well if a histopathological proof is needed particularly when the primary cancer site is not known or when there is a doubt with different brain expansive lesions (glioma, lymphoma, granuloma, etc.). Besides, the surgical resection can be very effective in large cerebellar metastases obstructing the cerebrospinal fluid flow and causing tonsillar herniation as it offers the possibility to the patient to better tolerate radiation therapy. Obviously, the surgical option should be considered only after a multidisciplinary discussion with the oncologist, the radiotherapist, the neurosurgeon, and the patient with his family as well taking into account the systemic control of the cancer and the estimated global survival. In these cases, a complete surgical resection appears to prolong survival and enhance the neurological functional outcome even in the era of radiosurgery [6]. The main keyword remains the appropriate multidisciplinary selection of the patients. In very selected cases, there is even a place to surgical resection in multiple brain metastases when one of these is life-threatening (especially for posterior fossa).

All adjuncts usually used in young adults can be used in the surgical treatment of brain metastases in the elderly: neuronavigation, cortical and subcortical stimulations, and awake surgery. The preoperative anesthetic preparation should mandatorily include cardiovascular and pulmonary assessments.

12.4 Role of Radiotherapy and Radiosurgery

Whole brain radiotherapy (WBRT) has been widely used during decades, prolonging survival but does not appear to be superior to surgical resection. Commonly 20–30 grays are delivered to the whole brain (with or without hippocampus sparing [7]) in 10–15 fractions. The number of fractions can be tailored to the status of the elderly patient, with an accelerated schema allowing very fragile old patients to better endure the radiation [8].

Stereotactic radiosurgery (SRS) is being increasingly used as an alternative to whole brain radiotherapy as it is supposed to have less toxicity particularly in elderly patients [2–4, 9] while it provides a local control of the disease. The neurotoxicity of radiation therapy may impact significantly the quality of life and the cognitive status in this elderly group of patients while their survival is prolonged with chemotherapies. Indeed, after 6–12 months following radiotherapy, elderly patients are exposed to radiation encephalopathy with subsequently subcortical dementia, gait disturbances, and urinary dysfunction mimicking chronic hydrocephalus and considerably altering the quality of life [10]. Recent randomized studies comparing WBRT plus SRS and SRS alone in patients harboring one to four brain metastases did not show significant differences in terms of survival, frequency of neurological deaths, and preservation of neurological status [11]. However, SRS appears to provide a local control while preserving the performance status and limiting the risk of radiation encephalopathy [12]. In fine, SRS alone may be considered in elderly patients having less than three to four metastases inferior to 3 cm of diameter either as an alternative or as an adjunct to WBRT.

Key Points

- The prognosis of elderly patients with brain metastases depends upon their performance status (Karnofsky Performance Score superior to 60) and the control of the extracranial cancer disease
- SRS should be considered in oligometastatic patients (one to four metastases) as an alternative or as an adjunct to classical WBRT. SRS alone is susceptible to preserve learning and memory functions when compared to SRS plus WBRT [13].
- Neurosurgical resection should be systematically discussed in cases of a unique large metastasis amenable to resection without significant neurological risk.
- The management of elderly patients with brain metastases should consider the local control of the disease, the systemic one, and their performance status scale at mid- and long term as the global survival is being prolonged with the use of systemic targeted therapies and new chemotherapies (Figs. 12.1, 12.2, 12.3, 12.4, 12.5, and 12.6).

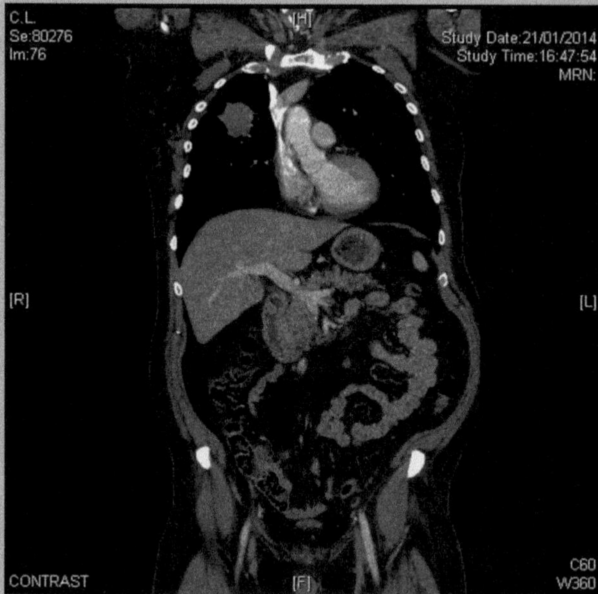

Fig. 12.1 Lung cancer is one of the most common provider of brain metastases particularly the small-cell cancer

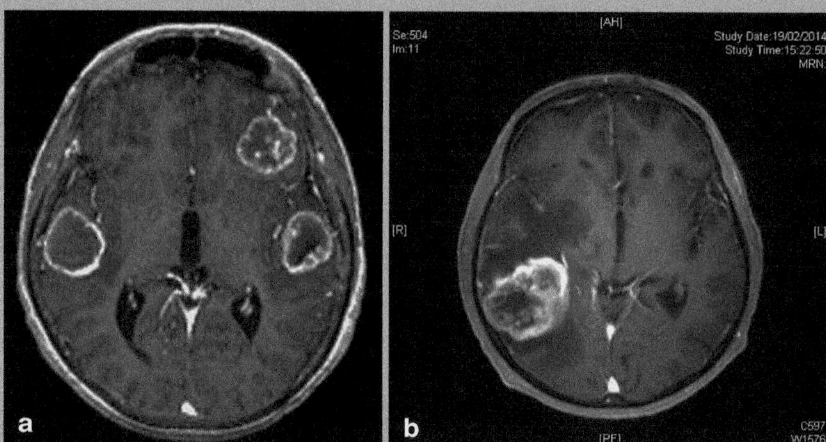

Fig. 12.2 Multiple brain metastases are not amenable to surgery except if there is a need for histological proof (**a**), while neurosurgical resection remains a good option for large unique metastasis (**b**)

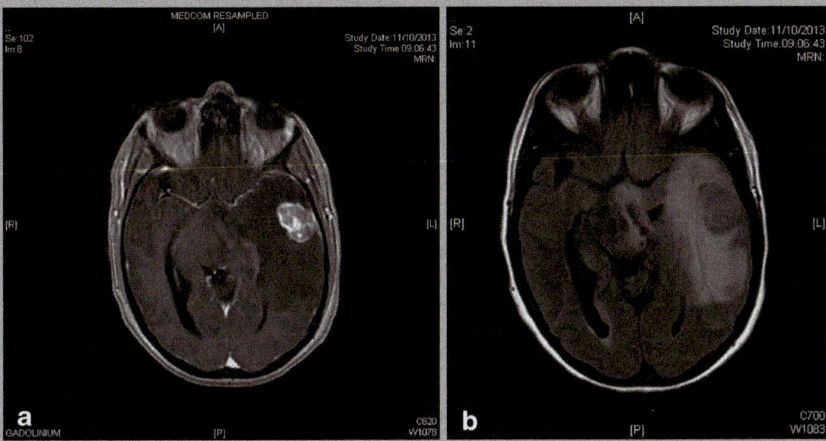

Fig. 12.3 Left temporal lobe unique metastasis (kidney cancer) (**a**) with a very extensive life-threatening edema (**b**)

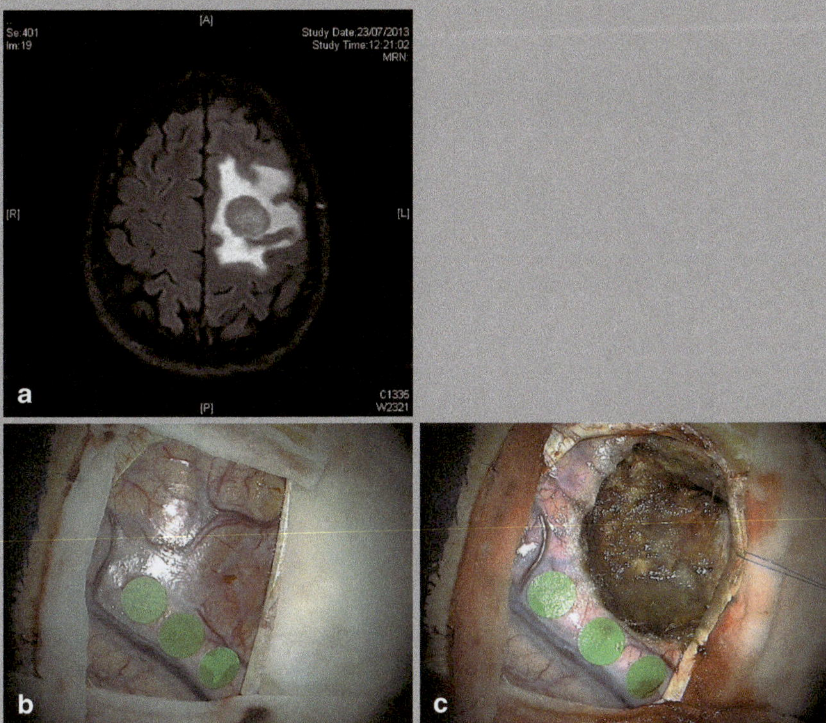

Fig. 12.4 Rolandic left metastasis with extensive edema without primitive cancer identified (**a**), requiring therefore surgical resection with an awake technique and cortical stimulation to identify the motor cortex (*green pastilles*) (**b**) allowing total removal without neurological deficit (**c**)

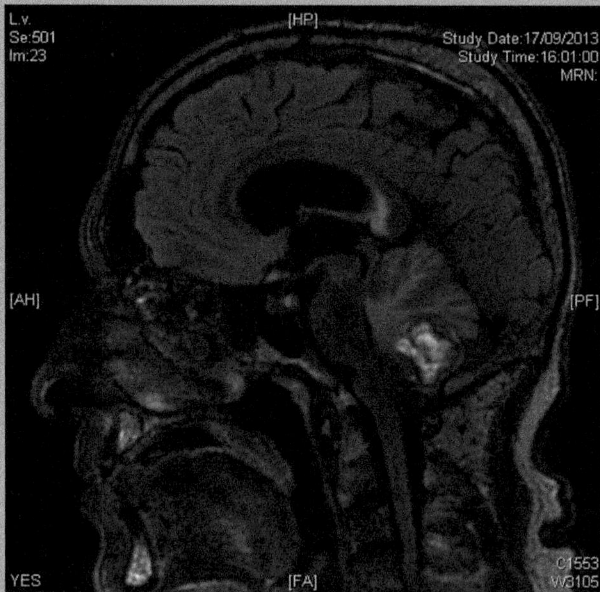

Fig. 12.5 Cerebellar life-threatening unique metastasis optimal for surgical resection because of tonsillar herniation

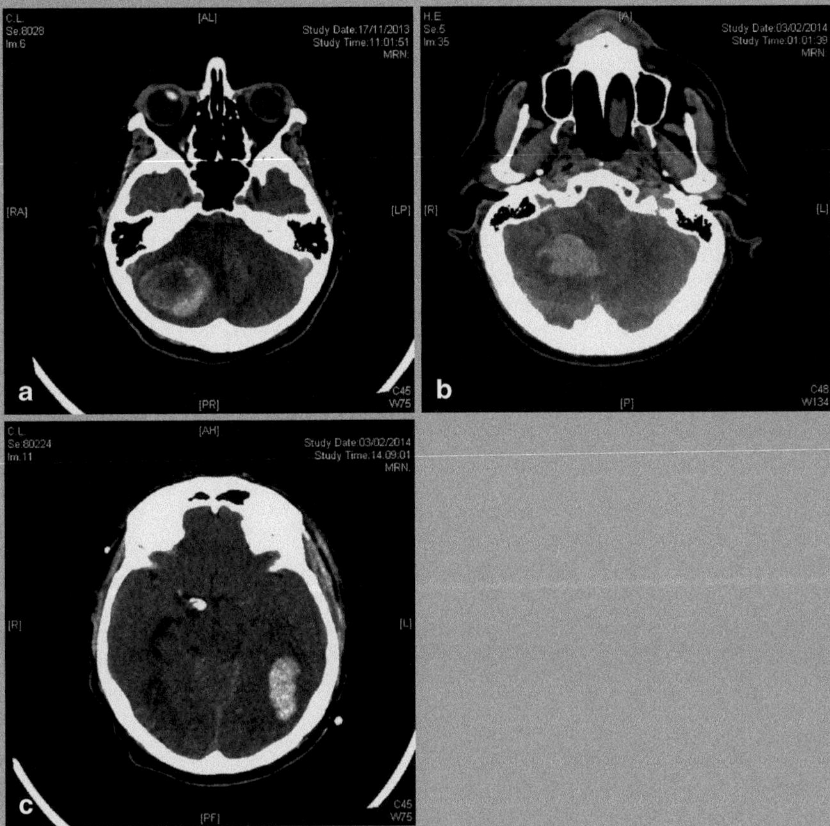

Fig. 12.6 Examples of brain metastases revealed in an acute pseudo-stroke presentation revealing melanoma (**a**), kidney (**b**), and thyroid (**c**) cancers

References

1. Rades D, Pluemer A, Veninga T, Schild SE (2008) Comparison of different treatment approaches for one to two brain metastases in elderly patients. Strahlenther Onkol 184:565–571
2. Evers JN et al (2014) A new score predicting survival prognosis after whole-brain radiotherapy alone for brain metastases in elderly patients. Anticancer Res 34:2455–2458
3. Nieder C, Thamm R, Astner ST, Geinitz H, Molls M (2007) Is whole-brain radiotherapy effective and safe in elderly patients with brain metastases? Oncology 72:326–329
4. Noel G et al (2005) Linac stereotactic radiosurgery: an effective and safe treatment for elderly patients with brain metastases. Int J Radiat Oncol Biol Phys 63:1555–1561
5. Park J-Y et al (2015) Gamma knife radiosurgery for elderly patients with brain metastases: evaluation of scoring systems that predict survival. BMC Cancer 15:54
6. Hatiboglu MA, Wildrick DM, Sawaya R (2013) The role of surgical resection in patients with brain metastases. Ecancermedicalscience 7:308

7. Oskan F et al (2014) Hippocampus sparing in whole-brain radiotherapy. A review. Strahlenther Onkol 190:337–341
8. Rades D et al (2011) Shorter-course whole-brain radiotherapy for brain metastases in elderly patients. Int J Radiat Oncol Biol Phys 81:e469–e473
9. Minniti G et al (2013) Stereotactic radiosurgery in elderly patients with brain metastases. J Neurooncol 111:319–325
10. Crossen JR, Garwood D, Glatstein E, Neuwelt EA (1994) Neurobehavioral sequelae of cranial irradiation in adults: a review of radiation-induced encephalopathy. J Clin Oncol 12:627–642
11. Aoyama H, Tago M, Shirato H, Japanese Radiation Oncology Study Group 99-1 (JROSG 99-1) Investigators (2015) Stereotactic Radiosurgery With or Without Whole-Brain Radiotherapy for Brain Metastases: Secondary Analysis of the JROSG 99-1 Randomized Clinical Trial. JAMA Oncol 1:457–464
12. Patil CG et al (2012) Whole brain radiation therapy (WBRT) alone versus WBRT and radiosurgery for the treatment of brain metastases. Cochrane Database Syst Rev 12;(9):CD006121. doi:10.1002/14651858.CD006121.pub3.
13. Chang EL et al (2009) Neurocognition in patients with brain metastases treated with radiosurgery or radiosurgery plus whole-brain irradiation: a randomised controlled trial. Lancet Oncol 10:1037–1044

Part IV

Spinal Diseases

Degenerative Spine Disease 13

Christian Ewald and Albrecht Waschke

13.1 General Principles

13.1.1 Introduction

Degenerative spinal disease (DSD) is a typical problem of the elderly patient. Against the background of the ongoing demographic change, neuro-, orthopedic-, and spine surgeons are more and more confronted with this topic and the concomitant clinical and economic problems.

Especially in elderly patients, the management of degenerative spinal pathologies is challenging, and "evidence-based" guidelines or treatment recommendations are barely available or lack completely [1, 2].

To illustrate this development, there are some data based on the *Diagnosis-Related Groups (DRG) system* in Germany, in which degenerative spinal pathologies like stenosis, spondylosis, and disc herniation as the main hospital diagnosis were coded 2005 in 156.333 patients >65 years and 2014 in 254.329 patients [3]. These numbers underline the future importance of this topic in spinal surgery.

In elderly patients diagnosis and therapy are often complicated by age-related problems like concomitant cardiovascular, cerebral, and/or endocrinologic disturbances. Osteoporosis and a decreased physical and mental performance are additional factors which have to be considered when a treatment concept is planned.

With this chapter we want to summarize the pathophysiological mechanisms and to describe diagnostic and therapeutic pathways based on the published scientific data and on our own practical and experimental experiences.

C. Ewald (✉) • A. Waschke
Department of Neurosurgery, Städtisches Klinikum Brandenburg GmbH,
Hochtstr. 29, 14770 Brandenburg an der Havel, Germany
e-mail: c.ewald@klinikum-brandenburg.de; Albrecht.waschke@med.uni-jena.de

© Springer International Publishing Switzerland 2017

M. Berhouma, P. Krolak-Salmon (eds.), *Brain and Spine Surgery in the Elderly*,
DOI 10.1007/978-3-319-40232-1_13

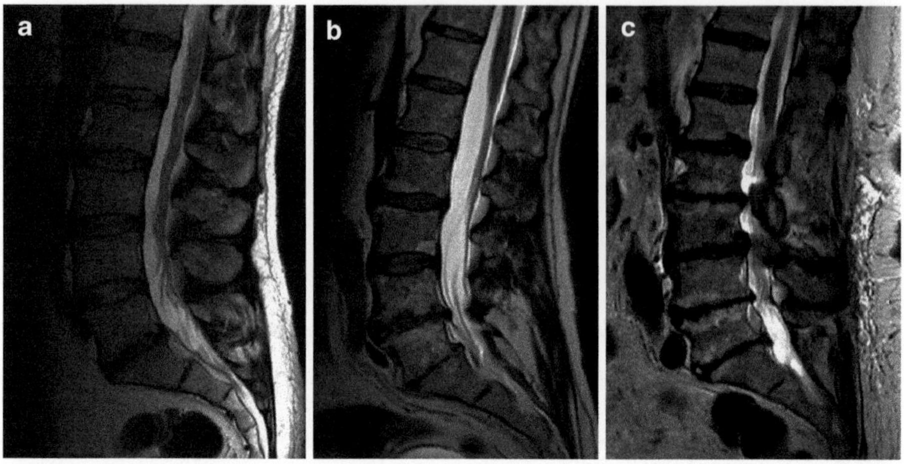

Fig. 13.1 Figure illustrates the physiological aging process of the lumbar spine. A T2-weighted sagittal MRI of an asymptomatic 15-year- (**a**), 50-year- (**b**), and 80-year (**c**)-old patients shows the typical changes like fluid and consecutive height loss of the discs and progressive narrowing and also deformation of the spinal canal

13.1.2 Age-Related Spine Degeneration

More than 75 % of the population in the Western industrialized countries experience back pain at least once during their lifetime. The concomitant temporary disability represents an enormous socioeconomic burden. In this context, one should be aware that there is a difference between normal age-related degenerative changes and "pathological" degeneration, which is associated with neck and back pain. A high percentage of individuals (between 15 and 70 %) with more or less pronounced signs of disc degeneration never experience relevant symptoms.

Degenerating "spondylosis" or spinal osteoarthritis is the most common alteration of the aging spine. This condition seems to be inevitable, with osteophytes (bone spurs) arising circumferentially from the margin of the vertebral body usually accompanied by a height reduction of the associated disc as the typical radiological sign (Fig. 13.1). In the historical context, the term "spondylosis" was created to differ between degenerative changes of the anterior column (vertebral body and intervertebral disc) and those of the facet joints (osteoarthritis). However, up to now it has come clear that age-related changes in the anterior column and aseptic osteoarthritis of the synovial joints have the same origin; they coexist and are closely interrelated.

13.1.2.1 Disc Degeneration

The degenerative changes of the whole spine are finally only a physiological reaction on the ongoing aging process. Already in the early adulthood, degeneration begins with a fluid loss within the discs which lead to a continuous height loss of the spinal segment (Fig. 13.2).

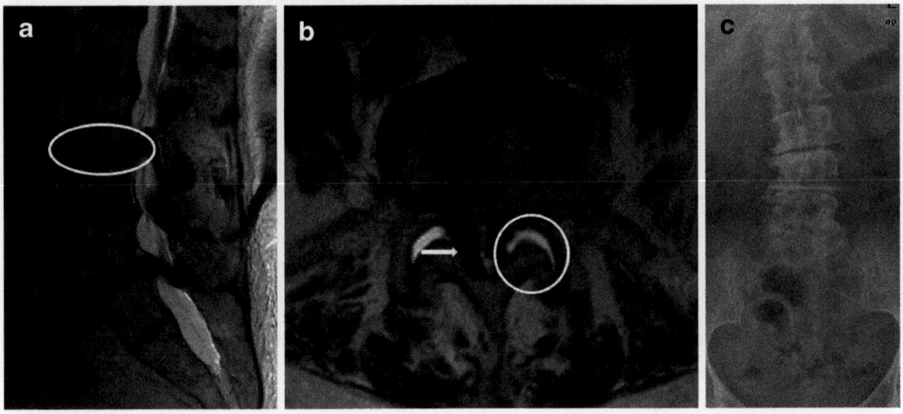

Fig. 13.2 Figure shows the typical radiological features of lumbar spine degeneration with disc bulging (**a**) ligamentum flavum hypertrophy (**b**, *arrow*), facet joint arthrosis (**b**, *circle*), and degenerative scoliosis (**c**)

The "motion segment" or "functional spinal unit" is defined as the spinal disc with the adjacent vertebral body, the facet joints, and the surrounding ligaments.

Concerning the degeneration process, different stages can be defined:

Juvenile disc

- Normal disc height and gel-like appearance (hydration) of the nucleus pulposus.
- Cartilage end plates are thick and resistant.

Adult disc

- Disc height normal, but nucleus pulposus less hydrated.
- Cartilage end plates are thinned.

Degeneration (early stage)

- Nucleus pulposus consolidated and filled with fibrous tissue
- Annulus fibrosus and nucleus pulposus not well demarcated yet

Degeneration (advanced stage)

- Annulus fibrosus with tears, nucleus with deep clefts
- Sclerosis of the bony end plates

Degeneration (end stage)

- Intervertebral disc completely degenerated
- End plates with marked sclerosis

13.1.2.2 End Plates

During the aging process, changes in the end plates become more and more evident, such as:

- Fissure formation
- Fractures
- Horizontal clefts
- Increased vascular penetration
- Calcification and sclerosis

Based on MRI findings and histological correlations, end plate changes have been classified by Modic into three types [4]. During the last years, Modic changes have been extensively used to identify the causes of nonspecific low back pain. In this context, Modic type I changes were associated with unspecific low back pain. Modic changes are very common in the lumbar spine. However, they are also found in the thoracic and cervical spine and they are listed below:

Type I

- Low signal in T1 and high signal in T2-weighted images. These changes are associated with vascularized granulation tissue within the subchondral bone indicating an ongoing active degeneration.

Type II

- High signal in T1- and T2-weighted images indicating a fatty replacement of the adjacent bone marrow.

Type III

- Low signal in T1- and T2-weighted images indicating subchondral bone sclerosis.

13.1.2.3 Facet Joints

The facet joints, also called zygapophyseal joints, are paired synovial articulations between the posterior elements of any adjacent vertebrae. The altered biomechanical situation promotes arthritic changes of these joints and the ligamenta flava (Fig. 13.2). Together with the disc bulging, a successive stenosis of the spinal canal and the lateral recesses results. These pathoanatomical changes occur within the whole spine but with slight regional differences. Spine areas with an increased mobility like the cervical and the lumbar spine are in particular susceptible for progressive degeneration with a predilection of the segments C5/C6 and C6/C7 as well as L4/L5 and L5/S1.

They are an essential part of the posterior column and are classified according to Fujiwara et al. [5]:

Grade 0: normal
Grade 1: moderately compressed with osteophytes

Grade 2: subchondral sclerosis and osteophytes
Grade 3: large osteophytes, no joint gap left

Degenerative changes in the facet joints combined with disc degeneration can lead to a compression of nerve roots in the lateral recess, but also a central 360 °stenosis is possible. Although there is some evidence that disc degeneration usually precedes facet joint osteoarthritis, the grade of disc degeneration does not correlate with that of the facet joint.

13.1.2.4 Vertebral Body

The bony components, namely, the corpus vertebrae, are mainly responsible for the static stability of the spinal column. Aging of the vertebral bodies is generally characterized by a decreased structural strength, mainly due to osteoporosis. Osteoporosis manifests as a general skeletal disorder, whose main feature is the reduced bone mass combined with microarchitectural changes within the bone tissue and a subsequently elevated fracture risk.

The prevalence of osteoporosis in Western Europe is estimated around 45 % for women and around 20 % for men, respectively, older than 70 years [6].

According to the operational definition of the WHO in 1994, osteoporosis is present if the bone mineral density (BMD) measured by dual X-ray absorptiometry (DXA) bone densitometry at the lumbar spine differs more than –2.5 standard deviations from the mean value of a healthy female between 20 and 29 years. The difference of the BMD values in comparison to this indicated as standard deviations is the so-called *T*-score. This definition can be used for men older than 50 years of age as well.

However, for the daily praxis in spine surgery, *T*-scores play a rather limited role. Of much more relevance are the absolute values of the BMD. These values can be determined by quantitative computed tomography (QCT). In contrast to DXA, the CT calculates the physical density value for each voxel (specified in mg/cc) allowing to asses an absolute value of the bone mineral density. Furthermore, mechanical parameters of the respective bone area are captured better by QCT [7].

In consequence, BMD values from QCT measurements must not be specified as T-scores, nor are they comparable to DXA values. Based on our own experience, implant anchoring (especially pedicle screws, but anterior cervical plates, too) is significantly decreased below a BMD of 100 mg/cc. In these cases an additional augmentation of the respective implant should be considered, or, alternatively, instrumentation should be expanded over multiple segments.

The increased bone fragility can induce osteoporotic fractures which lead to a bulging of the disc into the vertebral body, to kyphotic deformity, and to a loss of the sagittal balance (see below). The end stage is characterized by a so-called fish vertebra (totally collapsed vertebral body with discs bulging into the end plates).

13.1.2.5 Sagittal Balance

The ongoing degeneration comprising vertebral bodies, intervertebral discs, ligaments, and facet joints is the pathophysiological correlate for a secondary degenerative instability of the spine. Multisegmental deformities in the sagittal (kyphosis, degenerative spondylolisthesis) as well as in the coronal (scoliosis) plane with additional rotatory misalignment are possible (Fig. 13.2). In upright position the following aspects are important for a balanced state:

- Coronal balance
- Sagittal balance
- Sagittal profile
- Muscle tension bending

Coronal balance is defined by a plumb line that does not deviate off the intergluteal groove. Sagittal balance is closely correlated with lumbar and cervical lordosis as well as thoracic kyphosis. A thoracic kyphosis of 20–60° is usually considered as normal [8]. The normal range for cervical lordosis (C2–C7) is 20–60° [9]. In the lumbar spine, the last two segments (L4/L5 and L5/S1) contribute about two thirds of the whole lumbar lordosis (L1–S1). In standing position, a plumb line from the center of C7 should be centered over the first sacral segment [10]. Patients with chronic low back pain and lumbar degenerative disease often present with modifications of the sagittal balance and are mostly featured by anterior sagittal imbalance, loss of lumbar and cervical lordosis, and an increase of pelvic tilt [11]. The spinal muscles must counteract this imbalance and thereby fatigue, possibly resulting in severe pain. The anterior imbalance has a great impact because it increases the risk of progressive thoracic kyphosis.

13.1.3 Clinical Symptoms

Degenerative changes of the spine provoke a lot of different clinical symptoms. But especially in elderly patients, the typical clinical features are often masked by a lot of possible comorbidities. On the other side – as mentioned above – spine degeneration is a physiological phenomenon and not each radiological abnormality has to be treated as a symptomatic degenerative pathology. So only the matching correlation of the clinical and radiological features can be the base for a successful treatment plan.

Two important pathogenetic causes for symptoms in degenerative spine disease have to be mentioned:

- The arthritic changes of the facet joints, together with an optional increased mobility of the segment leading to local pain.
- The degenerative narrowing of the spinal canal compromises the adjacent neural structures with radicular pain and optional neurological deficits reaching from mild sensory disturbances to severe tetraparesis in cases of a cervical myelopathy.

13.1.4 Diagnostics

The diagnostic algorithm for potential degenerative spinal changes is always based on three consecutive columns irrespective from the affected section of the spine:

1. Patients history
2. Clinical examination
3. Radiological procedures

13.1.4.1 Patient's History

An exact and not only spine-related evaluation of the patient's history, especially in elderly patients, is mandatory because only the synopsis of clinical and radiological findings define further diagnostic and therapeutic measures. The initial questionnaire should include pain characteristics (burning, stabbing, movement dependency, etc.), duration and distribution (mono-/poly-/pseudoradicular?), possible neurological (motoric, sensory, vegetative) disturbances, and possible other preexisting comorbidities including cardiovascular, cerebral, and neoplastic pathologies. An osteoporosis is often known.

Special "red flags" which require urgent diagnostics can be ruled out during the first interview; these are:

- Severe neurological deficits including vegetative disturbances, possibly indicating a relevant compression of neural structures
- Fever, progressive pain, and/or immunological deficits, indicating a possible infectious pathology (spondylodiscitis, intraspinal abscess, or empyema)
- Trauma history, suggesting a fracture, sometimes even a sudden onset of the symptoms can be the clinical correlate of a spontaneous osteoporotic fracture
- History of a malignoma, with a spinal tumor or metastasis

In these cases, even when there are no relevant deficits, further diagnostics have to be scheduled within hours or days to not overlook potential spinal cord – or even life-threatening pathologies.

13.1.4.2 Clinical Examination

The following clinical examination has to be performed not only as "symptom-related check" but rather as a complete "whole body examination" focusing on neurological but also on orthopedic and on medical abnormalities. Systemic CNS problems like ischemia, neurodegenerative diseases, normal pressure hydrocephalus, and chronic inflammatory CNS diseases can be causative for the symptoms of the patient. Also cardiovascular pathologies like peripheral arterial disease (PAD) and even myocardial infarction can mimic lumbar or cervical radiculopathy. There is a relevant coincidence of spine degeneration and cox- and gonarthrosis, and an exact examination can reveal the pain causing the problem.

Apart from the body check, a (neuro-)psychological evaluation can be helpful, especially in cases of a planned operative treatment. So a possible psychopathological component of the pain on the one hand and neurocognitive deficits in cases of neurodegenerative diseases on the other hand can be determined. During the last years, the psychological pre- and postinterventional state of the patient has been recognized as an important and even prognostic factor within the treatment concept of degenerative spine disease.

13.1.4.3 Radiological Procedures

In symptomatic patients a targeted radiological examination is necessary. So the causative pathology can be named, additional diagnostic procedures can be scheduled, and, in the end, a treatment concept can be established.

But one always has to bear in mind that the sole radiological detection of degenerative spine changes is not sufficient to indicate specific therapeutic measures. As mentioned before, there has to be always a correlation between clinical symptoms and the radiological findings. Terms like "absolute" or "relative" spinal stenosis only describe the radiological image; they do not reflect the clinical relevance and should be avoided in this context. The diameter of the spinal canal does neither reflect the clinical symptoms nor it even allows a prognostic statement before and after treatment [12].

The most important diagnostic tools are:

- Magnetic resonance tomography (MRI)
- Standard radiographs (flexion/extension/standing)
- Computed tomography (CT)

The gold standard for the detection of degenerative spine changes in the cervical but also in the lumbar area is the magnetic resonance tomography (MRI). The sensitivity concerning lumbar degenerative pathologies is described between 87 and 96 % with a specifity between 75 and 86 % [13]. In the cervical spine, the data are comparable. Routinely, the examination has to be performed as T1- and T2-weighted sequence in sagittal and transversal orientation. Changes of the discs, the bone, the ligaments, and the facet joints are visible as well as abnormalities concerning the regional alignment of the vertebral column in all three orientations. Furthermore, the MRI allows an exact assessment of intra- and sometimes even extraspinal pathologies. It shows the neural structures like spinal cord, cauda equina, and nerve roots and their potential contact to the surrounding structures. In special cases, when a tumor or an infection is suspected, contrast enhanced imaging is necessary.

Nevertheless, the native standard radiograph in two orientations (anterior-posterior and lateral) of the spine still has its place in the diagnostic of degenerative spine disease. In cases of an unclear history, it can rule out fractures or osteolytic changes. Changes in the alignment possibly indicate a relevant instability which can be definitely diagnosed with an X-ray in standing position and/or under flexion/extension. In selected patients films of the whole spinal column can be necessary to assess reactive changes in distant spine sections [13].

The domain of the computed tomography is the delineation of bone. Fractures, osteolysis, and genuine spondylolisthesis can be located exactly, and discoligamental changes ("soft disc") can be distinguished from osteophytes ("hard disc"). In the context of a scheduled surgical intervention, a preoperative depiction of the vertebrae is reasonable, especially when an additional instrumentation is planned.

Against this background the evaluation of the bone density, especially in elderly patients, becomes more and more important. Quantitative computed tomography (qCT) is a good option to get an exact value of the bone mineral density. According to our experience, a BMD of lower than 100 mg/cc is an indication for an additional cement augmentation or an extension of the instrumentation. A myelography today is only in exceptional cases indicated, e.g., in patients with a ferromagnetic implant or when a mobility-dependent compression of neuro structures especially in the cervical spine are needed.

13.1.4.4 Additional Diagnostics

Additional electrophysiological examinations help to rule out some of the differential diagnosis, e.g., neurodegenerative diseases, inflammatory radiculopathies, nerve compression syndromes, and other mono-/polyneuropathies.

Electromyography and sensory evoked potentials can define the clinical relevant level in cases of a multisegmental spinal stenosis. In the cervical spine, subclinical myelin affection can be determined with the motor evoked potential as the most sensitive and prognosis relevant technique even when clinically evident neurological deficits have not yet occurred [14, 15].

To confirm or to rule out other reasons for the complaints, more technical examinations might be necessary. So in cases of a suspected peripheral arterial occlusive disease, an angiologic assessment with ultrasound evaluation of the ABI (ankle-brachial index) has to follow. Degenerative or traumatic changes in shoulder, hip, or knee – if clinically suspected – require specific radiological examinations.

Laboratory tests can be path breaking in cases of an infection and in autoimmune diseases. When a systemic CNS infection or a chronic inflammatory CNS process seems possible, a spinal tap is indicated.

13.2 Cervical Spine

13.2.1 Cervical Disc Herniation

Cervical disc herniation is the result of an extrusion of the nucleus pulposus through tears in the annulus fibrosus with mechanical irritation of cervical nerve roots or the spinal cord in consequence.

The main causes of disc herniation are age-related changes of the intervertebral disc making the annulus fibrosus susceptible to fissuring and tearing. Cervical radiculopathy due to disc herniation usually occurs during early stages of motion segment degeneration and mainly affects individuals in the fourth and fifth decades of life. Thus, in contrast to younger patients, pure "soft disc protrusions" are rare in elderly patients. If present, they are generally not the only pathology; in fact, they are frequently associated with further degenerative changes. These combined lesions are usually detectable as the so-called hard disc (that means calcified) protrusion in combination with bony spurs at the edges of the vertebral body and osteophytes. Furthermore, there are almost always degenerative changes of the uncovertebral joint with a concomitant uncoforaminal stenosis leading to additional compression of the segmental nerve root. The irritation of the spinal nerve may be pronounced either in

Table 13.1 Table depicts the clinical signs of cervical radiculopathy

Root syndrome	Pain radiation	Reference muscle	Reflex loss
C5	Shoulder, upper arm	Deltoid	–
C6	Radial side of forearm	Biceps, brachioradialis	Biceps, brachioradialis
C7	Whole forearm, mainly second/third finger, chest	Triceps	Triceps
C8	Ulnar side of forearm	Abductor digiti minimi, interossei	Trömner

the dorsal or in the recurrent ramus. The pathophysiology of radiculopathy involves both mechanical deformation and chemical irritation of the nerve roots. This results in a dermatome-associated distribution of the radiating pain.

13.2.1.1 Clinical Symptoms

The clinical symptoms occur for direct compression of the segmental spinal nerve (radicular pain) and the rear longitudinal ligament (dull pain), sometimes even presenting as so-called pseudoradicular pain. This kind of pain can be differentiated from radicular pain insofar, as dermatomal or myotomal allocation is not or only inaccurately possible. In the first line, pseudoradicular pain originates from the joint capsule: It is suspected that degenerative changes of the disc promote a change of the facet joint position so that tension on the joint capsule induces neck pain in consequence. On the other hand, pseudoradicular pain is the result of continuous innervation of the dorsal ramus which provokes muscular pain as well.

In addition to that, the muscle tone of the paraspinal muscles is partly controlled by receptors in the joint capsule resulting in a spontaneous pain in the affected muscles. This pain can be reproduced by pressure on so-called trigger points. In contrast, pressure on the posterior longitudinal ligament by disc protrusion rather leads to dull neck pain, often with a gradual onset. If there is real compression of a segmental spinal nerve, a radicular pain syndrome is the typical result. The pain radiates (into the shoulder, forearm, and chest) with a strict dermatome- and myotome-associated distribution (Table 13.1). The extent of compression correlates to some degree with the pain level. In advanced stages, paresis and atrophy of the depending muscles are possible.

13.2.2 Cervical Spondylotic Myelopathy (CSM)

Narrowing of the spinal canal by a disc herniation or osteophytes can lead to severe neurological deficits because of a direct compromise of the spinal cord resulting in the clinical syndrome of myelopathy. The most common cause for cervical myelopathy in the elderly is cervical spondylosis. Ossification of the posterior longitudinal ligament (OPPL), trauma, or tumors is seen much less frequent as a cause for cervical myelopathy in the elderly.

The pathophysiology of CSM is related to static, dynamic, and vascular factors.

13.2.2.1 Static Factors

The normal sagittal diameter of the subaxial cervical spinal canal varies between 14 and 22 mm. Normally, the spinal cord occupies about three-quarters of the size of the spinal. A narrowing of the spinal canal (static factor) results from cervical spondylosis, disc degeneration, osteophyte formation, and hypertrophy of the facet joints and the yellow ligament. Development of cervical myelopathy is more frequent in patients with a congenitally narrow spinal canal.

13.2.2.2 Dynamic Factors

Flexion and extension of the cervical spine can result in lengthening and consecutive stretching of the spinal cord over vertebral osteophytes, which may lead to a chronic injury of the myelon. Extension of the cervical spine leads to folding of the yellow ligament with dorsal compression of the cord combined with anterior compression due to posterior disc bulging. If disc degeneration in combination with degenerative instability is present, the resulting translative movement may lead to further compression of the spinal cord and consecutive increase of strain and shear forces applied on the cord.

13.2.2.3 Vascular Factors

The corticospinal tract is very vulnerable to ischemia undergoing demyelinization, much more if the spinal canal is narrowed: a compressed spinal cord certainly does not tolerate hypoperfusion. Reversely, a spinal cord with diminished perfusion will not tolerate compression as well.

The following mechanisms of injury to the vascular system of the spinal cord are known:

- Direct compression of the anterior spinal artery
- Torsion and tension of the anterior sulcal arteries with reduced blood flow in the transverse perforating vessels causing ischemia and degeneration of the gray and medial white matter (typically in the early stage of CSM)
- Compression of segmental vessels in the neural foramen
- Interruption of liquor circulation

Apoptosis seems to be the fundamental process in the pathogenesis of CSM [16]. Segmental changes of the comprised segment are presumably the result of neuronal loss due to apoptosis, and the early apoptotic loss of oligodendrocytes is supposed to cause degeneration of the long corticospinal tracts.

13.2.2.4 Clinical Symptoms

The clinical symptoms correlate with the affected region of the cervical spine, but there is no correlation between the extent of compression and the clinical symptoms. In most cases, symptoms are developing slowly. Initial symptoms comprise numb and clumsy hands, compromising fine motor skills (like fastening buttons, sorting coins, etc.), followed by gait ataxia, especially in the dark in the later stages of the disease. Muscle weakness affects primarily the triceps muscle, the little hand muscles, and the proximal

Table 13.2 Nurick grading system [17]

Grading	Signs of myelopathy	Gait	Daily activities/working
0	No	Normal	No limitations
1	Yes	Normal	No limitations
2	Yes	Slight disturbance	No limitations
3	Yes	Significant disturbance	Limitations
4	Yes	Only with support	Not possible
5	Yes	Wheel chair/bedridden	Not possible

hip flexors (iliopsoas muscle). If CSM is ongoing, spastic gait, hyperreflexia, pathological reflexes (Babinski, Gordon, Oppenheimer), and sensory/vibratory deficits are detectable. Bladder and sphincter function may be impaired as well in the chronic stage of a CSM. The Lhermitte sign (pain on sudden head flexion causing electrical sensations along the spine) is positive in only a few patients which rather have an acute stenosis. One always has to keep in mind that multiple comorbidities of elderly patients (diabetes mellitus, chronic kidney disease, polyneuropathy, Parkinson's disease, system atrophies) can mask the initial and often mild symptoms of a CSM.

For observation of the clinical course as well as for scientific reasons, numerous scales have been introduced. The Nurick grading systems is based on gait abnormalities and was introduced in 1972 (Table 13.2).

The Japanese Orthopedic Association proposed a grading system (JOA score) by recording motor function of upper and lower extremities, trunk, and bladder function. The JOA score is widely used in the scientific literature [18]. Furthermore, in Europe the European Myelopathy Score was developed in 1994 [19].

There are some patients with neck pain as the predominant symptom which is part of the so-called spondylotic syndrome. These patients often complain about recurrent episodes of position-dependent neck pain, which is aggravated with motion. Upon request, they report on aggravation in the night and early morning. The neck pain is often accompanied by episodes of vertigo, dizziness, and vegetative symptoms. As well, headaches are a frequent concomitant symptom.

13.2.2.5 Diagnostics

Imaging

Both cervical root compression syndromes as a result of cervical disc herniation and cervical myelopathy are first of all clinical diagnoses. In most cases, an exact history and examination allows the diagnosis of radiculopathy and myelopathy. Root compression syndromes are characterized by the typical referred pain (see above) following dermatomal and myotomal distribution. In contrast to radiculopathy, a myelopathic syndrome generally begins subtly with numb, clumsy, and sometimes painful hands.

Imaging studies are helpful but sometimes confusing, because in nearly every patient older than 60 years of age, degenerative changes are detectable.

As earlier mentioned, the MRI has become the gold standard for the visualization of degenerative pathologies of the cervical spine. Image quality is excellent regarding soft tissue contrast and differentiation, whereas there are some limitations regarding bony tissue and bony alterations. Disc herniations are visualized with high sensitivity. The

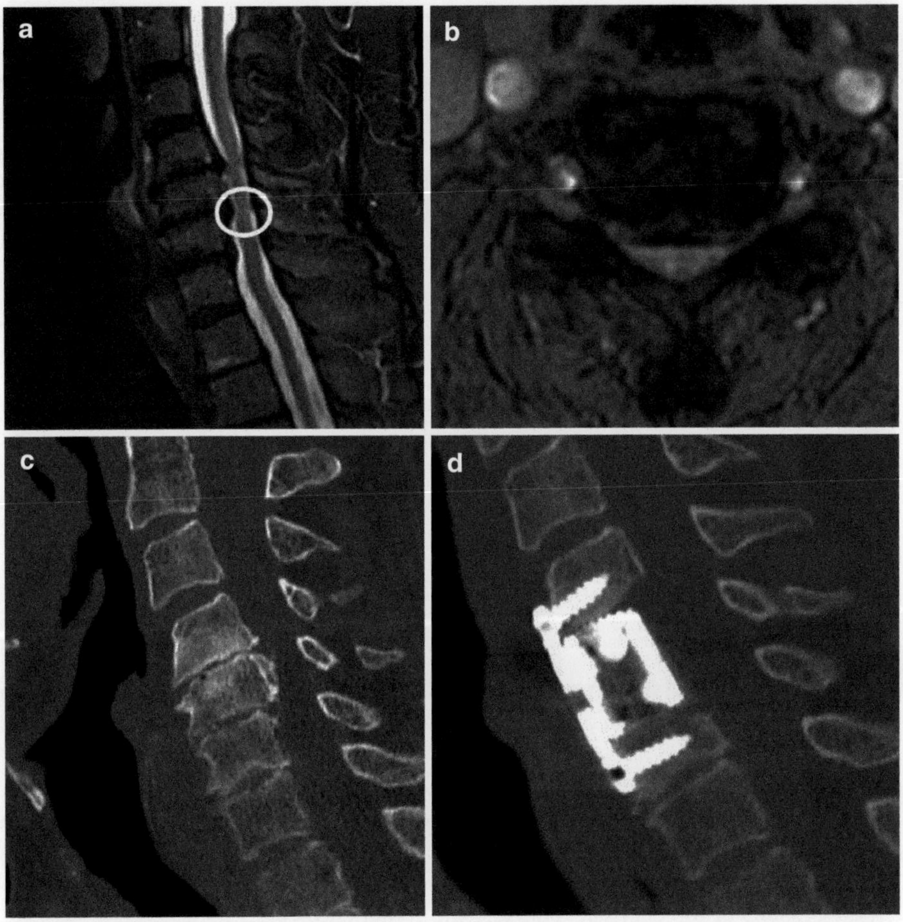

Fig. 13.3 Figure shows the MRI and CT scans of a patient suffering from a cervical spondylotic myelopathy. MRI preoperatively visualizes the narrowing of the spinal canal (**a**, **b**) and even a "radiologic myelopathy" at the level of C5/C6 (*circle*); CT reveals bony changes as the main problem (**c**). Note that the compression originates from ventral. CT after surgery shows the implant in the correct position (**d**)

different sequences can detect the stages of degeneration. In contrast to younger people, the T2- weighted sequences show the herniation mostly as iso- or hypointense because of the advanced degeneration process of the nucleus in elderly. T1- weighted images with contrast enhancement may differentiate between a sequestrated nucleus and scarred changes. If the herniation is subacute, the prolapse sometimes enhances in the periphery. The same also applies for the nerve root. Oblique sequences (90° to the long axis of the foramen) are helpful to visualize the neuroforamen and its content, especially in cases of long-lasting uncoforaminal degeneration processes with nerve root impingement. In patients suffering from myelopathy, the MRI may show the typical signal intensity changes, first and foremost the T2 hyperintensity within the spinal cord, which are sometimes called "radiological myelopathy" (Fig. 13.3). The prognostic significance of these changes remains unclear.

In addition to the MRI, CT scans are helpful especially for the planning of a surgical intervention. Bony changes, facet joint degeneration, uncoforaminal stenosis, and osteophytes are very well detectable. Furthermore, spontaneously fused segments are visualized with sufficient certainty.

In selected patients the CT can be done with additional myelography of the spinal canal. In the pre-MRI era, this imaging modality was the only one to visualize the spinal cord and the nerve roots in relation to the osseous structures of the cervical spine. In the present time, there are only two indications for post-myelography CT: if patients have contraindications for MRI (pacemaker, neurostimulators or other metallic implants etc.) and if additional information from dynamic images (flexion, extension) and its effects to nerve root and spinal cord compression is needed.

Standard radiographs of the cervical spine provide additional information about sagittal alignment, sagittal balance, and bony structures. They can be performed under flexion and extension to get further information about alignment changes and a potentially aggravated spondylolisthesis, but the value of these images remains controversial. The same applies for oblique radiographs to visualize the neural foramen. Normally, these images are of little use, because the CT provides more exact information about bony structures, neural foramen stenosis, and facet joint osteoarthritis.

Neurophysiologic Assessment

If the clinical picture is not clear or there is only little correlation of the clinical and radiological findings, additional electrophysiological assessment may be helpful. The question to be answered by electrophysiological diagnostics is whether a lesion is chronic or acute and which segment is the mostly involved one. Disadvantageous of all electrophysiology are frequent false-positive findings, especially in elderly patients. There is often a subclinical polyneuropathy which interferes with the electrodiagnostics of the cervical roots and the spinal cord.

For cervical root compression syndromes, the electromyography (EMG) of cervical myotomes including neck muscles plays a certain role. Acute root lesions show denervation activity (positive sharp waves, fibrillations) in the dependent muscles. Additionally, sensory nerve conduction studies may prove a preganglionic lesion, if the sensory nerve action potential is reproducible in clinical areas with subjective sensory loss.

For diagnosis of CSM, the EMG is of little relevance. In this context, evoked potentials (somatosensory and motor evoked potentials – SSEP, MEP) may have some importance. Tibial nerve SSEP abnormalities correlate with the extent of spinal cord damage in CSM [20]. In order to obtain a high sensitivity, both somatosensory and motor evoked potentials should be recorded on all limbs with a special attention to segmental cervical and cervico-medullary responses [21].

Differential Diagnosis

The following differential diagnoses have to be taken into account regarding degenerative cervical pathologies with nerve root or spinal cord compression in elderly people:

- Tumors (intradural/extradural)
- Inflammatory disorders
- Coronary heart disease!
- Compression syndromes of peripheral nerves and plexus brachialis
- Rheumatoid arthritis
- Shoulder girdle disorders (impingement syndrome, tendinitis, rotator cuff tear)
- Chronic inflammatory CNS diseases (Lyme disease, multiple sclerosis
- Neurodegenerative diseases

  Seldom

Amyotrophic lateral sclerosis
Paraneoplastic
Toxic/metabolic causes
Acute idiopathic transverse myelitis
Vascular pathologies (malformation, cavernoma)
Drug induced
Viral infections

13.2.3 Therapy

13.2.3.1 Nonsurgical Treatment

The treatment decision depends from patient symptoms and his individual psychological strain ("pain is a private problem") as well as on the underlying pathology and on the patient's general condition and comorbidities. Furthermore, the natural history of the disease has to be acknowledged, and the expected outcome of the treatment has to be weighed against its risks and benefits considering the natural history.

As in younger patients, conservative treatment approaches are justified if there is no relevant neurologic deficit or rather no deficit can be expected in the near future. Cervical root compression syndromes often respond very well to a combination of local heat application and oral medication. Heat application leads to local hyperemia and relaxation of neck and shoulder muscles. Oral medication is applied with NSAID as the main column (Fig. 13.7). The use of soft collars in the acute phase is unclear. At least, there is no evidence-based recommendation pro or contra [22]. Local injections may be helpful in the early stage, but there is no even evidence for a long-term benefit neither for lidocaine IM nor for anesthetic nerve blocks including steroids [23, 24].

There is moderate evidence that spinal manipulation and mobilization are superior to general practitioner management concerning short-term pain reduction, but the effect of spinal manipulation is similar compared to high-technology rehabilitative exercises in the short- and long-term follow-up [25, 26].

13.2.3.2 Surgical Treatment

Indication

In the vast majority of degenerative cervical spine pathologies in elderly, a surgical approach is only justified if there has been an appropriate conservative treatment effort [27]. But nevertheless in some cases, an operative treatment, even in elderly people, is indicated. But before considering a surgical treatment, some criteria should be full filled for cervical disc herniation [28]:

- Evidence of nerve root compression because of the herniation.
- Signs and symptoms concordant with the compressed nerve root.
- If there is a progressive motor deficit, indication for surgery is corroborated.

In patients suffering from cervical spondylotic myelopathy, one has to bear in mind that the primary goal of every treatment (nonsurgical and surgical) is the prevention of further progression of the disease. Communicating this message to the patient prior to surgery is one of the keys to a successful treatment. If patients are informed about realistic goals, chances, and risks of the planned surgery, disappointment can be avoided from the beginning.

Surgery for CSM is generally indicated if there are:

- Progressive myelopathy or progressive neurologic deficits
- Evidence of spinal cord compression
- Progressive kyphosis in combination with myelopathy

The debate concerning the question, whether anterior or posterior approaches should be chosen for surgical management, is currently ongoing. The controversy on which of the two approaches is appropriate must always be related to the target pathology. That's why it is important to recognize whether the compression originates anterior or posterior from the neural structures. In consequence, the pathology should be treated where it is (Figs. 13.3, 13.4, and 13.5). Thus, an anterior cord or nerve root compression is generally better targeted from an anterior approach (Fig. 13.3) and multisegmental or purely posterior compression from a posterior approach (Fig. 13.5). Furthermore, the following points have to be considered:

- How is the sagittal profile of the cervical spine?
  - If there is a kyphosis, how much kyphosis is present? If present, is the kyphosis fixed or can it be reduced? For fixed or severe kyphosis (>10 ° C2-C7), anterior approaches are advantageous. If posterior approaches are necessary, pedicle screw instrumentation should be considered [29].

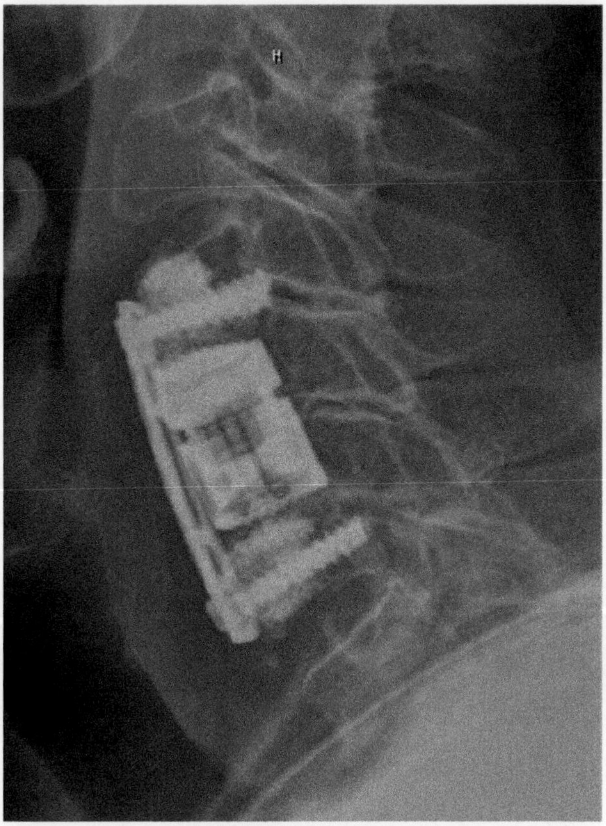

Fig. 13.4 Figure shows cement augmentation of cervical body screw after corpectomy C5 in a patient with a severe osteoporosis

- How is the bone quality (one of the most important questions when dealing with surgical approaches to CSM in elderly!)?
  - If bone quality is not sufficient (generally, if BMD is <100 mg/cc, see page 5) and more than one segment is involved, dorsal procedures (if possible with pedicle screw instrumentation) or circumferential fusion are probably advantageous. If corporectomy and plating is necessary in a patient with reduced bone quality, additional cement augmentation may be considered [30].
- Is there instability?
  - If present (clinical and/or radiological) think about fusion. Non-fusion procedures (like laminoplasty) are contraindicated.
- How many segments are involved?
  - For mono- or bisegmental pathologies, anterior approaches are suitable. If three or more segments are involved, dorsal procedures or circumferential approaches are preferable.

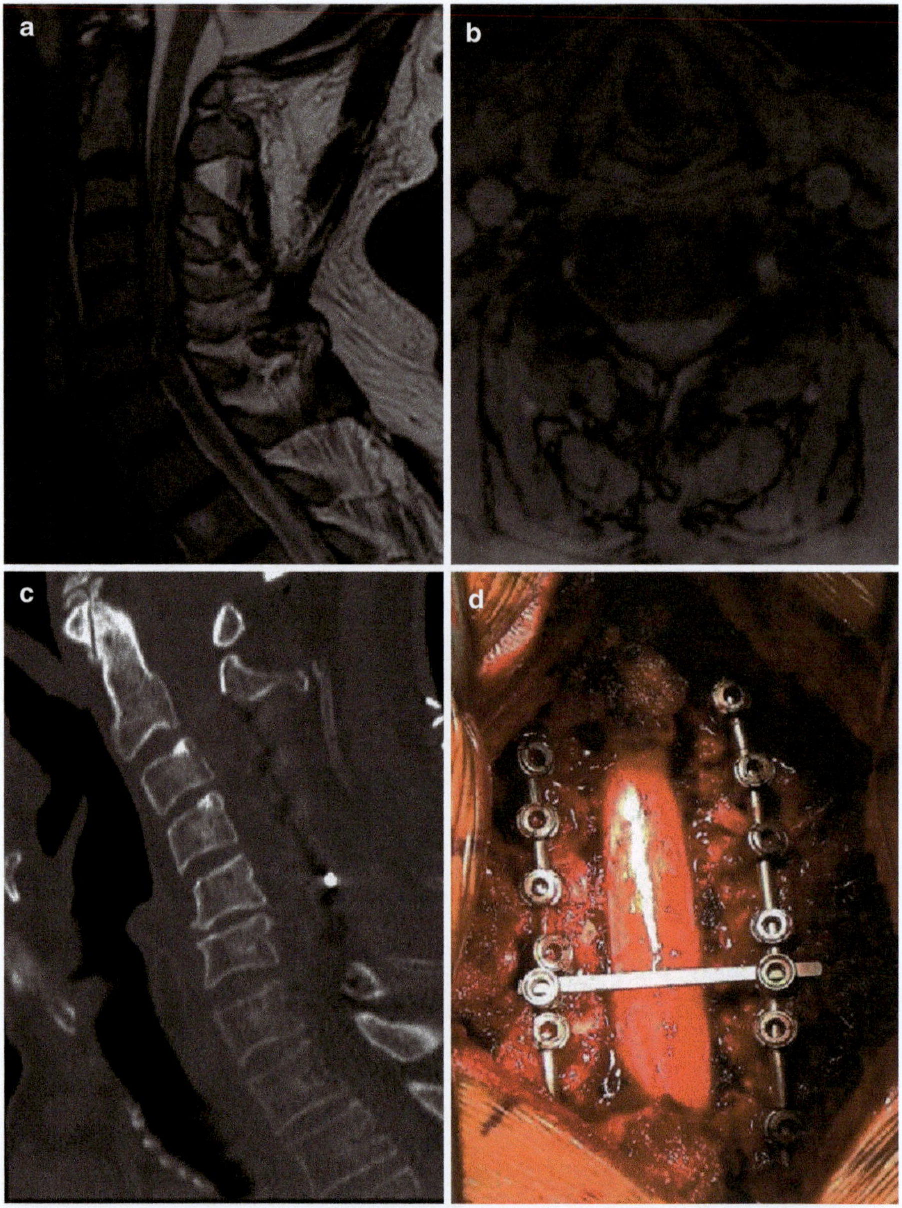

Fig. 13.5 Figure shows the case of a 66-year-old patient suffering from a cervical myelopathy caused by a multilevel cervical degenerative stenosis (**a, b**). (**c**) Shows the postoperative CT after multilevel laminectomy; (**d**) shows the intraoperative situation with the decompressed dural sleeve and the instrumentation with massa lateralis screws. Note the slight kyphosis of the cervical spine after the operation (**c**)

Table 13.3 Summarizes advantages and disadvantages of the different surgical approaches to the cervical spine

Ventral procedures	Advantage	Disadvantage
Anterior cervical discectomy and fusion (ACDF), if appropriate with additional plating	Decompression directly from anterior Preservation of the vertebral body Easy and safe for simple mono- or bisegmental disc herniations Feasible for multiple segments if bone quality is sufficient	Complex surgery, if multiple stenotic segments are involved; problematic, if marked bony spurs are present High-risk surgery if spinal canal is very narrow Nonunion if multiple segments are involved Hardware failure (plate dislocation, cage subsidence) in case of reduced bone quality
Corpectomy with plating (Figs. 13.3 and 13.4)	Sufficient decompression Restoration of sagittal profile is possible	Complex surgery Considerable nonunion rate Contraindicated if bone quality is bad Long operation time
Dorsal procedures		
Posterior foraminotomy (Frykholm)	Fast Low morbidity	Suitable only for lateral soft disc herniation
Laminectomy	Safe and easy Effective Suitable for multiple segments	Secondary instability (Swan neck deformity) Indirect decompression
Laminectomy with instrumentation (massa lateralis/pedicle screws) and fusion (Fig. 13.5)	Effective Avoidance of secondary deformity Restoration of sagittal profile is possible to some extent	Hardware failure (in particular if massa lateralis screws are used in combination with reduced bone quality) Complex surgery (if pedicle screws are used)
Laminoplasty	Motion preservation (theoretically)	Complex surgery Progressive limitation of cervical range of motion No proof of superiority Neck pain
Combined procedures		
	Effective Appropriate in case of reduced bone quality Best results for severe kyphosis	Complex! Normally two-step surgery Long operation times Enormous strain for patients

13.2.3.3 Surgical Techniques

Several surgical techniques are available to treat degenerative pathologies in the cervical spine, and they are used complementary in the daily clinical practice. First, the initial goal is to decompress the neural structures without causing instability. If instability is present or had been generated by surgery, instrumentation and fusion is indicated. These principles are similar to those of the surgical treatment of younger people (Table 13.3).

13.3 Lumbar Spine

13.3.1 Lumbar Disc Herniation

Isolated lumbar disc herniation is a rather rare entity in elderly patients; in fact it's often part of a multisegmental degeneration process leading to lumbar spinal stenos (see below). Nevertheless, it has to be mentioned as a possible cause of radicular symptoms considering that, even in cases of multisegmental stenosis, the treatment of a concomitant sequestrated disc herniation might be more successful than a multilevel fusion and decompression procedure.

Depending from the site of herniation, different symptoms can occur. One can differ between medial, mediolateral, and lateral pulposus prolapses with the spinal canal including the dural sleeve and the nerve roots as the leading structures. Furthermore, an up – and downward – sequestration is possible. These anatomical specialties define the complaints of the patient and have to be considered when assessing the symptoms of the patients.

13.3.1.1 Clinical Symptoms

The typical symptom of a lumbar disc herniation is the radicular "sciatic" pain possibly combined with sensory or motor disturbances. Like in the cervical spine, the distribution of pain and possible neurological deficits can define the affected nerve root (Table 13.4).

Table 13.4 Illustrates the clinical signs of lumbar nerve root compression

Root syndrome	Pain radiation	Reference muscle	Reflex loss
L3	Medial thigh	Iliopsoas, thigh adductors	Adductor
L4	Ventral thigh, medial lower leg, medial ankle	Quadriceps femoris	Patellar
L5	Lateral leg, lateral ankle, back of the foot, first toe	Extensor hallucis longus, gluteus medius	Tibialis posterior
S1	Back of the leg, heel, lateral foot last toe	Gastrocnemius	Achilles

In correlation with the different possible pathoanatomy of the disc herniation, one can state out a clinical, pathoanatomical combination: so medial and mediolateral extrusions normally affect the lower nerve root in cases of downward (caudal) sequestration; in cases of an upward (cranial) sequestration, the upper nerve root is affected. Patients with a lateral/extraforaminal disc herniation also suffer from symptoms of the upper nerve root. For example, a mediolateral disc herniation L4/L5 upward sequestration provokes an L4 radiculopathy, while the same location but with downward sequestration leads to an L5 clinic. An extraforaminal herniation leads to an L4 radiculopathy as well.

Typically, the symptoms aggravate during coughing, sneezing, and pressing.

13.3.2 Lumbar Spinal Stenosis

The more frequent problem in elderly patients, compared to isolated disc herniation, is the uni- and multilevel lumbar spinal stenosis. As mentioned above the ongoing degeneration leads to a multilevel narrowing of the spinal canal and a possible misalignment of the whole spinal column.

13.3.2.1 Clinical Symptoms

The typical symptoms of the degenerative lumbar spinal stenosis in the elderly are the radicular pain and more often the so-called spinal claudication.

Spinal claudication comprises a symptom complex including back and (pseudo-) radicular pain into the lower extremities. Typically, the complaints aggravate during standing and walking leading to a progressive reduction of the walking distance. Flexing the spine with widening of the spinal canal allows a clinical differentiation from peripheral artery disease (PAD). Patients suffering from spinal claudication tolerate uphill walking better than downhill walking, and bicycle riding is better possible than walking. This is in contrast to patients with a PAD whose complaints will often aggravate even when they ride a bicycle.

Concerning the exact anamnesis and the diagnostic tools, we refer to the chapter above.

13.3.3 Differential Diagnosis

As mentioned above the spectrum of clinical symptoms in elderly patients suffering from lumbar degenerative spinal changes is manifold, and the list of possible differential diagnosis is long. On the other side, an exact anamnesis and an extensive clinical examination can rule out a lot of possible pitfalls. So the personal contact and the personal examination are mandatory and of particular interest.

Possible differential diagnoses are:

- Vascular claudication
- Cox-/gonarthrosis

- Psychological disorders
- Cervical/thoracic degenerative disc disease
- Metabolic or inflammatory neuropathies
- Osteoporotic vertebral fractures

Seldom

Spinal infections/tumors
Myelopathy
Cerebrovascular or cerebrospinal lesions
Spinal dysplasias
Myopathy
Chronic inflammatory CNS diseases (Lyme disease, multiple sclerosis, etc.)
Bone necrosis of the femoral head
Hip fracture
Retroperitoneal/pelvic processes with affection of the lumbosacral plexus
Thrombosis
Aortic aneurysms

Against this background one has to consider that the possible differential diagnosis can occur even together with the lumbar problem. So an additional vascular occlusive disease is described in up to 26 % of the patients with comparable data concerning a coxarthrosis. Osteopenia and osteoporosis are reported in up to 100 % of the patients [31–33].

Nevertheless, the typical symptoms of degenerative spine disease are obvious in elderly patients as well, and a competent treatment in these cases is mandatory to prevent immobilization-caused complications which might lead to severe and sometimes life-threatening complications (e.g., thrombosis, pneumonia).

13.3.4 Therapy

Only the symptomatic patient has to be treated! In the lumbar spine, an abnormal radiological picture is not an indication neither for a conservative nor for a surgical intervention.

When the complaints of the patients require a treatment, different therapeutic options have to be considered. The therapeutic spectrum reaches from pain medication "on demand" to extensive dorsoventral operations. There are only a few valid studies with respect to this, but during the last year, the first data focusing on elderly patients were published [34]. But still there are no overall accepted guidelines or standards, and the management has to remain an individually based one, bearing in mind the problems of the elderly patients.

In general, a conservative treatment is considered in patients with mild complaints and/or severe comorbidities hindering a surgical approach.

After reviewing the data, a marginal evidence for the surgical versus the conservative management can be stated out [35–38] including one analysis study considering

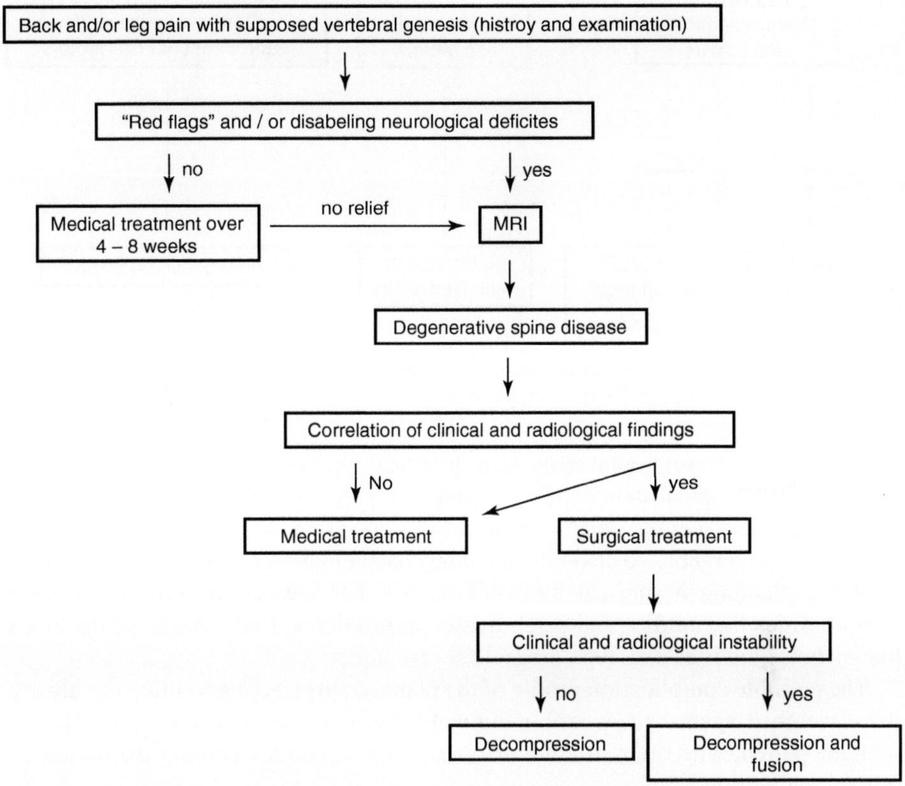

Fig. 13.6 Figure summarizes the diagnostic and therapeutic algorithm for lumbar degenerative spine disease

only elderly people [34]. Nevertheless, different surgical techniques (decompression/fusion/interspinous devices, etc.) and a different follow-up make an objective assessment difficult, and the correct treatment are still under discussion [39].

A clear indication for a surgical treatment are disabling neurological deficits (paresis/paralysis). In cases of severe deficits or especially vegetative disturbances, the indication for surgery has to be scheduled eventually as emergency.

When there are no neurological deficits and pain is the "only" symptom, the treatment concept is a more individual one, based on the constriction of live quality and the psychological strain of the individual patient. An objectification of the indication for surgery in these patients is difficult. The walking distance as a parameter might help. Some pain-, quality of life-, and spine-related scoring systems like short form 36 (SF-36) [40], Oswestry Disability Index [41], and the visual analog scale can be useful as well; anyway, these parameters have to be recorded during the follow-up to have objective and reproducible parameters even for post hoc and scientific analysis of the treatment strategy.

Especially when a surgical treatment is considered, a strict correlation between clinical symptoms and radiological findings is mandatory!

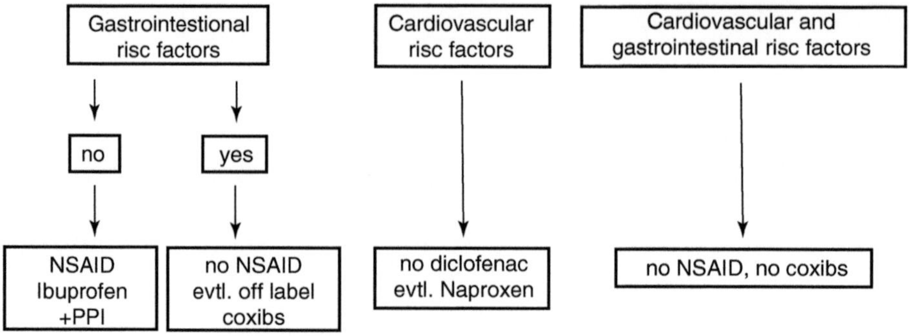

Fig. 13.7 Figure illustrates the actual, personal recommendations for the use of NSAID (Modified according to [43])

A relevant neuroforaminal stenosis, a short history of complaints, predominant leg pain, and neurological deficits are described as predictors for a positive outcome. Nonsmokers also seem to benefit more from an operation, so that it is recommended by some spine surgeons to cease the nicotine consummation before surgery [42].

When planning a surgical intervention, one has always to consider possible comorbidities like cardio- and cerebrovascular problems. Endocrinologic disorders like diabetes mellitus can, e.g., promote severe infections.

The possible complication profile of the planned surgical intervention has always to be weighed against the possible clinical benefit. This has to be communicated with the patient who often has an unrealistic expectation concerning the prognosis of the intervention.

The diagnostic and treatment algorithm is summarized in Fig. 13.6.

13.3.4.1 Nonsurgical Treatment

The conservative treatment concepts are based on the supposed painful pathophysiological mechanisms including an aseptic inflammation and reactive muscular disorders. It comprises medical and physiotherapeutic measures which in the majority of the cases indeed have a reproducible pain-alleviating effect sometime lasting for a long time. Unfortunately, robust evidence-based guidelines are lacking again.

The most popular analgesic substances are nonsteroidal anti-inflammatory drugs (NSAID) which are the basis of a medical analgesic therapy. But especially in elderly people, one has to consider the cardiovascular and gastrointestinal situation.

The most established agents like ibuprofen and naproxen (and aspirin, too) are available on the counter in most countries, but there is still a remarkable risk for gastrointestinal and also cardiac side effects. Actually naproxen is considered to be the at least harmful product with respect to cardiovascular side effects (Fig. 13.7). Proton pump inhibitors (PPI) are mandatory in these patients [43].

COX-2 inhibitors (coxibs) as "off label" option even influence the cardiovascular system. So, coronary artery and cerebrovascular diseases are contraindications as well. These facts often hinder a sufficient analgesic treatment. On the other side, the use of corticosteroids or stronger analgesics including metamizole or opioids,

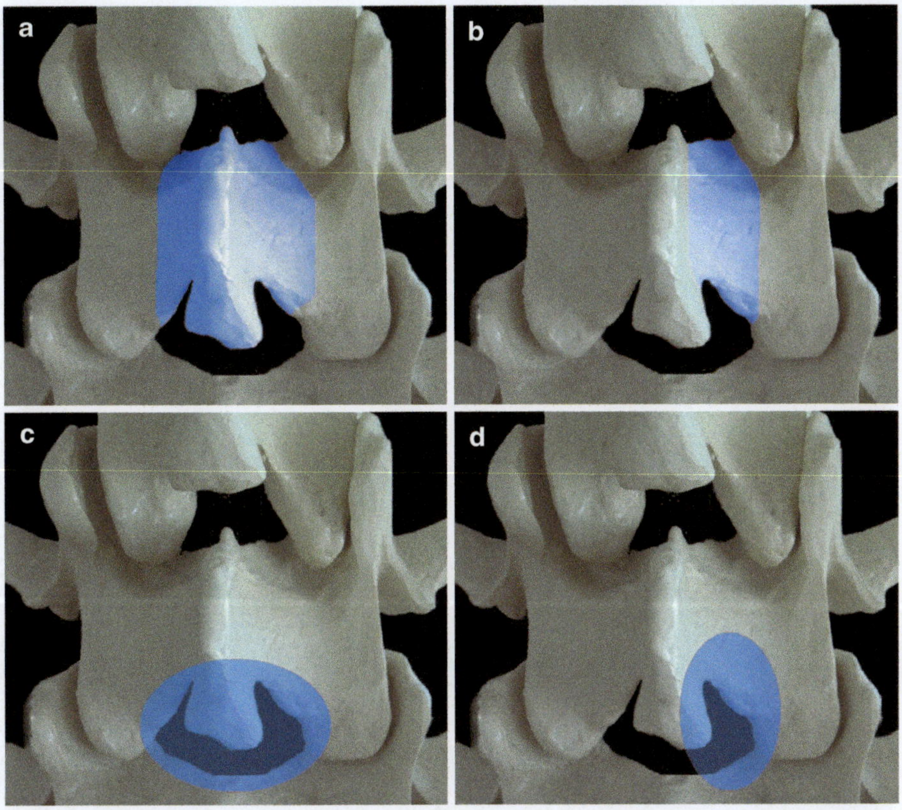

Fig. 13.8 Figure illustrates the possible techniques of spinal canal decompression with laminectomy (**a**), hemilaminectomy (**b**), interlaminar fenestration with undercutting (**c**), interlaminar fenestration (**d**)

antidepressive drugs, and other central-acting drugs like pregabalin and gabapentin as analogues of ɣ-aminobutyric acid is under critical discussion [37, 44, 45].

Local injections including facet joint infiltration, epidural local anesthesia, and/or steroid injections may help in some cases, but up to now, there are not enough data to demonstrate a reproducible long-term pain-reducing effect [46–48].

The most important column in the conservative management of degenerative spine disease, especially in elderly patients, remains the physiotherapeutic treatment. The possible measures include muscle-relaxing techniques like massages and local heat application in the acute stadium and a consequent outpatient-based physiotherapeutic guidance to strengthen the thoracolumbar muscle bending so that the patient regains and particularly preserves his motility [43].

Taken together, the conservative treatment of disabling low back pain in elderly pain is challenging with an interdisciplinary approach including spine surgeon, general practitioner, pain therapist, and physiotherapist required.

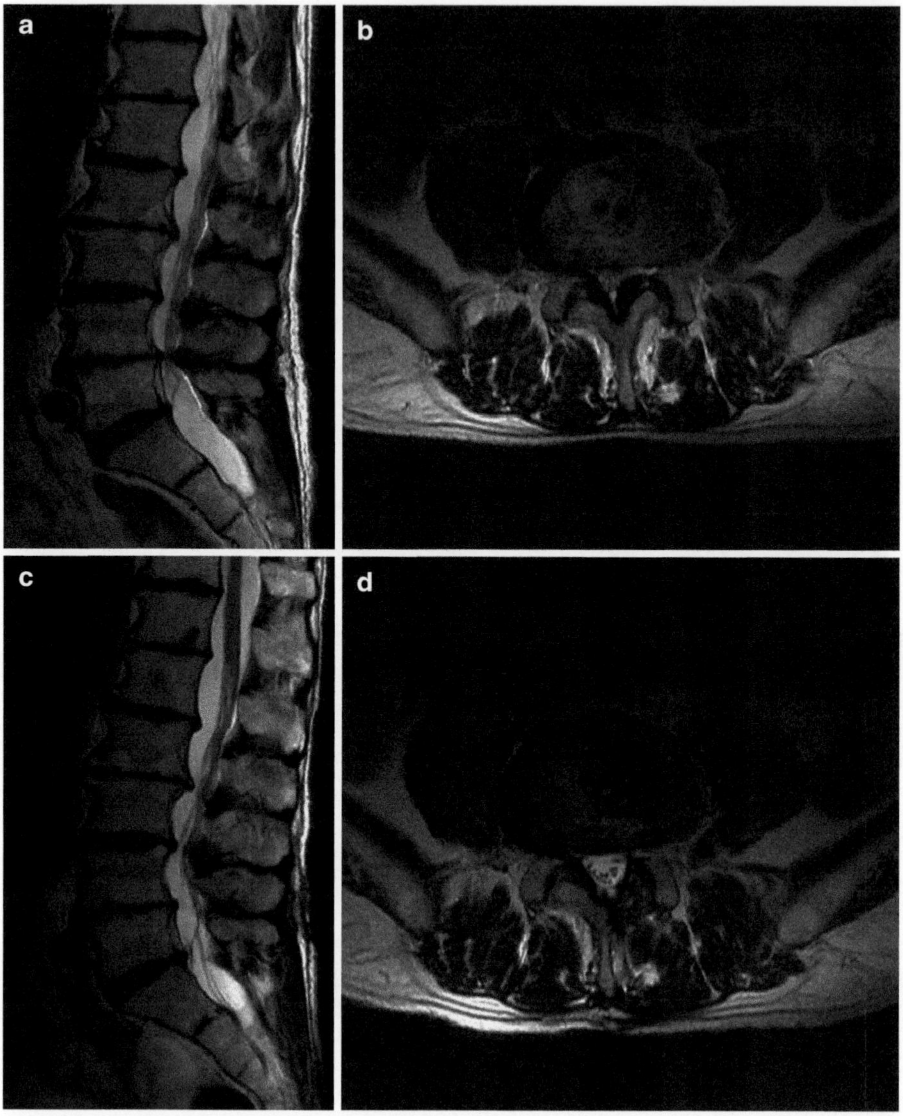

Fig. 13.9 This is an example for a sole decompression procedure (interlaminar fenestration) at the level L4/L5 on the left side in a patient suffering from one-sided sciatic pain. Presented are the pre- (**a**, **b**) and postoperative (**c**, **d**) MRI pictures

13.3.4.2 Surgical Treatment

Concerning the operative treatment of lumbar degenerative spine disease, the surgeon should always keep in mind the maxim "*as extensive as necessary, as minimal as possible*."

Decompression

As mentioned above the operative treatment aims in the first line on the decompression of the neural structures mean the dural sleeve and the adjacent nerve roots. In cases of a relevant instability, an additional fusion can be necessary (see below)

Possible techniques for decompression at lumbar levels are laminectomy, hemilaminectomy, and uni- or bilateral interlaminar fenestration, sometimes with undercutting to the contralateral side (Fig. 13.8). Laminectomy leads to a loss of the dorsal bending so that by now it's considered a destabilizing procedure which nowadays should be avoided. On the other side, hemilaminectomy and interlaminar fenestration allow a wide decompression with preservation of the relevant structures like facet joints and interspinous ligaments (Fig. 13.9).

The complication rate of a sole decompression at the lumbar spine is considerable. There are prospective data focusing on elderly patients describing complications in 18 % of the procedures. The most striking problems were dural leaks (9 %) but without clinical relevance and deep wound infections [39, 49]. Cardiovascular comorbidities can lead to additional pre-, peri-, and postoperative complications, so possible operative procedures require a clear indication and a strict anesthesiologic and cardiologic evaluation, before surgery is scheduled.

Another problem is sometimes an insufficient decompression leaving a clinical relevant remnant stenosis. The reoperation rate after decompression is reported with 11 % after 10 years [50].

Instrumentation and Fusion

An additive instrumentation together with fusion procedures is an established measure within the treatment spectrum of degenerative lumbar spine diseases. But unfortunately there are up to now no overall accepted guidelines which clearly define the indication for such a more extensive procedure. An abundance of available devices has lead to a more and more uncritical and not scientifically based use of screws, rods, cages, hooks, and so on.

Nevertheless, there is a good evidence for an additional fusion in cases of a genuine spondylolisthesis. In all other cases, an additional fusion in elderly and often polymorbid patients is barely scientifically underlined.

Furthermore, most spine surgeons go together that in case of a clinically and radiographically evident instability, a fusion procedure is also indicated. Painful degenerative scoliosis, translational instabilities, and even the degenerative olisthesis are examples for that. Another indication for an additional fusion is a manifest instability after decompression procedures.

The most popular technique is the instrumented intercorporal fusion which can be performed as ALIF (anterior lumbar interbody fusion), PLIF (posterior lumbar interbody fusion), or TLIF (transforaminal lumbar interbody fusion). Intraoperative distraction and the possibility of extended bony decompression within the fused levels lead to a relief of the nerval structures without a potential loss of stability.

On the other side, one has to consider the possible complication of an additional fusion procedure. Compared to simple decompression, there is a relevant increased operation time with an increased blood loss which might be problematic especially

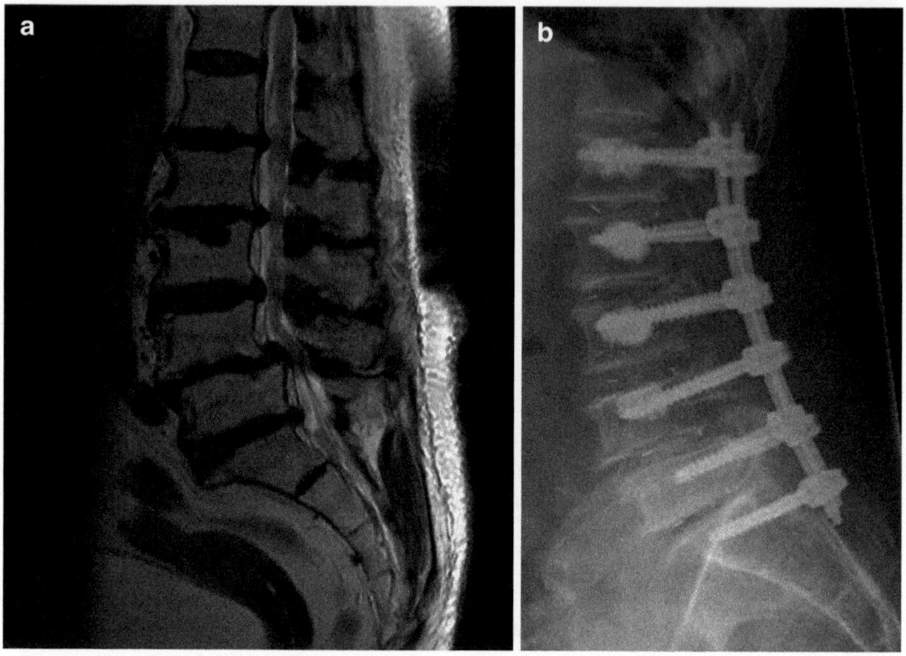

Fig. 13.10 Figure shows an MRI of a 69-year-old woman suffering from a severe bilateral lumbosciatic pain syndrome. She was unable to walk. MRI (**a**) revealed a multilevel spinal stenosis including a degenerative olisthesis at L4/L5. Surgical treatment comprised multilevel decompression and cement-augmented posterior lumbar interbody fusion

in cases of relevant comorbidities. The rate of medical problems and wound healing problems is higher in older patients. The bad bone quality represents always a problem which is sometimes hard to handle. A preoperative quantification of the bone mineral density is mandatory, and in cases of a manifest osteoporosis with a BMD <100 mg/cc, an additional augmentation of the instrumentation has to be considered (Fig. 13.10). The problem of adjacent level degeneration including adjacent level fractures is still not completely understood.

Interspinous and Dynamic Devices

In contrast to the complete immobilization of a fused segment with the possible adjacent level degeneration, there are some new devices which have been developed under the presumption that abnormal motion induces pain. So preservation of the "normal" motion range was the first-line objective. Dynamic fixation systems and interspinous devices have been developed allowing a decompression on the one side and a motion-preserving (partial) fixation on the other. These devices should reduce the intradiscal pressure, they should release the facet joints, and they should widen the spinal canal and neuroforamina by distraction. The significance of these techniques has not yet been defined completely. Up to now the clinical benefit seems to be comparable with decompression procedures but with an elevated risk of complications including fractures and material dislocation [51, 52].

13.3.5 Prognosis

Despite the up to now moderate evidence for an operative treatment of degenerative lumbar spine diseases, one has to consider that there is an reoperation rate of up to 15 % [50, 53–55] during follow-up for "complications" like recurrent disc herniation, restenosis, and adjacent level degeneration.

During the last years, we learned from a lot of high-quality studies that extent of the stenosis and different operative technique is of less importance compared to the psychological state and the expectations of the patient [56–58]. This has to be considered when planning a surgical therapy. The patient has to be informed honestly about the possible results of the operation – surgery targets to the correction of an unstable spine or on the decompression of neural structures and not on a reversal or a cure of the degeneration process! So local pain in this context is still realistic even after an operative treatment, a fortiori in cases of a multilevel disease. So, in conclusion, diagnosis and treatment of degenerative lumbar spine disease require – especially in elderly people – a multidisciplinary approach of course considering pathoanatomical and pathophysiological specialties but even more the psychological situation including pain sensation and the expectations of the individual patients. Only when all this goes together, an acceptable result for all involved parties can be achieved.

References

1. Allen RT, Rihn JA, Glassman SD et al (2009) An evidence-based approach to spine surgery. Am J Med Qual 24(6 Suppl):15–24
2. Watters WC 3rd, Baisden J, Gilbert TJ et al (2008) Degenerative lumbar spinal stenosis: an evidence-based clinical guideline for the diagnosis and treatment of degenerative lumbar spinal stenosis. Spine J 8(2):305–310
3. Statistisches Bundesamt (2016) Gesundheit, Diagnosedaten der Patienten und Patientinnen in Krankenhäusern. Statistisches Bundesamt, Wiesbaden. https://www.destatis.de. Contacted on 23 Mar 2016
4. Modic MT, Steinberg PM, Ross JS et al (1988) Degenerative disk disease: assessment of changes in vertebral body marrow with MR imaging. Radiology 166(1 Pt 1):193–199
5. Fujiwara A, Tamai K, An HS et al (2000) The effect of disc degeneration and facet joint osteoarthritis on the segmental flexibility of the lumbar spine. J Spinal Disord 13(5):444–450
6. Hadji P, Klein S, Gothe H et al (2013) The epidemiology of osteoporosis--Bone Evaluation Study (BEST): an analysis of routine health insurance data. Dtsch Arztebl Int 110(4):52–57
7. Martin DE, Severns AE, Kabo JM (2004) Determination of mechanical stiffness of bone by pQCT measurements: correlation with non-destructive mechanical four-point bending test data. J Biomech 37(8):1289–1293
8. Bernhardt M, Bridwell KH (1989) Segmental analysis of the sagittal plane alignment of the normal thoracic and lumbar spines and thoracolumbar junction. Spine 14(7):717–721

9. Grob D, Frauenfelder H, Mannion AF (2007) The association between cervical spine curvature and neck pain. Eur Spine J16(5):669–678
10. Jackson RP, McManus AC (1994) Radiographic analysis of sagittal plane alignment and balance in standing volunteers and patients with low back pain matched for age, sex, and size. A prospective controlled clinical study. Spine 19(14):1611–1618
11. Barrey C, Roussouly P, Le Huec JC et al (2013) Compensatory mechanisms contributing to keep the sagittal balance of the spine. Eur Spine J 22(Suppl 6):834–841
12. Moojen WA, Schenck CD, Nijeholt GJ et al (2015) Preoperative MR imaging in patients with intermittent neurogenic claudication: relevance for diagnosis and prognosis. Spine [Epub ahead of print]
13. Wassenaar M, van Rijn RM, van Tulder MW et al (2012) Magnetic resonance imaging for diagnosing lumbar spinal pathology in adult patients with low back pain or sciatica: a diagnostic systematic review. Eur Spine J 21(2):220–227. Bess S, Protopsaltis TS, Lafage V et al (2016) Clinical and radiographic evaluation of adult spinal deformity. Clin Spine Surg 29(1):6–16
14. Tanaka N, Nakanishi K, Fujimoto Y et al (2009) Clinical results of cervical myelopathy in patients older than 80 years of age: evaluation of spinal function with motor evoked potentials. J Neurosurg Spine 11((4):421–426
15. Nakanishi K, Tanaka N, Kamei N et al (2014) Electrophysiological evidence of functional improvement in the corticospinal tract after laminoplasty in patients with cervical compressive myelopathy: clinical article. J Neurosurg Spine 21(2):210–216
16. Kim DH, Vaccaro AR, Henderson FC et al (2003) Molecular biology of cervical myelopathy and spinal cord injury: role of oligodendrocyte apoptosis. Spine J 3(6):510–519
17. Nurick S (1972) The pathogenesis of the spinal cord disorder associated with cervical spondylosis. Brain 95(1):87–100
18. Hirabayashi K, Satomi K (1988) Operative procedure and results of expansive open-door laminoplasty. Spine 13(7):870–876
19. Herdmann J, Linzbach M, Krzan M (1994) The European myelopathy score. In: Baucher B, Brock M, Klinger M (eds) Advances in neurosurgery. Springer, Berlin, pp 266–268
20. Yu YL, Jones SJ (1985) Somatosensory evoked potentials in cervical spondylosis. Correlation of median, ulnar and posterior tibial nerve responses with clinical and radiological findings. Brain 108(Pt 2):273–300
21. Nove-Josserand A, Andre-Obadia N, Mauguiere F (2002) Cervical spondylotic myelopathy: motor and somatosensory evoked potentials, clinical and radiological correlation. Rev Neurol 158(12 Pt 1):1191–1197
22. Kongsted A, Qerama E, Kasch H et al (2007) Neck collar, "act-as-usual" or active mobilization for whiplash injury? A randomized parallel-group trial. Spine 32(6):618–626
23. Peloso PM, Gross AR et al (2006) Medicinal and injection therapies for mechanical neck disorders: a Cochrane systematic review. J Rheumatol 33(5):957–967
24. Gross AR, Peloso PM, Galway E et al (2013) Physician-delivered injection therapies for mechanical neck disorders: a systematic review update (non-oral, non-intravenous pharmacological interventions for neck pain). Open Orthop J 20(7):562–581
25. Bronfort G, Haas M et al (2004) Efficacy of spinal manipulation and mobilization for low back pain and neck pain: a systematic review and best evidence synthesis. Spine J 4(3):335–356
26. Gross AR, Hoving JL, Haines TA et al (2004) A Cochrane review of manipulation and mobilization for mechanical neck disorders. Spine 29(14):1541–1548
27. Fouyas IP, Statham PF, Sandercock PA (2002) Cochrane review on the role of surgery in cervical spondylotic radiculomyelopathy. Spine 27(7):736–747
28. Carette S, Fehlings MG (2005) Clinical practice. Cervical radiculopathy. N Engl J Med 353(4):392–399
29. Abumi K (2015) Cervical spondylotic myelopathy: posterior decompression and pedicle screw fixation. Eur Spine J 24(Suppl 2):186–196

30. Waschke A, Walter J, Duenisch P et al (2013) Anterior cervical intercorporal fusion in patients with osteoporotic or tumorous fractures using a cement augmented cervical plate system: first results of a prospective single-center study. J Spinal Disord Tech 26(3):E112–E117
31. Imagama S, Matsuyama Y, Sakai Y et al (2011) An arterial pulse examination is not sufficient for diagnosis of peripheral arterial disease in lumbar spinal canal stenosis: a prospective multicenter study. Spine 36(15):1204–1210
32. Saito J, Ohtori S, Kishida S et al (2012) Difficulty of diagnosing the origin of lower leg pain in patients with both lumbar spinal stenosis and hip joint osteoarthritis. Spine 37(25): 2089–2093
33. Lee BH, Moon SH, Kim HJ et al (2012) Osteoporotic profiles in elderly patients with symptomatic lumbar spinal canal stenosis. Indian J Orthop 46(3):279–284
34. Rihn JA, Hilibrand AS, Zhao W et al (2015) Effectiveness of surgery for lumbar stenosis and degenerative spondylolisthesis in the octogenarian population: analysis of the Spine Patient Outcomes Research Trial (SPORT) data. J Bone Joint Surg Am 97(3):177–185
35. Atlas SJ, Keller RB, Wu YA et al (2005) Long term outcomes of surgical and nonsurgical management of lumbar spinal stenosis; 8 to 10 year results from the maine lumbar spine study. Spine 30(8):936–943
36. Chang Y, Singer DE, Wu YA et al (2005) The effect of surgical and nonsurgical treatment on longitudinal outcomes of lumbar spinal stenosis over 10 years. J Am Geriatr Soc 53:785–792
37. Atlas SJ, Elitto A (2006) Spinal stenosis: surgical versus nonsurgical treatment. Clin Orthopad Relat Res 443:198–207
38. Lurie JD, Tosteson TD, Tosteson A et al (2015) Long-term outcomes of lumbar spinal stenosis: eight-year results of the Spine Patient Outcomes Research Trial (SPORT). Spine 40(2):63–76
39. Zaina F, Tomkins-Lane C, Carragee E et al (2016) Surgical versus non-surgical treatment for lumbar spinal stenosis. Cochrane Database Syst Rev 29:1
40. RAND cooperation, Santa Monica USA. http://www.rand.org/health/surveys_tools/mos/mos_core_36item_survey.html. Contacted on 4 Apr 2016
41. Fairbank JC, Pynsent PB (2000) The Oswestry Disability Index. Spine 25:2940–2953
42. Pearson A, Lurie J, Tosteson TD et al (2012) Who should have surgery for spinal stenosis? Treatment effect predictors in SPORT. Spine 21:1791–1802
43. Nationale Versorgungsleitlinie Kreuzschmerz (2015). www.leitlinien.de/mdb/downloads/nvl/kreuzschmerz/kreuzschmerz-1aufl-vers5-lang.pdf. Last contact on 5 Apr 2016
44. van Tulder MW, Koes B, Malmivaara A (2006) Outcome of non-invasive treatment modalities on back pain: an evidence-based review. Eur Spine J 15(Suppl 1):64–81
45. Markman JD Frazer ME, Rast SA et al (2015) Double-blind, randomized, controlled, crossover trial of pregabalin for neurogenic claudication. Neurology 84(3):265–272 (3)
46. Brown LL (2012) A double-blind, randomized, prospective study of epidural steroid injection vs. the mild(®) procedure in patients with symptomatic lumbar spinal stenosis. Pain Pract 12(5):333–341
47. Cohen SP, Hanling S, Bicket MC et al (2015) Epidural steroid injections compared with gabapentin for lumbosacral radicular pain: multicenter randomized double blind comparative efficacy study. BMJ 16:350
48. Racoosin JA, Seymour SM, Cascio L et al (2015) Serious neurologic events after epidural glucocorticoid injection-the FDA's risk assessment. N Engl J Med 374:2299–2301 (1)
49. Jakola AS, Sørlie A, Gulati S et al (2010) Clinical outcomes and safety assessment in elderly patients undergoing decompressive laminectomy for lumbar spinal stenosis: a prospective study. BMC Surg 10:34
50. Jansson KG, Nemeth G, Granath F et al (2005) Spinal stenosis re-operation rate in Sweden is 11% at 10 years – a national analysis of 9,664 operations. Eur Spine J 14:659–663
51. Moojen WA, Arts MP, Jacobs WC et al (2015) IPD without bony decompression versus conventional surgical decompression for lumbar spinal stenosis: 2-year results of a double-blind randomized controlled trial. Eur Spine J 24(10):2295–2305

52. Lønne G, Johnsen LG, Rossvoll I et al (2015) Minimally invasive decompression versus x-stop in lumbar spinal stenosis: a randomized controlled multicenter study. Spine 40(2):77–85
53. Chotai S, Parker SL, Sivaganesan A et al (2015) Effect of complications within 90 days on patient-reported outcomes 3 months and 12 months following elective surgery for lumbar degenerative disease. Neurosurg Focus 39(6):E8
54. Leven D, Passias PG, Errico TJ et al (2015) Risk factors for reoperation in patients treated surgically for intervertebral disc herniation: a subanalysis of eight-year SPORT data. J Bone Joint Surg Am 97(16):1316–1325
55. Gerling MC, Leven D, Passias PG et al (2016) Risk factors for reoperation in patients treated surgically for lumbar stenosis: a subanalysis of the 8 year data from the SPORT trial. Spine 41:901–909 [Epub ahead of print]
56. Lurie JD, Henderson ER, McDonough CM et al (2016) The effect of expectations on treatment outcome for lumbar intervertebral disc herniation. Spine 41:803–809
57. Nerland US, Jakola AS, Solheim O et al (2015) Minimally invasive decompression versus open laminectomy for central stenosis of the lumbar spine: pragmatic comparative effectiveness study. BMJ 1:350
58. Overdevest G, Vleggeert-Lankamp C, Jacobs W et al (2015) Effectiveness of posterior decompression techniques compared with conventional laminectomy for lumbar stenosis. Eur Spine J 24(10):2244–2263

Spinal Injuries of the Elderly

14

Christopher D. Witiw, Laureen D. Hachem,
and Michael G. Fehlings

14.1 Introduction

Presently, we are in the midst of a global demographic transition. Worldwide, average life expectancy has increased from 46.5 years in 1950 to 66.0 in the year 2000 and is thought to reach 76 years by 2045. The number of people aged 65 years or older is projected to increase by 140 % between 2006 and 2030 [1], and the "oldest old" (aged 85 years or older) is projected to increase 151 % over this period [2]. This general demographic transition is being translated into an observed shift in age patterns for individuals with traumatic spinal injuries. The mean age at injury has increased nearly 10 years between the 1970s and 2000s, and this has led to a substantial change in the practice patterns of spinal neurosurgeons [3].

The aged population is at a greater risk of sustaining traumatic injury to the spine than their younger counterparts. The reasons are multifactorial. Sensorineural function declines with age. Reduced vision and hearing contribute to a diminished

C.D. Witiw, MD
Division of Neurosurgery, Department of Surgery, University of Toronto,
Toronto, ON, Canada
e-mail: christopher.witiw@mail.utoronto.ca

L.D. Hachem
Faculty of Medicine, University of Toronto, Toronto, ON, Canada
e-mail: laureen.hachem@mail.utoronto.ca

M.G. Fehlings, MD, PhD, FRCSC, FACS (✉)
Division of Neurosurgery, Department of Surgery, University of Toronto,
Toronto, ON, Canada

Head Spinal Program, McEwen Centre for Regenerative Medicine, Toronto Western Hospital,
University Health Network, 399 Bathurst Street, 4WW-449, Toronto, ON, Canada M5T 2S8

Department of Surgery, Halbert Chair in Neural Repair and Regeneration, University of
Toronto, Toronto, ON, Canada
e-mail: Michael.Fehlings@uhn.on.ca

© Springer International Publishing Switzerland 2017

M. Berhouma, P. Krolak-Salmon (eds.), *Brain and Spine Surgery in the Elderly*,
DOI 10.1007/978-3-319-40232-1_14

ability to recognize and avoid environmental hazards. Furthermore, impaired balance and gait, compounded by reduced strength and flexibility, place elderly individuals at risk for falls. While more likely to be involved in a trauma, older individuals are also at higher risk of injury. Underlying degenerative spinal stenosis and osteoporosis of the vertebrae place the spinal cord at higher risk of compressive forces from the surrounding osteoligamentous structures of the spinal column. The prognosis following a spinal injury is also lessened with age. Decline in physiological reserve may be further exacerbated by coexisting medical conditions and polypharmacy. Synergistic relations between all of these factors make management of traumatic spinal cord injury (SCI) in the elderly a particular challenge.

With this chapter, we aim to provide an up-to-date review of the relevant considerations for spinal neurosurgeons involved with the management of an elderly individual following traumatic injury to the spine. The first two sections focus on the features of traumatic injury and management considerations that differ between the elderly population and those in younger cohorts. The three subsequent sections deal with specific injuries common to the elderly, namely, odontoid fractures, traumatic central cord syndrome (TCCS), and vertebral compression fractures (VCRs). The final section concludes with a synopsis of the available evidence pertaining to the outcomes of elderly individuals. Common decision-making challenges will be highlighted, and areas of ongoing controversy are discussed. This should serve to raise awareness of certain pitfalls and facilitate appraisal of the continuing influx of new clinical data in this increasingly relevant and ever-changing area of spinal neurosurgery.

14.2 Unique Features of Spine and Spinal Cord Injury in the Elderly

Patterns of traumatic injury to the spine differ between the elderly and their younger counterparts. This is owed primarily to differences in traumatic mechanism and age-related changes to the spinal column. An understanding of the factors that influence spinal injuries in the elderly along with the unique features of these injuries is essential for appropriate diagnosis and management and is the focus of this section.

14.2.1 Patterns of Injury

Injuries in the elderly often result from a relatively minor trauma [4]. Falls represent the leading etiology of acute SCI in this population [3]. These injuries are on the rise in developed countries and appear to be linked with the shifting population demographics [5]. This mechanism is in contrast to the more common high-energy mechanisms found in younger cohorts such as motor vehicle collisions, violence, and recreational sports (Fig. 14.1).

Falls in the elderly often lead to high cervical injuries and rarely result in injury at the thoracic and lumbar levels that are more commonly associated with

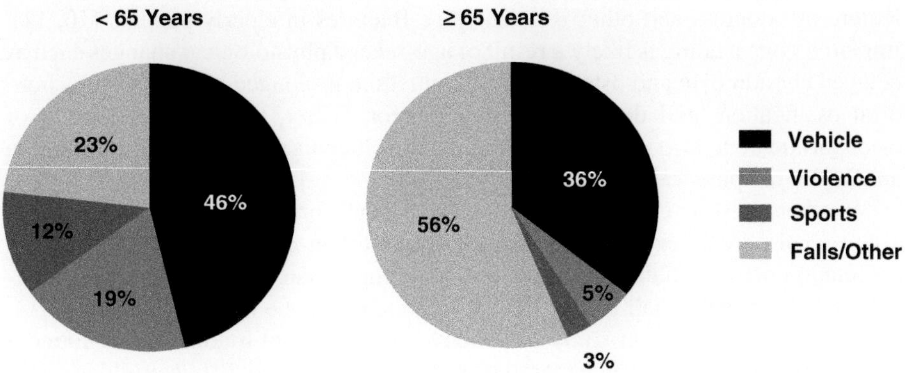

Fig. 14.1 Etiology of traumatic spinal cord injury by age in a cohort of patients (n=6132) from the NSCISC database. The majority of spinal cord injuries in elderly patients 65 years of age or older (n=328) were due to falls. In contrast, the most common cause of spinal cord injury in patients under the age of 65 (n=5800) was motor vehicle accidents (Figure derived from the data of Putzke et al. [4])

Table 14.1 Common spinal injury patterns in the elderly

Injury	Physiological predisposition
Odontoid fracture	Decreased subaxial cervical spine mobility
Central cord syndrome	Cervical spondylosis and resulting spinal canal stenosis
Vertebral compression fracture	Osteoporosis of the vertebral cones

high-energy forces and found in younger populations. In fact, the incidence of high cervical SCI has more than doubled in the USA since the 1970s, attributable in part to a greater incidence of fall-related spinal injuries [3].

Age-related changes to the spine predispose the elderly to specific injury patterns (Table 14.1). Degenerative changes throughout the subaxial cervical spine lead to rigidity and leave the atlantoaxial region as the segment of greatest mobility in elderly patients. As such, atlantoaxial injuries are more commonly seen in the elderly compared to younger individuals where enhanced mobility of the subaxial cervical spine can dissipate external forces [6–8]. Furthermore, cervical spondylosis and stenosis in the aging spine predispose to TCCS, precipitated by a hyperextension injury. Decreased bone quality of the vertebral bodies due to osteoporotic changes predisposes elderly individuals to vertebral compression fractures even with only minimal trauma. Compression fractures often result in segmental kyphotic deformity, and the altered alignment increases the fracture risk of adjacent vertebrae [9].

14.2.2 Fracture Healing and Recovery

Osteoporotic changes and age-related bone loss in the elderly lead to predictable changes in healing patterns after spine fractures. Bony nonunion is a common feature of odontoid and other isolated spine fractures in elderly patients [10, 11]. Impaired bone healing is likely a result of age-related physiological changes such as delayed chondrocyte and osteoblast differentiation, prolonged period of endochondrial ossification, and decreased vascularization [12, 13]. Decreased quality of osteoporotic bone also presents challenges for achieving adequate surgical fixation and fusion of spine fractures.

Whether age-related changes within the spinal cord itself influence recovery after spinal cord injury remains unclear. Postmortem analyses have revealed an association between older age and loss of small myelinated fibers in the corticospinal tract along with small neurons in the intermediate zone of the ventral horn [14, 15]. Despite this, a recent study of patients who sustained traumatic SCI found a similar extent of myelin degeneration and axonal survival between elderly and young patients [16]. Nevertheless, anatomical changes of the aging spinal cord may impact long-term regeneration and recovery after SCI, and thus further investigation is necessary.

Box 14.1: Summary of Unique Features of Spine and Spinal Cord Injuries in the Elderly

- Spine injuries in the elderly are often due to low-energy mechanisms (commonly falls) and frequently lead to injuries of the high cervical spine.
- Reduced cervical spine mobility may enhance susceptibility to C1–C2 injuries in elderly individuals.
- Age-related, degenerative cervical spinal stenosis predisposes to traumatic central cord syndrome in the elderly population
- Decreased bone quality leads to delayed union of fractures.

14.3 Unique Considerations When Managing the Elderly with Spinal Trauma

All patients, including the elderly, with acute spinal cord injury should be assessed and managed in the immediate period with a systematic approach in accordance with the Advanced Trauma Life Support Guidelines [17]. Information gathering is of particular importance in elderly patients during the initial assessment. Whenever possible, relevant past medical history and current medications should be recorded. Coexisting conditions become more prevalent with advanced age [18]. These factors must be considered as they may alter management. Additionally, geriatric patients may have preestablished wishes pertaining to the aggressiveness of desired intervention, and these should be taken into account whenever possible. Within this section, we review the important factors of initial assessment and management of an elderly individual following a traumatic spinal injury.

14.3.1 Airway Protection and Ventilation

Adequate oxygen delivery to the spinal cord helps mitigate the local ischemic effects resulting from secondary injury mechanisms, and sufficient blood oxygenation is imperative [19]. Supplemental oxygen should be administered immediately in the acute setting, but vigilance for an induced decrement in respiratory drive should be considered in the setting of an elderly individual with preexisting respiratory pathology such as chronic obstructive pulmonary disease.

Those with high cervical SCIs are at high risk for respiratory failure, owing to dysfunction of the muscles of respiration caused by the injury. Establishment of a definitive airway and subsequent positive pressure ventilation should be considered early in the setting of impending airway compromise or respiratory failure. The potential for dentures to act as a source of airway obstruction in this population should not be overlooked. If airway protection is required, a rapid sequence induction is considered the standard of care [20]. During this process, neuromuscular blockade with succinylcholine should be avoided in any elderly individual with a history of neuromuscular disease or prolonged immobilization because of the recognized risk of a dangerous hyperkalemic response [21]. A non-depolarizing neuromuscular blocking agent such as rocuronium should be selected instead.

14.3.2 Hemodynamic Support

Current guidelines suggest aggressive arterial blood pressure monitoring and medical management including admission to a critical care unit. A general mean arterial blood pressure target between 85 and 90 mmHg should be maintained for 1 week following an SCI [22]. Close monitoring is of particular importance for the elderly, who may experience unanticipated adverse events relating to comorbid conditions and underlying cardiac abnormalities. Geriatric patients may be more susceptible to fluid overload due to limited cardiac reverse, and cautious administration of crystalloid solutions is necessary. Moreover, prolonged administration of vasoactive agents to induce hypertension may place unanticipated strain on an already weakened heart. A careful balance between maintenance of spinal cord perfusion and the risk of an acute coronary event must be achieved in this vulnerable population. These patients may also be at risk for hypotensive episodes because of prior administration of antihypertensive medications, and this should be taken into account when formulating a strategy for hemodynamic support.

14.3.3 Cardiac Arrhythmias

Patients with high cervical SCIs are at high risk for cardiac arrhythmias that require intervention [23]. The risk may be exacerbated in the elderly population because of underlying cardiac abnormalities. Symptomatic bradycardia should be treated upfront with atropine to ensure adequate cardiac output. If heart rate and symptoms are refractory to atropine, aminophylline [24] or temporary pacing should be considered.

14.3.4 Corticosteroid Administration

The role for steroid administration remains controversial for any patient with acute SCI [25]. The primary concern with administration is the elevated risk of adverse events. In particular, the National Acute Spinal Cord Injury Study (NASCIS) III trial found significantly higher incidence of severe pneumonia and a higher incidence of severe sepsis that approached significance in those receiving methylprednisolone sodium succinate (MPSS) following a 48-h protocol [26]. We contend that, in general, steroid administration should remain an option for individuals with cervical SCI, but because of the risk of complications and potential comorbidities in the elderly population, we do not routinely administer MPPS to elderly individuals.

14.3.5 Other Comorbid Diseases

Underlying medical comorbidities are commonly found in this population, and a careful history of prior diagnoses and current medications is critical. Underlying cardiac arrhythmias or hypercoagulable states may necessitate anticoagulation, and the risk of thromboembolism must be weighed against the need for hemostasis in the setting of trauma. A history of long-standing diabetes reduces bone quality and thus results in delayed fracture and wound healing [27]. Nutritional deficiencies also lead to similar impairment in fracture repair [28, 29]. These medical comorbidities in the elderly also impart unique considerations when deciding on treatment goals. Surgical intervention may be contraindicated in patients with a high burden of comorbid disease as the risks of perioperative mortality outweigh the potential risks of fracture nonunion or prolonged immobilization associated with conservative treatment.

Box 14.2: Summary of Unique Considerations When Managing the Elderly with Spinal Trauma

- Supplemental oxygen should be administered in the acute setting, but vigilance for induced respiratory drive from preexisting pulmonary conditions is critical.
- A mean arterial blood pressure target between 85 and 90 mmHg should be maintained for 1 week in elderly individuals with spinal cord injury; however, a balance between spinal cord perfusion and cardiac strain must be established.
- The risk of cardiac arrhythmias in elderly with high cervical spinal cord injury may be elevated because of underlying cardiac abnormalities.
- A careful history of medical conditions and current medications should be obtained as early as possible.
- When managing any elderly individual with a preexisting condition that necessitates anticoagulation, an appropriate balance between thromboembolic risk and the need for hemostasis should be sought.

14.4 Geriatric Odontoid Fractures

Odontoid fractures are the most common cervical spine injury in the elderly [30]. Despite this, optimal treatment remains controversial. Anatomical and physiological changes of the aging spine make the management of odontoid fractures particularly challenging. This section will outline the clinical presentation, classification, evidence for management, and predictors of treatment outcomes for geriatric odontoid fractures.

14.4.1 Clinical Presentation

As low-energy falls are the principal mechanism of injury in the elderly, geriatric odontoid fractures are not typically associated with concomitant spine or ligamentous injuries [31, 32]. Neurological deficits are relatively uncommon but may be seen in the context of significant posterior displacement of the bone, attributable to a hyperextension injury [32–34]. More commonly, patients present with neck pain or limitation in neck mobility and in some cases may even be asymptomatic. Nevertheless, a complete clinical and radiographic assessment is required to assess fracture severity, neurological impairment, and any associated injuries.

14.4.2 Management

Fracture pattern predominates in the treatment decision process. CT imaging is the best radiographic modality for assessment of fracture pattern, degree of bone displacement, and identification of concurrent fractures. Upon review of the cervical spinal CT, these fractures are classified into three distinct types according to the commonly used Anderson and D'Alonzo system (Fig. 14.2) [35]. Type I fractures are uncommon and involve an oblique fracture through the upper portion of the odontoid process. Type II fractures are the most common and occur in the odontoid process at the junction with the axis body. Type III fractures extend into the body of C2 and have wider cancellous fracture surfaces. It is generally agreed that patients with types I and III fracture patterns may be safely managed with cervical orthosis unless there is evidence of spinal cord injury or clear instability [36, 37]. Conversely, there is substantial controversy over the optimal treatment of type II geriatric odontoid fractures.

14.4.2.1 Surgical Management

Recent studies have demonstrated improved outcomes with operative management compared to conservative treatment. In a retrospective analysis of 322 patients over 65 years of age with type II odontoid fractures, Chapman et al. found that surgical treatment significantly increased 30-day survival and there was a trend toward decreased long-term mortality, compared with nonsurgical management [38]. A subgroup analysis of the data suggested that although nonunion in the

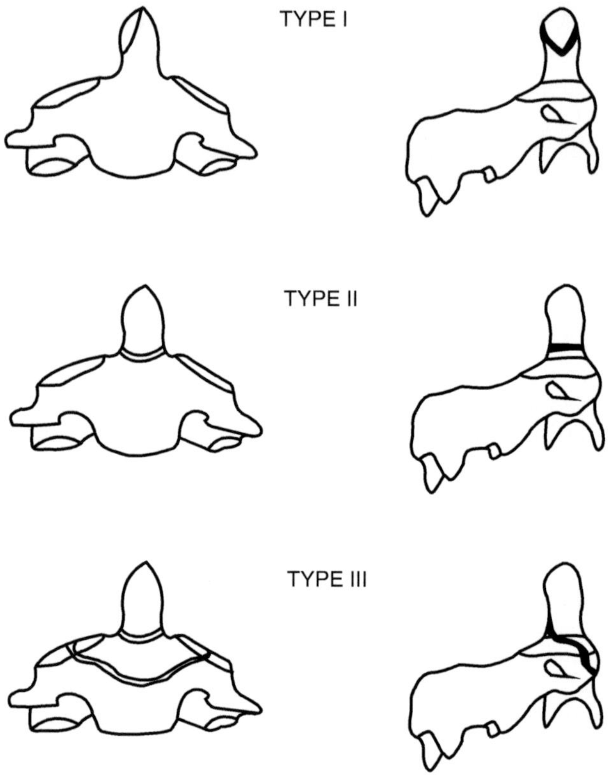

Fig. 14.2 Anderson and D'Alonzo classification of fractures of the odontoid process (Reproduced with permission; Anderson and d'Alonzo [35])

nonoperative group did not portend worse clinical outcomes at 12 months, the majority of these patients (7 out of 11) required delayed surgical intervention [39]. Vaccaro et al. conducted the only prospective study to date comparing operative and nonoperative management for geriatric odontoid fractures. This study included 159 patients 65 years of age or older, of which 101 were treated surgically and 58 conservatively (most commonly cervical collar, $n=47$). Surgical treatment was associated with significant improvements in disability and health-related quality of life, along with a trend toward decreased mortality compared to nonsurgical treatment [40]. Recently, a large systematic review examining 21 articles published between 2000 and 2015 found short- and long-term mortality were significantly lower in patients >60 years who underwent surgical treatment with no difference in the rate of complications (Fig. 14.3) [41]. Given the current evidence, it is reasonable to consider operative management in elderly patients with type II odontoid fractures who are able to tolerate surgery.

Modern surgical management of odontoid fractures involves either anterior odontoid screw fixation or posterior C1–C2 instrumented fusion. Generally odontoid screw fixation is not recommended in the elderly population, attributable in large part to the prevalence of clinical factors in this population which prevent adequate anterior fixation including osteoporosis, pathologic fractures, impaired bone

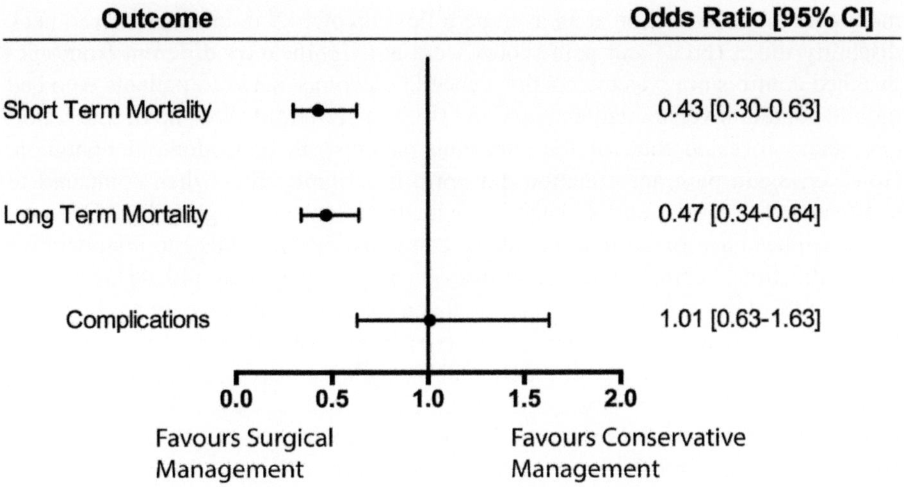

Fig. 14.3 Mortality and complication rate in geriatric patients with type II odontoid fractures treated surgically versus conservatively. Forest plot showing the odds ratio for short-term mortality, long-term mortality, and complication based on a meta-analysis from 21 articles containing a total of 1233 patients (Figure derived from the data of Schroeder et al. [41])

healing, cervical kyphosis, and cervical spondylosis [6, 42, 43]. In a retrospective study of 29 consecutive patients (age >65 years), Andersson et al. reported higher rates of complications leading to treatment failure in patients who underwent anterior screw fixation compared with posterior C1–C2 fusion [44]. Conversely, data from a recent systematic review found no significant difference in mortality or complication rate between the approaches [41]. This may suggest that elderly patients, who are appropriately selected patients, may achieve similar outcomes with an odontoid screw fixation.

14.4.2.2 Nonsurgical Management

If nonsurgical management is undertaken, cervical immobilization may be achieved through either a rigid cervical collar or halo brace. Substantial concern has been expressed regarding the potential complications of prolonged immobilization associated with either means of immobilization. Both devices are poorly tolerated in patients over the age of 60; halo braces, in particular, lead to increased risks of pneumonia, respiratory problems, and cardiac arrests [45, 46]. This has caused many to favor cervical collars for the purpose of cervical immobilization [47]. However, a recent systematic review including data from six studies published since 2000 found no significant differences in complication and short-term mortality [41].

While it has been shown that conservative treatment in the elderly yields high rates of nonunion compared to surgical management, there is some data to suggest that nonunion is not necessarily associated with a poor outcome. In a cohort study of 34 elderly patients with minimally displaced (<50 % displacement) type II odontoid fractures treated with rigid cervical collar for 12 weeks, 70 % of patients had mobile odontoid nonunion at an average follow-up of 14.9 months. However, neck disability index (NDI) and pain scores were not significantly different from age-matched controls nor was there a difference in outcomes between patients who had mobile nonunion versus stable nonunion [10]. Longer-term follow-up of this cohort (>4 years) revealed that, of the surviving patients, all had odontoid nonunion. However, again pain and function did not differ significantly when compared to age-matched controls, and satisfaction with treatment was high [11]. Moreover, recent studies have found that the rate of complications secondary to nonoperative immobilization is comparable to that from surgical management [40, 41].

All of this lends support to the notion that a stable bony union may not be a necessary treatment goal in the elderly with type II odontoid fractures [48]. However, much concern remains over the potential for delayed myelopathy from fracture instability or SCI from a subsequent traumatic event. Those treated conservatively should have frequent follow-up assessments including repeat flexion-extension radiographs to monitor for potential progression of instability. In the face of controversial evidence, the risks of treatment-related complications must be carefully considered in the clinical context of each individual patient.

14.4.2.3 Limitations of the Current Evidence

The limitations of the currently available evidence regarding the management of geriatric odontoid fractures preclude definitive treatment guidelines. The majority of data has been derived from level 3 or 4 studies with small cohorts and retrospective designs. Moreover, little information is provided on the criteria for surgical or nonsurgical candidacy, thus making it difficult to delineate potential useful predictors of treatment response. Inclusion and exclusion criteria vary widely between studies, and as such direct comparisons of treatment outcomes must be made with caution. Large prospective studies aiming to address the current limitations are necessary to provide further data to guide treatment decisions. Given the current available evidence, we support surgical intervention if deemed safe and appropriate by all members of the team responsible for the care of the elderly individual including the primary spinal surgeon and if this is in accordance with the wishes of the individual themselves and their family.

14.4.3 Predictors of Treatment Response and Clinical Outcomes

There is a paucity of data on the clinical outcomes and predictors of treatment response of odontoid fractures in the elderly. Woods et al. found that the burden of comorbid illness, as measured by Charlson comorbidity score, has a significant influence on survival after odontoid fractures in the elderly regardless of treatment modality [49]. In a multicenter prospective cohort study of 159 patients who are 65 years and older with type II odontoid fractures, Fehlings et al. found that older age, male sex, initial nonsurgical treatment, and baseline neurological system comorbidity were associated with poor response to treatment [50]. Patel et al. estimated the mortality risk to be almost five times higher in patients presenting with a type II odontoid fracture associated with neurological deficits compared to those without any deficits [51]. Although odontoid nonunion has shown no correlation with clinical outcome in multiple studies, there still remains concern over the risk of delayed myelopathy, and thus further data from long-term studies is necessary.

Box 14.3: Summary of Geriatric Odontoid Fractures

- Odontoid fractures are the most common cervical spine injury in the elderly.
- Types I and III injuries, generally, may be managed without surgical intervention, but the optimal management of type II injuries is controversial.
- Surgical management may reduce mortality in the elderly but should only be undertaken if in accordance with the wishes of the individual and their family and deemed safe and appropriate by the primary surgeon and all other members of the medical team.
- Prolonged immobilization, particularly with the use of a halo brace, may lead to complications in the elderly. This may be reduced by the use of hard cervical collars, but the evidence is not definitive.
- Nonunion does not necessarily correlate with poor neurological and functional outcomes.
- Very old patients have high morbidity and mortality regardless of treatment type.

14.5 Traumatic Central Cord Syndrome

TCCS was first described by Schneider et al. in the 1950s [52]. It is the most common type of incomplete SCI and is of particular relevance to the elderly population because it is within this group where the majority of these injuries occur. Despite the commonality, controversy regarding optimal management persists. Most pertains to the role and timing of surgical intervention. This section will focus on the clinical presentation and the factors that a practitioner must consider when managing an elderly individual with a TCCS.

14.5.1 Clinical Presentation

TCCS classically presents in an elderly individual with underlying cervical canal stenosis from spondylotic processes, who sustains a hyperextension-type neck injury. Often the mechanism may seem fairly innocuous; however, the extent of spinal canal narrowing and degenerative osteoligamentous changes (Fig. 14.4) can lead to profound neurological injury.

The distribution of neurological injury is such that the upper extremities are more severely affected than the lower. Generally, the fine motor function of the

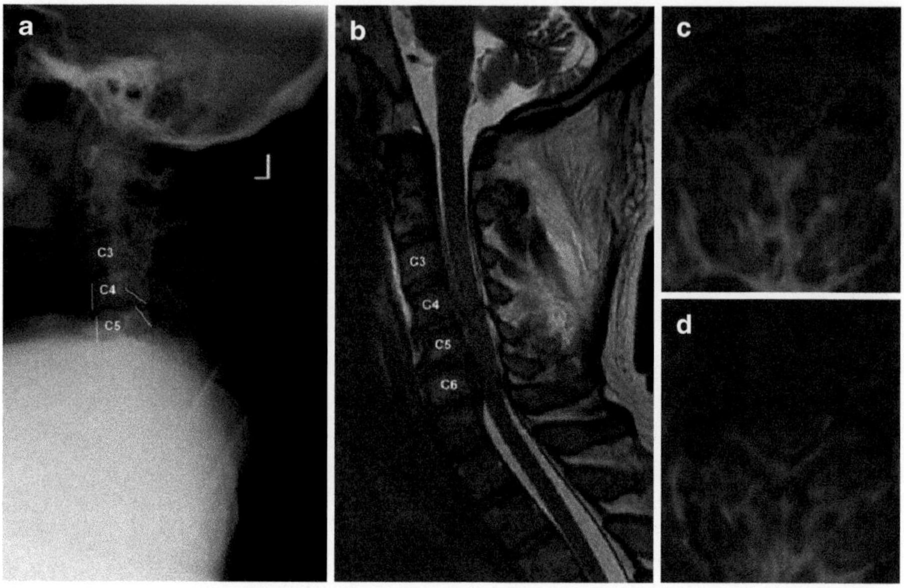

Fig. 14.4 Traumatic instability at C4/C5 secondary to a fall from standing height. (**a**) Radiographic evidence of facet subluxation at C4/C5; (**b**) sagittal T2-weighted magnetic resonance (MR) image of the same patient demonstrating cervical spinal canal stenosis from spondylosis; (**c**) axial MR image at the level of the C4/C5 interspace demonstrating spinal canal stenosis and spinal cord compression; (**d**) axial MR image at the C5/C6 interspace demonstrating similar findings to panel **c**

upper extremities is most involved. The clinical symptomatology has been formally classified as an incomplete SCI with a total lower extremity motor score of 10 or more points higher than the total upper extremity motor score on the American Spinal Injury Association (ASIA) Impairment Scale [53]. The severity of injury may range from limited hand weakness to complete quadriparesis with only sacral sparing. Bladder, bowel, and sexual dysfunction may be present in severe cases.

14.5.2 Management

Initial management should be in keeping with that of any incomplete spinal cord injury [22]. However, practitioners must remain mindful of the unique considerations when managing the elderly with spinal trauma that were described earlier in this chapter.

14.5.2.1 Surgical Decision-Making

Surgical decision-making for those with TCCS is often challenging. Many do not have evidence of overt spinal column instability and spontaneous neurological improvement may be observed. It is generally agreed that surgical intervention is necessary in all cases where TCCS is associated with unstable injury to the spinal column or intervertebral disk herniation. Conversely, some question if surgical intervention is warranted in cases where TCCS results from the classic mechanism of hyperextension in the setting of cervical spondylosis without evidence of instability. A 2013 systematic review of the literature found four articles that compared surgical to conservative management in patients with TCCS [54]. All were small, single center retrospective studies. Three demonstrated superiority of surgery to conservative management in terms of neurological recovery; however, the study populations were heterogeneous and included unstable traumatic injuries. Generally, we favor surgical intervention for any patient with radiographic evidence of cervical spinal cord compression and neurological deficits on clinical examination.

14.5.2.2 Timing of Surgical Intervention

Once the decision is made for surgical intervention, further controversy exists surrounding optimal timing. A 2015 systematic review aimed to address this identified a total of nine studies. Low level evidence suggested early surgery (within 24 h of injury) was associated with significantly greater improvements in ASIA motor scores and functional independence at 1 year when compared to delayed surgery [55]. Further evidence indicates that those with surgery within 2 weeks of the injury had a greater score on the modified Japanese Orthopedic Association scale and a greater rate of recovery [55]. However, presently there is no class I studies available to guide decision-making, and the current studies are limited by a lack of uniform diagnostic criteria, small sample sizes, and heterogeneous patient populations.

There is a need for high-quality prospective studies aimed to address this in elderly individuals with TCSS. The Comparing Surgical Decompression Versus Conservative Treatment in Incomplete Spinal Cord Injury (COSMIC) trial (ClinicalTrials.gov Identifier: NCT01367405) holds promise. This randomized, multicenter controlled study is designed to compare the clinical outcome of early (<24 h) surgical versus conservative strategy which was initiated in 2013 [56]. The inclusion criteria are not exclusively limited to the elderly population, but given the general demographics, it is likely that this data will provide helpful information specific to elderly individuals.

Until higher-quality evidence is available, we suggest that those with TCCS who have severe neurological deficits (ASIA C or worse) should have decompression within 24 h if there is any magnetic resonance imaging evidence of ongoing spinal cord compression or unstable osteoligamentous injury. Those with less severe neurological injury should undergo decompressive surgery, but the timeframe for this can be expanded to 1 week as the evidence for surgical intervention within 24 h is not as compelling.

14.5.3 Age Effect on Recovery

As with many other injuries, the prognosis for recovery after a TCCS is lessened with advancing age [57]. The current evidence from smaller, single center cohorts suggest that elderly individuals have higher mortality, less ability to achieve ambulatory status, and independence in self-care and bowel and bladder function [58, 59]. These findings are supported by a multicenter, matched cohort study into the effect of age on recovery potential which found recovery was significantly lessened for elderly individuals [60]. In all, prognosis for recovery appears to be age dependent and is less optimistic for older individuals.

Box 14.4: Summary of Central Cord Syndrome in the Elderly

- High-quality evidence is lacking for the role and timing of surgical intervention for traumatic central cord syndrome.
- We suggest that any patient with a neurological exam of ASIA Grade C or worse should have surgery within 24 h of injury, but a timeframe of within 1 week is appropriate for those with less severe neurological injury.
- Age appears to influence recovery and prognosis is lessened in elderly individuals.

14.6 Vertebral Compression Fractures

Vertebral compression fractures (VCFs) are an insufficiency fracture involving the anterior column of vertebrae. These are the most common type of facture associated with osteoporosis [61]. Recent estimates suggest an annual incidence of 1.5 million in the USA, and it is thought that approximately 25 % of postmenopausal women will be affected by a VCF during their lifetime [62]. Direct medical costs have been estimated to exceed $1 billion annually [61].

The greatest risk factor for sustaining a VCF is a prior history of fragility fracture, but others include age over 64 years, low bone mineral density, weak grip strength, female gender, a maternal history of a fragility fracture, and a sedentary lifestyle [63]. Presently there is ongoing debate regarding the optimal course of management, and options generally include conservative therapy or percutaneous intervention with vertebroplasty or kyphoplasty. The aim of this section is to review the common clinical presentation of VCFs and review the current evidence available to guide management.

14.6.1 Clinical Presentation

Individuals with VCFs may present with a wide spectrum of symptomatology. Neurological impairment for spinal cord compression is rare and suggests a more concerning pathology such as malignancy or infection. Many present without any symptoms. Instead these fractures are diagnosed incidentally on radiographs for other indications. However, others may present with severe, debilitating pain. Commonly, pain is exacerbated by activity and relieved with rest. Focal tenderness over the affected vertebrae is often present. The natural history is similarly variable. Many will report substantial improvement in pain and function over a period of days with minimal intervention, while others will remain incapacitated for prolonged durations.

14.6.2 Conservative Management

The goals of treatment are pain relief, mobilization, restoration of function, and prevention of subsequent deformity. Treatment for osteoporosis should be initiated, and individuals should be referred on to the appropriate medical specialty services to ensure adequate medical management and risk factor reduction.

14.6.2.1 Analgesics

Generally conservative therapy initially includes narcotic analgesia when deemed necessary and appropriate. However, caution should be used in the administration of narcotics to elderly individuals as substantial adverse effects may be encountered such as cognitive changes, constipation, and, most concerning, respiratory depression.

14.6.2.2 External Orthosis

The role for external orthosis in patients with VCFs is to improve pain symptoms and reduce the risk of progressive segmental kyphotic deformity at the facture site. Unfortunately, these braces are frequently poorly tolerated in the elderly, and cognitive deficits may further exacerbate this and reduce the likelihood of compliance. Recently a randomized study was conducted where patients with VCFs were distributed between management with ridged brace, soft brace, or no brace. At 12-week follow-up, the disability scores for those who did not receive a brace were not inferior to those who received a soft or a rigid brace, and change in back pain and radiographic anterior body compression were similar among all groups [64]. We assess the role for external orthosis on a case-by-case basis and only suggest this treatment modality if the individual finds pain relief and is likely to be compliant. Conservative management is generally continued until sufficient mobilization is achieved and pain symptoms have mitigated to the point of tolerability. We encourage the discontinuation of opioid analgesics as soon as these criteria have been achieved in an effort to avoid the associated potential for adverse outcomes.

14.6.3 Surgical Management

The role for traditional open surgical intervention for VCFs in the elderly is limited. The indications for open surgical intervention and fusion include the evidence of neurological deficit on clinical examination or progressive debilitating deformity, both of which are relatively uncommon. Conversely, percutaneous fluoroscopic guided vertebroplasty or kyphoplasty are frequently performed. Vertebroplasty acts to stabilize the fracture by infusing polymethylmethacrylate (PMM) into the vertebral body, while kyphoplasty incorporates the same technique except infusion of the PMM is preceded by inflation of a balloon within the fractured vertebral body to create additional space. Proponents of kyphoplasty suggest this technique reduces the risk of PMM extravasation from the vertebral body [65].

Two recent meta-analyses have compared percutaneous intervention with conservative management. Anderson et al. found a nonsignificant difference in back pain scores at early (<12 weeks) assessment but a significant reduction in these scores at later follow-up (6–12 months) [66]. This finding was further supported by another meta-analysis by Guo et al. which identifies an improved effect in pain reduction at short-, mid-, and long-term follow-up. However, there appeared to be no significant difference in physical function and quality of life between either treatment modality [67].

Overall it appears that percutaneous intervention for VCFs may be associated with an improvement in pain symptoms which may correspond in a reduced time for functional independence, but high-quality data is much needed before any definitive recommendations may be provided [68]. Presently we base recommendations for percutaneous intervention on an individual basis after discussions with the patient and family.

Box 14.5: Summary of Vertebral Compression Fractures in the Elderly

- Vertebral compression fractures are the most common type of facture associated with osteoporosis.
- Options for conservative management include analgesics, external spinal orthosis, and early mobilization.
- Current data supports that management without a brace after vertebral compression fracture has no inferior effect on pain and disability outcomes when compared to soft or rigid bracing.
- Options for surgical intervention primarily include vertebroplasty and kyphoplasty. Both have shown a greater effect in back pain reduction when compared with conservative management; however, there is no clear evidence of significant improvement in physical function and quality of life.

14.7 Outcomes of Spine and Spinal Cord Injury in the Elderly

The use of objective outcome measures has facilitated quantitative assessment of recovery after spine injuries and has enabled identification of unique challenges faced by elderly patients recovering from these injuries. This section will outline the clinical outcomes in the elderly within the following domains: neurological recovery, functional recovery, survival, and quality of life.

14.7.1 Neurological Recovery

Initial motor and sensory deficits at the time of injury are often less severe in the elderly compared to younger patients due to a higher incidence of low-energy mechanisms. In a retrospective study of 3481 patients with SCI, Fassett et al. found that a significantly greater proportion of patients 70 years of age or older presented with milder neurological injuries (ASIA C and D) compared with patients less than 70 years of age [69]. In keeping with general findings, elderly individuals have a greater likelihood of neurological recovery from incomplete SCI [70, 71].

There is some evidence to suggest that the extent of neurological recovery in elderly patients is similar to that of younger patients. An analysis of 485 patients from the NASCIS II trial found that age did not significantly affect motor and sensory recovery within 1 year following SCI [16]. Moreover, there was no significant difference between elderly patients compared to younger patients in terms of myelin degeneration or axonal survival in sensory, motor, and autonomic spinal cord tracts on postmortem analysis. Similar results have also been reported in other retrospective studies [72, 73]. It has been shown that elderly patients have a higher incidence of neuropathic pain after SCI when compared to younger patients [74, 75].

14.7.2 Functional Recovery

Following traumatic SCI, elderly patients are more likely to develop medical complications such as pneumonia, gastrointestinal bleeding, and pulmonary emboli compared to younger patients, all of which may in turn prolong the course of functional recovery [76]. Penrod et al. found that only 41 % of elderly patients were ambulatory after TCCS compared to 97 % in younger patients. Increased risk of pressure ulcers following SCI is also a major concern among the elderly [77].

Data from the NASCIS III trial found reduced physical and cognitive Functional Independence Measure (FIM) scores in elderly patients at 6 weeks after SCI compared to younger patients; however, functional recovery between 6 weeks and 1 year was not different between the two groups [72]. In contrast, Aito et al. report decreased FIM scores in elderly patients with TCCS both at the time of discharge from rehabilitation and at 18-month follow-up [75]. An analysis of 6132 patients from the National Spinal Cord Injury Statistical Center (NSCISC) database also found that functional recovery remained lower in older patients with chronic SCI (>1 year) [4].

14.7.3 Mortality

There is overwhelming evidence to suggest that age is a strong predictor of early mortality after spinal injury even after adjusting for potential confounders. An analysis of the data from the NASCIS III trial found that elderly patients had a 38.6 % mortality rate at 1 year after SCI compared to 3.1 % in younger patients after acute traumatic SCI with most deaths occurring within 6 weeks of injury [72]. Similar results were obtained from an analysis of NASCIS II trial data [16]. Fassett et al. found an almost eightfold increase in mortality in elderly patients with SCI compared to younger patients [69]. DeVivo et al. found that survival 2 years after SCI was 59 % in elderly patients (>60 years) compared to 85–95 % in younger patients (age 16–60) [76].

Spinal column injuries that leave the spinal cord intact appear to carry more favorable outcomes than those with associated neurological injury. Golob et al. report significantly lower mortality in elderly patients with isolated cervical spine fractures without SCI compared to those with traumatic cervical spine fractures affecting the spinal cord [78].

The extent to which therapeutic interventions can alter the course of mortality is highly dependent on patient age. A retrospective analysis of 640 elderly patients (age ≥65 years) with cervical spine fractures found operative treatment reduced mortality at 3 months and 1 year post-injury in patients 65–74 years old but had no survival benefit in patients 75–84 years and increased mortality in those over the age of 85 [79].

The high mortality rate seen among elderly patients after spine or spinal cord injuries is likely a result of multiple factors including reduced functional status, increased rates of complications, and a high burden of preexisting comorbid disease. Furlan et al. found that the primary causes of death within the first year after SCI in the elderly were cardiac arrhythmias, respiratory complications, and coagulation problems [16].

14.7.4 Quality of Life

Data specifically pertaining to quality of life among elderly patients with spinal injuries is much needed. Putzke et al. found that elderly patients with SCI report worse overall life satisfaction, perceived physical health, and overall handicap compared to younger patients [4]. Barrett et al. found those who sustained an SCI at or after the age of 60 years had higher self-reported handicap in the domains of physical independence and social integration than those who were less than 60 years at the time of injury [80].

14.7.5 Implications for Clinical Practice

Despite the potential for motor and sensory improvement in elderly patients with spinal cord injuries, functional recovery is limited and mortality rates are high. Neurological recovery in the elderly may translate less readily into clinically meaningful improvements in disability, due to decreased functional reserve and preexisting burden of comorbid disease. These considerations should be factored into pretreatment discussions with patients themselves and their family members. Realistic goals of care should be established at the earliest possible time during the clinical course following injury, but reassessment of such goals and reestablishment of prognostic estimates should be made if unanticipated changes are encountered. Informed discussions such as this serve to calibrate expectations, and more prognosis-based research studies will enhance this important communication.

Box 14.6: Summary of Outcomes in Elderly Patients with Spine or Spinal Cord Injuries

- Incomplete spinal cord injuries are more common in the elderly compared to younger patients, and initial neurological deficits are often less severe.
- The extent of neurological recovery after SCI may not be significantly affected by age.
- Functional deficits after spinal injuries often persist in elderly patients, but elderly patients may benefit from rehabilitation strategies aimed at improving functional independence
- Spinal injuries carry high mortality rates in the elderly.

Conclusions

The present global demographic transition leaves a substantial set of management considerations to those responsible for the care of elderly patients with spinal injury. Numerous preexisting medical conditions and confounding pharmacotherapy must be identified early and managed appropriately. Overall prognosis is generally lessened with advanced age, and conversations between surgeons and the patients themselves and their families are critical to the provision of appropriate care. Data continues to emerge that will help guide clinical decision-making, and many of the current assumptions may change. Neurosurgeons must stay apprised of this ever-changing evidence-based landscape, and this chapter should serve to help establish a foundation upon which to incorporate new data as it emerges.

References

1. Krug EG, Dahlberg LL, Mercy JA, Zwi AB, Lozano R (2002) World report on violence and health. Lancet 360:1083–1088
2. Bengtson VL, Lowenstein A (2003) Global aging and its challenge to families. Transaction Publishers, New York
3. Devivo MJ (2012) Epidemiology of traumatic spinal cord injury: trends and future implications. Spinal Cord 50(5):365–372
4. Putzke JD, Barrett JJ, Richards JS, DeVivo MJ (2003) Age and spinal cord injury: an emphasis on outcomes among the elderly. J Spinal Cord Med 26(1):37–44
5. Lee BB, Cripps RA, Fitzharris M, Wing PC (2014) The global map for traumatic spinal cord injury epidemiology: update 2011, global incidence rate. Spinal Cord 52(2):110–116
6. Elgafy H, Dvorak MF, Vaccaro AR, Ebraheim N (2009) Treatment of displaced type II odontoid fractures in elderly patients. Am J Orthop (Belle Mead NJ) 38(8):410–416

7. Malik SA, Murphy M, Connolly P, O'Byrne J (2008) Evaluation of morbidity, mortality and outcome following cervical spine injuries in elderly patients. Eur Spine J 17(4):585–591
8. Lomoschitz FM, Blackmore CC, Mirza SK, Mann FA (2002) Cervical spine injuries in patients 65 years old and older: epidemiologic analysis regarding the effects of age and injury mechanism on distribution, type, and stability of injuries. AJR Am J Roentgenol 178(3):573–577
9. Ferguson SJ, Steffen T (2003) Biomechanics of the aging spine. Eur Spine J 12(Suppl 2):S97–S103
10. Molinari RW, Khera OA, Gruhn WL, McAssey RW (2012) Rigid cervical collar treatment for geriatric type II odontoid fractures. Eur Spine J 21(5):855–862
11. Raudenbush B, Molinari R (2015) Longer-term outcomes of geriatric odontoid fracture non-union. Geriatr Orthop Surg Rehabil 6(4):251–257
12. Lu C, Miclau T, Hu D et al (2005) Cellular basis for age-related changes in fracture repair. J Orthop Res 23(6):1300–1307
13. Lu C, Hansen E, Sapozhnikova A, Hu D, Miclau T, Marcucio RS (2008) Effect of age on vascularization during fracture repair. J Orthop Res 26(10):1384–1389
14. Terao S, Sobue G, Hashizume Y, Shimada N, Mitsuma T (1994) Age-related changes of the myelinated fibers in the human corticospinal tract: a quantitative analysis. Acta Neuropathol 88(2):137–142
15. Terao S, Sobue G, Hashizume Y, Li M, Inagaki T, Mitsuma T (1996) Age-related changes in human spinal ventral horn cells with special reference to the loss of small neurons in the intermediate zone: a quantitative analysis. Acta Neuropathol 92(2):109–114
16. Furlan JC, Bracken MB, Fehlings MG (2010) Is age a key determinant of mortality and neurological outcome after acute traumatic spinal cord injury? Neurobiol Aging 31(3):434–446
17. Committee on Trauma, American College of Surgeons (2012). ATLS: Advanced Trauma Life Support Program for Doctors (9th ed.). Chicago. American College of Surgeons
18. Milzman DP, Boulanger BR, Rodriguez A, Soderstrom CA, Mitchell KA, Magnant CM (1992) Pre-existing disease in trauma patients: a predictor of fate independent of age and injury severity score. J Trauma 32(2):236–243; discussion 243–234
19. Stevens RD, Bhardwaj A, Kirsch JR, Mirski MA (2003) Critical care and perioperative management in traumatic spinal cord injury. J Neurosurg Anesthesiol 15(3):215–229
20. Bonhomme V, Hans P (2009) Management of the unstable cervical spine: elective versus emergent cases. Curr Opin Anaesthesiol 22(5):579–585
21. Martyn JA, Richtsfeld M (2006) Succinylcholine-induced hyperkalemia in acquired pathologic states: etiologic factors and molecular mechanisms. Anesthesiology 104(1):158–169
22. Aarabi B, Hadley MN, Dhall SS et al (2013) Management of acute traumatic central cord syndrome (ATCCS). Neurosurgery 72(Suppl 2):195–204
23. Bilello JF, Davis JW, Cunningham MA, Groom TF, Lemaster D, Sue LP (2003) Cervical spinal cord injury and the need for cardiovascular intervention. Arch Surg 138(10):1127–1129
24. Pasnoori VR, Leesar MA (2004) Use of aminophylline in the treatment of severe symptomatic bradycardia resistant to atropine. Cardiol Rev 12(2):65–68
25. Fehlings MG, Wilson JR, Cho N (2014) Methylprednisolone for the treatment of acute spinal cord injury: counterpoint. Neurosurgery 61(Suppl 1):36–42
26. Bracken MB, Shepard MJ, Holford TR et al (1997) Administration of methylprednisolone for 24 or 48 hours or tirilazad mesylate for 48 hours in the treatment of acute spinal cord injury. Results of the Third National Acute Spinal Cord Injury Randomized Controlled Trial. National Acute Spinal Cord Injury Study. JAMA 277(20):1597–1604
27. Kayal RA, Tsatsas D, Bauer MA et al (2007) Diminished bone formation during diabetic fracture healing is related to the premature resorption of cartilage associated with increased osteoclast activity. J Bone Miner Res 22(4):560–568
28. Maier GS, Seeger JB, Horas K, Roth KE, Kurth AA, Maus U (2015) The prevalence of vitamin D deficiency in patients with vertebral fragility fractures. Bone Joint J 97-b(1):89–93
29. Einhorn TA, Bonnarens F, Burstein AH (1986) The contributions of dietary protein and mineral to the healing of experimental fractures. A biomechanical study. J Bone Joint Surg Am 68(9):1389–1395

30. Ryan MD, Henderson JJ (1992) The epidemiology of fractures and fracture-dislocations of the cervical spine. Injury 23(1):38–40
31. Hanigan WC, Powell FC, Elwood PW, Henderson JP (1993) Odontoid fractures in elderly patients. J Neurosurg 78(1):32–35
32. Muller EJ, Wick M, Russe O, Muhr G (1999) Management of odontoid fractures in the elderly. Eur Spine J 8(5):360–365
33. Ryan MD, Taylor TK (1993) Odontoid fractures in the elderly. J Spinal Disord 6(5):397–401
34. Scheyerer MJ, Zimmermann SM, Simmen HP, Wanner GA, Werner CM (2013) Treatment modality in type II odontoid fractures defines the outcome in elderly patients. BMC Surg 13:54
35. Anderson LD, D'Alonzo RT (1974) Fractures of the odontoid process of the axis. J Bone Joint Surg Am 56(8):1663–1674
36. Chiba K, Fujimura Y, Toyama Y, Fujii E, Nakanishi T, Hirabayashi K (1996) Treatment protocol for fractures of the odontoid process. J Spinal Disord 9(4):267–276
37. Ryken TC, Hadley MN, Aarabi B et al (2013) Management of isolated fractures of the axis in adults. Neurosurgery 72(Suppl 2):132–150
38. Chapman J, Smith JS, Kopjar B et al (2013) The AOSpine North America Geriatric Odontoid Fracture Mortality Study: a retrospective review of mortality outcomes for operative versus nonoperative treatment of 322 patients with long-term follow-up. Spine 38(13):1098–1104
39. Smith JS, Kepler CK, Kopjar B et al (2013) Effect of type II odontoid fracture nonunion on outcome among elderly patients treated without surgery: based on the AOSpine North America geriatric odontoid fracture study. Spine (Phila Pa 1976) 38(26):2240–2246
40. Vaccaro AR, Kepler CK, Kopjar B et al (2013) Functional and quality-of-life outcomes in geriatric patients with type-II dens fracture. J Bone Joint Surg Am 95(8):729–735
41. Schroeder GD, Kepler CK, Kurd MF et al (2015) A systematic review of the treatment of geriatric type II odontoid fractures. Neurosurgery 77(Suppl 4):S6–S14
42. Osti M, Philipp H, Meusburger B, Benedetto KP (2011) Analysis of failure following anterior screw fixation of Type II odontoid fractures in geriatric patients. Eur Spine J 20(11):1915–1920
43. Nourbakhsh A, Shi R, Vannemreddy P, Nanda A (2009) Operative versus nonoperative management of acute odontoid Type II fractures: a meta-analysis. J Neurosurg Spine 11(6):651–658
44. Andersson S, Rodrigues M, Olerud C (2000) Odontoid fractures: high complication rate associated with anterior screw fixation in the elderly. Eur Spine J 9(1):56–59
45. Majercik S, Tashjian RZ, Biffl WL, Harrington DT, Cioffi WG (2005) Halo vest immobilization in the elderly: a death sentence? J Trauma 59(2):350–356; discussion 356–358
46. Lennarson PJ, Mostafavi H, Traynelis VC, Walters BC (2000) Management of type II dens fractures: a case–control study. Spine (Phila Pa 1976) 25(10):1234–1237
47. Joaquim AF, Patel AA (2015) Surgical treatment of Type II odontoid fractures: anterior odontoid screw fixation or posterior cervical instrumented fusion? Neurosurg Focus 38(4):E11
48. Koech F, Ackland HM, Varma DK, Williamson OD, Malham GM (2008) Nonoperative management of type II odontoid fractures in the elderly. Spine (Phila Pa 1976) 33(26):2881–2886
49. Woods BI, Hohl JB, Braly B, Donaldson W 3rd, Kang J, Lee JY (2014) Mortality in elderly patients following operative and nonoperative management of odontoid fractures. J Spinal Disord Tech 27(6):321–326
50. Fehlings MG, Arun R, Vaccaro AR, Arnold PM, Chapman JR, Kopjar B (2013) Predictors of treatment outcomes in geriatric patients with odontoid fractures: AOSpine North America multi-centre prospective GOF study. Spine (Phila Pa 1976) 38(11):881–886
51. Patel A, Smith HE, Radcliff K, Yadlapalli N, Vaccaro AR (2012) Odontoid fractures with neurologic deficit have higher mortality and morbidity. Clin Orthop Relat Res 470(6):1614–1620
52. Schneider RC, Cherry G, Pantek H (1954) The syndrome of acute central cervical spinal cord injury; with special reference to the mechanisms involved in hyperextension injuries of cervical spine. J Neurosurg 11(6):546–577
53. van Middendorp JJ, Hosman AJ, Pouw MH, Van de Meent H (2009) ASIA impairment scale conversion in traumatic SCI: is it related with the ability to walk? A descriptive comparison with functional ambulation outcome measures in 273 patients. Spinal Cord 47(7):555–560

54. Dahdaleh NS, Lawton CD, El Ahmadieh TY et al (2013) Evidence-based management of central cord syndrome. Neurosurg Focus 35(1):E6
55. Anderson KK, Tetreault L, Shamji MF et al (2015) Optimal timing of surgical decompression for acute traumatic central cord syndrome: a systematic review of the literature. Neurosurgery 77(Suppl 4):S15–S32
56. Bartels RH, Hosman AJ, van de Meent H et al (2013) Design of COSMIC: a randomized, multi-centre controlled trial comparing conservative or early surgical management of incomplete cervical cord syndrome without spinal instability. BMC Musculoskelet Disord 14:52
57. Roth EJ, Lawler MH, Yarkony GM (1990) Traumatic central cord syndrome: clinical features and functional outcomes. Arch Phys Med Rehabil 71(1):18–23
58. Penrod LE, Hegde SK, Ditunno JF Jr (1990) Age effect on prognosis for functional recovery in acute, traumatic central cord syndrome. Arch Phys Med Rehabil 71(12):963–968
59. Lenehan B, Street J, O'Toole P, Siddiqui A, Poynton A (2009) Central cord syndrome in Ireland: the effect of age on clinical outcome. Eur Spine J 18(10):1458–1463
60. Cifu DX, Seel RT, Kreutzer JS, McKinley WO (1999) A multicenter investigation of age-related differences in lengths of stay, hospitalization charges, and outcomes for a matched tetraplegia sample. Arch Phys Med Rehabil 80(7):733–740
61. Burge R, Dawson-Hughes B, Solomon DH, Wong JB, King A, Tosteson A (2007) Incidence and economic burden of osteoporosis-related fractures in the United States, 2005–2025. J Bone Miner Res 22(3):465–475
62. Alexandru D, So W (2012) Evaluation and management of vertebral compression fractures. Perm J 16(4):46–51
63. Albrand G, Munoz F, Sornay-Rendu E, DuBoeuf F, Delmas PD (2003) Independent predictors of all osteoporosis-related fractures in healthy postmenopausal women: the OFELY study. Bone 32(1):78–85
64. Kim HJ, Yi JM, Cho HG et al (2014) Comparative study of the treatment outcomes of osteoporotic compression fractures without neurologic injury using a rigid brace, a soft brace, and no brace: a prospective randomized controlled non-inferiority trial. J Bone Joint Surg Am 96(23):1959–1966
65. Eck JC, Nachtigall D, Humphreys SC, Hodges SD (2008) Comparison of vertebroplasty and balloon kyphoplasty for treatment of vertebral compression fractures: a meta-analysis of the literature. Spine J 8(3):488–497
66. Anderson PA, Froyshteter AB, Tontz WL Jr (2013) Meta-analysis of vertebral augmentation compared with conservative treatment for osteoporotic spinal fractures. J Bone Miner Res 28(2):372–382
67. Guo JB, Zhu Y, Chen BL et al (2015) Surgical versus non-surgical treatment for vertebral compression fracture with osteopenia: a systematic review and meta-analysis. PLoS One 10(5):e0127145
68. Goldstein CL, Chutkan NB, Choma TJ, Orr RD (2015) Management of the elderly with vertebral compression fractures. Neurosurgery 77(Suppl 4):S33–S45
69. Fassett DR, Harrop JS, Maltenfort M et al (2007) Mortality rates in geriatric patients with spinal cord injuries. J Neurosurg Spine 7(3):277–281
70. Hagen EM, Aarli JA, Gronning M (2005) The clinical significance of spinal cord injuries in patients older than 60 years of age. Acta Neurol Scand 112(1):42–47
71. Gulati A, Yeo CJ, Cooney AD, McLean AN, Fraser MH, Allan DB (2011) Functional outcome and discharge destination in elderly patients with spinal cord injuries. Spinal Cord 49(2):215–218
72. Furlan JC, Fehlings MG (2009) The impact of age on mortality, impairment, and disability among adults with acute traumatic spinal cord injury. J Neurotrauma 26(10):1707–1717
73. Seel RT, Huang ME, Cifu DX, Kolakowsky-Hayner SA, McKinley WO (2001) Age-related differences in length of stays, hospitalization costs, and outcomes for an injury-matched sample of adults with paraplegia. J Spinal Cord Med 24(4):241–250
74. Werhagen L, Budh CN, Hultling C, Molander C (2004) Neuropathic pain after traumatic spinal cord injury--relations to gender, spinal level, completeness, and age at the time of injury. Spinal Cord 42(12):665–673

75. Aito S, D'Andrea M, Werhagen L et al (2007) Neurological and functional outcome in traumatic central cord syndrome. Spinal Cord 45(4):292–297
76. DeVivo MJ, Kartus PL, Rutt RD, Stover SL, Fine PR (1990) The influence of age at time of spinal cord injury on rehabilitation outcome. Arch Neurol 47(6):687–691
77. New PW, Epi MC (2007) Influence of age and gender on rehabilitation outcomes in nontraumatic spinal cord injury. J Spinal Cord Med 30(3):225–237
78. Golob JF Jr, Claridge JA, Yowler CJ, Como JJ, Peerless JR (2008) Isolated cervical spine fractures in the elderly: a deadly injury. J Trauma 64(2):311–315
79. Harris MB, Reichmann WM, Bono CM et al (2010) Mortality in elderly patients after cervical spine fractures. J Bone Joint Surg Am 92(3):567–574
80. Barrett JJ, Putzke JD, Richards JS (2002) Early versus late onset of spinal cord injury among the elderly. J Clin Psychol Med 9(3):219–226

Extradural Vertebral Tumors in the Elderly

15

Ryan J. Filler, Timothy T. Roberts, and Edward C. Benzel

15.1 Introduction

Extramedullary, extradural spinal tumors present with relative frequency in the elderly, the vast majority of which are attributable to metastatic disease. Primary bony lesions such as plasmacytoma, multiple myeloma, chordoma, and chondrosarcoma are also known to disproportionately afflict the elderly spine. Benign lesions such as hemangiomas, enchondromas, bone islands, and bone infarcts are also relatively common, as are insufficiency fractures, infectious and inflammatory processes, and metabolic sequelae that can mimic tumorous disease.

This chapter reviews the most frequent causes of extradural spinal tumors in the elderly. In addition to a discussion of the most common metastatic, primary benign, and primary malignant spinal lesions, the essential principles of diagnosis, workup, and both nonoperative and operative management are considered.

R.J. Filler
Albany Medical College, Albany, NY, USA

T.T. Roberts
Department of Neurosurgery, Center for Spine Health, Neurological Institute, Cleveland Clinic, Cleveland, OH, USA

E.C. Benzel, MD (✉)
Department of Neurosurgery, Center for Spine Health, Neurological Institute, Cleveland Clinic, Cleveland, OH, USA

Cleveland Clinic, Department of Neurological Surgery, Center for Spine Health, 9500 Euclid Ave S40, Cleveland, OH 44195, USA
e-mail: benzele@ccf.org

© Springer International Publishing Switzerland 2017

M. Berhouma, P. Krolak-Salmon (eds.), *Brain and Spine Surgery in the Elderly*,
DOI 10.1007/978-3-319-40232-1_15

15.2 Metastatic Spinal Tumors

15.2.1 Epidemiology

There are 1.2 million new cases of metastatic disease in the USA annually. Symptomatic spinal metastases are present in 10–30 % of these cases and are the presenting symptom of malignant disease in 12–20 % of cases [1, 2]. The spine is the third most common site of metastases in the body, following the liver and lungs. It is the most common skeletal location for metastatic disease.

The most common lesions to metastasize to the spine are breast, prostate, lung, renal cell, and thyroid cancers. Each of these are discussed individually below. The incidence of spinal metastases has been slowly increasing, likely due to the improved survival of cancer patients and possibly due to advancements in diagnostic technologies. Spinal metastases are present in approximately 30 % of autopsied cancer patients [3]. Overall, 68–70 % of spinal metastases manifest within the thoracic spine, 16–22 % in the lumbosacral spine, and 8–15 % in the cervical spine [4].

15.2.2 Breast Cancer

Worldwide, breast cancer is the most commonly diagnosed malignancy, with over a million cases annually and the leading cause of female cancer death. In the USA, it is the most diagnosed cancer in females and the second leading cause of female cancer death with over 230,000 diagnoses annually and over 40,000 deaths, though mortality rates have declined since the 1970s [5, 7, 8]. North America, Australia/New Zealand, and western and northern Europe have a higher incidence of breast cancer than Asia and sub-Saharan Africa [6].

Breast cancer reportedly metastasizes to the spine in 16–37 % of cases [9]. In one study, upon autopsy, 70–90 % of patients with breast cancer had bone metastases present [10, 11].

Breast cancer can be classified with respect to expression of estrogen receptor (ER), progesterone receptor (PR), and overexpression and/or amplification of human epidermal growth factor-2 receptor (HER2). Receptor status is generally considered to have some prognostic value. ER-negative cancers appear to have higher recurrence rates in the first 5 years as compared to ER-positive cancers [12]; however beyond 5 years, the recurrence rate for ER-negative cancers is approximately zero, while the recurrence rate for ER-positive cancers remains at approximately 0.5–2 %. HER2 overexpression is typically unfavorable; however its value as a prognostic indicator is greatly dependent on treatment options [13, 14].

15.2.3 Prostate Cancer

Globally, prostate cancer is the second most diagnosed cancer in males, with over a million cases and over 300,000 deaths in 2012 [15]. In 2016, it is estimated that there will be over 180,000 cases and over 26,000 deaths in the USA [5]. An American male has a 16 % chance of developing prostate cancer over the course of his lifetime but only a 2.9 % chance of dying from prostate cancer. There is a higher incidence among blacks than among whites in the USA [16]. Most cases of prostate cancer never become clinically significant; upon autopsy prostate cancer is present in 30 % of 55-year-old men and approximately 60 % of 80-year-old men [17]. Clinically, prostate cancer can range from small benign, well-differentiated tumors to highly aggressive fatal tumors. Prognosis is highly dependent on the extent of the tumor at diagnosis; patients with localized tumors have a 5-year relative survival rate of 100 %, whereas for patients with distant metastases the rate is 31.9 % [16].

The lumbosacral spine is the primary site of metastasis in prostate cancer, receiving 9–15 % of metastases [9]. Prostate metastases are classically osteoblastic (bone forming); however they are also accompanied by increases in the rate of bone resorption [18, 19].

15.2.4 Lung Cancer

In 2012, lung cancer affected 1.8 million people globally and resulted in 1.6 million deaths [20]. In the USA, lung cancer affects 225,000 patients and causes more than 160,000 deaths annually [5]. By 1985, lung cancer was the leading cause of cancer death in men and women. Though mortality rates have declined in recent years, due to a decrease in smoking [21], over 90 % of all lung cancers are due to cigarette smoking, making it the primary risk factor for developing lung cancer [22]. Lung cancer represents approximately 12–15 % of metastatic spinal disease [9].

The terms lung cancer and bronchogenic carcinoma describe malignancies that develop in the airways or pulmonary parenchyma. Small cell lung cancer (SCLC) or non-small cell lung cancer (NSCLC) makes up approximately 95 % of all lung cancer cases. Lung cancer metastases in bone are often accompanied by symptoms such as back pain, chest pain, and/or pain in the extremities. About 20 % of NSCLC patients and 30–40 % of SCLC patients have bone metastases [23]. They are more commonly osteolytic than osteoblastic [24]. Figure 15.1 depicts metastatic lung cancer in a 60-year-old male with an extensive tobacco use history. The patient first presented with acute left-sided upper and lower extremity weakness, due to tumorous spinal cord compression at around the C7 level.

15.2.5 Renal Cell Cancer

Renal cell carcinoma (RCC) accounts for 80–85 % of primary kidney cancer. Renal cell carcinoma is the most common cancer of the kidneys and occurs in the renal cortex. Transitional cell carcinomas, occurring in the renal pelvis, account for another 8 %, while other parenchymal tumors like collecting duct tumors, renal sarcomas, and oncocytomas are uncommon.

The incidence of renal cell carcinoma varies throughout the world with the highest recorded rates in the Czech Republic and North America [25, 26]. In the USA,

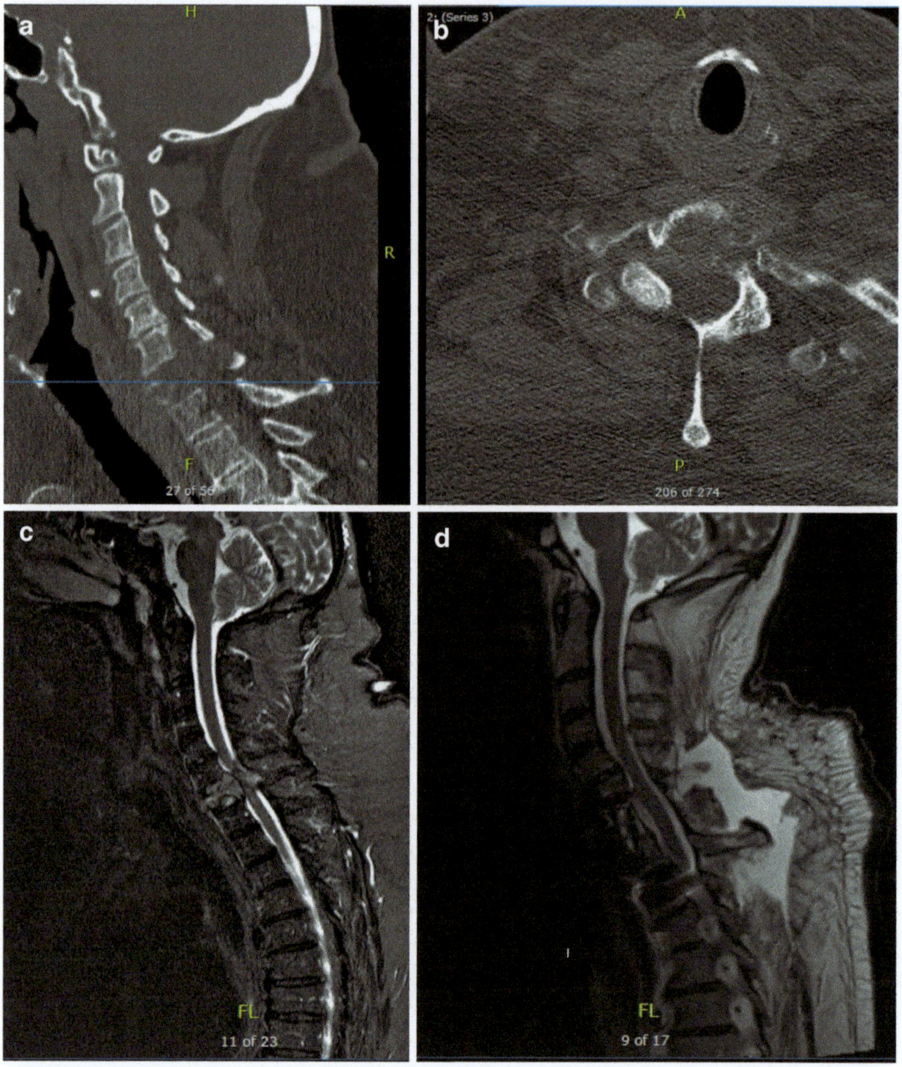

Fig. 15.1 Sagittal (**a**) and axial (**b**) CT images of a 60-year-old male with metastatic non-small cell lung cancer. There is extensive tumorous erosion of the C7 vertebral body, with fracture instability of the cervical spine and compression of the spinal cord, best seen on the sagittal STIR MRI (**c**). The patient underwent staged C7 anterior corpectomy, C6–T1 cage placement, and instrumented fusion, followed by a posterior C7 laminectomy with C5–T3 instrumentation 5 days later. An MRI obtained shortly postoperatively (**d**) demonstrates the spinal cord decompression as well as postoperative seroma formation which spontaneously resolved

there are 63,000 new diagnoses and nearly 14,000 deaths annually from RCC [5]. It affects men twice as commonly as women and, in the USA, is less prevalent in Asian Americans and Pacific Islanders compared with American Indians, Hispanics, Whites, and African Americans [28, 32]. RCC primarily affects older individuals, typically those between the ages of 60 and 80, with a median diagnosis age of 64; it is uncommon in patients below 40 years of age [29–31].

Because RCC can remain asymptomatic for long periods, approximately a quarter of patients diagnosed with RCC already have distant metastases and/or advanced regional cancer [27]. Stage at diagnosis is an important prognostic factor; one study showed that RCC patients whose cancer was detected incidentally, prior to the onset of symptoms, had significantly better 5-year survival rates compared to patients whose RCC symptomatic at diagnosis [33].

Patients with recurrent RCC have been observed to have bone metastases in 16–31 % of cases [34, 35]. Rates of spinal metastases have been estimated at 3–6 % [9]. Renal cell carcinomas also have one of the highest recurrence rates of 40–50 % following resection [9].

15.2.6 Thyroid Cancer

The American Cancer Society estimates that in 2015, about 62,000 new cases of thyroid cancer will be diagnosed (47,000 in women and 15,000 in men) and that approximately 2000 patients will die from thyroid cancer. Thyroid cancer tends to affect younger people compared to other types of cancer; roughly two-thirds of cases are diagnosed in individuals under 55 years of age [21, 36, 37]. Thyroid follicular epithelial-derived cancers can generally be classified into three types: papillary, follicular, and anaplastic. Papillary- and follicular-type cancers are considered differentiated, whereas anaplastic cancer is undifferentiated and is thought to arise from differentiated types [38, 39].

Papillary thyroid cancer has a lower mortality rate than follicular type cancer which is typically more aggressive, has more distant metastases, and affects older patients than papillary type cancer. Important prognostic factors are size of the primary tumor, presence of metastases, age at diagnosis, and sex, women typically having a better prognosis [40, 41].

Thyroid cancers metastasize to the spine, forming lytic lesions, approximately 4 % of the time [9, 40]. In one study of 887 thyroid carcinoma patients at a single institution, 5 % of patients had bone metastases with 52 % of these lesions occurring in the vertebrae. In this series, the male to female ratio was 1:3, multiple bone lesions were more common than single bone lesions (57 % and 43 % respectively), and the prevalence of bone metastases was higher in follicular-type thyroid carcinoma (14.5 %) than in papillary type (2.7 %) [42]. A different study found that over 80 % of bone metastases from differentiated thyroid tumors (follicular and papillary type) occur in the red marrow of the axial skeleton [43].

15.2.7 Other Metastatic Diseases and Prognostic Factors

Essentially any malignant lesion can metastasize to the spine. Other types of tumors observed to metastasize to vertebrae include various gastrointestinal tumors including pancreatic and hepatocellular carcinoma, as well as melanoma, and urinary tract/bladder cancers. The histopathology and tumor grade have substantial prognostic implications. Generally speaking, GI and lung (both small cell and non-small cell) carry extremely poor prognoses, while breast, prostate, and most thyroid cancers carry relatively favorable prognoses. The presence of visceral metastases in addition to vertebral metastatic disease is an extremely poor prognostic factor with one study demonstrating 23.5 months survival without visceral disease versus 5.8 months for concomitant visceral metastases [44]. Advanced age (>60 years), neurological deficits, electrolyte abnormalities such as hypercalcemia, number of affected vertebrae, as well as the location of lesions in the upper cervical spine have also been identified as poor prognostic factors [45].

15.3 Primary Spinal Benign Tumors

15.3.1 Hemangioma

Hemangiomas are vascular intraosseous lesions. While they classically remain contained within the cancellous vertebral bodies, extraosseous extension has been observed. Hemangiomas are most common found in the thoracic and lumbar spine and are thought to be present in up to 10 % of all people [46]. Hemangiomas are typically asymptomatic and are often found incidentally when imaging patients for other reasons. Symptomatic lesions occur in 1 % of patients or fewer. When lesions are symptomatic, patients may present with back pain or neurological deficits; pathologic fractures, spontaneous epidural bleeding, and spinal stenosis have been reported. Aggressive hemangiomas have potential to compress the spinal cord and/or spinal roots. Lesions detected incidentally may not produce symptoms for years but can become painful after a time in some patients. Lesions requiring intervention at the time of diagnosis have reported recurrence rates of approximately 29 % within 2 years [46].

15.3.2 Aneurysmal Bone Cyst

Aneurysmal bone cysts (ABCs) are blood-filled cavities comprising 1.4 % of all primary bone tumors and 15 % of all primary spine tumors [47]. Most ABCs occur in patients between the ages of 10 and 20 years but can present throughout life. Females have a slightly greater prevalence [48]. Most ABCs occur in the posterior spinal elements of the thoracic and lumbar spine. In 30–40 % of cases, multiple contiguous vertebrae are affected [49]. In most cases, pain develops slowly and gradually in the affected area, and upon presentation a spinal mass or deformity may be palpable. While ABCs are often slow growing and are benign, they do not resolve spontaneously. Surgical intervention is often the preferred treatment option [47]. Patients with neurological deficits may benefit from decompression. Recurrence rates depend on the completeness of resection; intralesional resection techniques can have recurrence rates of up to 30 %, whereas complete marginal resection has a recurrence rate of approximately 10 %; given their proximity to spinal elements and other critical structures, however, marginal resection is not always possible [49].

15.3.3 Giant Cell Tumor

Giant cell tumors (GCT) comprise 5–8 % of primary bone tumors, though only 2–5 % of these occur in the spine [50]. GCTs occur in males and females equally and affect the vertebral bodies of cervical, thoracic, and lumbar divisions with similar frequency [51]. GCT lesions are typically detected in patients 20–50 years of age, which is relatively late for most primary bone tumors. GTCs may grow aggressively, complicating management. The most common presentation is back pain with possible radicular pain. They are usually diagnosed at an advanced state and can cause spinal cord compression and associated symptoms. In one study of 24 patients with spinal GCT, all had back pain and half had neurological deficits [51]. En bloc excision with wide margins is recommended for thoracic and lumbar tumors [51, 52], whereas embolization may be preferable for sacral lesions [53]. Rates of local recurrence for en bloc excision are relatively high, at approximately 25 % [52]. Incomplete resections produce recurrence rates of 25–50 % [51, 54]. Despite the fact that tumors are technically benign, GTCs have been known to metastasize to the lungs. In peripheral bony lesions, this occurs in 1–2 % of patients; however, lung metastatic rates from spinal involvement may occur in up to 13 % of patients [55].

15.3.4 Osteoid Osteoma and Osteoblastoma

Osteoid osteoma and osteoblastoma are small, bone-forming tumors that most commonly affect children. These benign lesions share identical osteoblastic bone-forming histology and are differentiated based on size: 15–20 mm diameter for osteoid osteoma and greater than 20 mm for osteoblastoma. Both lesions classically cause night "aching" pain associated with prostaglandin production. For this reason, symptoms may respond exquisitely to oral NSAID administration.

Osteoid osteoma comprise approximately 10 % of primary bone tumors [56, 57], with over 50 % of them occurring in the long leg bones. Approximately 10 % of lesions occur in the spine. Osteoid osteoma and osteoblastoma are peculiar in that they have a strong predilection for appearing within the posterior elements, including the pedicles, laminae, pars, and spinous processes [56]. Patients typically present with back pain which can be present for years before presentation and is classically worse at night [56]. The average patient age is 19 years, and >80 % of cases are detected prior to 30 years of age. Osteoid osteomas affect males more frequently and are the most common cause of painful scoliosis in young people [58]. Typically, they do not produce neurological symptoms.

Osteoblastoma is a bone-forming tumor related to osteoid osteoma, but they tend to be larger and more aggressive. Highly uncommon, they comprise 1–5 % of primary bone tumors, with 28–36 % being in the spine [59]. Spinal osteoblastoma typically occurs in the posterior elements of the vertebrae, but growth into the vertebral body is seen in larger tumors. They are more prevalent in the lumbar spine [59]. The average age at diagnosis is between 20 and 24 years of age, though it has been reported in patients age 1–72 years [56]. The ratio of affected males to females is 2:1. Neurological deficits are reported in 32 % of spinal osteoblastoma patients [60], and 10–15 % of patients may have an associated aneurysmal bone cyst (ABC) [56]. Prognosis depends on completeness of resection; recurrence ranges between 10 and 24 % [59]. Complications due to spinal cord necrosis, spinal cord compression, and malignant conversion to sarcoma (rare) are known to occur [61].

15.3.5 Chondroblastoma

Chondroblastoma is a benign cartilage-forming tumor that develops in the epiphysis of growing bones [62–64]. Chondroblastoma accounts for 5 % of benign bone tumors and 1–2 % of all primary bone tumors [65–67]. Like its bone-forming relative, osteoblastoma, chondroblastoma is chiefly a disease of young people with an average age at diagnosis of less than 20 years. Reported age of presentation ranges from 2 to 73 years [68–70, 72, 73]. Males are approximately twice as likely as females to develop chondroblastoma [65, 66, 68–71]. Chondroblastoma are exceptionally rare in the spine, comprising only 0.5–1 % of all cases [74]. One study, examining chondroblastoma of the spine specifically, found only 20 reported cases in the literature [74]. In these cases, chondroblastoma was encountered more frequently in cervical and thoracic spine than in lumbar and sacral spine. The vertebral body and posterior elements were affected in most patients, and the tumor had invaded the spinal canal in approximately two-thirds of patients. Males were 2–3 times more likely to be affected than females, and the average age at diagnosis was about 29 years, with a range of 5–62 years [74]. Chondroblastoma of the spine in elderly patients (65 years and older) is extremely rare.

15.4 Primary Spinal Malignant Tumors

15.4.1 Osteosarcoma

Osteogenic sarcoma or osteosarcomas are primary malignant tumors of malignant osteoid-producing cells [75–77]. While osteosarcoma typically affects children and young adults, they can occur in older populations. In the elderly, especially, osteosarcomas are frequently regarded as secondary tumors caused by the sarcomatous transformation of irradiated tissues or in patients with Paget's disease. Secondary transformation has also been known to occur in patient with fibrous dysplasia, enchondromatosis, bone infarcts, and other bone lesions [78]. Osteosarcoma arising in adults is more likely to affect the spine, as opposed to osteosarcoma in children. Males are more likely to be affected than females, as are Caucasians compared to other races [78]. In the USA, the majority of osteosarcomas affecting patients over the age of 60 are of secondary origin [79]. Compared to primary osteosarcomas, secondary osteosarcomas have poor prognoses, with a 5-year disease-free survival rate of 17 % [79–81].

15.4.2 Chondrosarcoma

Chondrosarcomas are a diverse group of malignant bone tumors characterized by their production of chondroid (cartilaginous) matrix [82]. Chondrosarcoma represent 20–27 % of primary malignant bony tumors and are the third most common primary malignant bone tumor after myeloma and osteosarcoma [83, 84]. Approximately 30 % of chondrosarcomas occur in the axial skeleton [86]. Compared to many bone tumors, chondrosarcomas typically affect the elderly, with a median patient age of 51 years [87]. There is also a slight male predominance [87].

The natural history of chondrosarcoma varies significantly with the grade of the lesion. Ninety percent of chondrosarcoma are considered conventional, and 90 % of these are classified as low-to-intermediate grade [85]. While conventional, low-grade chondrosarcomas have slow growth and limited metastatic potential, these tumors typically do not respond well to radiation or chemotherapy. High-grade chondrosarcomas, which account for the other 5–10 % of conventional chondrosarcoma as well as some of the non-conventional rarer forms, possess high metastatic potential and substantially poorer prognoses following resection alone [85]. Chemotherapy and radiation therapy have demonstrated efficacy against some of these rarer aggressive tumors.

15.4.3 Chordoma

Chordomas are rare primary bone tumors arising from primitive notochord remnants of the axial skeleton. Embryonically, the notochord develops into the intervertebral disk material. Therefore, these lesions only appear midline along the axial skeleton in the skull and spine. Approximately 35 % of chordomas arise in the skull base, 50 % in the sacrum, 5 % in the cervical spine, and 10 % in the thoracic and lumbar spine. Chordomas account for 1–4 % of primary osseous tumors and have an incidence of less than 0.1 per 100,000 people per year. Like chondrosarcoma, they disproportionally affect older individuals. In one study the median age at diagnosis was 62 [91], and there is a slight male predominance. Chordomas are characterized as exhibiting slow but aggressive local growth, a relatively low to late metastatic potential, and a high frequency of recurrence [88–90, 92, 93]. Metastases, when present, often occur in soft tissue, lymph nodes, liver, bone, lung, and skin and are reported to occur in 40–60 % of patients over the course of their illness [95–98]. Because chordomas are derived from ectodermal tissue, they are not technically considered true sarcomas, even though they are often clinically classified as such since they are primary osseous tumors [94].

15.4.4 Multiple Myeloma

Multiple myeloma is a lesion cause by the neoplastic proliferation of plasma cells that produce excessive amounts of monoclonal immunoglobulin. This hypercellular proliferation in the bone marrow often results in bony destruction, characterized by radiographic osteolytic "punched-out" lesions, pathologic fractures, and neurological compression.

In the USA, multiple myeloma represents 1 % of all cancers and over 10 % of blood cancers [5]. It has an incidence of about four to five cases per 100,000 inhabitants, which is similar to Europe [99–101]. Prevalence depends in part on ethnicity; people of African descent are two to three times more likely to be affected than whites, while people of Japanese and Mexican decent are less likely that Caucasians to be affected. Males are 1.4 times more likely than females to develop the cancer [102–105]. Multiple myeloma is most common in older adults with a median age at diagnosis of 66 years. Less than 10 % of patients are younger than 50 years at the time of diagnosis [102, 106]. There is a familial component to multiple myeloma; the relative risk of developing the disease is 3.7 times higher for an individual if a first-degree relative is affected [107].

In the spine, multiple myeloma can cause compression of the spinal cord and/or spinal roots most commonly due to the formation of an extramedullary plasmacytoma or due to structural changes resulting from pathologic fractures of vertebral bodies. These symptoms occur in approximately 5 % of multiple myeloma patients.

15.4.5 Lymphoma

Primary non-Hodgkin lymphoma of bone (PLB) is a rare disease that usually presents as one or more destructive bone lesions. It represents less than 2 % of lymphomas in adults [108], 3–7 % of primary bone tumors [109, 110], and 3–5 % of extranodal non-Hodgkin lymphomas [111, 112]. PLB predominantly affects older adults; 92 % of PLB patients are over 30 years of age and 56 % are over 60 years [113, 115]. Males are affected 1.2–1.8 times more frequently than females [113–116]. The axial skeleton is affected in 63 % of cases as compared to the appendicular skeleton which is affected in 37 % of cases [113]. Five-year survival rates are generally above 70 % with use of multi-agent chemotherapy [116–121].

15.5 Tumorlike Conditions of the Spine

15.5.1 Fibrous Dysplasia

Fibrous dysplasia (FD) is a benign developmental disorder of bone characterized by the replacement of mature lamellar cancellous bone with immature fibro-osseous tissue [123]. This results in regions of poorly formed trabeculae that are weak and prone to fracture. FD represents 7 % of benign osseous tumors. While the disease typically affects young people, it can present throughout life. Males and females are equally affected [122, 123]. There is a monostotic form of fibrous dysplasia, which affects typically one region of a single bone, and a polyostotic form, which can affect multiple regions of multiple bones. The monostotic form accounts for 75–80 % of FD cases [124]. The polyostotic form may be associated with other cutaneous and/or endocrine disorders, such as McCune-Albright syndrome [125, 126].

Fibrous dysplasia in the spine is uncommon, especially in the monostotic form [126–128, 130]. One study of individuals with McCune-Albright syndrome) found that 7 % of patients had fibrous lesions in the cervical spine and 14 % in the lumbar spine [131]. A different study of patients with polyostotic fibrous dysplasia, ranging from 4 to 80 years (average age 25 years), found that 63 % of patients had spinal involvement. Most of the lesions occurred in the posterior elements of the spine, most commonly in the thoracolumbar vertebrae and less commonly in the cervical and sacral divisions [129]. There have been reported cases of patients who have had malignant transformation of fibrous dysplastic spinal lesions [127, 132].

15.5.2 Paget's Disease

Paget's disease of bone, formerly known as osteitis deformans, produces single (monostotic) or multiple (polyostotic) areas of overgrown bone that is brittle and hypervascularized, caused by excessive, disordered bone remodeling. Many patients are asymptomatic, and diagnosis is frequently made incidentally, often through findings of elevated alkaline phosphatase or through unrelated radiographic studies. Paget's disease of bone is relatively common in older individuals of affected populations, with an estimated prevalence between 2.3 and 9 % and a slightly greater preponderance among males [132, 133]. According to autopsy studies, approximately 3–4 % of people over 50 years of age show evidence of Paget's disease. Affected populations occur commonly in England, Scotland, Central Europe, Greece, and regions settled by immigrants from those areas [132, 134–138]. Paget's disease is uncommon in individuals from Scandinavia and Asia [132, 139–142]. Secondary osteosarcoma may develop in pagetic bone in an estimated 0.2–1 % of patients. Secondary osteosarcoma from Paget's is notoriously aggressive and often fatal [143–147]. The spine is considered the second most common location of Paget's disease [148–154]. Typically, pagetic spine lesions are part of the polyostotic form of the disease; monostotic Paget's disease rarely affects the spine [155]. In a study of patients with Paget's disease in the spine, it was found that 62 % of patients had lesions of the lumbar spine and 8.2 % had cervical lesions, with half of those cases affecting the second vertebral body (C2) [156].

15.5.3 Infectious Diseases of the Spine

Vertebral osteomyelitis typically refers to a bacterial infection of the vertebral body, whereas discitis refers to an infection of the intervertebral disk material. These two terms are frequently used interchangeably, as most infections encountered in the clinical setting involve both the disk space and the surrounding bony structures. A less commonly employed term, pyogenic spondylitis, more accurately describes both processes.

Vertebral bodies typically become infected via hematogenous spread of bacteria, and less commonly fungi or other pathogens, from a distant source [161]. Alternately, vertebral osteomyelitis may occur due to iatrogenic introduction of infectious agents through surgery and injection or from nearby soft tissue infection [157]. The intervertebral disk space adjacent to the infected vertebral body often becomes infected. The intervertebral disk is considered one of the most avascular structures in the human body and is therefore especially susceptible to bacterial growth and growth of other organisms.

Vertebral osteomyelitis is a relatively common disease that affects older adults, typically over 50 years. It becomes more prevalent with increasing age [158, 162]. Males are affected about twice as frequently as females. Two studies investigating the incidence of vertebral osteomyelitis reported rates of 1:250,000 and 1:450,000 [159, 160]. Risk factors include bacterial endocarditis, intravenous drug abuse, immunodeficiency, and diabetes. Degenerative spine disease may also increase one's risk; however its association may just be coincidental with increasing age. Vertebral osteomyelitis may arise as a complication of translumbar aortography, discography, chemonucleolysis, epidural catheter placement, lumbar puncture, myelography, and epidural and facet joint injections [163, 164].

Spinal tuberculosis (TB), also known as Pott's disease, is classically manifest by osteolytic, caseating thoracolumbar vertebral body lesions that result in anterior wedging or collapse into a focal kyphosis. Substantial improvements in antibiotics and stabilization techniques have drastically decreased the incidence and morbidity of Pott's disease in Western nations. However, the disease remains prevalent in many developing regions where drug-resistant TB is major and ongoing epidemic. Elderly patients, especially those from developing nations, may have sequelae of skeletal TB.

15.5.4 Brown Tumor

Osteitis fibrosa cystica (OFC), also referred to as a "brown tumor," is a rare consequence of severe, untreated primary or secondary hyperparathyroidism. Females are more commonly affected than males, with symptoms most often manifesting the fifth and sixth decades of life. Radiographically, tumors appear as well-demarcated osteolytic lesions. On gross inspection, lesions have a characteristic fibrous dark brown appearance owing to their high hemosiderin content [168]. Lesions may resolve when the underlying metabolic defect is corrected.

15.5.5 Eosinophilic Granuloma

Eosinophilic granulomas (EG) are benign lesions of bone that affect approximately five to six per million individuals annually in the USA. While EG is primarily encountered in pediatric patients, the disease can be encountered in adulthood. EG are the most benign and most common manifestation of the spectrum of diseases known as Langerhans cell histiocytosis (LCH), formerly known as histiocytosis X. This broad range of multisystem conditions can range in severity form being completely benign to being fatal in infancy. The range of often bizarre-presenting symptoms (exophthalmos, skin lesions, pituitary dysfunction, bony lesions) is caused by tumorous growths with identical histological features [165].

Adult patients with LCH lesions of the spine most frequently present with localized neck and/or back pain and stiffness. In children, vertebra plana, or the "pancake"-like flattening of the vertebral body, may be pathognomonic presentation of LCH; however, vertebra plana from EG is seldom seen in adults [165]. Over 50 % of all bony EG lesions occur in the spine. The vertebral bodies of thoracic spine are most commonly affected, followed by the lumbar and then cervical spines. Neurological involvement has been found to occur in as many as two-thirds of adult EG patients [165].

15.6 Diagnosis of Spinal Lesions

15.6.1 History

A detailed and thorough medical history is essential to evaluating elderly patients with back- or neck-related complaints. Axial back or neck pain is the most common presenting complaint of patients with spinal metastases (85–96 % of patients) [166]. Axial pain due to metastases is often difficult to distinguish from pain due to other causes, though progressive, nonmechanical, unrelenting night pain frequently characterizes metastatic disease in the spine. However, mechanical pain should not rule out a diagnosis of metastatic disease. Pain may develop without any apparent causal event or following a minor trauma and is likely due to stimulation of nociceptors and/or mechanical compromise of vertebrae, including fracture.

Providers must carefully characterize the pain, identifying its location, severity, duration, periodicity, and identify alleviating and exacerbating factors. A common complaint of patients with tumorous lesions is radicular pain related to spinal root or spinal cord compression. Neurological symptoms classically develop after the onset of axial pain.

"Red flag" symptoms should be carefully and specifically assessed, including the presence of constitutional symptoms including recent, unintended weight loss, night pain, night sweats, or unexplained general malaise.

Next, carefully and thorough past medical and surgical history should be acquired. Most importantly, does the patient have a history of malignancy, including treatments for skin lesions? Metastatic lesions may be asymptomatic and are frequently detected incidentally from imaging studies of the patient's primary malignancy [167]. Providers should assess whether patient with known cancer histories received treatments such as radiation, chemotherapy, or other medical or surgical procedures. Risk factors for malignancy should also be assessed, including history of tobacco use, alcohol consumption, family history of cancer, and occupational exposures.

15.6.2 Physical Exam

Physical examination of the spine should include inspection, range of motion, regions of tenderness (especially over bony as opposed to muscular prominences), and deformity. Gait analysis should be performed. Bilateral upper and lower extremities should be assessed for strength, sensation, and reflexes. Neurological defects from root compression may result in focal weakness, sensory loss, and/or blunted reflexes. Spinal cord compression can result in myelopathy, including sensory disturbances, imbalance, loss of fine motor control, hyperreflexia, loss of bowel and bladder control, and weakness.

When metastatic disease is known or suspected, a thorough examination of possible primary sites such as the thyroid, abdomen, rectum, prostate, and breasts should be performed. Multidisciplinary assessment is often necessary to confidently rule out malignancy.

For patients with a single osseous lesion and without any known primary malignancy, primary bone tumors should be considered in the differential diagnosis [167]. Spine providers should not neglect other skeletal areas typically associated with metastatic disease, including, but not limited to, the proximal humerus, hip, distal femur, and proximal tibia. Accompanying pain in these regions should be carefully evaluated for metastatic disease.

15.6.3 Imaging

Plain radiographs are often the starting point for identifying lesions. Although advanced imaging modalities are often employed, much diagnostic information can be gleaned from a simple AP and lateral radiograph series. Aside from identifying the size and location of a lesion, radiographs can determine if a lesion is blastic (radiodense) or lytic (radiolucent). Several types of lesions have characteristic appearances on plain radiographs and may confidently be diagnosed with mere orthogonal plain films. Other lesions require additional advanced imaging such as MRI and CT to narrow the differential diagnosis, as well as for staging, biopsy planning, and operative planning purposed.

Several characteristics on both plain film and CT are suggestive of aggressive, malignancy. Poorly demarcated, large, lytic lesions with cortical involvement, without surrounding blastic rims are all suggestive of a quickly expanding, aggressive lesion. In elderly patients, such processes should be presumed malignant and likely metastatic until proven otherwise. If a solitary, concerning spinal lesion is found, workup generally involved an MRI with IV contrast of the entire spine; a CT with IV and PO contrast of the chest, abdomen, and pelvis; and a whole-body bone scan. Standing radiographs of the entire spine may be helpful in assessing mechanical stability.

15.6.4 Laboratory Studies

When a tumor is identified, laboratory studies may help differentiate the diagnosis. At a minimum, a complete blood cell count with differential and smear, a complete metabolic panel including calcium (including ionized), erythrocyte sedimentation rate, C-reactive protein, alkaline phosphatase (including bone specific), as well as prostate-specific antigen (PSA) (when applicable) should be obtained. Hypercalcemia can result when there is extensive bony lysis. Inflammatory markers are typically nonspecific but can be elevated with certain tumors (multiple myeloma) as well as inflammatory and infectious processes. Amylase and lipase may be elevated in certain GI tumors, as can PSA in prostate cancer.

15.6.5 Biopsy

Generally speaking, a biopsy must be obtained whenever a benign diagnosis is less than certain and almost always prior to invasive or highly morbid treatments, such as radiation or chemotherapy. If there is a known primary cancer with obvious metastatic disease, biopsy is not always necessary; however, the appearance of a spinal lesion in a patient with a distant history of a breast lumpectomy or similarly equivocal lesion, for example, should always be worked up as if it were a new primary lesion.

Biopsy of the vertebrae is often difficult, given its relative anatomic depth and the multitude of surrounding vulnerable and essential structures. Fine needle biopsy is rarely sufficient for tissue diagnosis and is not recommended for bony tumors. At a minimum, core needle biopsy or incisional biopsy is necessary for tissue diagnosis. When primary malignancy is suspected, special attention should be paid to the location of the biopsy tract, as such tracts will also need to be excised whenever feasible.

In patients with multiple spinal lesions, metastatic disease is the most likely etiology. In such cases, the most superficial and readily accessible tissue should be considered for biopsy. When incisional biopsy is performed, intraoperative frozen sectioning can be of great utility as pathologists can offer real-time insight into the histological nature of the lesion. This allows providers to make intraoperative decisions about whether they want to proceed with excision, perform a debulking, or even close and offer adjuvant treatments such as neoadjuvant chemotherapy or radiation.

15.6.6 Differential Diagnoses

In order to generative an appropriate differential diagnosis, a number of factors must be considered, including the age of the patient, the nature (benign versus malignant) of the lesion, and the location of the lesion (vertebral body versus posterior elements). It is also helpful to divide lesions into solitary bony lesions (monostotic) and multiple (polyostotic) categories [169]. Table 15.1 provides an outline of some of the more common mono- and polyostotic spinal lesions found in elderly populations. An essential fact to remember is that as many as 97 % of vertebral lesions found in patients over the age of 40 year of age are metastatic lesions. No symptomatic spinal lesion in an elderly person should be considered a primary tumor until the possibility of metastatic disease has been confidently ruled out.

Table 15.1 Common differential diagnoses for monostotic and polyostotic vertebral lesions in the elderly

	Monostotic lesion	Polyostotic lesions
Benign	Hemangioma	*Rare in elderly*
	Enchondroma Bone island	
Malignant	Chondrosarcoma	Metastatic disease
	Chordoma	Multiple myeloma
	Lymphoma	
Inflammatory	Bacterial discitis, osteomyelitis	Bacterial discitis, osteomyelitis
	TB (Pott's disease)	
Metabolic/other	Insufficiency fracture	Paget's Disease
	Bone infarctions	Osteitis fibrosa cystica (brown tumor)

15.7 Nonoperative Management

Indications for operative and nonoperative treatments for spinal tumors vary on many factors. First, the nature of the disease should be considered: is the tumor benign or malignant—or might it not be a tumorous condition at all, but a metabolic, inflammatory, or infectious process? Second, does the lesion result in mechanic instability? Mechanical instability is a complicated and nuanced concept that is generally defined herein as the inability of the spine to undergo normal motion under normal physiologic loads. Instability may be produced by disk disease, bony lesions, pathological fractures, or impending fractures. Third, is the patient neurologically stable? Is the lesion causing spinal cord, conus medullaris, or nerve root compression? Next, the natural history of the lesion must be considered: is this an aggressive, rapidly progressive lesion, or is it slow growing and well contained? Finally, the overall health, prognosis, and desires of the patient and family must be considered—is the patient active, otherwise healthy, and wants every possible curative measure? Or is the patient suffering from multisystem disease and has multiple known metastases for a high-grade aggressive lesion? Such situations are rarely as "cut and dry" as presented here. As always, a clear, honest, and direct conversation with patients and family is paramount to optimizing patient satisfaction and quality of life.

15.7.1 Indications for Nonoperative Management

Nonoperative treatment modalities are broad in nature and purpose. They range from reassurance and observation, to far more aggressive medical modalities such as radiation and chemotherapy. Indications for nonoperative management are difficult to clearly define; indeed, the appropriateness of nonoperative care varies on a case-by-case basis. In very broad and general terms, tumorous lesions most amenable to nonoperative measures are those that are benign, slow-growing, and mechanically and neurologically stable. Additionally, patients with very poor prognoses or those medically unfit for surgery may be amenable to nonoperative measures.

15.7.2 Observation

Lesions most amenable to periodic observation and reassurance are benign, slow-growing lesions. Often, these are found incidentally. The most common benign, incidental lesions in elderly populations include hemangiomas, lipomas, bone infarctions, bone islands, and enchondromas. Other benign conditions which less commonly present in the elderly include neurofibromas, fibrous dysplasia, osteofibrous dysplasia, eosinophilic granuloma, and aneurysmal bone cysts. Unless these are symptomatic or they are severely compromising mechanical stability, observation and reassurance may be appropriate.

15.7.3 Bracing

Bracing is a means of using external pressures to stabilize the spine. Bracing may be indicated in certain circumstances to stabilize severely mechanically unstable lesions in patients who are too medically unstable or who do not wish to undergo internal stabilization procedures. Commonly used braces range from rigid cervical collars to thoracolumbar (TL), thoracolumbosacral (TLS), and cervicothoacolumbosacral (CTLS) orthoses. Casting, halo traction, and other customized orthoses may be indicated in limited circumstances. LSOs have been found to be largely ineffective at reducing lumbar motion and may even create an undesirable lever arm at the lumbosacral junction [170]. As should always be the case, the duration of bracing should be determined prior to institution, since in most cases spine stability will only diminish with time. A brace, if used, perhaps should be considered for the duration of the patient's life. This has significant integument and quality of life implications. Hence, the use of bracing may be of limited or questionable utility in most patients.

15.7.4 Medical Therapies

Bisphosphonate therapy is indicated in certain tumorous conditions. Benign conditions such as Paget's disease may be managed with bisphosphonates, which have been found to decrease bone turnover, disease severity, as well as subjective pain scores, among other surrogate markers [171]. Bisphosphonates may also be used as an adjuvant to treatments for certain metastatic bony disease. Much of the bone destruction that occurs with secondary bone metastases comes from the combination of osteoclast activation and osteoblast inhibition. In multiple myeloma, for example, a cascade of irregular cytokine and interleukin activity results in the rapid resorption of bone. Bisphosphonates inhibit these osteoclast-mediated functions and have been demonstrated in certain high-dose IV formulations to significantly decrease the rate of skeletal-related events, such as pathologic fractures, compression fractures, and hypercalcemia, as well as decrease the need for radiation in patients with breast cancer and multiple myeloma, among other cancers [172].

Radiation is classically reserved for malignant and certain metastatic diseases in unresectable locations. Radiation is also classically indicated in instances of spinal cord impingement due to metastatic disease. Some lesions are especially susceptible to radiation, including multiple myeloma and breast carcinomas [168]. Many types of metastatic and other primary tumors, however, are radioresistant; and some patients have received maximal doses of radiation. In such instances, surgery and other interventions may be necessary [173].

Recently, stereotactic radiation, or the use of multiple radiation sources from different angles that converge at the intended site, can treat focal lesions with better precision than conventional radiation. Stereotactic radiation techniques demonstrate unprecedented local tumor control for radioresistant tumors and can be used in regions once deemed too vulnerable for conventional wider-field radiation [172].

Chemotherapy is classically indicated for metastatic disease. Lesions known to respond well to chemotherapy include thyroid cancers, osteosarcoma, and lymphoma [168, 172]. Steroids may also have the ability to reduce pain from metastatic spinal disease as well as to reduce vasogenic edema which can stabilize or improve neurogenic deficits associated with pathologic compression [172].

15.8 Operative Management

15.8.1 Primary Spinal Lesions

Like nonoperative treatments, operative indications for spine tumors depend on a wide variety of factors. In general, benign tumors that are symptomatic, rapidly growing, or causing structurally or neurologically instability, resection with or without reconstruction may be considered. For malignant tumors that are solitary or recurrent, resection with or without reconstruction may be considered. Radio- or chemo-resilient tumors may also be amenable to resection [168]. Finally, an inability to obtain tissue biopsy may be an indication for a single-stage excisional biopsy. Various types of excision and reconstructive procedures are discussed below.

15.8.2 Metastatic Spinal Lesions

Metastatic disease is by far the most common etiology for vertebral tumors in the elderly. Surgical indications for metastatic disease are a complicated and constantly evolving topic that must be addressed at the individual patient level. The classic adage that metastatic disease is treated with only with medical, not surgical means, is neither current nor applicable to the spine. While it remains true that surgery is rarely a "curative" approach to metastatic disease, spinal surgery for metastatic disease has several justified and evidenced indications. First, neurological compression from metastatic lesions is an indication for surgical decompression. Neurological compression occurs in up to 20 % of patients with metastatic spinal disease, substantially more than in patients with primary spinal lesions, either benign or malignant [168]. Compression most commonly occurs from pressure on the neural elements by growing metastatic lesions or from retropulsed bone and disk fragments after pathologic fractures. Most commonly, compressive lesions present first with back pain, followed by radicular pain or generalized sensory and/or motor disturbances caudal to the lesion. Bowel and bladder dysfunction can occur. Decompression of compressive lesions may require stabilization and reconstruction; these techniques are discussed below.

15.8.3 Operative Strategies

Staging of tumors and thorough preoperative planning is essential to spinal tumor surgery. It is worth noting the classic Enneking staging systems utilized in much orthopedic oncology do not technically apply to the spine, which does not feature the typical anatomic compartments found in the extremities. An alternate staging system has been suggested, consisting of four vertebral zones (I–IV) and the extent of tumor spread (A for interosseous, B for extraosseous, and C for distant spread) [168]. Table 15.2 depicts this anatomic tumor classification as well as its generally recommended approaches, stabilization considerations, and other relevant factors.

Intralesional excision is the processes by which a lesion is cut into and removed often in piecemeal from the inside. It is often accompanied by curettage, or the methodical scraping and debridement of the tumor walls. Intralesional excision is most appropriate for indolent and definitively benign tumors that have little chance of recurrence if trace residual tumorous matter is left behind (e.g., EG, ABC, osteoblastoma/osteoid osteoma). Intralesional techniques can also be used to debulk metastatic disease, especially when the residual tumorous matter is amenable to radiation or elimination by other means [168].

Marginal excision is the process by which a lesion is removed in a single piece with a minimal margin of healthy tissue surrounding it. Because marginal excision does not guarantee that small residual pockets of tumorous cells are not left behind, it is most appropriate for low-grade malignancies like prostate metastases or aggressive benign lesions such as giant cell tumors. Tumors that respond especially well to adjunctive therapies such as radiation may also be amenable to marginal excision, including breast cancer and plasmacytomas [168].

Wide excision is the process by which a lesion is removed in a single piece with a thick margin of surrounding healthy tissue. This technique has the lowest chance that trace amounts of tumor are left behind; however, it is also the most destructive and often requires sacrifice of healthy and often essential structures such as load-bearing bone, nerves, and vessels. Wide excision is reserved for highly malignant

Table 15.2 Anatomic zones for spinal tumors and their recommended surgical approaches and considerations

		Recommended approach	Stabilization considerations	Additional considerations
Zone				
I	Spinous process, pars, inferior facets	Posterior approach	Consider instrumented stabilization if multilevel, especially in cervical/thoracic spine to prevent kyphosis	Consider instrumentation if bilateral facet resection, as ~50 % resection risks iatrogenic spondylolisthesis
II	Superior facets, transverse processes, pedicles	Posterior and/or posterolateral approach	Consider instrumented stabilization if multilevel, especially in cervical/thoracic spine to prevent kyphosis	Consider instrumentation if bilateral facet resection, as ~50 % resection risks iatrogenic spondylolisthesis
III	Anterior ¾ of vertebral body	Anterior approach	Typically require some reconstruction efforts, with or without instrumentation	Extraosseous (B) lesions may involve great vessels, esophagus, trachea, and other vital structures. Preoperative planning is essential
IV	Posterior ¼ vertebral body and region anterior to dura	Combined anterior and posterior approach	Generally require complete en bloc resection	Most inaccessible lesions, requires extensive reconstruction
Extent				
A	Intraosseous			
B	Extraosseous			
C	Distal spread			

and/or aggressive lesions such as osteosarcoma, chordoma, and high-grade chondrosarcoma. All primary malignancies without known metastases should generally be considered candidates for wide excision, as this offers the best chance of disease-free survival. Solitary metastases may also be amenable to wide excision when the chance of survival is high [168].

Surgical decompression is a technique of removing compressive structures from around nerves of the spinal cord. Decompression can be either direct, by removing or debulking tumorous material from around neural structures or by removing retropulsed pathologic fracture fragments from the spinal canal, or indirect, as in removing the lamina and posterior elements to make room for the compressed spinal cord. Spinal cord compression is reported in up to 20 % of patients with widespread cancer [168]. Radiation therapy is often effective for reducing cord compression, especially for metastatic disease; however, many tumors are radioresistant or the presence of bony retropulsion precludes effective irradiation [173]. In such cases, operative decompression is often necessary [173].

Reconstruction is the processes by which excised tissues are replaced by a variety of grafts and/or implants. Although reconstruction is a complex and often a case-specific topic, some basic concepts are universal. First, the anterior, weight-bearing column of the spinal must be restored. An unsupported anterior column will inevitably collapse into kyphosis. Bony autograft or allograft and mechanical cages or spacers are often deployed to transfer loads across the void left by the evacuated pathologic tissue [174]. Second, the posterior tension band, formed normally by the spinous processes, interspinous ligaments, ligamentum flavum, and facet joints, among other structures, should be reconstructed or substituted for in order to prevent kyphotic deformity. This is especially true in the cervical and thoracic spine, where post-laminectomy kyphosis is a common and highly morbid phenomenon [168]. Fusion constructions with screw, hook, and rod instrumentation as well as a variety of suture/cable tensioning techniques are used to reestablish the posterior spinal tension band. Other important concepts include the importance of combining anterior and posterior approaches when working with both longer fusion constructions and soft, tumor-laden bone [174]. Finally, it is important to achieve bony fusion in relatively active patients with favorable prognoses (greater than 3–6 months), as implants will eventually fail unless relieved by bony union [168]. Table 15.2 outlines basic reconstruction and stabilization considerations based on tumor location and surgical approach. Figure 15.2 depicts preoperative and postoperative images from a 67-year-old male with metastatic prostate cancer of the mid-thoracic spine. The patient underwent multilevel decompression, tumor debulking, and instrumented fusion.

Vertebroplasty and kyphoplasty have also been described in the treatment of vertebral body tumors, both for mechanical stabilization and for decreasing axial pain. Vertebroplasty may be especially effective in patients with spinal plasmacytoma and multiple myeloma [175]. These techniques are contraindicated, however, in patients with severe loss of vertebral height (>75 %), spinal canal compromise due to epidural disease, posterior vertebral body tumor erosion, and significant involvement of three of more vertebral levels [174].

Conclusion

Extramedullary extradural spinal tumors in the elderly are relatively common. The vast majority of cases are secondary metastatic lesions, although both benign and malignant primary spinal lesions can occur in elderly populations. No symptomatic spinal lesion in an elderly person should be considered a primary tumor until the possibility of metastatic disease has been confidently excluded. The surgical indications for metastatic spinal disease have expanded substantially over the past few decades, with wider accepted indications for surgical decompression, stabilization, as well as tumor excision and resection.

As the population lives longer, more active lives, we are likely to see an increase in the number of patients presenting with—and seeking aggressive therapies for—a variety of primary and secondary spinal tumors. Hopefully, our collective surgical acumen and technologies will continue to evolve alongside these growing and all-but-inevitable demands.

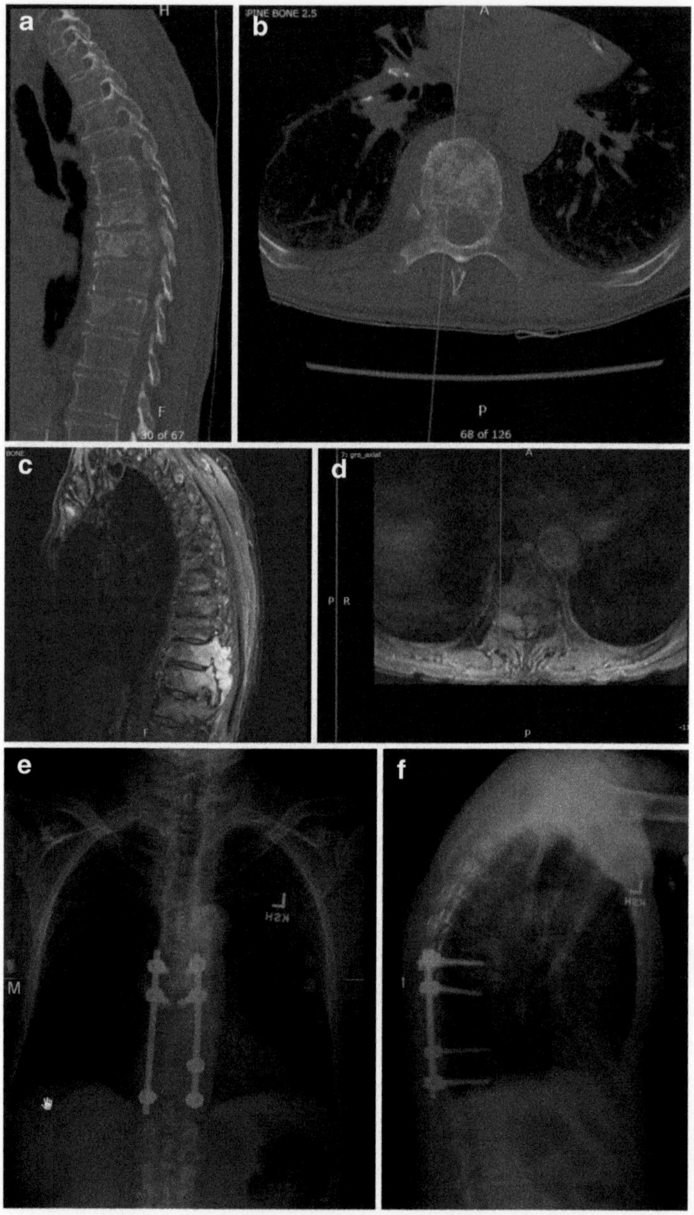

Fig. 15.2 Sagittal (**a**) and axial (**b**) CT images of a 67-year-old male with a known history of metastatic prostate cancer, previously treated with chemotherapy, androgen-modulation therapy, and irradiation. He presented with 3 weeks of progressive bilateral lower extremity weakness, and he had been in a bed-bound prior to intervention. Preoperative sagittal T2 (**c**) and axial STIR (**d**) imaging demonstrates tumorous invasion of the T10 vertebral body as well as partial involvement of the right-sided T11 body. He underwent a T10-T11 decompressive thoracic laminectomy, tumor debulking, and segmental instrumented fusion of T8–12 with cement pedicle screw augmentation (**e**, AP postoperative plain standing radiograph; **f**, lateral postoperative plain standing radiograph). The right-sided pedicle screw did not gain sufficient purchase in tumor-laden body and was removed immediately after attempted placement. Postoperatively, the regained ambulatory ability with minimal use of an assistive device until his eventual expiration 5 months postoperative

References

1. Tatsui H, Onomura T, Morishita S, Oketa M, Inoue T (1996) Survival rates of patients with metastatic spinal cancer after scintigraphic detection of abnormal radioactive accumulation. Spine 21:2143–2148
2. Schiff D, O'Neill BP, Suman VJ (1997) Spinal epidural metastasis as the initial manifestation of malignancy: clinical features and diagnostic approach. Neurology 49:452–456
3. Ortiz Gomez JA (1995) The incidence of vertebral body metastases. Int Orthop 19:309–311
4. Brihaye J, Ectors P, Lemort M, Van Houtte P (1988) The management of spinal epidural metastases. Adv Tech Stand Neurosurg 16:121–176
5. Siegel RL, Miller KD, Jemal A (2016) Cancer statistics. CA Cancer J Clin 66:7
6. Torre LA, Bray F, Siegel RL et al (2015) Global cancer statistics. CA Cancer J Clin 65:87
7. Siegel R, Naishadham D, Jemal A (2013) Cancer statistics. CA Cancer J Clin 63:11
8. Kohler BA, Sherman RL, Howlader N et al (2015) Annual Report to the Nation on the Status of Cancer, 1975-2011, featuring incidence of breast cancer subtypes by race/ethnicity, poverty, and state. J Natl Cancer Inst 107:48
9. Constans JP, de Divitiis E, Donzelli R, Spaziante R, Meder JF, Haye C (1983) Spinal metastases with neurological manifestations: review of 600 cases. J Neurosurg 59:111–118
10. Bubendorf L, Schöpfer A, Wagner U et al (2000) Metastatic patterns of prostate cancer: an autopsy study of 1,589 patients. Hum Pathol 31:578
11. Lee YT (1983) Breast carcinoma: pattern of metastasis at autopsy. J Surg Oncol 23:175
12. Colzani E, Liljegren A, Johansson AL et al (2011) Prognosis of patients with breast cancer: causes of death and effects of time since diagnosis, age, and tumor characteristics. J Clin Oncol 29:4014
13. Harris L, Fritsche H, Mennel R et al (2007) American Society of Clinical Oncology 2007 update of recommendations for the use of tumor markers in breast cancer. J Clin Oncol 25:5287
14. Wolff AC, Hammond ME, Schwartz JN et al (2007) American Society of Clinical Oncology/College of American Pathologists guideline recommendations for human epidermal growth factor receptor 2 testing in breast cancer. J Clin Oncol 25:118
15. Humphrey PA (2014) Cancers of the male reproductive organs. In: Stewart BW, Wild CP (eds) World cancer report. World Health Organization, Lyon
16. Ries LAG, Melbert D, Krapcho M et al (eds) (2007) SEER cancer statistics review, 1975-2004. National Cancer Institute, Bethesda
17. Bell KJ, Del Mar C, Wright G et al (2015) Prevalence of incidental prostate cancer: a systematic review of autopsy studies. Int J Cancer 137:1749
18. Gleave ME, Coupland D, Drachenberg D et al (1996) Ability of serum prostate-specific antigen levels to predict normal bone scans in patients with newly diagnosed prostate cancer. Urology 47:708
19. Smith MR, Cook RJ, Coleman R et al (2007) Predictors of skeletal complications in men with hormone-refractory metastatic prostate cancer. Urology 70:315
20. Brambilla E, Travis WD (2014) Lung cancer. In: Stewart BW, Wild CP (eds) World cancer report. World Health Organization, Lyon
21. Jemal A, Simard EP, Dorell C et al (2013) Annual Report to the Nation on the Status of Cancer, 1975-2009, featuring the burden and trends in human papillomavirus (HPV)-associated cancers and HPV vaccination coverage levels. J Natl Cancer Inst 105:175
22. Alberg AJ, Samet JM (2003) Epidemiology of lung cancer. Chest 123:21S
23. Toloza EM, Harpole L, McCrory DC (2003) Noninvasive staging of non-small cell lung cancer: a review of the current evidence. Chest 123:137S
24. Schumacher T, Brink I, Mix M et al (2001) FDG-PET imaging for the staging and follow-up of small cell lung cancer. Eur J Nucl Med 28:483
25. Znaor A, Lortet-Tieulent J, Laversanne M et al (2015) International variations and trends in renal cell carcinoma incidence and mortality. Eur Urol 67:519
26. Chow WH, Dong LM, Devesa SS (2010) Epidemiology and risk factors for kidney cancer. Nat Rev Urol 7:245

27. Garnick MB (1998) Primary neoplasms of the kidney. In: Brady HR, Wilcox CS (eds) Therapy in nephrology and hypertension: a companion to Brenner and Rector's the kidney. WB Saunders, Philadelphia
28. Siegel R, Ward E, Brawley O, Jemal A (2011) Cancer statistics, 2011: the impact of eliminating socioeconomic and racial disparities on premature cancer deaths. CA Cancer J Clin 61:212
29. Siemer S, Hack M, Lehmann J et al (2006) Outcome of renal tumors in young adults. J Urol 175:1240
30. Thompson RH, Ordonez MA, Iasonos A et al (2008) Renal cell carcinoma in young and old patients – is there a difference? J Urol 180:1262
31. Cook A, Lorenzo AJ, Salle JL et al (2006) Pediatric renal cell carcinoma: single institution 25-year case series and initial experience with partial nephrectomy. J Urol 175:1456
32. Siegel R, Naishadham D, Jemal A (2012) Cancer statistics, 2012. CA Cancer J Clin 62:10
33. Gudbjartsson T, Thoroddsen A, Petursdottir V et al (2005) Effect of incidental detection for survival of patients with renal cell carcinoma: results of population-based study of 701 patients. Urology 66:1186
34. Baloch KG, Grimer RJ, Carter SR, Tillman RM (2000) Radical surgery for the solitary bony metastasis from renal-cell carcinoma. J Bone Joint Surg Br 82:62
35. Kollender Y, Bickels J, Price WM et al (2000) Metastatic renal cell carcinoma of bone: indications and technique of surgical intervention. J Urol 164:1505
36. American Cancer Society: thyroid cancer. http://www.cancer.org/Cancer/ThyroidCancer/DetailedGuide/thyroid-cancer-key-statistics. Accessed on 14 Mar 2016
37. Ries LAG, Melbert D, Krapcho M et al (2006) SEER cancer statistics review 1975-2004. National Cancer Institute, Bethesda
38. Chen AY, Jemal A, Ward EM (2009) Increasing incidence of differentiated thyroid cancer in the United States, 1988-2005. Cancer 115:3801
39. American Thyroid Association (ATA) Guidelines Taskforce on Thyroid Nodules and Differentiated Thyroid Cancer, Cooper DS, Doherty GM et al (2009) Revised American Thyroid Association management guidelines for patients with thyroid nodules and differentiated thyroid cancer. Thyroid 19:1167
40. Grebe SK, Hay ID (1995) Follicular thyroid cancer. Endocrinol Metab Clin North Am 24:761
41. Mazzaferri EL, Jhiang SM (1994) Long-term impact of initial surgical and medical therapy on papillary and follicular thyroid cancer. Am J Med 97:418
42. Wu K, Hou S-M, Huang T-S, Yang R-S (2008) Thyroid carcinoma with bone metastases: a prognostic factor study. Clin Med Oncol 2:129–134
43. Muresan MM, Olivier P, Leclère J, Sirveaux F, Brunaud L, Klein M, Zarnegar R, Weryha G (2008) Bone metastases from differentiated thyroid carcinoma. Endocr Relat Cancer 15(1):37–49
44. Weigel B, Maghsudi M, Neumann C et al (1999) Surgical management of symptomatic spinal metastases: postoperative outcome and quality of life. Spine (Phila Pa 1976) 24:2240
45. Hadjipavlou A, Kakavelakis K, Korovessis P, Simmons JW (2012) Prognostic factors, surgical outcomes, and guidelines for managing metastatic spine cancer. In: Benzel EC (ed) Spine surgery: techniques, complication avoidance, and management, 3rd edn. Elsevier-Saunders, Philadelphia. pp 1049–1061. Pastushyn AI, Slin'ko EI, Mirzoyeva GM (1998) Vertebral hemangiomas: diagnosis, management, natural history and clinicopathological correlates in 86 patients. Surg Neurol 50(6):535–547
46. Nguyen JP, Djindjian M, Gaston A et al (1987) Vertebral hemangiomas presenting with neurologic symptoms. Surg Neurol 27(4):391–397
47. Saccomanni B (2008) Aneurysmal bone cyst of spine: a review of literature. Arch Orthop Trauma Surg 128(10):1145–1147, http://dx.doi.org/10.1007%2Fs00402-007-0477-6
48. Gasbarrini A, Cappuccio M, Donthineni R, Bandiera S, Boriani S (2009) Management of benign tumors of the mobile spine. Orthop Clin North Am 40(1):9–19
49. Hay MC, Paterson D, Taylor TK (1978) Aneurysmal bone cysts of the spine. J Bone Joint Surg Br 60(3):406–411

50. Mendenhall WM, Zlotecki RA, Scarborough MT, Gibbs CP, Mendenhall NP (2006) Giant cell tumor of bone. Am J Clin Oncol 29(1):96–99
51. Sanjay BK, Sim FH, Unni KK, McLeod RA, Klassen RA (1993) Giant-cell tumours of the spine. J Bone Joint Surg Br 75(1):148–154
52. Martin C, McCarthy EF (2010) Giant cell tumor of the sacrum and spine: series of 23 cases and a review of the literature. Iowa Orthop J 30:69–75
53. Lackman RD, Khoury LD, Esmail A, Donthineni-Rao R (2002) The treatment of sacral giant-cell tumours by serial arterial embolisation. J Bone Joint Surg Br 84(6):873–877
54. Hart RA, Boriani S, Biagini R, Currier B, Weinstein JN (1997) A system for surgical staging and management of spine tumors: a clinical outcome study of giant cell tumors of the spine. Spine (Phila Pa 1976) 22(15):1773–1783
55. Donthineni R, Boriani L, Ofluoglu O, Bandiera S (2009) Metastatic behaviour of giant cell tumour of the spine. Int Orthop 33(2):497–501
56. Jackson RP, Reckling FW, Mants FA (1977) Osteoid osteoma and osteoblastoma: similar histologic lesions with different natural histories. Clin Orthop Relat Res 128:303–313
57. Swee RG, McLeod RA, Beabout JW (1979) Osteoid osteoma: detection, diagnosis, and localization. Radiology 130(1):117–123
58. Pettine KA, Klassen RA (1986) Osteoid-osteoma and osteoblastoma of the spine. J Bone Joint Surg Am 68(3):354–361
59. Berry M, Mankin H, Gebhardt M, Rosenberg A, Hornicek F (2008) Osteoblastoma: a 30-year study of 99 cases. J Surg Oncol 98(3):179–183
60. Kroon HM, Schurmans J (1990) Osteoblastoma: clinical and radiologic findings in 98 new cases. Radiology 175(3):783–790
61. Kunze E, Enderle A, Radig K, Schneider-Stock R (1996) Aggressive osteoblastoma with focal malignant transformation and development of pulmonary metastases: a case report with a review of literature. Gen Diagn Pathol 141(5–6):377–392
62. Jaffe HL, Lichtenstein L (1942) Benign chondroblastoma of bone: reinterpretation of the so-called calcified or chondro-matous giant cell tumors. Am J Pathol 18:969–991
63. Bloem JL, Mulder JD (1985) Chondroblastoma: a clinical and radiological study of 104 cases. Skeletal Radiol 14:1–9
64. Kurt AM, Unni KK, Sim FH, McLeod RA (1989) Chondroblastoma of bone. Hum Pathol 20:965–976
65. Schajowicz F, Gallardo H (1970) Epiphysial chondroblastoma of bone: a clinicopathological study of sixty-nine cases. J Bone Joint Surg Br 52(2):205–226
66. Dahlin DC, Ivins JC (1972) Benign chondroblastoma: a study of 125 cases. Cancer 30(2):401–413
67. Unni KK, Inwards CY (2010) Chondromyxoid fibroma. In: Unni KK, Inwards CY (eds) Dahlin's bone tumors, 6th edn. Wolters Kluwer/Lippincott Williams & Wilkins, Philadelphia, pp 50–59
68. Springfield DS, Capanna R, Gherlinzoni F, Picci P, Campanacci M (1985) Chondroblastoma: a review of seventy cases. J Bone Joint Surg Am 67(5):748–755
69. de Silva MV, Reid R (2003) Chondroblastoma: varied histologic appearance, potential diagnostic pitfalls, and clinicopathologic features associated with local recurrence. Ann Diagn Pathol 7(4):205–213
70. Lin PP, Thenappan A, Deavers MT, Lewis VO, Yasko AW (2005) Treatment and prognosis of chondroblastoma. Clin Orthop Relat Res 438:103–109
71. Sailhan F, Chotel F, Parot R, SOFOP (2009) Chondroblastoma of bone in a pediatric population. J Bone Joint Surg Am 91(9):2159–2168
72. Ramappa AJ, Lee FY, Tang P, Carlson JR, Gebhardt MC, Mankin HJ (2000) Chondroblastoma of bone. J Bone Joint Surg Am 82(8):1140–1145
73. Suneja R, Grimer RJ, Belthur M et al (2005) Chondroblastoma of bone: long-term results and functional outcome after intralesional curettage. J Bone Joint Surg Br 87(7):974–978
74. Ilaslan H, Sundaram M, Unni KK (2003) Vertebral chondroblastoma. Skeletal Radiol 32(2):66–71

75. Huvos A (1991) Bone tumors: diagnosis, treatment, prognosis, 2nd edn. WB Saunder, Philadelphia
76. Sissons HA (1976) The WHO classification of bone tumors. Recent Results Cancer Res (54):104–108
77. McKenna R, Schwinn C, Soong K et al (1966) Sarcomas of the osteogenic series (osteosarcoma, chondrosarcoma, parosteal osteogenic sarcoma, and sarcomata arising in abnormal bone): an analysis of 552 cases. J Bone Joint Surg Am 48:1
78. Mirabello L, Troisi RJ, Savage SA (2009) Osteosarcoma incidence and survival rates from 1973 to 2004: data from the surveillance, epidemiology, and end results program. Cancer 115:1531
79. Author unknown. Post radiation osteosarcoma. Accessed at http://www.bonetumor.org/tumors-unknown-type/post-radiation-osteosarcoma-post-radiation-sarcoma
80. Campanacci M (2013) Bone and soft tissue tumors: clinical features, imaging, pathology and treatment. Springer Science & Business Media, New York, pp 500–502
81. Huvos AG (1986) Osteogenic sarcoma of bones and soft tissues in older persons. A clinicopathologic analysis of 117 patients older than 60 years. Cancer 57:1442
82. Hogendoorn PCW, Bovee JM, Nielsen GP (2013) Chondrosarcoma (grades I-III), including primary and secondary variants and periosteal chondrosarcoma. In: Fletcher CDM, Bridge JA, Hogendoorn PCW, Mertens F (eds) World Health Organization classification of tumours of soft tissue and bone, vol 5, 4th edn. IARC, Lyon, p 264
83. Dorfman HD, Czerniak B (1995) Bone cancers. Cancer 75:203
84. Murphey MD, Walker EA, Wilson AJ et al (2003) From the archives of the AFIP: imaging of primary chondrosarcoma: radiologic-pathologic correlation. Radiographics 23:1245
85. Angelini A, Guerra G, Mavrogenis AF et al (2012) Clinical outcome of central conventional chondrosarcoma. J Surg Oncol 106:929
86. Giuffrida AY, Burgueno JE, Koniaris LG et al (2009) Chondrosarcoma in the United States (1973 to 2003): an analysis of 2890 cases from the SEER database. J Bone Joint Surg Am 91:1063
87. York JE, Berk RH, Fuller GN et al (1999) Chondrosarcoma of the spine: 1954 to 1997. J Neurosurg 90:73
88. Stacchiotti S, Casali PG, Lo Vullo S et al (2010) Chordoma of the mobile spine and sacrum: a retrospective analysis of a series of patients surgically treated at two referral centers. Ann Surg Oncol 17:211
89. York JE, Kaczaraj A, Abi-Said D et al (1999) Sacral chordoma: 40-year experience at a major cancer center. Neurosurgery 44:74
90. Osaka S, Kodoh O, Sugita H et al (2006) Clinical significance of a wide excision policy for sacrococcygeal chordoma. J Cancer Res Clin Oncol 132:213
91. Ferraresi V, Nuzzo C, Zoccali C et al (2010) Chordoma: clinical characteristics, management and prognosis of a case series of 25 patients. BMC Cancer 10:22
92. Jemal A, Siegel R, Ward E, Murray T, Xu J, Thun MJ (2007) Cancer statistics, 2007. CA Cancer J Clin 57(1):43–66
93. Chugh R, Tawbi H, Lucas DR, Biermann JS, Schuetze SM, Baker LH (2007) Chordoma: the nonsarcoma primary bone tumor. Oncologist 12(11):1344–1350
94. Peña CE, Horvat BL, Fisher ER (1970) The ultrastructure of chordoma. Am J Clin Pathol 53(4):544–551
95. Mirra JM, Della Rocca C, Nelson SD, Mertens F (2002) Chordoma. In: Fletcher CD, Unni K, Mertens F (eds) Pathology and genetics of tumours of soft tissue and bone. IARC Press, Lyon, pp 316–317
96. Higinbotham NL, Phillips RF, Farr HW, Hustu HO (1967) Chordoma. Thirty-five-year study at Memorial Hospital. Cancer 20(11):1841–1850
97. Catton C, O'Sullivan B, Bell R, Laperriere N, Cummings B, Fornasier V, Wunder J (1996) Chordoma: long-term follow-up after radical photon irradiation. Radiother Oncol 41(1):67–72

98. Chambers PW, Schwinn CP (1979) Chordoma. A clinicopathologic study of metastasis. Am J Clin Pathol 72(5):765–776
99. Phekoo KJ, Schey SA, Richards MA et al (2004) A population study to define the incidence and survival of multiple myeloma in a National Health Service Region in UK. Br J Haematol 127:299
100. Sant M, Allemani C, Tereanu C et al (2010) Incidence of hematologic malignancies in Europe by morphologic subtype: results of the HAEMACARE project. Blood 116:3724
101. Smith A, Howell D, Patmore R et al (2011) Incidence of haematological malignancy by sub-type: a report from the Haematological Malignancy Research Network. Br J Cancer 105:1684
102. Kyle RA, Gertz MA, Witzig TE et al (2003) Review of 1027 patients with newly diagnosed multiple myeloma. Mayo Clin Proc 78:21
103. Waxman AJ, Mink PJ, Devesa SS et al (2010) Racial disparities in incidence and outcome in multiple myeloma: a population-based study. Blood 116:5501
104. Shirley MH, Sayeed S, Barnes I et al (2013) Incidence of haematological malignancies by ethnic group in England, 2001-7. Br J Haematol 163:465
105. Huang SY, Yao M, Tang JL et al (2007) Epidemiology of multiple myeloma in Taiwan: increasing incidence for the past 25 years and higher prevalence of extramedullary myeloma in patients younger than 55 years. Cancer 110:896
106. Bladé J, Kyle RA (1998) Multiple myeloma in young patients: clinical presentation and treatment approach. Leuk Lymphoma 30:493
107. Lynch HT, Sanger WG, Pirruccello S et al (2001) Familial multiple myeloma: a family study and review of the literature. J Natl Cancer Inst 93:1479
108. Dubey P, Ha CS, Besa PC et al (1997) Localized primary malignant lymphoma of bone. Int J Radiat Oncol Biol Phys 37:1087
109. Limb D, Dreghorn C, Murphy JK, Mannion R (1994) Primary lymphoma of bone. Int Orthop 18:180
110. Hogendoorn PCW, Kluin PM (2013) Primary non-Hodgkin lymphoma of bone. In: Fletcher CDM, Bridge JA, Hogendoorn PCW, Mertens F (eds) WHO classification of tumours of soft tissue and bone, 4th edn. International Agency for Research on Cancer, Lyon, p 316
111. Freeman C, Berg JW, Cutler SJ (1972) Occurrence and prognosis of extranodal lymphomas. Cancer 29:252
112. Rosenberg SA, Diamond HD, Jaslowitz B, Craver LF (1961) Lymphosarcoma: a review of 1269 cases. Medicine (Baltimore) 40:31
113. Jawad MU, Schneiderbauer MM, Min ES et al (2010) Primary lymphoma of bone in adult patients. Cancer 116:871
114. Mulligan ME, McRae GA, Murphey MD (1999) Imaging features of primary lymphoma of bone. AJR Am J Roentgenol 173:1691
115. Cai L, Stauder MC, Zhang YJ et al (2012) Early-stage primary bone lymphoma: a retrospective, multicenter Rare Cancer Network (RCN) Study. Int J Radiat Oncol Biol Phys 83:284
116. Bruno Ventre M, Ferreri AJ, Gospodarowicz M et al (2014) Clinical features, management, and prognosis of an international series of 161 patients with limited-stage diffuse large B-cell lymphoma of the bone (the IELSG-14 study). Oncologist 19:291
117. Messina C, Ferreri AJ, Govi S et al (2014) Clinical features, management and prognosis of multifocal primary bone lymphoma: a retrospective study of the international extranodal lymphoma study group (the IELSG 14 study). Br J Haematol 164:834
118. Catlett JP, Williams SA, O'Connor SC et al (2008) Primary lymphoma of bone: an institutional experience. Leuk Lymphoma 49:2125
119. Power DG, McVey GP, Korpanty G et al (2008) Primary bone lymphoma: single institution case series. Ir J Med Sci 177:247
120. Ford DR, Wilson D, Sothi S et al (2007) Primary bone lymphoma – treatment and outcome. Clin Oncol (R Coll Radiol) 19:50

121. Alencar A, Pitcher D, Byrne G, Lossos IS (2010) Primary bone lymphoma – the University of Miami experience. Leuk Lymphoma 51:39
122. Chapurlat RD, Meunier PJ (2000) Fibrous dysplasia of bone. Ballieres Best Pract Res Clin Rheumatol 14:385–398
123. Dorfman HD, Czerniak B (1998) Fibroosseous lesions. In: Dorfman HD (ed) Bone tumors. Mosby, St. Louis, pp 441–491
124. Smith SE, Kransdorf MJ (2000) Primary musculoskeletal tumors of fibrous origin. Semin Musculoskelet Radiol 4:73–88
125. Albright F, Butler AM, Hampton AO, Smith P (1937) Syndrome characterized by osteitis fibrosa disseminata, areas of pigmentation and endocrine dysfunction, with precocious puberty in females. Report of five cases. N Engl J Med 216:727–746
126. Nabarro MN, Giblin PE (1994) Monostotic fibrous dysplasia of the thoracic spine. Spine 19:463–465
127. Riminucci M, Liu B, Corsi A, Shenker A, Spiegel AM, Robey PG, Bianco P (1999) The histopathology of fibrous dysplasia of bone in patients with activating mutations of the Gs alpha gene: site-specific patterns and recurrent histological hallmarks. J Pathol 187:249–258
128. Avimadje AM, Goupille P, Zerkak D, Begnard G, Brunais-Besse J, Valat JP (2000) Monostotic fibrous dysplasia of the lumbar spine. Joint Bone Spine 67:65–70
129. Leet AI, Magur E, Lee JS, Wientroub S, Robey PG, Collins MT (2004) Fibrous dysplasia in the spine: prevalence of lesions and association with scoliosis. J Bone Joint Surg Am 86(3):531–537
130. Wright JF, Stoker DJ (1988) Fibrous dysplasia of the spine. Clin Radiol 39:523–527
131. Harris WH, Dudley HR Jr, Barry RJ (1962) The natural history of fibrous dysplasia. An orthopaedic, pathological, and roentgenographic study. Am J Orthop 44:207–233
132. Altman RD, Bloch DA, Hochberg MC, Murphy WA (2000) Prevalence of pelvic Paget's disease of bone in the United States. J Bone Miner Res 15:461
133. Siris E, Roodman GD (2003) Paget disease section X. In: Favus MJ (ed) Primer on the metabolic bone diseases. ASBMR, Washington, DC, p 495
134. Gardner MJ, Guyer PB, Barker DJ (1978) Paget's disease of bone among British migrants to Australia. Br Med J 2:1436
135. Gómez Acotto C, Mautalen CA (2001) European origin of patients with Paget's disease of bone in the Buenos Aires area. Eur J Epidemiol 17:409
136. Gennari L, Di Stefano M, Merlotti D et al (2005) Prevalence of Paget's disease of bone in Italy. J Bone Miner Res 20:1845
137. Barker DJ, Chamberlain AT, Guyer PB, Gardner MJ (1980) Paget's disease of bone: the Lancashire focus. Br Med J 280:1105
138. Guyer PB, Chamberlain AT (1980) Paget's disease of bone in two American cities. Br Med J 280:985
139. Falch JA (1979) Paget's disease in Norway. Lancet 2:1022
140. Sridhar GR (1994) Paget's disease in India: is it truly rare? Natl Med J India 7:101
141. Yip KM, Lee YL, Kumta SM, Lin J (1996) The second case of Paget's disease (osteitis deformans) in a Chinese lady. Singapore Med J 37:665
142. Barker DJ (1981) The epidemiology of Paget's disease. Metab Bone Dis Relat Res 3:231
143. Wermers RA, Tiegs RD, Atkinson EJ et al (2008) Morbidity and mortality associated with Paget's disease of bone: a population-based study. J Bone Miner Res 23:819
144. Hansen MF, Seton M, Merchant A (2006) Osteosarcoma in Paget's disease of bone. J Bone Miner Res 21 Suppl 2:P58
145. Ralston SH, Langston AL, Reid IR (2008) Pathogenesis and management of Paget's disease of bone. Lancet 372:155
146. Mankin HJ, Hornicek FJ (2005) Paget's sarcoma: a historical and outcome review. Clin Orthop Relat Res 438:97
147. Deyrup AT, Montag AG, Inwards CY et al (2007) Sarcomas arising in Paget disease of bone: a clinicopathologic analysis of 70 cases. Arch Pathol Lab Med 131:942

148. Seitz S, Priemel M, Zustin J, Beil FT, Semler J, Minne H, Schinke T, Amling M (2009) Paget's disease of bone: histologic analysis of 754 patients. J Bone Miner Res 24:62–69
149. Altman RD (1980) Musculoskeletal manifestations of Paget's disease of bone. Arthritis Rheum 23:1121–1127
150. Meunier PJ, Salson C, Mathieu L, Chapuy MC, Delmas P, Alexandre C, Charhon S (1987) Skeletal distribution and biochemical parameters of Paget's disease. Clin Orthop Relat Res 217:37–44
151. Hadjipavlou A, Lander P (1991) Paget disease of the spine. J Bone Joint Surg Am 73:1376–1381
152. Mirra JM, Brien EW, Tehranzadeh J (1995) Paget's disease of bone: review with emphasis on radiologic features, part I. Skeletal Radiol 24:163–171
153. Mirra JM, Brien EW, Tehranzadeh J (1995) Paget's disease of bone: review with emphasis on radiologic features, part II. Skeletal Radiol 24:173–184
154. Davie M, Davies M, Francis R, Fraser W, Hosking D, Tansley R (1999) Paget's disease of bone: a review of 889 patients. Bone 24:11S–12S
155. Lewis RJ, Jacoes B, Marchisello PJ, Bullough PG (1977) Monostotic Paget's disease of the spine. Clin Orthop Relat Res 127:208–211
156. Pestka JM, Seitz S, Zustin J, Püschel K, Amling M, Barvencik F (2012) Paget disease of the spine: an evaluation of 101 patients with a histomorphometric analysis of 29 cases. Eur Spine J 21(5):999–1006
157. Berbari EF, Kanj SS, Kowalski TJ et al (2015) Infectious Diseases Society of America (IDSA) clinical practice guidelines for the diagnosis and treatment of native vertebral osteomyelitis in adults. Clin Infect Dis 61:e26
158. Sapico FL, Montgomerie JZ (1979) Pyogenic vertebral osteomyelitis: report of nine cases and review of the literature. Rev Infect Dis 1:754
159. Digby JM, Kersley JB (1979) Pyogenic non-tuberculous spinal infection: an analysis of thirty cases. J Bone Joint Surg Br 61:47
160. Beronius M, Bergman B, Andersson R (2001) Vertebral osteomyelitis in Göteborg, Sweden: a retrospective study of patients during 1990-95. Scand J Infect Dis 33:527
161. Pigrau C, Rodríguez-Pardo D, Fernández-Hidalgo N et al (2015) Health care associated hematogenous pyogenic vertebral osteomyelitis: a severe and potentially preventable infectious disease. Medicine (Baltimore) 94:e365
162. Cahill DW, Love LC, Rechtine GR (1991) Pyogenic osteomyelitis of the spine in the elderly. J Neurosurg 74:878
163. Falagas ME, Bliziotis IA, Mavrogenis AF, Papagelopoulos PJ (2006) Spondylodiscitis after facet joint steroid injection: a case report and review of the literature. Scand J Infect Dis 38:295
164. Hooten WM, Mizerak A, Carns PE, Huntoon MA (2006) Discitis after lumbar epidural corticosteroid injection: a case report and analysis of the case report literature. Pain Med 7:46
165. DiCaprio MR, Roberts TT (2014) The diagnosis and management of langerhans cell histiocytosis. J Am Acad Orthop Surg 22(10):643–652
166. Gilbert RW, Kim J-H, Posner JB (1978) Epidural spinal cord compression from metastatic tumor: diagnosis and treatment. Ann Neurol 3:40–51
167. White AP, Kwon BK, Lindskog DM, Friedlaender GE, Grauer JN (2006) Metastatic disease of the spine. J Am Acad Orthop Surg 14(11):587–598
168. Lewandrowski K, Anderson ME, McLain RF (2011) Tumors of the spine. In: Herkowitz HN, Garfin SR, Eismont FJ, Bell GR, Balderston RA (eds) Rothman and Simeone: the spine, 6th edn. Elsevier Saunders, Philadelphia, pp 1480–1512
169. Rosenbaum AJ, Roberts TT, Leonard G, DiCaprio MR (2014) The evaluation and management of polyostotic skeletal lesions. J Bone Joint Surg (Am) Rev 2(11):e3
170. Silva FE, Lehman Jr. RA, Lenke LG (2011) Bracing the spine. In: Herkowitz HN, Garfin SR, Eismont FJ, Bell GR, Balderston RA (eds) Rothman and Simeone: the spine, 6th edn. Elsevier Saunders, Philadelphia

171. Reid IR, Miller P, Lyles K, Fraser W, Brown JP, Saidi J, Mesenbrink P et al (2005) Comparison of a single infusion of zoledronic acid with risedronate for Paget's disease. N Engl J Med 353:898–908
172. Bradley Elder J, Vitaz TW, Bilsky TW (2012) Staging, classification, and oncologic approaches for metastatic tumors involving the spine. In: Benzel EC (ed) Spine surgery: techniques, complication avoidance, and management, 3rd edn. Elsevier-Saunders, Philadelphia, pp 1061–1080
173. Mesfin A, Buchowski JM, Gokaslan ZL, Bird JE (2015) Management of metastatic cervical spine tumors. J Am Acad Orthop Surg 23:38–46
174. Rose PS, Buchowski JM (2011) Metastatic disease in the thoracic and lumbar spine: evaluation and management. J Am Acad Orthop Surg 19:37–48
175. Cortet B, Cotton A, Boutry N et al (1996) Percutaneous vertebroplasty for osteolytic metastases and myeloma: effects of the percentage of lesion filling and the leakage of methylmethacrylate at clinical follow up. Radiology 200(2):525–530

Intramedullary Spinal Cord Tumors

16

Rajiv R. Iyer and George I. Jallo

Funding disclosure for this work: None.
Source of financial support and industry affiliations:

Rajiv R. Iyer, MD: None.
George I. Jallo, MD: None.

16.1 Introduction

As health care quality continues to improve and reach new limits, neurosurgeons are increasingly confronted with management dilemmas for disorders in the geriatric population. Some physicians hesitate to recommend surgery for elderly patients (>65 years), arguing that older age harbors higher surgical risk and may lead to functional compromise, therefore deferring to conservative treatment measures. However, throughout the years, reports have suggested that in elderly patients, good functional outcomes after surgery can result when patients are carefully selected and that age alone should not preclude surgical candidacy [2, 59].

Primary spinal cord tumors (SCTs) represent a small fraction (2–4 %) of central nervous system (CNS) tumors but, when encountered, can lead to significant morbidity and mortality [7, 31, 34]. These lesions are relatively rare with an overall incidence of approximately 0.2–1/100,000 and some reported incidences of up to 2.5/100,000 in the advanced age population [20, 58]. Primary SCTs are generally classified as extradural versus intradural. Intradural SCTs are further subdivided based on anatomic location in relation to the spinal cord as well as on histopathology. Intradural extramedullary (IDEM) tumors, such as nerve sheath tumors and meningiomas, lie external to the spinal cord, while intramedullary spinal cord tumors (IMSCTs) lie within the substance of the spinal cord and are derived from components of its cellular architecture.

R.R. Iyer, MD
Department of Neurosurgery, The Johns Hopkins University School of Medicine, Johns Hopkins All Children's Hospital, Baltimore, USA

G.I. Jallo, MD (✉)
Institute for Brain Protections Sciences, Johns Hopkins All Children's Hospital, 601 5th Street South, Suite 511, St. Petersburg, FL 33701, USA
e-mail: gjallo1@jhmi.edu

© Springer International Publishing Switzerland 2017

M. Berhouma, P. Krolak-Salmon (eds.), *Brain and Spine Surgery in the Elderly*,
DOI 10.1007/978-3-319-40232-1_16

While there is no classic clinical presentation of patients with IMSCTs, commonly, patients complain of axial back pain and radiculopathy, while other neurological symptoms vary based on tumor anatomy. In some cases, tumor-associated syringes may exist, and clinical features may include dissociative sensory loss and hemiparesis, with indolent neurological deterioration. Spasticity, myelopathy, and long tract signs, as well as bowel or bladder dysfunction, occur in later stages of the disease [1, 14, 30, 52]. Although IMSCTs are rare beyond the seventh decade of life, it is critical to understand their clinical characteristics in light of an increasing geriatric population given their potentially debilitating morbidity without intervention. The diagnosis of SCTs in elderly patients can be challenging, as symptoms can mimic features of other disorders such as pernicious anemia, degenerative disorders, or diabetes, and, thus, elderly patients in particular may present in advanced disease states [9, 35]. Given this diagnostic challenge, a high index of suspicion should be maintained for SCTs in those elderly patients who present with neurological complaints and objective findings on physical examination.

16.2 Incidence and Etiology

In the elderly population, primary glial tumors are the most frequently occurring IMSCT (80%), which are further subdivided into astrocytomas and ependymomas [25]. Unlike children, in whom IMSCTs are predominantly astrocytomas, the majority of IMSCTs in adults are ependymomas, with astrocytomas being second most common [12, 28]. Hemangioblastomas are less common, with an incidence of approximately 2–15% and a frequent association with von Hippel-Lindau (vHL) disease [41]. Other rare intramedullary lesions include subependymomas, lymphomas, gangliogliomas, dermoid cysts, lipomas, hamartomas, and, rarely, intramedullary metastases [46].

16.3 Ependymomas

Accounting for approximately 60% of IMSCTs found in adults, ependymomas are unencapsulated spinal cord lesions that are thought to be surgically amenable secondary to their well-demarcated borders and resection planes (Fig. 16.1) [13, 26, 28, 29]. Ependymomas are classified as subependymomas (WHO grade I), cellular ependymomas (WHO grade II), and anaplastic ependymomas (WHO grade III). Myxopapillary ependymomas (WHO grade I) are less common and are typically found in the lumbar cistern and filum terminale region [54]. Myxopapillary ependymomas are generally a separately considered disease process given their unique location and their ability to disseminate the CSF space, necessitating resection in an en bloc fashion. The majority of ependymomas are histologically benign with minimal infiltration of surrounding spinal cord tissue, and most lesions occur in the cervical and thoracic spine. Approximately two-thirds of ependymomas have an associated syrinx [56]. Importantly, there is also an association between spinal cord ependymomas and neurofibromatosis type II (NF-2), an autosomal dominant disorder resulting from deficiency of the "merlin" protein due to mutation of the *NF2* gene on chromosome 22 [3, 42].

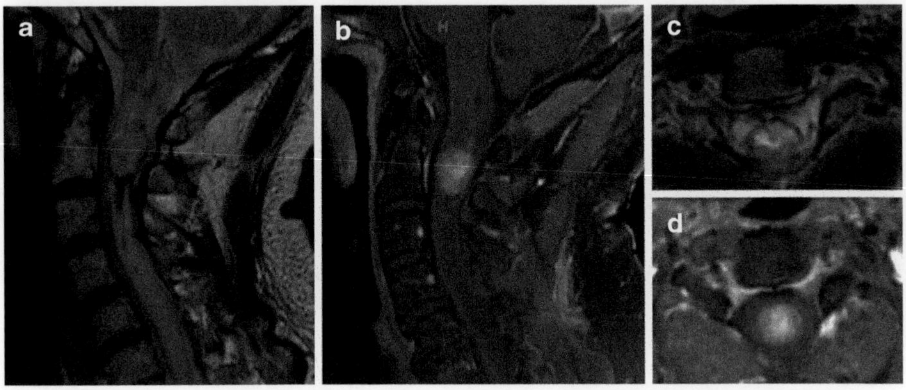

Fig. 16.1 Grade II cervical spine ependymoma. (**a**) Sagittal T2-weighted MRI. (**b**) Sagittal T1-weighted post contrast MRI. (**c**) Axial T2-weighted MRI. (**d**) Axial T1-weighted post contrast MRI

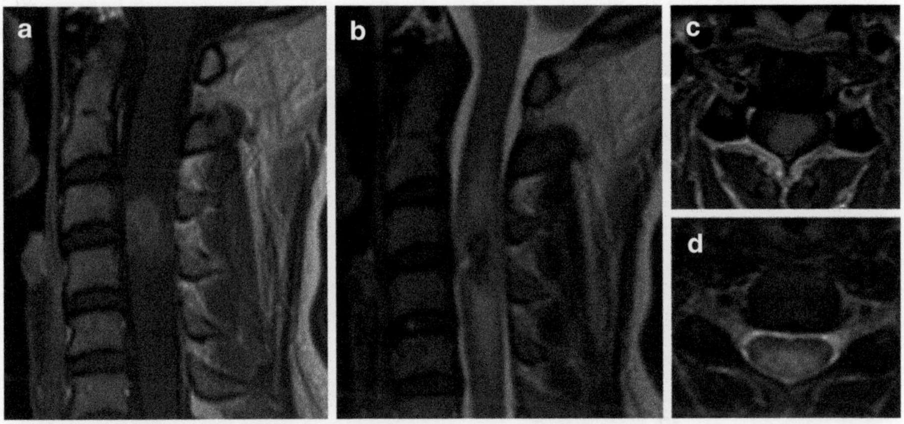

Fig. 16.2 Low-grade spinal astrocytoma. (**a**) Sagittal T1-weighted post contrast MRI. (**b**) Sagittal T2-weighted MRI. (**c**) Axial T1-weighted post contrast MRI. (**d**) Axial T2-weighted MRI

16.4 Astrocytomas

Spinal cord astrocytomas are the most common SCT in the pediatric population and the second most frequently encountered IMSCT in adults. Nevertheless, astrocytic tumors of the spinal cord are relatively rare entities, which make treatment paradigms difficult to define, especially for the advanced age population. In adults, most astrocytic tumors are low-grade lesions with less-defined borders secondary to their infiltrating nature (Fig. 16.2). Tumor-associated syringes are present in approximately 22 % of cases [56]. In the pediatric population, the vast majority of spinal cord astrocytomas are pilocytic. With increasing age, grade II fibrillary astrocytomas are more commonly found. It remains unclear whether an increased association with malignancy exists in these tumors in the advanced age population [20, 25, 30]. Across ages, patients with spinal cord glioblastoma multiforme (GBM) have a poor prognosis despite aggressive therapy with surgery and radiation therapy [37].

16.5 Hemangioblastomas

Hemangioblastomas are rare, benign, densely vascular lesions that occur both intracranially and in the spinal cord (Fig. 16.3). They occur in a sporadic, solitary fashion as well as in associated with vHL disease, an autosomal dominant inherited disorder that occurs as a result of a defect on chromosome 3p [55]. Approximately 40 % of spinal cord hemangioblastomas arise in the context of vHL [11]. Spinal cord hemangioblastomas occur rarely in the elderly population. Reports suggest that the mean age at first surgery in the vHL population is about 33 years, and only about 20 % of patients with sporadic spinal hemangioblastomas are over the age of 60 [18, 45, 63]. The majority of spinal cord hemangioblastomas arise from the dorsal or dorsolateral spinal cord surface and frequently present with symptoms of pain or sensory disturbances [38, 39]. Grossly, these are well-circumscribed lesions that allow for total resection. Syrinx formation is common and reported to be about 80 % [56]. Histologically, they consist of a network of thin-walled vascular channels and surrounding lipen-laden stroma that secretes growth factors such as vascular endothelial growth factor (VEGF) [62, 65]. Overall, surgical resection of symptomatic spinal cord hemangioblastomas is well tolerated, and in the clinical setting of vHL disease, patients must be followed for long-term neurological and radiographic monitoring [45].

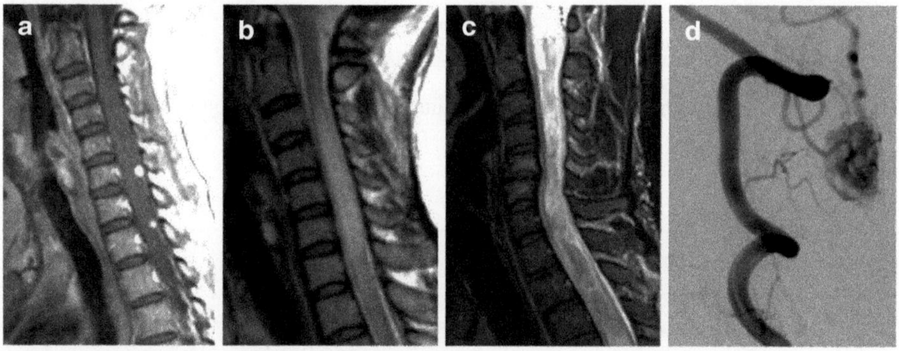

Fig. 16.3 Spinal hemangioblastoma. (**a**) Sagittal T1-weighted post contrast MRI. (**b**) Sagittal T2-weighted MRI. (**c**) Separate example of sagittal T2-weighted MRI demonstrating extensive syrinx. (**d**) Cerebral angiogram demonstrated feeding vessels for hemangioblastomas

16.6 Cavernous Malformations

Intramedullary cavernous malformations (CMs), or cavernomas, are angiographically occult lesions comprised of closely packed capillary-like sinusoidal vessels without intervening neural tissue. CMs arise throughout the CNS with the majority occurring intracranially. Intraspinal lesions account for approximately 5 % of all CMs, and they are best detected with MRI with a classic low-intensity hemosiderin ring on both T1- and T2-weighted imaging (Fig. 16.4) [5]. This MR appearance is thought to be due to micro hemorrhages and hemosiderin deposition over time. Patients with intraspinal CMs are typically screened for similar intracranial lesions because as many as 42 % of patients discovered to have an intraspinal cavernoma harbor similar intracranial pathology as well [10]. It is important to also recognize that patients with multiple CNS CMs may have the familial form of this disorder [53, 68]. CMs are uncommon in the elderly population, with less than 10 % of cases being reported in patients greater than 65 years of age and mean ages reported to be in the fourth or fifth decade of life [33, 64]. They most often occur in the cervical and thoracic spine, without a clear gender predilection. Clinical presentation can vary but common symptoms are those of sensory disturbances, myelopathy, and motor deficit [19, 40]. Patients may present acutely following hemorrhage or present with a chronic, indolent deterioration due to gliosis and increased edema over time [33]. Intramedullary CMs are generally amenable to surgical intervention as they have a classic mulberry-like appearance, with a hemosiderin rim and surrounding gliotic tissue that allows the surgeon to dissect the lesion away from normal tissue.

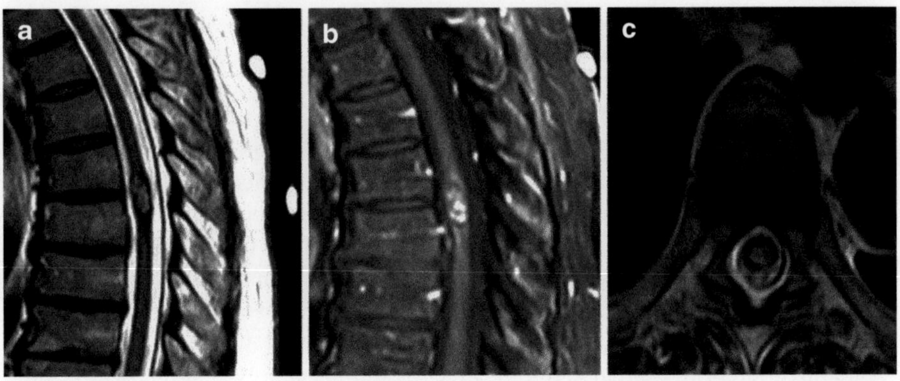

Fig. 16.4 Spinal cavernous malformation. (**a**) Sagittal T2-weighted MRI. (**b**) Sagittal T1-weighted post contrast MRI. (**c**) Axial T2-weighted MRI

16.7 Diagnostic Imaging

Magnetic resonance imaging (MRI) is the diagnostic modality of choice for IMSCTs, and expansile spinal cord lesions that typically exhibit gadolinium contrast enhancement are classic. Improvement in MR quality has led to its use as the gold standard imaging modality for IMSCTs. Preoperative planning is made easier by understanding the characteristic enhancing pattern of such lesions, tumor-associated syringes or edema, tumor proximity to the dorsal surface of the spinal cord, tumor laterality, and more.

Ependymomas typically lie in a central location in the spinal cord, while astrocytomas are typically more eccentrically located [6]. Astrocytomas and ependymomas are generally T1 isointense and T2 hyperintense, with difficult differentiation on T2-weighted imaging between tumor and surrounding edema or syrinx [50]. Gadolinium contrast enhancement is sharp and well circumscribed for ependymomas, consistent with the well-demarcated surgical planes used to dissect these lesions away from normal neural elements. Spinal astrocytomas demonstrate a patchier form of enhancement, with irregular and fuzzy borders between tumor and surrounding normal neural tissue, consistent with their infiltrating nature [50]. Some SCTs such as hemangioblastomas demonstrate unique features such as vascular flow voids on T2-weighted imaging, hypertrophic feeding vessels, and the presence of a large syrinx out of proportion to the tumor substance. These lesions may exhibit a small enhancing nodule with surrounding cyst or syrinx, thus aiding the surgeon in localization of the true tumor substance. Computed tomography (CT) myelography remains an adjunctive imaging modality for the diagnosis of intradural SCTs.

16.8 Surgical Technique

Operative techniques for IMSCTs in the elderly population do not vary significantly from those that are described in the literature [7, 13, 22]. After induction of anesthesia, patients are placed prone in a neutral position. The choice of the operating room table or head fixation depends upon the surgeon's preference. Through the entirety of the case, electrophysiological monitoring is performed using SSEPs and MEPs. A midline incision and subperiosteal dissection is performed, and a laminectomy or osteoplastic laminoplasty is performed extending one level above and below the lesion. Care is taken during the laminectomy to not disrupt the facet joints to prevent destabilization of the spinal column. Once the dura is exposed, intraoperative ultrasonography is performed to confirm tumor localization and to ensure adequate bony exposure for tumor resection [23]. A midline durotomy is performed and tenting sutures are placed to the lateral musculature. Intraoperative epidural leads may be placed for additional electrophysiological monitoring of the motor pathways [17]. This modality, known as the D-wave, represents the number of functioning fast-conducting corticospinal tract fibers within the spinal cord. Interpreted together with MEPs, D-wave measurement informs the surgeon when 50 % of these fibers have been affected, representing a threshold between likely transient versus prolonged motor deficit following surgery [32, 48, 51]. The operating microscope is used to inspect the spinal cord surface for abnormalities suggestive of underlying tumor. Identifying the midline may be challenging due to spinal cord rotation or asymmetry, but the presence of veins traveling toward the dorsal median sulcus may be helpful. A midline myelotomy is then performed with sufficient length to span the entire rostro-caudal extent of the tumor. Depending on tumor subtype, a well-demarcated plane between tumor and surrounding normal spinal cord tissue may or may not be present. Typically, with ependymomas, a well-defined interface between normal and tumor tissue can be used to carefully isolate the lesion without harmful manipulation of normal spinal cord tissue. Astrocytomas are typically more diffuse without a clear plane separating tumor from normal tissue. It is suggested that the presence of a syrinx may assist with definition of resection planes and thus lead to improved tumor resection, which holds especially true for ependymomas and hemangioblastomas but less so for diffusely infiltrative astrocytomas [56]. Tumor debulking can be performed with a contact laser probe or ultrasonic aspirator, with the goal of surgery being complete removal. Deliberately unresected tumor and subtotal resection (STR) may be appropriate when intraoperative monitoring heralds neurological deterioration [61]. After tumor resection is complete, meticulous hemostasis is achieved and a watertight dural closure is performed. Especially if an elderly patient has thinner or more porous dura, the risk of cerebrospinal fluid (CSF) leak may be higher, and the use of synthetic dural substitutes and fibrin glue is appropriate. If an osteoplastic laminoplasty was performed, miniplates are used to secure this in place, and multilayered closure of the fascia, soft tissues, and skin is carried out.

16.9 Operative Considerations/Outcomes

Over the past several decades, there has been a vast body of literature describing the international operative experience with IMSCTs [8, 13, 21, 27, 43, 61]. The standard of care for most IMSCTs is operative resection, which has become a safe and effective treatment choice with the advent of microsurgical techniques and intraoperative measurement such as motor evoked potentials (MEPs) and somatosensory evoked potentials (SSEPs). Even with the development of these operative tools, treatment of IMSCTs in the elderly patient population is controversial. Some clinicians believe that less aggressive treatment such as biopsy followed by radiation therapy is the favored approach over attempted gross total resection (GTR) due to the assumed risks of surgery such as neurological injury and functional loss.

Difficult clinical decision-making and controversy in elderly patients with IMSCTs is in part due to a dearth of literature guiding the management of these patients in particular. *Sandler* et al. in 1992 examined 21 patients with spinal cord astrocytomas, 15 of who received postoperative radiation therapy after surgical intervention. In this study, no general attempt was made to perform GTR, with over 50 % of patients undergoing laminectomy for biopsy without resection. At 5-year follow-up, survival was 68 %, with 80 % of deaths occurring as a result of local tumor recurrence. Of note, the three oldest patients in this study demonstrated tumor recurrence within the first year of diagnosis [57]. An alternate treatment approach described by *Shrivastava* et al. in 2005 examined surgical outcomes specifically in older patients that underwent more aggressive resection of IMSCTs and determined that age alone did not confer any additional risk with such intervention. Nearly one fourth of the patients analyzed in this study had undergone prior biopsy procedures and radiation therapy, and after intervention, GTR (>95 % tumor resection) or subtotal resection (STR; >80 % resection) was achieved in all 30 patients examined. At 10-year follow-up, 93 % of patients were alive, and of those surviving, McCormick grade (a measurement of functional status) improved in patients harboring low-grade tumors [61]. Similarly, *Hanbali* and colleagues in 2002 analyzed 26 patients who underwent surgery for low-grade ependymomas. In their study, five patients were >60 years of age, all of whom underwent surgery with intention of GTR. Follow-up was available for four out of five patients, with all patients either remaining at functional baseline or improving at 1-year follow-up [27]. Overall, these studies suggest that microscope-assisted and electrophysiologically guided surgical treatment of IMSCTs in older patients carries low morbidity and mortality. Radiation therapy for low-grade IMSCTs is also controversial. Although some studies maintain the safety of postoperative radiation therapy, among groups advocating an aggressive initial surgical approach with intended GTR, radiation therapy is generally reserved for aggressively infiltrating tumors, multifocal disease, and patients who are inappropriate surgical candidates [27, 36].

16.10 Postoperative Management

Following surgery for IMSCTs, patients are generally kept in a recumbent position for 24–48 h to prevent gravity-associated spinal fluid pressure on the newly approximated dural closure. A sub- or supra-fascial drain may be placed in order to monitor for CSF drainage from the wound and, if a dural leak is present, to create a CSF fistula to protect the incision from breakdown or leak. Especially in elderly patients, watertight dural closure and postoperative management to minimize CSF leak are critical. The use of an osteoplastic laminoplasty is thought to help reduce the risk of postoperative CSF leak and, thus indirectly, reduce hospital length of stay [44]. Physical therapy and mobilization occur in the period following recumbency, and perioperative steroids are generally quickly tapered. Improvements in transient postoperative deficits are often catalyzed by acute rehabilitation, which is especially critical in older patients for whom appropriate social and environmental support systems are paramount in achieving independence and higher functional status.

Post-laminectomy or post-laminoplasty kyphosis and spinal deformity are recognized phenomena following surgery for IMSCT resection. Primarily, this clinical scenario occurs in the pediatric population, with reported rates between 30 and 90 % [15, 49, 66, 67]. The issues of spinal deformity and instability following IMSCT surgery in adults are poorly defined, as data describing deformity rates are sparse [4,

47]. There has been some suggestion that extensive laminectomies for intradural tumor resection may be a risk factor in the development of symptomatic spinal instability at long-term follow-up [60]. Other studies suggest that in adult patients, post-laminectomy or laminoplasty deformity rates are only around 10% within 13–14 months of surgery [44]. During IMSCT resection in the elderly patient, intraoperative fusion is the exception, rather than the norm, as care is typically taken to preserve the facet joints during bony exposure. If, however, tumor extensiveness warrants wide decompression and pre-planned facet joint disruption, or if surgery occurs at a spinal junction, one must consider intraoperative instrumentation in order to prevent adverse future outcomes. While there are no data specifying the rates of instability following laminectomy or laminoplasty for IMSCT resection in the elderly patient population, trends toward fusion as an instability-preventing measuring is primarily geared toward younger patients [4]. Avoiding surgical fixation is likely beneficial for elderly patients undergoing spinal tumor resection, as it indirectly decreases intraoperative blood loss, length of anesthesia, and the ability to mobilize following surgery [16, 24].

References

1. Aghayev K, Vrionis F, Chamberlain MC (2011) Adult intradural primary spinal cord tumors. J Natl Compr Canc Netw 9:434–447
2. Amelot A, Balabaud L, Choi D, Fox Z, Crockard HA, Albert T, Arts CM, Buchowski JM, Bunger C, Chung CK, Coppes MH, Depreitere B, Fehlings MG, Harrop J, Kawahara N, Kim ES, Lee CS, Leung Y, Liu ZJ, Martin-Benlloch JA, Massicotte EM, Meyer B, Oner FC, Peul W, Quraishi N, Tokuhashi Y, Tomita K, Ulbricht C, Verlaan JJ, Wang M, Mazel C (2015) Surgery for metastatic spine tumors in the elderly. Advanced age is not a contraindication to surgery!. Spine J:S1529–9430(15). PMID: 26239762
3. Asthagiri AR, Parry DM, Butman JA, Kim HJ, Tsilou ET, Zhuang Z, Lonser RR (2009) Neurofibromatosis type 2. Lancet 373:1974–1986
4. Avila MJ, Walter CM, Skoch J, Abbasifard S, Patel AS, Sattarov K, Baaj AA (2015) Fusion after intradural spine tumor resection in adults: a review of evidence and practices. Clin Neurol Neurosurg 138:169–173
5. Barnwell SL, Dowd CF, Davis RL, Edwards MS, Gutin PH, Wilson CB (1990) Cryptic vascular malformations of the spinal cord: diagnosis by magnetic resonance imaging and outcome of surgery. J Neurosurg 72:403–407
6. Bourgouin PM, Lesage J, Fontaine S, Konan A, Roy D, Bard C, Del Carpio O'Donovan R (1998) A pattern approach to the differential diagnosis of intramedullary spinal cord lesions on MR imaging. AJR Am J Roentgenol 170:1645–1649
7. Brotchi J (2002) Intrinsic spinal cord tumor resection. Neurosurgery 50:1059–1063
8. Brotchi J, Fischer G (1998) Spinal cord ependymomas. Neurosurg Focus 4:e2
9. Bull FE, Dodge HW Jr, Hanlon DG, Sickert RC (1956) Tumor of the spinal cord; occurrence in patients with pernicious anemia and subacute combined sclerosis. J Am Med Assoc 162:707–709
10. Cohen-Gadol AA, Jacob JT, Edwards DA, Krauss WE (2006) Coexistence of intracranial and spinal cavernous malformations: a study of prevalence and natural history. J Neurosurg 104:376–381
11. Conway JE, Chou D, Clatterbuck RE, Brem H, Long DM, Rigamonti D (2001) Hemangioblastomas of the central nervous system in von Hippel-Lindau syndrome and sporadic disease. Neurosurgery 48:55–62; discussion 62–53

12. Cooper PR (1989) Outcome after operative treatment of intramedullary spinal cord tumors in adults: intermediate and long-term results in 51 patients. Neurosurgery 25:855–859
13. Cooper PR, Epstein F (1985) Radical resection of intramedullary spinal cord tumors in adults. Recent experience in 29 patients. J Neurosurg 63:492–499
14. Dang L, Liu X, Dang G, Jiang L, Wei F, Yu M, Wu F, Liu Z (2015) Primary tumors of the spine: a review of clinical features in 438 patients. J Neurooncol 121:513–520
15. de Jonge T, Slullitel H, Dubousset J, Miladi L, Wicart P, Illes T (2005) Late-onset spinal deformities in children treated by laminectomy and radiation therapy for malignant tumours. Eur Spine J 14:765–771
16. Deiner S, Silverstein JH (2011) Anesthesia for geriatric patients. Minerva Anestesiol 77:180–189
17. Deletis V, Sala F (2008) Intraoperative neurophysiological monitoring of the spinal cord during spinal cord and spine surgery: a review focus on the corticospinal tracts. Clin Neurophysiol 119:248–264
18. Deng X, Wang K, Wu L, Yang C, Yang T, Zhao L, Yang J, Wang G, Fang J, Xu Y (2014) Intraspinal hemangioblastomas: analysis of 92 cases in a single institution: clinical article. J Neurosurg Spine 21:260–269
19. Deutsch H, Jallo GI, Faktorovich A, Epstein F (2000) Spinal intramedullary cavernoma: clinical presentation and surgical outcome. J Neurosurg 93:65–70
20. Duong LM, McCarthy BJ, McLendon RE, Dolecek TA, Kruchko C, Douglas LL, Ajani UA (2012) Descriptive epidemiology of malignant and nonmalignant primary spinal cord, spinal meninges, and cauda equina tumors, United States, 2004–2007. Cancer 118:4220–4227
21. Epstein FJ, Farmer JP, Freed D (1992) Adult intramedullary astrocytomas of the spinal cord. J Neurosurg 77:355–359
22. Epstein FJ, Farmer JP, Freed D (1993) Adult intramedullary spinal cord ependymomas: the result of surgery in 38 patients. J Neurosurg 79:204–209
23. Epstein FJ, Farmer JP, Schneider SJ (1991) Intraoperative ultrasonography: an important surgical adjunct for intramedullary tumors. J Neurosurg 74:729–733
24. Garcia PS, Duggan EW, McCullough IL, Lee SC, Fishman D (2015) Postanesthesia care for the elderly patient. Clin Ther 37:2651–2665
25. Grimm S, Chamberlain MC (2009) Adult primary spinal cord tumors. Expert Rev Neurother 9:1487–1495
26. Guidetti B, Mercuri S, Vagnozzi R (1981) Long-term results of the surgical treatment of 129 intramedullary spinal gliomas. J Neurosurg 54:323–330
27. Hanbali F, Fourney DR, Marmor E, Suki D, Rhines LD, Weinberg JS, McCutcheon IE, Suk I, Gokaslan ZL (2002) Spinal cord ependymoma: radical surgical resection and outcome. Neurosurgery 51:1162–1172; discussion 1172–1164
28. Helseth A, Mork SJ (1989) Primary intraspinal neoplasms in Norway, 1955 to 1986. A population-based survey of 467 patients. J Neurosurg 71:842–845
29. Hoshimaru M, Koyama T, Hashimoto N, Kikuchi H (1999) Results of microsurgical treatment for intramedullary spinal cord ependymomas: analysis of 36 cases. Neurosurgery 44:264–269
30. Houten JK, Cooper PR (2000) Spinal cord astrocytomas: presentation, management and outcome. J Neurooncol 47:219–224
31. Jallo GI, Danish S, Velasquez L, Epstein F (2001) Intramedullary low-grade astrocytomas: long-term outcome following radical surgery. J Neurooncol 53:61–66
32. Jallo GI, Freed D, Epstein F (2003) Intramedullary spinal cord tumors in children. Childs Nerv Syst 19:641–649
33. Jallo GI, Freed D, Zareck M, Epstein F, Kothbauer KF (2006) Clinical presentation and optimal management for intramedullary cavernous malformations. Neurosurg Focus 21:e10
34. Jallo GI, Kothbauer KF, Epstein FJ (2001) Intrinsic spinal cord tumor resection. Neurosurgery 49:1124–1128

35. Khodadad G (1973) Common errors in the diagnosis of spinal meningiomas. Geriatrics 28:143–145
36. Linstadt DE, Wara WM, Leibel SA, Gutin PH, Wilson CB, Sheline GE (1989) Postoperative radiotherapy of primary spinal cord tumors. Int J Radiat Oncol Biol Phys 16:1397–1403
37. Liu A, Sankey EW, Bettegowda C, Burger PC, Jallo GI, Groves ML (2015) Poor prognosis despite aggressive treatment in adults with intramedullary spinal cord glioblastoma. J Clin Neurosci 22:1628–1631
38. Lonser RR (2014) Surgical management of sporadic spinal cord hemangioblastomas. World Neurosurg 82:632–633
39. Lonser RR, Weil RJ, Wanebo JE, DeVroom HL, Oldfield EH (2003) Surgical management of spinal cord hemangioblastomas in patients with von Hippel-Lindau disease. J Neurosurg 98:106–116
40. Lu DC, Lawton MT (2010) Clinical presentation and surgical management of intramedullary spinal cord cavernous malformations. Neurosurg Focus 29:E12
41. Mandigo CE, Ogden AT, Angevine PD, McCormick PC (2009) Operative management of spinal hemangioblastoma. Neurosurgery 65:1166–1177
42. Martuza RL, Eldridge R (1988) Neurofibromatosis 2 (bilateral acoustic neurofibromatosis). N Engl J Med 318:684–688
43. McCormick PC, Torres R, Post KD, Stein BM (1990) Intramedullary ependymoma of the spinal cord. J Neurosurg 72:523–532
44. McGirt MJ, Garces-Ambrossi GL, Parker SL, Sciubba DM, Bydon A, Wolinksy JP, Gokaslan ZL, Jallo G, Witham TF (2010) Short-term progressive spinal deformity following laminoplasty versus laminectomy for resection of intradural spinal tumors: analysis of 238 patients. Neurosurgery 66:1005–1012
45. Mehta GU, Asthagiri AR, Bakhtian KD, Auh S, Oldfield EH, Lonser RR (2010) Functional outcome after resection of spinal cord hemangioblastomas associated with von Hippel-Lindau disease. J Neurosurg Spine 12:233–242
46. Miller DJ, McCutcheon IE (2000) Hemangioblastomas and other uncommon intramedullary tumors. J Neurooncol 47:253–270
47. Montano N, Trevisi G, Cioni B, Lucantoni C, Della Pepa GM, Meglio M, Papacci F (2014) The role of laminoplasty in preventing spinal deformity in adult patients submitted to resection of an intradural spinal tumor. Case series and literature review. Clin Neurol Neurosurg 125:69–74
48. Morota N, Deletis V, Constantini S, Kofler M, Cohen H, Epstein FJ (1997) The role of motor evoked potentials during surgery for intramedullary spinal cord tumors. Neurosurgery 41:1327–1336
49. Papagelopoulos PJ, Peterson HA, Ebersold MJ, Emmanuel PR, Choudhury SN, Quast LM (1997) Spinal column deformity and instability after lumbar or thoracolumbar laminectomy for intraspinal tumors in children and young adults. Spine (Phila Pa 1976) 22:442–451
50. Parizel PM, Baleriaux D, Rodesch G, Segebarth C, Lalmand B, Christophe C, Lemort M, Haesendonck P, Niendorf HP, Flament-Durand J et al (1989) Gd-DTPA-enhanced MR imaging of spinal tumors. AJR Am J Roentgenol 152:1087–1096
51. Patton HD, Amassian VE (1954) Single and multiple-unit analysis of cortical stage of pyramidal tract activation. J Neurophysiol 17:345–363
52. Raco A, Esposito V, Lenzi J, Piccirilli M, Delfini R, Cantore G (2005) Long-term follow-up of intramedullary spinal cord tumors: a series of 202 cases. Neurosurgery 56:972–981; discussion 972–981
53. Rigamonti D, Hadley MN, Drayer BP, Johnson PC, Hoenig-Rigamonti K, Knight JT, Spetzler RF (1988) Cerebral cavernous malformations. Incidence and familial occurrence. N Engl J Med 319:343–347
54. Ruda R, Gilbert M, Soffietti R (2008) Ependymomas of the adult: molecular biology and treatment. Curr Opin Neurol 21:754–761

55. Samartzis D, Gillis CC, Shih P, O'Toole JE, Fessler RG (2015) Intramedullary spinal cord tumors: part I-epidemiology, pathophysiology, and diagnosis. Global Spine J 5:425–435
56. Samii M, Klekamp J (1994) Surgical results of 100 intramedullary tumors in relation to accompanying syringomyelia. Neurosurgery 35:865–873; discussion 873
57. Sandler HM, Papadopoulos SM, Thornton AF Jr, Ross DA (1992) Spinal cord astrocytomas: results of therapy. Neurosurgery 30:490–493
58. Schellinger KA, Propp JM, Villano JL, McCarthy BJ (2008) Descriptive epidemiology of primary spinal cord tumors. J Neurooncol 87:173–179
59. Schul DB, Wolf S, Krammer MJ, Landscheidt JF, Tomasino A, Lumenta CB (2012) Meningioma surgery in the elderly: outcome and validation of 2 proposed grading score systems. Neurosurgery 70:555–565
60. Sciubba DM, Chaichana KL, Woodworth GF, McGirt MJ, Gokaslan ZL, Jallo GI (2008) Factors associated with cervical instability requiring fusion after cervical laminectomy for intradural tumor resection. J Neurosurg Spine 8:413–419
61. Shrivastava RK, Epstein FJ, Perin NI, Post KD, Jallo GI (2005) Intramedullary spinal cord tumors in patients older than 50 years of age: management and outcome analysis. J Neurosurg Spine 2:249–255
62. Silver ML, Hennigar G (1952) Cerebellar hemangioma (hemangioblastoma); a clinicopathological review of 40 cases. J Neurosurg 9:484–494
63. Sun HI, Ozduman K, Usseli MI, Ozgen S, Pamir MN (2014) Sporadic spinal hemangioblastomas can be effectively treated by microsurgery alone. World Neurosurg 82:836–847
64. Vishteh AG, Sankhla S, Anson JA, Zabramski JM, Spetzler RF (1997) Surgical resection of intramedullary spinal cord cavernous malformations: delayed complications, long-term outcomes, and association with cryptic venous malformations. Neurosurgery 41:1094–1100; discussion 1100–1091
65. Wizigmann-Voos S, Breier G, Risau W, Plate KH (1995) Up-regulation of vascular endothelial growth factor and its receptors in von Hippel-Lindau disease-associated and sporadic hemangioblastomas. Cancer Res 55:1358–1364
66. Yao KC, McGirt MJ, Chaichana KL, Constantini S, Jallo GI (2007) Risk factors for progressive spinal deformity following resection of intramedullary spinal cord tumors in children: an analysis of 161 consecutive cases. J Neurosurg 107:463–468
67. Yeh JS, Sgouros S, Walsh AR, Hockley AD (2001) Spinal sagittal malalignment following surgery for primary intramedullary tumours in children. Pediatr Neurosurg 35:318–324
68. Zabramski JM, Wascher TM, Spetzler RF, Johnson B, Golfinos J, Drayer BP, Brown B, Rigamonti D, Brown G (1994) The natural history of familial cavernous malformations: results of an ongoing study. J Neurosurg 80:422–432

Intradural Extramedullary Spinal Tumors 17

Owoicho Adogwa and Richard G. Fessler

Although intradural tumors are uncommon, they should be considered in the differential diagnosis of patients presenting with back pain, radicular pain, sensorimotor deficits, or sphincter dysfunction. These tumors can be subclassified into extradural, intramedullary, and extramedullary spinal cord tumors on the basis of their anatomical relation to the spinal parenchyma. The heterogeneous cell composition of the intradural compartment allows the formation of neoplasms, arising from glial cells, neurons, and cells of spinal vasculature. In this chapter, we discuss the epidemiology, radiographic and histological characteristics, as well as the management of intradural extramedullary tumors.

17.1 Introduction

Primary tumors of the spinal cord are ten times less common than their intracranial counterparts and represent 2–4 % of all primary tumors of the central nervous system (CNS) [1, 2]. Notwithstanding the lower incidence of spinal cord tumors, the histopathology is similar to primary intracranial neoplasms [3, 4]. The majority of primary spinal cord tumors are classified as low grade according to the World Health Organization (WHO) pathology classification [5–7] (Figs. 17.1 and 17.2).

Spinal cord tumors are subdivided into three categories on the basis of their relationship to the thecal sac that surrounds the spinal spinal cord and cauda equina: extradural, intradural extramedullary, and intramedullary. Extradural tumors are the most common and primarily consist of systemic cancer metastases,

O. Adogwa
Department of Neurosurgery, Rush University Medical Center,
1725 W Harrison St., Suite 955, Chicago, IL, USA

R.G. Fessler (✉)
University of Chicago, Chicago, IL, USA
e-mail: rfessler@rush.edu

© Springer International Publishing Switzerland 2017

M. Berhouma, P. Krolak-Salmon (eds.), *Brain and Spine Surgery in the Elderly*,
DOI 10.1007/978-3-319-40232-1_17

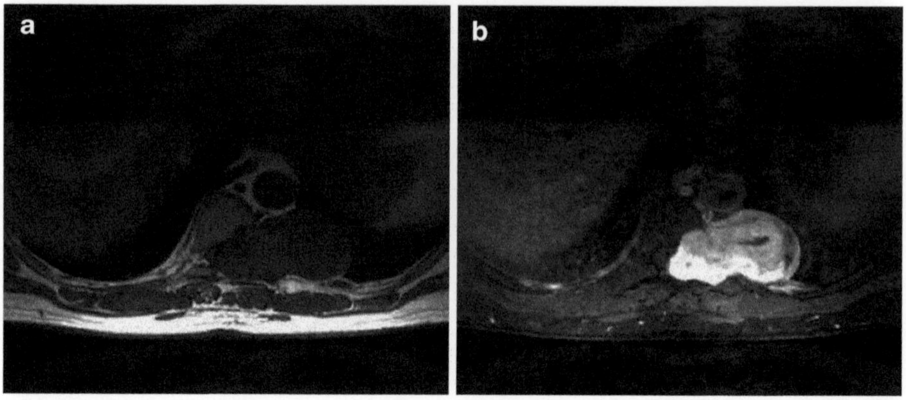

Fig. 17.1 Axial non-contrasted T1-weighted (**a**) and post-contrast (**b**) images of a thoracic dumbbell schwannoma

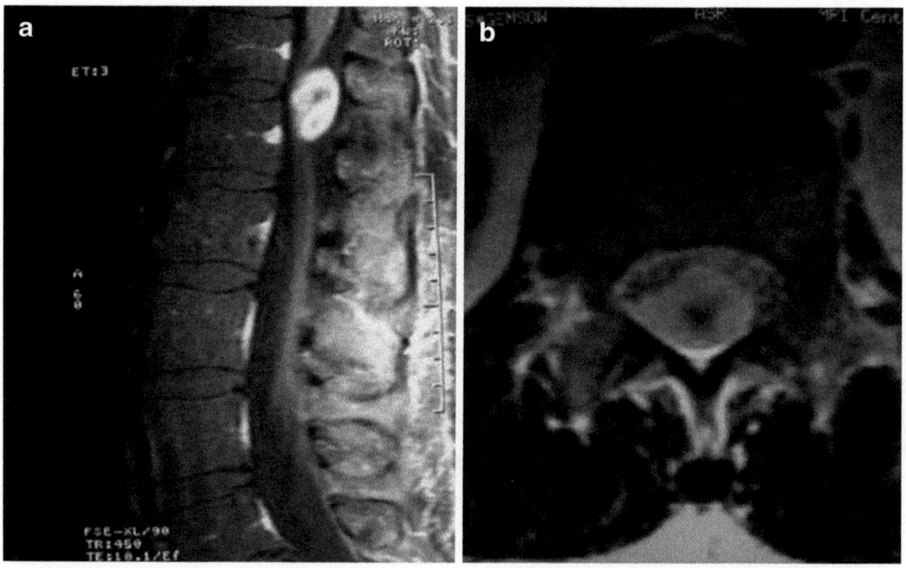

Fig. 17.2 Sagittal post-contrast T1-weighted (**a**) and axial non-contrasted T2-weighted (**b**) images of a lumbar intradural extramedullary nerve sheath tumor

resulting in epidural spinal cord compression, and are not discussed further in this chapter on primary intradural extramedullary spinal cord tumors [8]. Intradural extramedullary tumors are more common than intramedullary tumors, representing 80 % of all intradural tumors in adults and 65 % of all intradural tumors in children, with the most common tumors being schwannomas, meningiomas, and neurofibromas [4, 8–10]. Other tumor types, such as hemangiopericytoma, lipoma, paraganglioma, epidermoid cysts, and dermoid cysts, are less common. Intradural intramedullary spinal cord tumors (IMSCTs) constitute 20–30 % of all primary spinal cord tumors. About 90 % of IMSCTs are glial tumors, majority of which are ependymomas or astrocytomas [11–13]. Ependymomas represent about 60 % and astrocytomas 30 % [13, 14]. Of the intramedullary tumors with metastatic origins, 40–60 % and 14 % arise from primary neoplasms of the lung and breast, respectively [15–17] (Table 17.1).

Differentiation and diagnosis of spinal cord tumors are widely achievable through clinical examination and radiographic techniques. The clinical presentation is determined in part by the location of the tumor. Pain is the most common presenting symptom (72 %) and may manifest as back pain (27 %), radicular pain (25 %), or central pain (20 %) [18]. Motor disturbance is the next most common presenting symptom (55 %) followed by sensory loss (39 %; dermatomal, saddle, or segmental level) [18]. Sphincter disturbance is the least common presenting symptom seen in only 15 % of all patients [18].

MRI is the preferred method of radiographic assessment of intradural spinal tumors and can suggest histological subtype. Other radiographic modalities, such as CT and CT myelogram, are useful if contraindications to MRI exist. When tumors are suspected to have a vascular component, magnetic resonance angiogram (MRA) or spinal arteriogram can be beneficial. Histological examination of tumor after biopsy or surgical resection is useful to establish the histogenesis of intradural tumors in almost all cases.

17.2 Evaluation of the Patient with a Spinal Tumor

The evaluation of the patient with a known or suspected spinal tumor begins with a thorough history and physical examination. Patients with vertebral column tumors most frequently present with back pain but may also manifest spinal deformity, neurologic symptoms, and systemic symptoms related to malignancy. Elderly patients with intradural tumors infrequently have radicular or back pain but may present with neurologic deficit from spinal cord or root compromise.

The radiologic evaluation of the patient with a spinal tumor includes MRI for nearly all lesions. CT is particularly helpful for spinal column tumors in assessing the degree of vertebral bone destruction and osteopenia as well as for surgical planning. CT myelography may be useful in patients who are unable to undergo MRI. Plain and dynamic radiographs should also be obtained to assess deformity and instability. Radioisotope bone scanning is highly sensitive for spinal column tumors that demonstrate osteolytic or osteoblastic activity and is most frequently used when searching for small lesions, such as osteoid osteoma, or for metastases in patients with known malignancy. Finally, angiography delineates the vascular supply of a tumor and may also be used to perform embolization to reduce intraoperative blood loss from hypervascular lesions, such as an aneurysmal bone cyst, hemangioma, renal cell carcinoma, melanoma, or chordoma.

Table 17.1 Intradural extramedullary tumors

Tumor	Prevalence (%)	Location	Radiology MR	Treatment	Prognosis
Meningioma	50	Cervical/thoracic	T1, iso; T2, hyper	Resection	Good
			Contrast enhancing		
Schwannoma	25	Thoracic > cervical	T1, iso/hypo; T2, hyper	Resection	Good
			Contrast enhancing		
Neurofibroma	25	Thoracic, lumbar	Solid or plexiform	Resection	Good
			T1, hypo; T2, hyper		
			Contrast enhancing		
MPNST	Rare	No predilection	Rapid growth on serial MR, contrast enhancing	Resection/RT/CT	Poor
Leptomeningeal metastasis	Common	Lumbar	T1, iso	Intrathecal CT	Poor
			Contrast enhancing		
Paraganglioma	Rare	No predilection	T1, iso; T2, hyper	Resection	Fair
			Contrast enhancing		
Myxopapillary	Most common	Cervical, thoracic	T1, iso/hypo	Surgery; RT/CT	Good
Ependymoma			T2, hyper	If unresectable	
			Contrast enhancing		
Mesenchymal lipomas	Rare	Lumbar	T1, hyper	Surgery	Good
			T2, hyper		
			STIR, hypo		
			Non-enhancing		
Dermoid	Rare	Lumbar	T1, hypo	Surgery	Good
			T2, hyper		
			FLAIR, hyper		
			STIR, hypo		
			DWI, bright		
			Non-enhancing		
Epidermoid	Rare	Lumbar	T1, hypo/hyper	Surgery	Good
			T2, hyper		
			FLAIR, hyper		
			STIR, hypo		
			DWI, moderately bright		
			Non-enhancing		

17.3 Incidence and Etiology

17.3.1 Nerve Sheath Tumors

Nerve sheath tumors (NSTs) are categorized as neurofibromas or schwannomas. Although histological and immonuhistochemistry studies support a common Schwann cell origin for both tumor types, each of these tumor types displays distinct clinicopathological characteristics during the formation of intradural, extramedullary spinal tumors and as such merits separate consideration.

NSTs account for about 23–25 % of intradural spinal cord tumors in adults and about 14 % in pediatric patients [15–17]. The peak incidence of NSTs is between the fourth through sixth decade of life, with no gender predilection [19]. Schwannomas are more common than neurofibromas and usually present as solitary tumors that occur proportionally throughout the spinal canal. Neurofibromas often show multiplicity, especially when associated with neurofibromatosis type 1.

The majority of nerve sheath tumors arise from a dorsal root although neurofibromas represent a higher proportion of ventral root tumors [20]. Most spinal NSTs (75–80 %) reside intradurally, but about 30 % of these tumors extend through the dural root sleeve as a dumbbell-shaped tumor with intradural and extradural components [20]; 10 % of spinal NSTs are located extramedullary and 1 % are located intramedullary. Intradural nerve sheath tumors most commonly affect the lumbosacral region, but cervical and thoracic tumors have been reported as well. The intramedullary NSTs are thought to arise from the perivascular nerve sheaths that accompany penetrating spinal cord vessels. Although NSTs are generally regarded as benign neoplasms, they can be malignant in a few cases, where they are designated the term malignant peripheral nerve sheath tumors (MPNSTs). 0.7 % of spinal NSTs are malignant, resulting in an exceedingly poor prognosis (median overall survival of ~22 months), irrespective of cranial or spinal location [18].

On imaging, NSTs have an isointense signal on T1-weighted images (T1WI) and a hyperintense signal on T2-weighted images (T2WI), with variable enhancement ranging from a homogeneous to a peripheral ring-like enhancement, after contrast administration.

Surgical resection is the primary treatment for NSTs, which is obtainable in most cases. Subtotal resection of these tumors might be an option when the tumor is attached to the spinal cord or when the tumor exhibits an extradural component closely associated with vital structures, such as the vertebral artery in the cervical region. Radiotherapy and chemotherapy are usually reserved for tumors that have malignant histological characteristics. Tumor recurrence is less than 5 % and might have a high association with subtotal tumor removal.

17.3.1.1 Schwannoma

Schwannomas are the most common intradural extramedullary (IDEM) spinal tumors, representing 30 % of such lesions and occurring at a rate of approximately 0.3–0.4 cases per 100 000 persons per year [18, 21]. They are benign tumors (WHO grade I), although malignant subtypes exist and usually arise from the dorsal sensory roots [22, 23]. Patients usually present in the fourth through sixth decades. Topographically, spinal cord nerve sheath tumors are located in the upper cervical region (16 %), cervical cord (31 %), thoracic cord (22 %), conus medullaris (7 %), and cauda equina (24 %) [15, 17, 24, 25].

The majority are solitary and sporadic; however, there is an association with NF2 [26]. Patients with NF2 often have multiple schwannomas and have high risk for malignant transformation [26]. The NF2 protein is thought to be a member of the ERM family of proteins, which is responsible for linking cytoskeletal components with proteins of the cell membrane that regulate cytoskeletal dynamics and cell-to-cell communication [15, 16]. Mutations in *NF2* may lead to the development of vestibular schwannomas (classically bilateral tumors of cranial nerve XIII), neurofibromas, ependymomas, gliomas, and meningiomas [9, 10, 15].

Schwannomas are either discovered incidentally or patients present with mild sensory symptoms consisting of shooting pain or paresthesias with nerve palpation; spontaneous pain can occur, but is uncommon.

On MRI, schwannomas appear as solid tumors in the dorsal sensory root region, with displacement of the spinal cord, conus medullaris, or filum terminale. Two thirds of schwannomas are slightly iso- to hypointense on T1WI and hyperintense on T2WI. Nearly all show intense enhancement following contrast administration. Enhancement patterns are homogeneous in 67 %, mildly inhomogeneous in 10 %, and heterogeneous with areas of intratumoral cystic degeneration in 22 %. Peritumoral edema is present in 37 %. Hemorrhage and calcification are not usually present [19, 23, 26].

Grossly, schwannomas appear as smooth globoid masses that do not enlarge the nerve but are suspended eccentrically from it with a discrete attachment. Histologically, they consist of elongated bipolar cells with fusiform, darkly staining nuclei arranged in a compact interlacing fascicles with a tendency toward palisade formation. Antoni A areas are more compact stellate-shaped cells while Antoni B areas are a loosely arranged pattern [25, 27, 28].

Especially in the elderly asymptomatic patient, schwannomas may be followed with serial imaging given their usual benign behavior. For symptomatic patients or radiographically enlarging tumors, maximal safe surgical resection is the most effective treatment modality. In most cases, schwannomas have an easily identified plane of dissection, and thus gross total resection (GTR) is the primary form of treatment [17, 25, 26, 29, 30]. Surgery is associated with minimal morbidity and provides symptomatic relief, and with complete surgical en bloc resection, local control rates of 90–100 % have been reported. Adjuvant therapy is typically not recommended, and incompletely resected tumors should be followed with serial MR imaging given the benign growth and natural history of these tumors. Malignant schwannomas should be treated with postoperative radiotherapy, even if total resection was achieved. At present there are no compelling data to suggest a role for either chemotherapy or targeted therapy, notwithstanding recent reports of response of vestibular schwannomas to bevacizumab and epidermal growth factor receptor inhibitors. In elderly patients with poor functional reserve that are unable to undergo surgical resection, stereotactic radiosurgery is an option for these patients.

17.3.1.2 Neurofibroma

Neurofibromas are usually benign tumors (WHO grade I) that arise from peripheral nerves. Two types are recognized: general (solitary, circumscribed, or globular) and plexiform. Solitary neurofibromas are usually discretely localized, globular, or fusiform nodules. Plexiform neurofibromas are characterized by redundant loops of nerve fiber bundles and tumor tissue intermixed in a disorganized pattern that extends over multiple nerve roots [30–33]. Unlike Schwannomas, neurofibromas encase nerve roots rather than displacing them.

Neurofibromas appear to be more common in patients with neurofibromatosis type 1 (*NF1*), a condition that results from a mutation in the neurofibromin 1 gene located on chromosome 17q11 [8, 12, 14, 15, 25]. NF1 is thought to encode a protease involved in Ras-GTP phosphorylation, which reduces activation of downstream mitogen-activated protein kinases (MAPKs) involved in cell proliferation and survival [8, 12, 14, 15, 25]. NF1 mutations are associated with an increased risk for the development of malignant peripheral NSTs and of a set of diverse tumors, including carcinoid tumors, optic nerve gliomas, pheochromocytomas, and rhabdomyosarcomas [15, 16].

On imaging, spinal neurofibromas are often indistinguishable from schwannomas. They are most commonly fusiform in shape, unlike schwannomas, which tend to be characteristically round. They encase the nerve roots with fibers interwoven with nerve tissue, in contrast to schwannomas, which commonly displace the nerve root due to their asymmetric growth. They are generally hypointense on T1WI and hyperintense on T2WI, although a T2 hyperintense rim and central area of low signal may be seen. Moderate enhancement is usually seen post-contrast.

If asymptomatic, neurofibromas can be followed with serial MR imaging. Patients with symptomatic or enlarging solitary tumors should undergo surgical resection. GTR with minimal morbidity can be achieved. The clinical results following resection of a plexiform neurofibroma associated with NF1 are poor because GTR is rarely achieved. Plexiform neurofibromas may undergo malignant transformation (malignant peripheral nerve sheath tumor [MPNST]). Radiotherapy or chemotherapy is almost never employed for benign neurofibromas. Patients with NF1 may be at risk for malignant degeneration following radiotherapy [41]. Data on chemotherapy use is limited to MPNSTs and is usually Adriamycin based as with other soft tissue sarcomas.

17.4 Meningioma

Spinal meningiomas account for up to 50 % of intradural spinal neoplasms and are the most common spinal tumors in adults [8–10, 13]. They usually arise from meningothelial arachnoid cap cells embedded in the dura near the root sleeve, which accounts for their predominant lateral position [25, 27]. They may also arise from pia or dural fibroblasts, probably as a result of their mesodermal origin [8–10, 13]. Although intradural meningiomas are usually solitary lesions, multiplicity might be encountered when these tumors are associated with neurofibromatosis type 2. Although meningiomas can develop in any age group, the preponderance occurs in individuals between the fifth and seventh decades. The majority (~80 %) of spinal cord meningioma patients are women, and 70–80 % occur in the thoracic region [8–10, 13]. The female preponderance in the adult population is thought to be due to the effect of estrogen, although the exact mechanism remains unclear [15]. In men, spinal cord meningiomas are equally distributed between the cervical and thoracic cord. Overall, 15 % of spinal cord meningiomas occur in the cervical spine, 81 % in the thoracic spine, and 4 % in the lumbar spine [18, 19, 26, 34].

The vast majority are WHO grade I lesions [18, 19, 26, 34]. Genetic predisposition (NF2) and prior exposure to ionizing radiation are the only definite risk factors [18, 19, 26, 34]. Similar histological subtypes are observed in both intracranial and spinal meningiomas, including meningothelial, metaplastic, psammomatous, transitional, atypical, and clear cell types. The psammomatous, meningothelial, and transitional subtypes are the most common meningiomas of the spine and, for reasons that are unknown, show a lower risk for recurrence than their intracranial counterparts [18, 19, 26, 34]. Multiple genes have been associated with spinal meningiomas – complete or partial loss of chromosome 22 and of its associated gene *NF2* along with loss of 1p, 9p, and 10q has all been implicated [29].

Meningiomas are either discovered incidentally or present commonly with back pain (70 %), motor dysfunction (60 %), sensory disturbance (40 %), and incontinence (40 %) [18, 20, 21, 35].

Radiographically, plain films are usually normal. Calcification is very rare and may be present in 1–5 % of cases. Bone erosion is atypical. On MR scans, most appear isointense with the spinal cord on both T1WI and T2WI and lightly hyperintense on T2W/fluid-attenuated inversion recovery (FLAIR) images. Meningiomas display intense, homogeneous enhancement following contrast administration. Occasionally, densely calcified meningiomas are profoundly hypointense on MR and demonstrate minimal contrast enhancement [18, 20, 21, 35].

Surgery is the most effective treatment modality. Most intradural meningiomas are noninvasive, benign neoplasms, helping with gross total resection of the tumor.

In most cases, meningiomas have an easily identified plane of dissection, and thus GTR is the primary form of treatment [17, 25, 26, 29, 30]. With complete surgical en bloc resection, local control rates of 90–100 % have been reported; however, gross total resection is not always achieved mostly due to tumor location and the need to preserve neurological function. The tumor recurrence rate with total or subtotal resection is between 3 and 7 %. Atypical and anaplastic spinal meningiomas have a higher tumor recurrence rate though rarely metastasize. Radiotherapy could be considered after subtotal resection or recurrence of spinal meningiomas though data on its effectiveness remains sparse.

17.5 Ependymoma

About 40 % of spinal canal ependymomas arise within the filum terminale. Although filum terminale ependymomas can develop in any age group, the majority occurs in individuals between the third and fifth decades [19, 26]. There appears to be a gender predilection as they tend to occur in men slightly more often than in women.

Myxopapillary ependymomas are by far the most common histologic type encountered in the filum terminale. They are WHO grade I lesions and histologically consist of papillary arrangement of cuboidal or columnar tumor cells surrounding a vascularized core of hyalinized and poorly cellular connective tissue [19, 26]. Mucinous changes undergone by tumor cells distinguish them from variants of ependymomas.

Patients typically present with radicular symptoms, lower extremity sensorimotor deficits, and/or sphincter dysfunction.

Myxopapillary ependymomas are typically benign, well-circumscribed tumors. Radiographically, they appear as a circumscribed mass with hypointense signal on T1WI and hyperintense signal on T2WI. They demonstrate homogeneous enhancement following contrast administration. Histologically, myxopapillary ependymomas display ependymal rosettes or perivascular pseudorosettes, with the characteristic deposition of myxoid material around blood vessels.

Surgery is the preferred treatment option. GTR of myxopapillary ependymomas is feasible if the nerve roots in the cauda equina are not entrapped within the tumor. In situations where the neural elements are entrapped within the tumor, maximal safe resection or subtotal resection is the preferred option in order to minimize surgical morbidity. Focal fractionalized radiotherapy seems to be effective at improving neurological outcome and reducing tumor recurrence rate after subtotal tumor resection or piecemeal total excision. These tumors can seed to the spinal subarachnoid space, in which case broader field radiation is used, but this is uncommon. Although chemotherapy is sometimes started for recurrent or disseminated myxopapillary ependymomas, results are unconvincing.

17.6 Paraganglioma

Spinal paragangliomas are rare heterogeneous tumors of neural crest origin commonly found in the cauda equina and filum terminale [30–32]. They are usually benign, nonfunctioning, sympathetic tumors and histologically resemble extra-adrenal paraganglia [30–32]. Paragangliomas tend to occur in the fourth to fifth decades of life and show a male predominance. They appear to have a predilection for the cauda equina and lumbar regions, although intradural thoracic or cervical paragangliomas frequently occur.

Radiographically, they appear as well-circumscribed vascular tumors that are difficult to differentiate radiographically and clinically from filum terminale ependymomas [30–32]. They are hypointense to isointense on T1WI and hyperintense on T2WI. They characteristically produce a heterogeneous "salt and pepper" pattern after contrast administration. Hemorrhage and intratumoral vessels with flow voids are common features of this tumor [10, 19, 26]. Scanning using radiolabeled metaiodobenzylguanidine (mIBG), a noradrenaline analogue with uptake independent of catecholamine secretion, can allow visualization of paragangliomas. Histologically, paragangliomas display a highly vascularized tumor bed containing round and polygonal cells grouped in clusters called zellballen. Immunohistological methods to detect chromogranin and synaptophysin can be useful for diagnosis.

They are usually benign tumors and GTR is the preferred treatment. Although catecholamine-secreting spinal paragangliomas are uncommon, preoperative screening for a hyperadrenergic state is necessary, particularly in elderly patients, to prevent hypertensive crisis during tumor removal. Laboratory analysis may include fractionated plasma metanephrines and 24 h urine catecholamine and metanephrine tests. Where an elevation is found, a clonidine suppression test can be done. Recurrence rate after sub-total resection (STR) is less than 6 % and does not appear to be reduced by concomitant radiotherapy or chemotherapy. Although iodine-131-labeled mIBG can slow progression and improve remission rate for metastatic paragangliomas, efficacy in primary intradural paragangliomas remains unknown.

17.7 Leptomeningeal Metastases

Leptomeningeal metastases are a common complication of cancer. These tumors are commonly the result of drop lesions from intracranial metastasis. They may also represent drop lesions from intracranial neoplasms such as gliomas and medulloblastomas. Metastatic spread from intracranial lesions can involve dissemination of neoplastic cells through the cerebrospinal fluid (CSF), and multiple lesions are common. They occur most frequently in the thoracolumbar or thoracic spine and tend to present as localized pain and spinal tenderness. Patients may also present with a radicular pain pattern; motor and sensory deficits are common. Sphincter dysfunction is present in about 33 % of patients.

The diagnosis can be challenging; however, early diagnosis and aggressive treatment can prevent irreversible neurologic deficits. Diagnosis is usually established by the demonstration of malignant cells in the cerebrospinal fluid (CSF) or by the presence of enhancing tumor nodules on spinal MRI [31]. Leptomeningeal metastases may present with three different imaging patterns: (1) diffuse, thin, enhancing coating of the surface of the spinal cord and nerve roots; (2) multiple small enhancing nodules on the surface of the cord and/or nerve roots; and (3) as a single mass in the lowest part of the thecal sac [31]. Unenhanced T1-weighted images might be normal or demonstrate nodular lesions that are isointense to the spinal cord, whereas the contrast-enhanced images demonstrate significant enhancement.

Intradural extramedullary metastasis usually suggests advanced widespread progression of the systemic malignancy; aggressive surgical resection of lesions is usually not recommended. Treatment is, therefore, directed toward palliative and functional goals. Radiotherapy allows improvement in neurological function in a large population of patients. Adjuvant treatment with intravenous or oral corticosteroids can improve neurological function as well and provide symptomatic relief.

17.8 CNS Lipoma

Lipomas are congenital, benign tumors that are found infrequently in the intradural compartment. They arise from premature disjunction of the neural ectoderm from the cutaneous ectoderm and are frequently associated with spinal dysraphisms. They are typically seen in young patients, however, and can be infrequently seen in older patients [15, 19, 26, 29]. They are typically slow growing tumors and become symptomatic because of the mass effect from their size. Intradural extramedullary lipomas are frequently located in the lower thoracic and lumbosacral regions.

Patients typically present with dysesthetic sensory changes, pain, gait abnormalities, paresis, and incontinence. Radiographically, they are hyperintense on T1- and T2-weighted images and show signal hypointensity on fat-suppressed or STIR images. These lesions are non-enhancing on post-contrast MRI. Microscopically, lipomas consist of mature adipose cells and connective tissue.

Surgery is the preferred treatment, although timing of surgery remains a controversial topic. Furthermore, the absence of a cleavage plane and the intermingling of neural and fibrofatty tissue at the periphery of the tumor make GTR very challenging. Intraoperative electrophysiological stimulation with evoked EMG monitoring is often used to allow differentiation between the functional spinal cord and the tumor. When complete or near total resection is achieved, there is a 90 % long-term progression-free survival at 16 years compared with only 35 % at 10 years after subtotal resection. Unfortunately, the improvement of neurologic symptoms postoperatively is not universal.

17.9 Hemangiopericytoma

Intradural extramedullary hemangiopericytomas are uncommon neoplasms of the CNS with uncertain histogenesis. They are hypercellular tumors with frequent mitoses and necrosis seen on microscopic examination. Hemangiopericytomas have an aggressive clinical course with high recurrence rates. Accordingly, surgical resection is usually needed. Because of the notable vascularity of these tumors, preoperative embolization is often attempted. Radiotherapy has proven effective in reducing recurrence of intracranial hemangiopericytomas, but there is insufficient evidence relating to spinal locations.

17.10 Epidermoid Cysts

Epidermoid cysts are uncommon lesions that comprise less than 1 % of all spinal tumors. They are more frequent in children and are usually congenital neoplasms arising from heterotopic ectodermal cell implantation into the neural tube early in embryonic development. They can be acquired and are considered a late complication of lumbar puncture. Lumbar punctures with nonstyleted needles have been implicated and are thought to introduce epidermal elements into the spinal canal that slowly grows, resulting in an intradural extramedullary neoplasm.

Patients typically present with radicular pain, motor deficits, gait abnormalities, and, infrequently, sphincter dysfunction. Radiographically, imaging findings are variable. These tumors are usually iso- to hyperintense compared to CSF on all sequences. There is usually minimum enhancement with gadolinium.

17.11 Dermoid Cysts

Intradural dermoid tumors are considered one of the congenital midline cystic tumors. Dermoids are thought to originate from epithelial inclusions within the neural groove during development. These tumors most commonly affect the lumbosacral region, with rare reports of thoracic involvement. Although these tumors usually present in the first two decades of life, they can infrequently present in elderly patients. On gross appearance, they may have skin appendages such as hair follicles and glandular tissue, which helps differentiate them from epidermoids. Radiographically, they have a variable imaging appearance though are hypointense to hyperintense signal on T1-weighted images and isointense to hyperintense signal on T2-weighted images. Dermoids weakly enhance after contrast administration.

Gross total resection is preferred when possible, but adhesion to neural tissue can prevent aggressive techniques. When STR is performed, emptying of the cystic contents and removal of a portion of the capsule are advised. Dissemination of the cystic contents spontaneously or during tumor removal might produce a granulomatous meningitis treatable with corticosteroids. Recurrence of resected intradural dermoid cysts is uncommon, and malignant transformation is uncommon. Adjuvant radiotherapy or chemotherapy for non-operable or malignant cases has not been thoroughly studied.

17.12 Principles of Treatment

The objectives of the surgical treatment for any spinal tumor must be clearly defined and discussed with the patient. In some cases, diagnosis may be the primary goal, and for many extradural tumors, this can be accomplished by image-guided biopsy, with relatively high diagnostic accuracy. IDEM tumors, however, require open exploration to obtain a biopsy safely for diagnostic certainty.

For most IDEM tumors and a number of primary spinal column tumors, lasting cure is the goal of surgery. Numerous studies have demonstrated that negative margins with en bloc resection of primary malignant tumors of the spine significantly decrease recurrence rates and prolong survival [9, 10, 15]. The surgical approach must be tailored to meet this marginal goal.

Conversely, for most metastatic lesions, symptomatic relief and palliation are the most common goals of surgical intervention; therefore, the effects of any selected treatment on the patient's quality of life must be carefully considered. In fact, for carefully selected patients with spinal metastases, surgical intervention may offer the best chance of improved quality of life.

In addition to the goals of (1) diagnosis, (2) tumor removal for local control or cure, (3) circumferential spinal cord decompression, and (4) symptomatic pain relief, any approach to spinal tumors must take into account the stability of the spinal segments involved. Where indicated, treatment options should incorporate arthrodesis, deformity correction, and fixation for levels that have been destabilized by the tumor or by the treatment itself.

17.13 Surgery in Elderly Patients

Traditional open decompressive operations for spinal tumors can carry up to a 30% complication rate, including neurologic deterioration, severe medical complications, massive hemorrhage, wound infections and dehiscence, hardware complications, cerebrospinal fluid (CSF) leaks, and death. This is particularly relevant for elderly patients with poor functional reserve in whom surgery is being considered. Wound complications after open surgery can affect up to 40% of patients.

Typical open surgical approaches also have significant drawbacks. First, subperiosteal dissection is required; therefore, denervation and devascularization of the paraspinal musculature ensue. This iatrogenic injury has been shown to lead to significant diminishment in postoperative axial muscle strength and performance. Second, in addition to sacrificing the bony and ligamentous portions of the posterior tension band, open laminectomy in the cervical spine injures the semispinalis capitis and cervicis muscles, which are thought to provide the primary force for maintained extension of the head and cervical spine. These untoward effects can produce iatrogenic sagittal plane destabilization that may lead to a progressive spinal deformity, most frequently seen in the cervical spine. Also known as postlaminectomy kyphosis, such deformity may occur in up to 10–40% of adults after laminectomy and is most common after intradural tumor surgery. Such deformity has been shown to affect outcomes negatively.

17.14 Minimally Invasive Techniques

The motivation to develop minimally invasive strategies to treat spinal tumors in elderly patients is driven by the significant complication rates associated with established surgical approaches to neoplastic spinal disease. The factors that influence the decision to use minimally invasive techniques in the treatment of spinal tumors are the same as those affecting the decision to initiate surgical therapy in the first place, namely, life expectancy; health status of the patient; tumor type, location, and extent; symptomatology; prior therapies; and spinal stability. The indications for intervention are intractable pain, neurologic deficit, spinal deformity, need for diagnosis, and tumor cure or control. To that end, the primary objective of minimally invasive surgery is to reduce approach-related injury to normal spinal anatomy around the lesion of interest. Ultimately, this should translate into shorter operative times, reduced blood loss, shorter hospital stays, fewer complications, less postoperative pain, reduced medication use, decreased medical resource use, and faster recovery times.

17.15 Treatment of Intradural Extramedullary Tumors

Patients' preoperative neurologic status and tumor histopathology are the most important factors in determining long-term neurological and functional outcome after surgery for patients with IDEM spinal cord tumors. Surgical morbidity has been significantly improved by advances in minimally invasive surgery, microsurgical techniques, and intraoperative electrophysiological monitoring.

GTR remains the primary goal of treatment for most types of IDEM tumors. Intraoperatively, the ability to identify a tumor–spinal cord plane has been a guiding principle for successful tumor resectability. Some tumors have a cleavage plane that facilitates the resection; however, other more infiltrative tumors lacking a tumor–normal spinal cord interface, such as lipomas, may not have such a plane, making complete resection impossible. When a plane of dissection is absent, resection can be associated with poor surgical outcomes despite electrophysiological monitoring during the procedure.

The treatment of recurrent IDEM tumors is largely based on tumor histology and remains controversial. In cases of subtotal resection, patients should be routinely followed by serial MRI for evidence of tumor progression, and radiation therapy is offered to patients with recurrence or enlarging tumors. In the rare cases where the tumor has infiltrated the spinal cord parenchyma, radical resection results in high morbidity. Therefore, conservative tumor removal or tissue diagnosis followed by radiation therapy is common practice. Re-resection is offered to patients with recurring IDEM tumors, as most are amenable to safe, complete removal with a low recurrence rate.

17.16 Radiosurgery

Stereotactic radiosurgery (SRS) has also been used in the treatment of intradural tumors [4]. SRS typically has been used to treat IDEM nerve sheath tumors and meningiomas but has also been applied to some hemangioblastomas, paragangliomas, and hemangiopericytomas [5, 8]. In 75–100 % of benign IDEM tumors, growth arrest or a decrease in tumor size has been seen on follow-up imaging after SRS. In 2005, Bhatnagar and colleagues reported 45 cases of benign intradural tumors treated by SRS with the CyberKnife [36]. The median treatment time was 59 min. Tumor doses (80 % isodose line) ranged from 9 to 31 Gy, with a median of 16 Gy [36]. Symptomatic improvement was seen in 78 % of patients, and the local control rate with a median follow-up of 8 months was 96 %. No toxicity from the treatments was observed. Interestingly, 42 % of the lesions had undergone prior surgery, and 20 % had received prior external beam radiation therapy (EBRT) [20, 27, 36]. Although these types of studies show promise for this modality in the treatment of benign intradural tumors, dosing has yet to be defined, the follow-up periods are far too short for lesions with benign histology, and comparative studies are lacking. For the time being, SRS of benign intradural tumors should likely be reserved for those patients who are unable to undergo more definitive surgical treatment or for whom other treatments have failed. SRS may be of particular benefit in patients with phakomatoses and multiple tumors, such as neurofibromatosis and von Hippel–Lindau disease.

Conclusion

Although rare, intradural spinal cord tumors should be an important consideration in the differential diagnosis of the elderly patients presenting with back or radicular pain associated with neurologic deficits. Radiographic assessment combined with histological examination helps with the identification of the histogenesis of these tumors, which is vital when exploring surgical and adjuvant treatment options and patient management. Advances in minimally invasive and microsurgical techniques have facilitated complete resection and definitive treatment in some cases; however, for more infiltrative IDEM tumors, adjuvant radiotherapy may be required. Early diagnoses and aggressive definitive treatment, when possible, optimize the management of these tumors.

References

1. Mechtler LL, Nandigam K (2013) Spinal cord tumors: new views and future directions. Neurol Clin 31(1):241–268
2. Hirano K, Imagama S, Sato K et al (2012) Primary spinal cord tumors: review of 678 surgically treated patients in Japan. A multicenter study. Eur Spine J 21(10):2019–2026
3. Abdel-Wahab M, Etuk B, Palermo J et al (2006) Spinal cord gliomas: a multi-institutional retrospective analysis. Int J Radiat Oncol Biol Phys 64(4):1060–1071
4. Abul-Kasim K, Thurnher MM, McKeever P, Sundgren PC (2008) Intradural spinal tumors: current classification and MRI features. Neuroradiology 50(4):301–314
5. Adams H, Avendano J, Raza SM, Gokaslan ZL, Jallo GI, Quinones-Hinojosa A (2012) Prognostic factors and survival in primary malignant astrocytomas of the spinal cord: a population-based analysis from 1973 to 2007. Spine (Phila Pa 1976) 37(12):E727–E735
6. Alfieri A, Mazzoleni G, Schwarz A et al (2005) Renal cell carcinoma and intradural spinal metastasis with cauda equina infiltration: case report--part II. Spine (Phila Pa 1976) 30(2):260–262
7. Arima H, Hasegawa T, Togawa D et al (2014) Feasibility of a novel diagnostic chart of intramedullary spinal cord tumors in magnetic resonance imaging. Spinal Cord 52(10):769–773
8. Chamberlain MC, Tredway TL (2011) Adult primary intradural spinal cord tumors: a review. Curr Neurol Neurosci Rep 11(3):320–328
9. Bostrom A, Kanther NC, Grote A, Bostrom J (2014) Management and outcome in adult intramedullary spinal cord tumours: a 20-year single institution experience. BMC Res Notes 7:908
10. Brotchi J (2013) Intramedullary astrocytomas surgery in adult patients: the rationale for cautious surgery. World Neurosurg 80(5):e139–e140
11. Cooper PR, Epstein F (1985) Radical resection of intramedullary spinal cord tumors in adults. Recent experience in 29 patients. J Neurosurg 63(4):492–499
12. Cristante L, Herrmann HD (1994) Surgical management of intramedullary spinal cord tumors: functional outcome and sources of morbidity. Neurosurgery 35(1):69–74; discussion 74–66
13. DeWire M, Fouladi M, Turner DC et al (2015) An open-label, two-stage, phase II study of bevacizumab and lapatinib in children with recurrent or refractory ependymoma: a collaborative ependymoma research network study (CERN). J Neurooncol 123(1):85–91
14. Dudley RW, Torok MR, Gallegos DR et al (2015) Pediatric low-grade ganglioglioma: epidemiology, treatments, and outcome analysis on 348 children from the surveillance, epidemiology, and end results database. Neurosurgery 76(3):313–319; discussion 319; quiz 319–320
15. el-Mahdy W, Kane PJ, Powell MP, Crockard HA (1999) Spinal intradural tumours: part I – extramedullary. Br J Neurosurg 13(6):550–557
16. Goodwin CR, Sankey EW, Liu A et al (2015) A systematic review of clinical outcomes for patients diagnosed with skin cancer spinal metastases. J Neurosurg Spine 6:1–13
17. Gunther JR, Sato M, Chintagumpala M et al (2015) Imaging changes in pediatric intracranial ependymoma patients treated with proton beam radiation therapy compared to intensity modulated radiation therapy. Int J Radiat Oncol Biol Phys 93(1):54–63

18. Traul DE, Shaffrey ME, Schiff D (2007) Part I: spinal-cord neoplasms-intradural neoplasms. Lancet Oncol 8(1):35–45
19. Kalayci M, Cagavi F, Gul S, Yenidunya S, Acikgoz B (2004) Intramedullary spinal cord metastases: diagnosis and treatment – an illustrated review. Acta Neurochir (Wien) 146(12):1347–1354; discussion 1354
20. Spirig J, Fournier JY, Hildebrandt G, Gautschi OP (2011) [Spinal tumors – part 2: intradural tumors. Epidemiology, clinical aspects and therapy]. Praxis (Bern 1994) 100(14):849–856
21. Tan LA, Kasliwal MK, Wewel J, Fontes RB, O'Toole JE (2014) Minimally invasive surgery for synchronous, same-level lumbar intradural-extramedullary neoplasm and acute disc herniation. Neurosurg Focus 37(Suppl 2):Video 16
22. Lonser RR, Weil RJ, Wanebo JE, DeVroom HL, Oldfield EH (2003) Surgical management of spinal cord hemangioblastomas in patients with von Hippel-Lindau disease. J Neurosurg 98(1):106–116
23. Mataliotakis G, Perera S, Nagaraju S, Marchionni M, Tzerakis N (2014) Intradural extramedullary cavernoma of a lumbar nerve root mimicking neurofibroma. A report of a rare case and the differential diagnosis. Spine J 14(12):e1–e7
24. O'Toole JE, Eichholz KM, Fessler RG (2006) Minimally invasive approaches to vertebral column and spinal cord tumors. Neurosurg Clin N Am 17(4):491–506
25. Parsa AT, Chi JH, Acosta FL Jr, Ames CP, McCormick PC (2005) Intramedullary spinal cord tumors: molecular insights and surgical innovation. Clin Neurosurg 52:76–84
26. Kane PJ, el-Mahdy W, Singh A, Powell MP, Crockard HA (1999) Spinal intradural tumours: part II – intramedullary. Br J Neurosurg 13(6):558–563
27. Parsa AT, Lee J, Parney IF, Weinstein P, McCormick PC, Ames C (2004) Spinal cord and intradural-extraparenchymal spinal tumors: current best care practices and strategies. J Neurooncol 69(1-3):291–318
28. Quinones-Hinojosa A, Gulati M, Lyon R, Gupta N, Yingling C (2002) Spinal cord mapping as an adjunct for resection of intramedullary tumors: surgical technique with case illustrations. Neurosurgery 51(5):1199–1206; discussion 1206–1197
29. Karsy M, Guan J, Sivakumar W, Neil JA, Schmidt MH, Mahan MA (2015) The genetic basis of intradural spinal tumors and its impact on clinical treatment. Neurosurg Focus 39(2):E3
30. Raco A, Esposito V, Lenzi J, Piccirilli M, Delfini R, Cantore G (2005) Long-term follow-up of intramedullary spinal cord tumors: a series of 202 cases. Neurosurgery 56(5):972–981; discussion 972–981
31. Quraishi NA, Arealis G, Salem KM, Purushothamdas S, Edwards KL, Boszczyk BM (2015) The surgical management of metastatic spinal tumors based on an Epidural Spinal Cord Compression (ESCC) scale. Spine J 15(8):1738–1743
32. Rodrigues GB, Waldron JN, Wong CS, Laperriere NJ (2000) A retrospective analysis of 52 cases of spinal cord glioma managed with radiation therapy. Int J Radiat Oncol Biol Phys 48(3):837–842
33. Samartzis D, Gillis CC, Shih P, O'Toole JE, Fessler RG (2015) Intramedullary spinal cord tumors: part I-epidemiology, pathophysiology, and diagnosis. Global Spine J 5(5):425–435
34. Wolf M, Kloth JK, Hahnel S, Rehnitz C, Wiedenhofer B, Weber MA (2012) Radiological diagnostics of spinal tumors. Part 2: special diagnostics of intradural tumors and tumor-like lesions. Orthopade 41(8):608–617
35. Spirig J, Fournier JY, Hildebrandt G, Gautschi OP (2011) Spinal tumors – part 1: extradural tumors. Epidemiology, clinical aspects and therapy. Praxis (Bern 1994) 100(14):839–848
36. Bhatnagar AK, Gerszten PC, Ozhasaglu C et al (2005) CyberKnife Frameless Radiosurgery for the treatment of extracranial benign tumors. Technol Cancer Res Treat 4(5):571–576

Spinal Infections 18

Hideki Nagashima

18.1 Terminology and Pathogenesis

The term spinal infection includes spondylitis, vertebral osteomyelitis, discitis, spondylodiscitis, and epidural abscess, i.e., the terms listed are different because they occur in different anatomic locations. Since the nucleus pulposus is an avascular structure in adults, most spinal infections do not originate in the disk. Infection starts in the metaphyseal region of one vertebra, where pathogens lodge in end arterioles that form arcades with slow blood flow. After destruction of the end plate, infection then spreads into the disk. Pathogens reach the adjacent vertebra via the same mechanism [184].

In children, the nucleus pulposus is vascularized and supplied with nutrients from intermetaphyseal arteries, and pathogens can directly access the vascularized nucleus pulposus and invade two adjacent vertebrae via destruction of both end plates [34, 102]. In the third decade of life, the nucleus pulposus becomes avascular as these arteries degenerate [34]. Despite these differences in the pathogenesis of spinal infection between adults and children, the most common type of spinal infection is spondylodiscitis in both age groups. During disease progression, some spinal infections form abscesses, such as retropharyngeal, retromediastinal, and psoas abscesses [99]. An abscess in the spinal canal is an epidural abscess, which may cause neurologic deficits [30, 66, 177]. Paraspinal or epidural abscesses have been reported in 44 % of patients with spinal infections [117, 123, 136, 146, 191].

H. Nagashima, MD, DMSc
Department of Orthopedic Surgery, Faculty of Medicine, Tottori University, 36-1 Nishi-cho, Yonago, Tottori 683-8504, Japan
e-mail: hidekin@med.tottori-u.ac.jp

© Springer International Publishing Switzerland 2017

M. Berhouma, P. Krolak-Salmon (eds.), *Brain and Spine Surgery in the Elderly*,
DOI 10.1007/978-3-319-40232-1_18

18.2 Epidemiology and Etiology

Spinal infections are uncommon causes of neck, back, or low back pain, accounting for less than 0.01 % of cases in the primary care setting [24]. The incidence of spinal infections has been reported as 1 per 500,000–1 per 250,000 [1, 21, 25, 46, 77, 100]. The spine is the site of 2–16.7 % of all bone infections [25, 46, 60, 90, 123, 152, 153, 164]. Males are more vulnerable to spinal infections than females, with a male predominance of 55–75 % [24, 81, 115, 123, 137, 159, 166, 174]. Around 2000, the mean age of patients with spinal infection was approximately 60 years [24, 125]. A systematic review [123] that included 1008 patients demonstrated that the lumbar spine was the most frequently affected area (58 %), followed by the thoracic (30 %) and cervical (11 %) spine; 4 % of patients had multiple levels of involvement [24, 25, 30, 70, 103, 117, 123, 129, 136, 141, 143, 146, 176, 191]. In patients with multiple levels of involvement, the continuous form was observed approximately twice more often than the skipping form [123]. Multiple levels of involvement were observed more frequently in intravenous drug users than in nondrug users [123]. Some spinal infections involve only a single vertebra, usually with a collapsed vertebral body [117, 189], which is similar to an osteoporotic vertebral fracture. Moreover, spinal infections sometimes occur with underlying vertebral disorders such as osteoporotic fractures [116, 123]. If vertebroplasty or kyphoplasty is performed after a misdiagnosis of simple osteoporotic vertebral fracture, removal of bone cement is necessary to manage the spinal infection. Therefore, surgeons have to be aware of such possibilities, especially in the elderly.

The number of spinal infections seems to have increased since the 1990s as a result of more elderly individuals, longer life expectancy for patients with chronic debilitating diseases, increases in the number of immunocompromised hosts and intravenous drug users, and increased use of spinal instrumentation surgery and epidural catheters for pain treatment [2, 11, 14, 23, 24, 29, 30, 53, 61, 125, 143, 153, 163]. Easy access to advanced diagnostic tools such as magnetic resonance imaging (MRI) has also increased the number of patients with a definite diagnosis of spinal infection [14, 97, 125]. A retrospective analysis of patients with spinal infection during the past half century [125] demonstrated that patients became older, with a mean age of 38 years between 1956 and 1965 compared to 65 years between 1996 and 2005. In Japan, one study showed that 43.7 % of patients with pyogenic spondylitis between 1988 and 2005 were 65 years of age or older [190], and another study demonstrated that the proportion of patients over 80 years increased rapidly to 26.2 % over a period of 5 years since 2004 [126].

In the younger population, this increase has been correlated with the growing number of intravenous drug users [123, 143]. Among the elderly, the increased incidence of spinal infection is more closely related to an increased incidence of disorders with a predisposition for osteomyelitis (e.g., diabetes mellitus and peripheral vascular disease), surgical procedures (e.g., dental extraction, open heart surgery, and prosthetic joint replacement), increased use of intravenous access devices, genitourinary surgery, and urinary catheterization [35, 36, 145, 176]. Belzunegui et al. compared spinal infections between patients aged 63 years or over and those aged under 63 years and found intravenous drug addiction and human immunodeficiency virus infection in 10 % and 13 % of the younger group, respectively, compared to 0 % of the elderly group. In contrast, a significantly higher proportion of patients in the elderly group recently underwent surgery (20 %) than in the younger group (0 %) [11]. In spinal infection arising from intravenous access devices, nosocomial bacteremia becomes a serious issue [176].

A study from Japan demonstrated that the proportion of patients with spinal infection that are immunocompromised dramatically increased from 3 % between 1956 and 1965 to 53 % between 1996 and 2005 [125]. In 1997, Carragee reported that 40 % of patients were immunocompromised hosts [24]. Diabetes mellitus is the most common underlying medical disorder. Spinal infection is also frequently observed in patients with cancer undergoing chemotherapy, chronic steroid therapy, or dialysis [22]. Diabetes mellitus was observed in 7–36 % of patients with spinal infection [24, 83, 95, 104, 117, 123, 136, 141, 189]. After diabetes mellitus, cancer was observed in 3–15 %, rheumatoid arthritis in 2–8 %, and corticosteroid use in 2–7 % [24, 83, 95, 104, 117, 123, 136, 141, 189]. Other conditions included intravenous drug abuse (11 %), other immunosuppression (7 %), alcoholism (5 %), liver cirrhosis (4 %), and renal failure (4 %) [123].

The genitourinary tract is the most common source of spinal infection, especially in the elderly [187]. The genitourinary tract has been reported to be the primary site of infection in 17–30 % of patients with spinal infection [24, 123, 157, 158]. Infection from the genitourinary system may spread directly to the spine via Batson's plexus, which does not involve enterohepatic circulation [145]. The prevalence of genitourinary tract infections increases with aging, and elderly females have the highest prevalence. Asymptomatic infection is not rare in elderly females [132, 134]. The aging processes that contribute to physiological dysfunction, which leads to a high incidence of genitourinary tract infections in the elderly population, may include increased vaginal bacterial colonization due to low pH related to postmenopausal decreases in circulating estrogen levels; urinary incontinence, affecting 6–8 % of people aged over 64 years in the community and up to 31 % of patients in hospitals and long-term care; the presence of indwelling urinary catheters, frequently used in elderly residents of long-term care institutions; and the coexistence of comorbid conditions such as diabetes mellitus or cancer [27, 78, 130, 132].

After genitourinary tract infection, endocarditis accounted for 12 % [25, 103, 123, 136, 141, 143, 146] and meningitis for 4 % of spinal infections [117, 123, 143, 146]. Recently, there has been a dramatic increase in the number of patients with spinal infection among patients with endocarditis as well as intravenous drug abusers [92, 108, 140, 155, 179, 183].

18.3 Symptoms and Diagnosis

18.3.1 Symptoms

The symptoms of spinal infection are often nonspecific, which can distract the clinician from the possibility of infection and delay diagnosis. A systematic review [123] that included 1008 patients demonstrated that pain in the neck, back, or low back is the most common symptom, occurring in more than 90 % of patients [9, 24, 25, 30, 70, 103, 117, 129, 136, 141, 143, 146, 157, 176, 191]. Fever is present in only approximately half of patients at presentation [157]. Range of motion of the spine is limited, which is often ascribed to localized spinal pain associated with muscle spasm. Neurological deficits are present in approximately 17–32 % of patients [123, 157]. Risk factors for neurological deficits include diabetes mellitus, advanced age, rheumatoid arthritis, and a more cephalad level of infection [32, 49, 99, 119, 170].

18.3.2 Laboratory Findings

Elevated erythrocyte sedimentation rate (ESR) is the most consistent laboratory finding supporting the diagnosis of spinal infection [46, 153]. Elevated white blood cell (WBC) count is not a constant finding [86, 153]. Elevated ESR has been reported in 70–100 % of patients with spinal infection, compared with only 13–60 % of patients with increased WBC [51, 70, 150, 157]. C-reactive protein (CRP) is also helpful in the diagnosis of spinal infection (Table 18.1). CRP increases 4–6 h after the onset of infection and peaks at 36–50 h [82]. On the other hand, changes in ESR are slower, with gradual increases over several days after onset and peaking in 7–8 days [82]. Other than infection, inflammatory diseases also elevate both CRP and ESR; therefore, elevated CRP and ESR do not constitute definitive evidence of infection. Plasma procalcitonin (PCT) has been reported to be a useful biomarker for differentiating between bacterial infection and systemic inflammatory disease [172]. The normal range of PCT is below 0.05 ng/mL, and patients with any bacterial infection have PCT greater than 0.5 ng/mL [7, 79].

Compared to pyogenic spinal infection, spinal infection with *Mycobacterium tuberculosis* is associated with milder increases in ESR, WBC, and CRP (Table 18.1). Interferon-γ release assays such as QuantiFERON® and T-SPOT® are helpful for diagnosing spinal infection with *Mycobacterium tuberculosis* [89, 167].

18.3.3 Imaging Studies

One of the problems with spinal infection is delayed diagnosis, despite recent advantages in imaging, microbiologic, and histopathologic techniques [93]. Sapico and Montgomerie found that diagnosis was delayed for more than 3 months after the onset of symptoms in approximately half of patients [157]. Most of this delay is due to the 2–4 week period after disease onset needed for characteristic changes to become evident on plain radiographs [3, 43, 112, 149, 157, 179]. The earliest radiographic finding is narrowing of the disk space, present in 74 % of patients. Destructive changes, such as lytic changes of the end plate or anterior vertebral body adjacent to the disk, which become evident 3–6 weeks after onset (Fig. 18.1), are the next most common finding [157]. In spinal infection with *Mycobacterium tuberculosis*, initial radiographs already show bony changes such as vertebral body atrophy [48].

Table 18.1 Differences in laboratory data among elderly patients with pyogenic versus tubercular spinal infection

Gender (age, years)	Male (79)	Female (81)
Pathogen	*Staphylococcus aureus*	*Mycobacterium tuberculosis*
RBC (/μL)	3,730,000	2,840,000
Hgb (g/dL)	11.6	9.1
WBC (/μL)	17,000	2,850
Neutrophils (%)	80.0	76.7
Lymphocytes (%)	11.0	18.9
CRP (mg/dL)	30.91	2.96

RBC red blood cell, *Hgb* hemoglobin, *WBC* white blood cell, *CRP* C-reactive protein
Normal range
RBC, $4.0–5.7 \times 10^6$/μL (males) and $3.6–5.1 \times 10^6$/μL (females)
Hgb, 12.0–17.0 g/dL (males) and 11.0–15.0 g/dL (females)
WBC, 3300–8800/μL
Neutrophil, 36.0–70.0 %
Lymphocyte, 22.0–53.0 %
CRP, <0.20 mg/dL

MRI is helpful for early diagnosis. Findings can be observed just 3–5 days after the onset of infection with a sensitivity of 96 % and a specificity of 93 % [121, 173]. In the elderly, it is difficult to observe initial findings of spinal infection on plain radiographs since they can have a variety of degenerative findings, such as spondylophytes and decreased disk space height. Therefore, physicians should order MRI immediately when evaluating a patient with suspected spinal infection, especially if the patient is elderly (Fig. 18.2). Characteristic MRI findings include decreased signal intensity of the vertebral bodies and the involved disk on T1-weighted images and increased signal changes of these structures and disappearance of intranuclear cleft of the involved disk on T2-weighted images (Fig. 18.1) [38, 121]. Gadolinium-enhanced MRI is also helpful, especially for evaluating the presence of abscess and the area of inflammation. In spinal infection with *Mycobacterium tuberculosis*, MRI sometimes initially shows normal disk height and signal. In contrast, a subligamentous abscess can already be apparent on the initial imaging study [165]. Paraspinal abscesses tend to be larger in spinal infection associated with *Mycobacterium tuberculosis* than in pyogenic infections; therefore, when a large rim of enhancement is observed on gadolinium-enhanced MRI, the possibility of spinal infection with *Mycobacterium tuberculosis* is higher [88]. Despite the accuracy of MRI, bacteriologic examination of involved tissues is essential for confirming the diagnosis [50, 99, 128].

^{99m}Tc bone scans are very sensitive for spinal infection, detecting at least 90 % of cases [121] and becoming positive within the first 2 or 3 days of acute spinal infection [3, 43, 112, 113, 148, 149, 157, 179–181]. However, they are less specific. The addition of a ^{67}Ga isotope to the ^{99m}Tc bone scan may improve specificity to 100 % [121]. One disadvantage of these scans is that they are less available when a prompt examination is required.

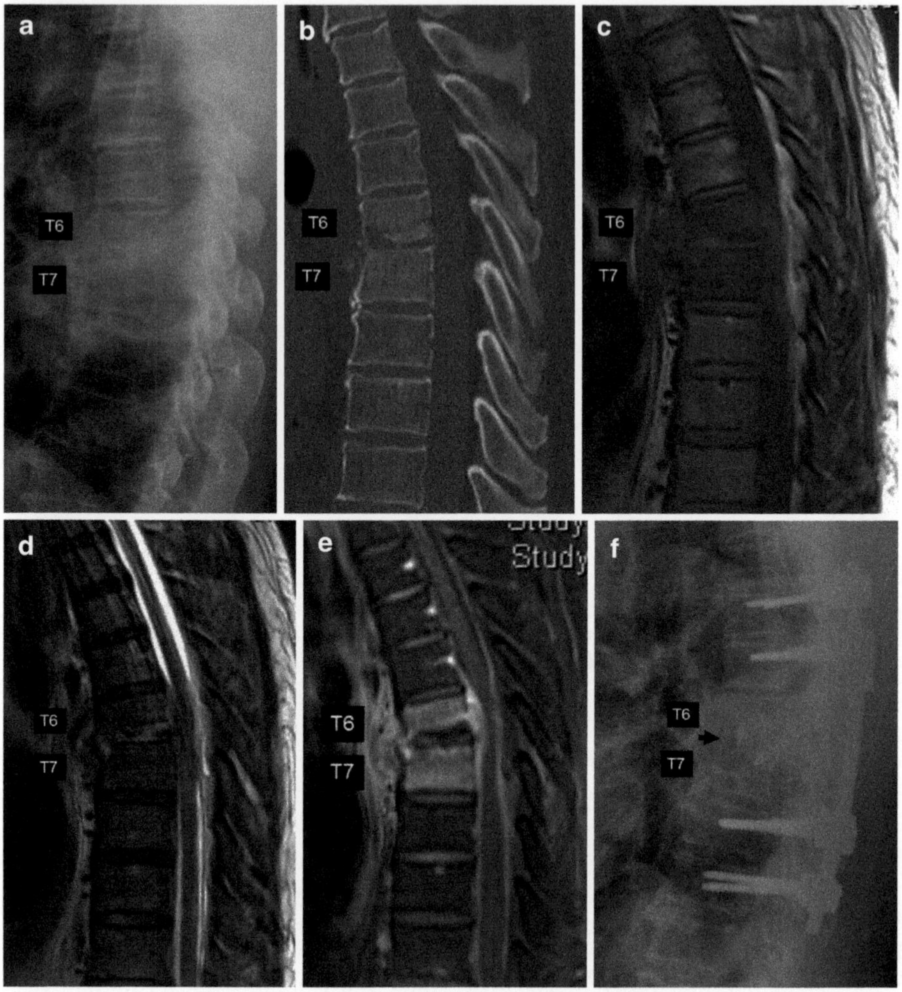

Fig. 18.1 A 78-year-old male with T6–T7 spinal infection with *Staphylococcus aureus*. A lateral plain radiograph shows reduced disk space height and obscured end plates between T6 and T7 (**a**). Reconstructed computed tomogram demonstrate destruction of the anteroinferior part of the T6 vertebral body (**b**). T1-weighted magnetic resonance images (MRI) show decreased signal intensity of the T6–T7 disk and vertebral bodies (**c**) and increased signal changes on T2-weighted images (**d**). Epidural and paraspinal inflammation is clearly visualized on gadolinium-enhanced MRI (**e**). This patient presented with sudden onset of incomplete paraplegia. He underwent a one-stage operation consisting of anterior radical debridement, autologous strut bone grafting (*arrow*), and posterior stabilization (**f**) (From Nagashima H (2016) Treatment strategies for spinal disorders in the elderly. Seikeigeka 67:471–478)

18.3.4 Bacteriologic Identification

To select appropriate antibiotics, organism detection is very important. In a patient with spinal infection suspected based on laboratory data and imaging studies, specimens must be collected from the locus of infection in addition to blood cultures

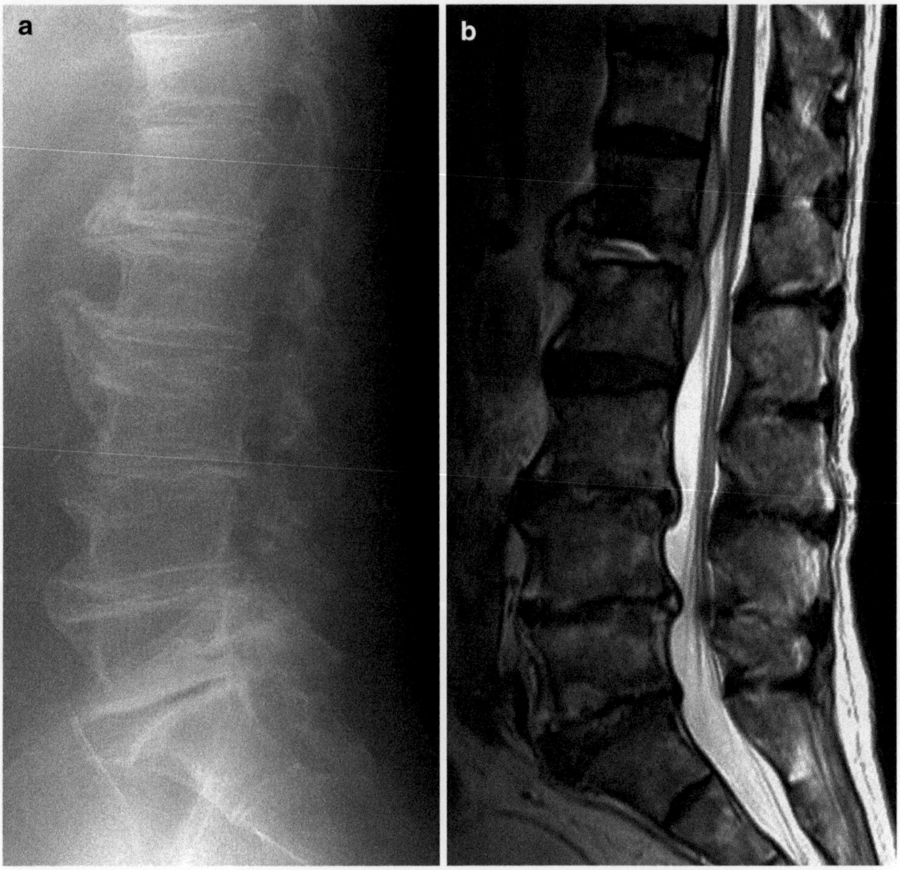

Fig. 18.2 An 83-year-old male with L1–L2 spinal infection by methicillin-resistant *Staphylococcus aureus*. A lateral plain radiograph showed multilevel degenerative findings, such as spondylophytes and the reduced height of disk space, without any findings of spinal infection (**a**). T2-weighted magnetic resonance images show increased signal changes of L1/L2 disk with epidural abscess (**b**)

before antibiotics are administered [42, 67, 125, 137]. In some suspected cases of *Mycobacterium tuberculosis* spinal infection or with a history of urinary tract infection, sputum or urine cultures are also helpful.

Some authors have noted a low incidence of positive blood cultures in patients with pyogenic osteomyelitis [156], while others state that blood cultures may yield positive results early as most of acute osteomyelitis occurred through hematogenous spread [35]. Indeed, blood cultures have been reported to result in isolation of the pathogen in 20–59 % of patients [68, 81, 123, 137]. To rule out contamination, two or three sets of blood culture should be collected for an hour.

Specimens from the locus of infection are usually collected using computed tomography (CT)-guided percutaneous needle biopsy or needle biopsy under fluoroscopy. Recently, CT-guided percutaneous needle biopsy became a standard practice in almost all hospitals [42]. CT-guided or open biopsy yields the causative organism more often than blood cultures [123]. The rate of pathogen detection from disk body aspirate varies from 41–90 % [15, 16, 24, 26, 28, 33, 42, 52, 85, 111, 120, 123, 126, 137, 188]. If a psoas abscess is present, the rate of pathogen detection is significantly higher, even when it is not accessible for puncture or drainage [42]. If cultures of blood and collected specimens are negative and clinical suspicion for spinal infection remains high, a second biopsy is recommended [42, 107]. In patients who have received antibiotics before biopsy, diagnostic rates are significantly lower [42]. A patient is sometimes referred after failed antibiotic therapy [171]. In such cases, a second biopsy should be performed to identify pathogens 1 or 2 weeks after the cessation of antibiotics, although the detection rate is still estimated to be low [42]. When multiple biopsies cannot detect a pathogen, open biopsy is an option. Open biopsy is reported to yield more positive results than percutaneous biopsy [31, 111].

Overall, a causative organism for spinal infection is identified from the blood or locus of infection in 67–100 % of patients [9, 24, 25, 30, 70, 103, 117, 123, 129, 136, 141, 143, 146, 176, 191]. When both are positive, there has been a 100 % concordance rate for pathogens identified from blood cultures and vertebral cultures [137]. Biopsy is necessary when a polymicrobial infection is suspected, since blood cultures often detect only one pathogen [117]. In the studies reviewed, a single organism was isolated from 85 % of patients, whereas polymicrobial infection was reported in 9 % of patients [9, 24, 25, 30, 70, 103, 117, 123, 129, 136, 141, 143, 146, 176, 191].

Since isolation of mycobacterial species from specimens usually takes 6–8 weeks, polymerase chain reaction (PCR), which detects mycobacterial DNA or RNA, has been used for rapid identification [13, 41]. PCR becomes positive even during the inactive phase since it can detect dead mycobacterium.

Even in elderly patients, antimicrobial therapy should not be started before a direct tissue culture has been obtained, since CT-guided needle biopsy is safe and effective [9, 12, 138, 169, 179, 185]. When CT-guided needle biopsy is negative, open biopsy should proceed if empiric antimicrobial therapy is not effective.

18.3.5 Pathogens

In patients with spinal infections, the prevalence of Gram-positive bacteria ranges from 26–93 %, while Gram-negative bacilli are isolated less often (range, 5–56 %) [70, 117, 123]. *Staphylococcus aureus* is the most commonly isolated pathogen, accounting for 32–84 % of patients [17, 21, 29, 51, 60, 70, 117, 123, 137, 143, 150, 156, 158, 176, 189], followed by *Streptococcus* species (range, 0–24 %) [24, 25, 30, 70, 103, 117, 123, 129, 136, 141, 143, 146, 176, 189, 191]. *Staphylococcus epidermidis* is typically considered an organism with low pathogenicity, but it has been recognized as a cause of spinal infections associated with implants such as pacemakers, sternal wires, prosthetic joints, and other prosthetic materials [6]. However, there has been a case report of an 84-year-old man with spontaneous spinal infection due to *Staphylococcus epidermidis* [80], and some studies have shown that *Staphylococcus epidermidis* is a frequently isolated pathogen in elderly and immunocompromised hosts [24, 70, 117].

Pseudomonas aeruginosa is a Gram-negative bacillus that rarely causes spinal infections, except in immunocompromised hosts or hospitalized patients on long-term antibiotic therapy for other conditions [21, 129, 179]. Patzakis et al. studied causative pathogens for spinal infection among intravenous drug users [143]. They found that *Pseudomonas aeruginosa* was the predominant etiologic organism (38 %), and *Staphylococcus aureus* had a relatively low prevalence (17 %). On the other hand, in another study of 15 intravenous drug users, 11 were positive for *Staphylococcus aureus*, and only one yielded *Pseudomonas aeruginosa* [24]. Graham and coworkers demonstrated that the average age of patients with hematogenous spinal infection due to Gram-negative bacilli was 76.5 years (range, 64–88 years) with a male-to-female ratio of 7:3. All of these patients had conditions that predisposed them to infection [68].

As described above, elderly individuals have the highest prevalence of genitourinary tract infections. *Escherichia coli* is the most common organism in elderly women with bacteriuria, with an incidence of 85.7–87.0 % [18, 19, 131, 133, 134]. Asymptomatic patients with this organism are not rare. Almost all of these patients do not require treatment. *Escherichia coli* and *Proteus* species are more likely pathogens in the elderly due to hematogenous seeding from the genitourinary tract [24, 156–158, 175]. Another reason for the high incidence of spinal infections with Gram-negative bacteria in the elderly is the possibility of nosocomial intravenous cannula-related sepsis in hospitalized patients [176]. Spine specialists have to be aware of the importance of the urinary tract in the pathogenesis of spinal infection [73, 74]. The preponderance of these pathogens might be predicted in elderly patients with spinal infection [175].

Some studies have demonstrated that methicillin-resistant *Staphylococcus aureus* (MRSA) accounts for 45–61 % of *Staphylococcus aureus* isolates in patients with spinal infections [8, 44, 70, 125, 142, 189], of which 27–40 % were nosocomial *Staphylococcus aureus* strains, and 1–50 % were community-acquired strains [33, 67, 189]. Another study found that methicillin-resistant *Staphylococcus aureus* or *epidermidis* was detected approximately 2.5 times more frequently in patients over 80 years than in patients 80 years or younger [126]. Although there has been only one report on spinal infections in patients over 80 years, age >65 years has been reported as a risk factor for drug-resistant *Streptococcus pneumoniae* in patients with pneumonia [28, 56, 135]. Therefore, elderly patients may be more susceptible to spinal infection with drug-resistant pathogens.

18.4 Management

18.4.1 Antibiotic Therapy

Before the development and availability of antibiotics, the mortality rate for spinal infection was high, ranging from 25–70 % [71, 99]. The prognosis of spinal infection has dramatically improved in the antibiotic era. However, inappropriate treatment could lead to a poor outcome. Since antibiotics form the basis of treatment for spinal infection, the selection of appropriate agents is extremely important. In addition to antibiotics, nonsurgical treatment includes spinal immobilization with external support, such as a thoracolumbosacral orthosis.

When a pathogen is identified from blood cultures or cultures from the locus of infection, appropriate antibiotic selection involves consideration of antimicrobial susceptibility and penetration into spinal tissues. The optimal duration of parenteral antimicrobial therapy and subsequent oral therapy remains controversial. High rates of readmission after short courses of therapy highlight the need for an adequate duration of parenteral antibiotic therapy [137]. Sapico and Montgomerie suggest that appropriate prolonged high-dose antimicrobial therapy is necessary until ESR reaches 50 % of the level at presentation [158]. Some authors have proposed 6–8 weeks of parenteral antibiotic therapy alone, while others have advocated 6–8 weeks of parenteral antibiotic therapy followed by oral therapy for 2 months or more [14, 24, 45, 47, 51, 141]. This lack of consensus is due to recent recommendations for managing spinal infection based on descriptive studies and expert opinion [67]. Some recent reviews [1, 66, 123, 177] still cite a paper published before 1980 [157] that showed that less than 4 weeks of parenteral antibiotics was associated with failure rates of up to 25 %. Some papers still recommend intravenous antibiotics for 4–6 weeks followed by oral therapy for an additional 2–6 weeks [25, 70, 117, 136, 146, 156]. However, antibiotic therapy has advanced considerably since the 1980s, and many types of antibiotics, especially strong oral antibiotics, have become available, which allows for intravenous therapy for less than 4 weeks. Oral antibiotics alone can effectively manage spinal infection in some patients [25, 117, 136].

Clindamycin, fluoroquinolones, macrolides, rifampicin, fusidic acid, metronidazole, and linezolid can reach therapeutic levels in the bone. β-Lactam antibiotics and glycopeptides achieve moderate levels, and aminoglycosides diffuse poorly into the bone [67]. Vancomycin, gentamicin, tobramycin, clindamycin, and teicoplanin can penetrate reasonably well into the nucleus pulposus [37, 162]. Fluoroquinolones such as ciprofloxacin have an excellent in vitro activity against a broad spectrum of bacteria [168] and can be used to treat Gram-negative osteomyelitis [57]. Ciprofloxacin inhibits topoisomerase IV and DNA gyrase, which are essential for bacterial DNA replication, transcription, repair, and recombination [118]. Furthermore, fluoroquinolones have excellent oral bioavailability and reach adequate bone concentrations for treating osteomyelitis even when administered orally [151]. Another fluoroquinolone, moxifloxacin, has been shown to be highly active against Gram-positive microorganisms, anaerobes, and *Mycobacterium tuberculosis* [4, 20, 40, 64, 84, 178]. Oral moxifloxacin also has demonstrated excellent bioavailability and can achieve high plasma and bone concentrations [112]. Rifampicin also has excellent oral bioavailability and a high tissue penetration index [101], but it is always used with other antibiotics due to the rapid development of resistance. Combination therapy with fluoroquinolones has been shown to be effective in the treatment of bone infections [33]. Although there are no consensus guidelines for the treatment of hematogenous spinal infection with Gram-negative bacilli, oral ciprofloxacin has been shown to be safe and effective as a standard parenteral agent, with success rates of greater than 80% [62, 106].

For spinal infection with *Mycobacterium tuberculosis*, a three-drug regimen from isoniazid (INH), rifampin (RMP), pyrazinamide (PZA), streptomycin (STM), and ethambutol (EMB) for 6–9 months is used. In general, INH, RMP, and EMB are used together. During the first month, four agents, for example, INH, RMP, PZA, and EMB, are commonly indicated. The reason for using a multidrug regimen is the potential for the development of resistance to a single drug. During antitubercular therapy, physicians have to monitor for adverse effects such as vestibulocochlear nerve damage with STM, optic neuritis with EMB, and peripheral neuritis with INH.

In patients with negative culture findings, antibiotics selection should be guided by a history of prior infection, such as urinary tract infection or cholecystitis. Without such a history, broad-spectrum antibiotics can be used.

Treatment failure is suspected when ESR is greater than 50 mm/h and CRP is greater than 2.75 mg/dL 4 weeks after the initiation of antibiotic therapy [189]. In contrast, a 50% or more reduction in the CRP level each week is indicative of a good response [33, 67].

18.4.2 Surgical Management

The indications for surgical treatment include progressive neurologic deficits due to spinal cord compression or epidural abscess, severe destruction of end plates with mechanical instability or segmental deformity, imminent risk of neurologic deficits, refractoriness to conservative treatment with prolonged high CRP and ESR, large abscess with fever or sepsis, negative cultures, and unbearable pain [47, 54, 61, 94, 147, 161]. Some patients have spinal infection and malignancy that require prompt chemotherapy. Since conservative treatment for spinal infection requires prolonged antibiotic therapy and there is no guarantee that the spinal infection would be controlled only with antibiotics, early surgical treatment is an alternative in such cases [127].

Radical debridement followed by autologous strut bone grafting, proposed by Hodgson and Sock in the early 1950s [76], has been considered the gold standard surgical treatment for spinal infection for many years. It is carried out via a thoracotomy or the extrapleural approach for the thoracic spine or a retroperitoneal approach for the lumbar spine (Fig. 18.1). The anterior approach allows for direct access to sufficiently debride infected tissues, as well as stabilization with bone grafting. Laminectomy only is contraindicated because it may lead to neurologic deterioration and increased spinal instability [49, 55, 87]. Costotransversectomy for the thoracic spine can enable abscess drainage, but a good recovery from neurological deficits cannot be expected [49].

The addition of posterior instrumentation to anterior debridement and strut bone grafting has been reported to be safe and associated with faster and more complete fusion and better correction (Fig. 18.1) [24, 69, 72]. Until the 1980s, however, the direct application of foreign materials in the infected area had been considered contraindicated since infection could not be brought under control due to biofilm formation. Since Oga et al. reported in 1993 that biofilm-covered colonies of *Mycobacterium tuberculosis* are very rare, anterior instrumentation at the same time as anterior debridement has become widely used to treat spinal infection with *Mycobacterium tuberculosis* [1, 21, 139]. Recently, this technique was also used to treat pyogenic spinal infection [72]. Gorensek et al. recommended posterior instrumentation and anterior column reconstruction through a single posterior approach because there is substantially less blood loss than in previous studies [65, 96, 154]. A number of studies have shown that it is safe to use titanium cages, which do not increase the rate of infection recurrence [39, 54, 72, 109, 154]. Degradative enzymes do not exert adverse effects on their structural integrity in an infected area [72, 98, 171]. Although there have been only few reports, polyetheretherketone (PEEK) cages could be used for anterior column reconstruction with successful outcomes in pyogenic spinal infection [65, 122, 144, 182]. In contrast, some patients have had postoperative recurrent infection necessitating the removal of implants [171]. Spine surgeons must be aware of this possibility.

In their study of elderly and debilitated patients undergoing anterior debridement and bone graft for compressive myelopathy due to pyogenic spinal infection, Gepstein et al. concluded that this approach provides a high probability of cure, despite a patient's advanced age and poor general health [63]. However, the risks and benefits must be evaluated before embarking on such an invasive surgery. In the elderly and patients in poor general condition, two-stage surgical treatment consisting of initial posterior instrumentation and subsequent debridement and bone grafting has been proposed [59, 75, 114]. After 2–3 months to allow for sufficient immobilization after posterior instrumentation, anterior debridement and bone grafting are performed as the second procedure. Some patients with faster bone union and pain resolution after the first procedure can avoid the second procedure [114]. Therefore, in elderly patients with spinal infection, posterior instrumentation only could be an alternative surgical option. If it provides dramatic pain relief, observation can be reasonable. If pain is not sufficiently relieved and there is a possibility of progressive deformity, additional anterior debridement and bone grafting could be scheduled (Fig. 18.3).

18.5 Prognosis

The mortality rate of patients with spinal infection ranges from 2–17% [9, 24, 25, 30, 110, 123, 129, 136, 141, 143, 146, 160, 176, 186, 191]. A 32% relapse rate has been described in the literature [30, 70, 117, 123, 136, 141, 143, 146, 176]. Most deaths were due to *Staphylococcus aureus*, despite appropriate antibiotic treatment [123, 136, 143, 146, 176]. On radiographs, approximately half of patients achieved fusion at the level of the infected disk by 5 years, and in the others fibrous ankylosis was observed [5, 58, 91, 124, 157].

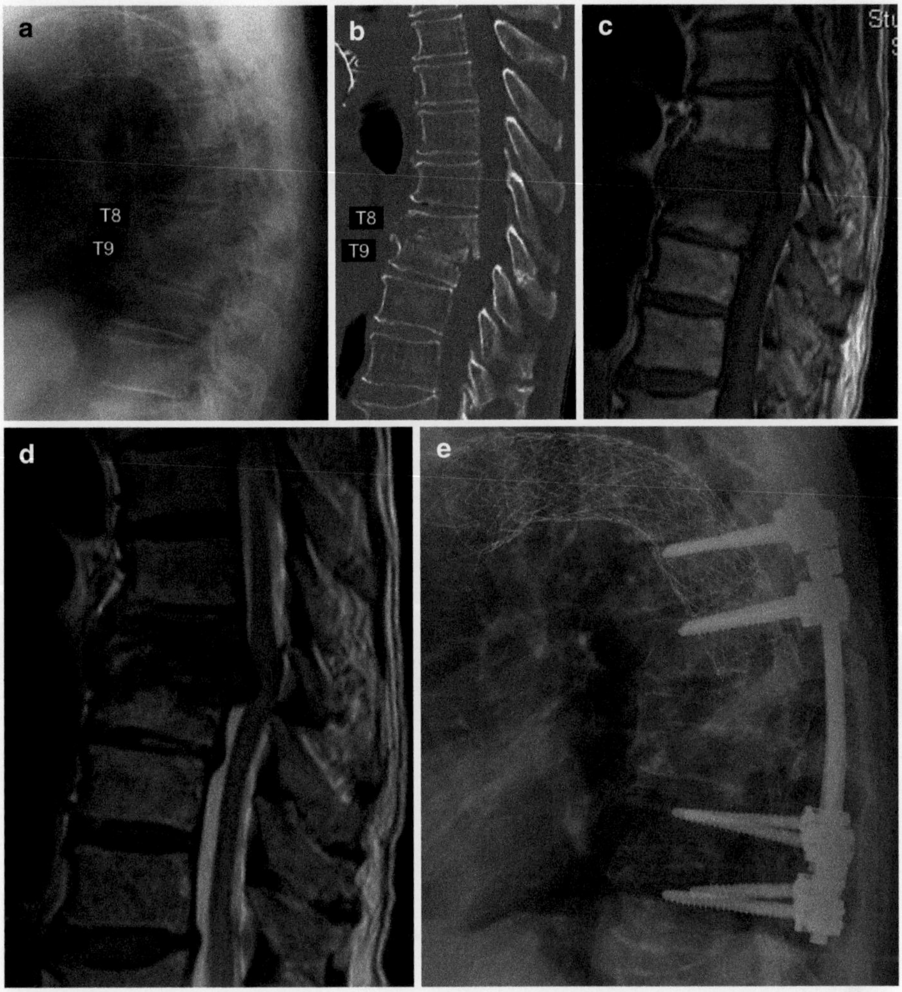

Fig. 18.3 An 81-year-old male with spinal infection at T8–T9. Endovascular stent grafting was performed for thoracic aortic aneurysm 2 years prior to the onset of spinal infection. Antibiotics were administered without any attempt to isolate the causative pathogen at the previous hospital. After he was referred to our hospital, computed tomography (CT)-guided percutaneous biopsy was performed 1 week after the cessation of antibiotics, but no pathogens could be detected. A lateral plain radiograph (**a**) and reconstructed CT images (**b**) demonstrate destruction of the T8 and T9 vertebral bodies and a kyphotic deformity. Magnetic resonance images show spinal infection at the T8–T9 level with the compression and signal change of the spinal cord (**c**, **d**). Since this patient had reduced pulmonary and cardiac function, laminectomy and posterior instrumentation with local bone grafting were performed (**e**). It provided dramatic relief of pain, so additional anterior procedure was not scheduled

During the progression of spinal infection, abscess or edema formation can destroy vertebrae or cause neurologic dysfunction [30, 66, 177] that lead to long-term disability. Rates of disability as high as 31 % have been reported after a mean follow-up of 6.5 years [117]. Moreover, 27 % of patients with spinal infection had complications that seriously affected their quality of life [123]. Subjective disability in activities of daily living was observed in 32 % of patients with spinal infection and in 55 % of patients with postoperative pyogenic spinal infection [30, 85]. Neurologic dysfunction was observed in 5 % of patients with spinal infection, and, of those, 39 % complained of slight or moderate pain 1 year after treatment [10]. Other report demonstrated severe chronic pain in 8 % of patients and neurological dysfunction in 13 % after more than 2 years of follow-up [24]. Independent predictors of long-term disability include neurological impairment at the time of diagnosis, time to diagnosis ≥8 weeks, and immunocompromised hosts [166]. Recent improvements in the management of spinal infection and the availability of MRI for earlier diagnosis might lead to lower rates of disability than in previous series [166].

O'Daly et al. conducted a retrospective study to assess long-term functional outcome after spinal infection. They found that adverse outcomes were observed in 66 % of patients, despite only 17 % having an objective persistent neurologic deficit during long-term follow-up [137]. Even in patients with what appears to be full recovery and no neurologic deficits at follow-up, SF-36 scores never returned to the same level as in an age-matched normative population [137]. Persistence of pain after the eradication of infection is known to have a significant negative effect on psychological and functional status [105]. Surgical and nonsurgical patients have a similar incidence of adverse outcomes [137].

Predisposing factors to paralysis include advanced age, diabetes mellitus, more cephalad level of infection, and *Staphylococcus aureus* infection [49]. However, another study demonstrated that outcomes in elderly patients with spinal infection were similar to those in younger patients [11].

References

1. Acosta FL Jr, Chin CT, Quinones-Hinojosa A, Ames CP, Weinstein PR, Chou D (2004) Diagnosis and management of adult pyogenic osteomyelitis of the cervical spine. Neurosurg Focus 17:E2
2. Acosta FL Jr, Galvez LF, Aryan HE, Ames CP (2006) Recent advances: infections of the spine. Curr Infect Dis Rep 8:390–393
3. Adatepe MH, Powell OM, Isaacs GH, Nichols K, Cefola R (1986) Hematogenous pyogenic vertebral osteomyelitis: diagnostic value of radionuclide bone imaging. J Nucl Med 27:1680–1685
4. Aldridge KE, Ashcraft DS (1997) Comparison of the in vitro activities of Bay 12–8039, a new quinolone, and other antimicrobials against clinically important anaerobes. Antimicrob Agents Chemother 41:709–711
5. Ambrose GB, Alpert M, Neer CS (1966) Vertebral osteomyelitis. A diagnostic problem. JAMA 197:619–622
6. Archer GL (1990) Staphylococcus epidermidis and other coagulase negative staphylococci. In: Mandell GL, Douglas RG, Bennett JE (eds) Principles and practice of infectious diseases. Churchill Livingstone, New York, pp 1511–1518
7. Arkader R, Troster EJ, Lopes MR, Junior RR, Carcillo JA, Leone C, Okay TS (2006) Procalcitonin does discriminate between sepsis and systemic inflammatory response syndrome. Arch Dis Child 91:117–120
8. Barber M (1961) Methicillin-resistant staphylococci. J Clin Pathol 14:385–393
9. Bateman JL, Pevzner MM (1995) Spinal osteomyelitis: a review of 10 years' experience. Orthopedics 18:561–565

10. Belzunegui J, Del Val N, Intxausti JJ, De Dios JR, Queiro R, Gonzalez C, Rodriguez-Valverde V, Figueroa M (1999) Vertebral osteomyelitis in northern Spain. Report of 62 cases. Clin Exp Rheumatol 17:447–452
11. Belzunegui J, Intxausti JJ, De Dios JR, Del Val N, Rodriguez Valverde V, Gonzalez C, Queiro R, Figueroa M (2000) Haematogenous vertebral osteomyelitis in the elderly. Clin Rheumatol 19:344–347
12. Bender CE, Berquist TH, Wold LE (1986) Imaging-assisted percutaneous biopsy of the thoracic spine. Mayo Clin Proc 61:942–950
13. Berk RH, Yazici M, Atabey N, Ozdamar OS, Pabuccuoglu U, Alici E (1996) Detection of Mycobacterium tuberculosis in formaldehyde solution-fixed, paraffin-embedded tissue by polymerase chain reaction in Pott's disease. Spine (Phila Pa 1976) 21:1991–1995
14. Beronius M, Bergman B, Andersson R (2001) Vertebral osteomyelitis in Goteborg, Sweden: a retrospective study of patients during 1990–95. Scand J Infect Dis 33:527–532
15. Bhagat S, Mathieson C, Jandhyala R, Johnston R (2007) Spondylodiscitis (disc space infection) associated with negative microbiological tests: comparison of outcome of suspected disc space infections to documented non-tuberculous pyogenic discitis. Br J Neurosurg 21:473–477
16. Bontoux D, Codello L, Debiais F, Lambert de Cursay G, Azais I, Alcalay M (1992) Infectious spondylodiscitis. Analysis of a series of 105 cases. Rev Rhum Mal Osteoartic 59:401–407
17. Borowski AM, Crow WN, Hadjipavlou AG, Chaljub G, Mader J, Cesani F, vanSonnenberg E (1998) Interventional radiology case conference: the University of Texas Medical Branch. Percutaneous management of pyogenic spondylodiskitis. AJR Am J Roentgenol 170:1587–1592
18. Boscia JA, Kobasa WD, Knight RA, Abrutyn E, Levison ME, Kaye D (1986) Epidemiology of bacteriuria in an elderly ambulatory population. Am J Med 80:208–214
19. Boscia JA, Kobasa WD, Knight RA, Abrutyn E, Levison ME, Kaye D (1987) Therapy vs no therapy for bacteriuria in elderly ambulatory nonhospitalized women. JAMA 257:1067–1071
20. Brueggemann AB, Kugler KC, Doern GV (1997) In vitro activity of BAY 12–8039, a novel 8-methoxyquinolone, compared to activities of six fluoroquinolones against Streptococcus pneumoniae. Haemophilus influenzae, and Moraxella catarrhalis. Antimicrob Agents Chemother 41:1594–1597
21. Butler JS, Shelly MJ, Timlin M, Powderly WG, O'Byrne JM (2006) Nontuberculous pyogenic spinal infection in adults: a 12-year experience from a tertiary referral center. Spine (Phila Pa 1976) 31:2695–2700
22. Cahill DW, Love LC, Rechtine GR (1991) Pyogenic osteomyelitis of the spine in the elderly. J Neurosurg 74:878–886
23. Calderone RR, Larsen JM (1996) Overview and classification of spinal infections. Orthop Clin North Am 27:1–8
24. Carragee EJ (1997) Pyogenic vertebral osteomyelitis. J Bone Joint Surg Am 79:874–880
25. Chelsom J, Solberg CO (1998) Vertebral osteomyelitis at a Norwegian university hospital 1987–97: clinical features, laboratory findings and outcome. Scand J Infect Dis 30:147–151
26. Chew FS, Kline MJ (2001) Diagnostic yield of CT-guided percutaneous aspiration procedures in suspected spontaneous infectious diskitis. Radiology 218:211–214
27. Childs SJ, Egan RJ (1996) Bacteriuria and urinary infections in the elderly. Urol Clin North Am 23:43–54
28. Clavo-Sanchez AJ, Giron-Gonzalez JA, Lopez-Prieto D, Canueto-Quintero J, Sanchez-Porto A, Vergara-Campos A, Marin-Casanova P, Cordoba-Dona JA (1997) Multivariate analysis of risk factors for infection due to penicillin-resistant and multidrug-resistant Streptococcus pneumoniae: a multicenter study. Clin Infect Dis 24:1052–1059
29. Collert S (1977) Osteomyelitis of the spine. Acta Orthop Scand 48:283–290
30. Colmenero JD, Jimenez-Mejias ME, Sanchez-Lora FJ, Reguera JM, Palomino-Nicas J, Martos F, Garcia de las Heras J, Pachon J (1997) Pyogenic, tuberculous, and brucellar vertebral osteomyelitis: a descriptive and comparative study of 219 cases. Ann Rheum Dis 56:709–715

31. Colmenero JD, Jimenez-Mejias ME, Reguera JM, Palomino-Nicas J, Ruiz-Mesa JD, Marquez-Rivas J, Lozano A, Pachon J (2004) Tuberculous vertebral osteomyelitis in the new millennium: still a diagnostic and therapeutic challenge. Eur J Clin Microbiol Infect Dis 23:477–483
32. Cooppan R, Schoenbaum S, Younger MD, Freidberg S, D'Elia J (1976) Vertebral osteomyelitis in insulin-dependent diabetics. S Afr Med J 50:1993–1996
33. Cottle L, Riordan T (2008) Infectious spondylodiscitis. J Infect 56:401–412
34. Coventry MB, Ghormley RK, Kernohan JW (1945) The intervertebral disc: its microscopic anatomy and pathology: part I. anatomy, development, and physiology. J Bone Joint Surg Am 27:13
35. Cunha BA (2002) Osteomyelitis in elderly patients. Clin Infect Dis 35:287–293
36. Currie MS (1992) Immunosenescence. Compr Ther 18:26–34
37. Currier BL, Banovac K, Eismont FJ (1994) Gentamicin penetration into normal rabbit nucleus pulposus. Spine (Phila Pa 1976) 19:2614–2618
38. Dagirmanjian A, Schils J, McHenry M, Modic MT (1996) MR imaging of vertebral osteomyelitis revisited. AJR Am J Roentgenol 167:1539–1543
39. Dai LY, Chen WH, Jiang LS (2008) Anterior instrumentation for the treatment of pyogenic vertebral osteomyelitis of thoracic and lumbar spine. Eur Spine J 17:1027–1034
40. Dalhoff A, Petersen U, Endermann R (1996) In vitro activity of BAY 12–8039, a new 8-methoxyquinolone. Chemotherapy 42:410–425
41. Daniel TM (1990) The rapid diagnosis of tuberculosis: a selective review. J Lab Clin Med 116:277–282
42. de Lucas EM, Gonzalez Mandly A, Gutierrez A, Pellon R, Martin-Cuesta L, Izquierdo J, Sanchez E, Ruiz E, Quintana F (2009) CT-guided fine-needle aspiration in vertebral osteomyelitis: true usefulness of a common practice. Clin Rheumatol 28:315–320
43. Devereaux MD, Hazelton RA (1983) Pyogenic spinal osteomyelitis--its clinical and radiological presentation. J Rheumatol 10:491–493
44. Diekema DJ, Pfaller MA, Schmitz FJ, Smayevsky J, Bell J, Jones RN, Beach M (2001) Survey of infections due to Staphylococcus species: frequency of occurrence and antimicrobial susceptibility of isolates collected in the United States, Canada, Latin America, Europe, and the Western Pacific region for the SENTRY Antimicrobial Surveillance Program, 1997–1999. Clin Infect Dis 32(Suppl 2):S114–S132
45. Dietze DD Jr, Fessler RG, Jacob RP (1997) Primary reconstruction for spinal infections. J Neurosurg 86:981–989
46. Digby JM, Kersley JB (1979) Pyogenic non-tuberculous spinal infection: an analysis of thirty cases. J Bone Joint Surg Br 61:47–55
47. Dimar JR, Carreon LY, Glassman SD, Campbell MJ, Hartman MJ, Johnson JR (2004) Treatment of pyogenic vertebral osteomyelitis with anterior debridement and fusion followed by delayed posterior spinal fusion. Spine (Phila Pa 1976) 29:326–332; discussion 332
48. Doub HP, Badgley CE (1932) The roentgen signs of tuberculosis of the vertebral body. Am J Radiol 27:11
49. Eismont FJ, Bohlman HH, Soni PL, Goldberg VM, Freehafer AA (1983) Pyogenic and fungal vertebral osteomyelitis with paralysis. J Bone Joint Surg Am 65:19–29
50. Eismont FJ, Green BA, Brown MD, Ghandur-Mnaymneh L (1987) Coexistent infection and tumor of the spine. A report of three cases. J Bone Joint Surg Am 69:452–458
51. Emery SE, Chan DP, Woodward HR (1989) Treatment of hematogenous pyogenic vertebral osteomyelitis with anterior debridement and primary bone grafting. Spine (Phila Pa 1976) 14:284–291
52. Enoch DA, Cargill JS, Laing R, Herbert S, Corrah TW, Brown NM (2008) Value of CT-guided biopsy in the diagnosis of septic discitis. J Clin Pathol 61:750–753
53. Espersen F, Frimodt-Moller N, Thamdrup Rosdahl V, Skinhoj P, Bentzon MW (1991) Changing pattern of bone and joint infections due to Staphylococcus aureus: study of cases of bacteremia in Denmark, 1959–1988. Rev Infect Dis 13:347–358

54. Fayazi AH, Ludwig SC, Dabbah M, Bryan Butler R, Gelb DE (2004) Preliminary results of staged anterior debridement and reconstruction using titanium mesh cages in the treatment of thoracolumbar vertebral osteomyelitis. Spine J 4:388–395
55. Fellander M (1975) Paraplegia in spondylitis: results of operative treatment. Paraplegia 13:75–88
56. Ferrara AM (2007) A brief review of moxifloxacin in the treatment of elderly patients with community-acquired pneumonia (CAP). Clin Interv Aging 2:179–187
57. Fraimow HS (2009) Systemic antimicrobial therapy in osteomyelitis. Semin Plast Surg 23:90–99
58. Frederickson B, Yuan H, Olans R (1978) Management and outcome of pyogenic vertebral osteomyelitis. Clin Orthop Relat Res 131:160–167
59. Fukuta S, Miyamoto K, Masuda T, Hosoe H, Kodama H, Nishimoto H, Sakaeda H, Shimizu K (2003) Two-stage (posterior and anterior) surgical treatment using posterior spinal instrumentation for pyogenic and tuberculotic spondylitis. Spine (Phila Pa 1976) 28:E302–E308
60. Garcia A Jr, Grantham SA (1960) Hematogenous pyogenic vertebral osteomyelitis. J Bone Joint Surg Am 42-a:429–436
61. Gasbarrini AL, Bertoldi E, Mazzetti M, Fini L, Terzi S, Gonella F, Mirabile L, Barbanti Brodano G, Furno A, Gasbarrini A, Boriani S (2005) Clinical features, diagnostic and therapeutic approaches to haematogenous vertebral osteomyelitis. Eur Rev Med Pharmacol Sci 9:53–66
62. Gentry LO, Rodriguez GG (1990) Oral ciprofloxacin compared with parenteral antibiotics in the treatment of osteomyelitis. Antimicrob Agents Chemother 34:40–43
63. Gepstein R, Folman Y, Lidor C, Barchilon V, Catz A, Hallel T (1992) Management of pyogenic vertebral osteomyelitis with spinal cord compression in the elderly. Paraplegia 30:795–798
64. Goldstein EJ, Citron DM, Hudspeth M, Hunt Gerardo S, Merriam CV (1997) In vitro activity of Bay 12–8039, a new 8-methoxyquinolone, compared to the activities of 11 other oral antimicrobial agents against 390 aerobic and anaerobic bacteria isolated from human and animal bite wound skin and soft tissue infections in humans. Antimicrob Agents Chemother 41:1552–1557
65. Gorensek M, Kosak R, Travnik L, Vengust R (2013) Posterior instrumentation, anterior column reconstruction with single posterior approach for treatment of pyogenic osteomyelitis of thoracic and lumbar spine. Eur Spine J 22:633–641
66. Govender S (2005) Spinal infections. J Bone Joint Surg Br 87:1454–1458
67. Grados F, Lescure FX, Senneville E, Flipo RM, Schmit JL, Fardellone P (2007) Suggestions for managing pyogenic (non-tuberculous) discitis in adults. Joint Bone Spine 74:133–139
68. Graham SM, Fishlock A, Millner P, Sandoe J (2013) The management gram-negative bacterial haematogenous vertebral osteomyelitis: a case series of diagnosis, treatment and therapeutic outcomes. Eur Spine J 22:1845–1853
69. Graziano GP, Sidhu KS (1993) Salvage reconstruction in acute and late sequelae from pyogenic thoracolumbar infection. J Spinal Disord 6:199–207
70. Hadjipavlou AG, Mader JT, Necessary JT, Muffoletto AJ (2000) Hematogenous pyogenic spinal infections and their surgical management. Spine (Phila Pa 1976) 25:1668–1679
71. Hatch ES (1931) Acute osteomyelitis of the spine. Report of case with recovery. Review of the literature. New Orleans Med Surg J 83:13
72. Hee HT, Majd ME, Holt RT, Pienkowski D (2002) Better treatment of vertebral osteomyelitis using posterior stabilization and titanium mesh cages. J Spinal Disord Tech 15:149–156; discussion 156
73. Henriques CQ (1958) Osteomyelitis as a complication in urology; with special reference to the paravertebral venous plexus. Br J Surg 46:19–28
74. Henson SW Jr, Coventry MB (1956) Osteomyelitis of the vertebrae as the result of infection of the urinary tract. Surg Gynecol Obstet 102:207–214
75. Hirakawa A, Miyamoto K, Masuda T, Fukuta S, Hosoe H, Iinuma N, Iwai C, Nishimoto H, Shimizu K (2010) Surgical outcome of 2-stage (posterior and anterior) surgical treatment using spinal instrumentation for tuberculous spondylitis. J Spinal Disord Tech 23:133–138

76. Hodgson AR, Stock FE (1956) Anterior spinal fusion a preliminary communication on the radical treatment of Pott's disease and Pott's paraplegia. Br J Surg 44:266–275
77. Hopkinson N, Stevenson J, Benjamin S (2001) A case ascertainment study of septic discitis: clinical, microbiological and radiological features. QJM 94:465–470
78. Iqbal P, Castleden CM (1997) Management of urinary incontinence in the elderly. Gerontology 43:151–157
79. Irwin AD, Carrol ED (2011) Procalcitonin. Arch Dis Child Educ Pract Ed 96:228–233
80. Isenberg Y, Parada JP (2010) Spontaneous vertebral osteomyelitis due to Staphylococcus epidermidis. J Med Microbiol 59:599–601
81. Jaramillo-de la Torre JJ, Bohinski RJ, Kuntz C t (2006) Vertebral osteomyelitis. Neurosurg Clin N Am 17(339–51):vii
82. Jaye DL, Waites KB (1997) Clinical applications of C-reactive protein in pediatrics. Pediatr Infect Dis J 16:735–746; quiz 746–7
83. Jensen AG, Espersen F, Skinhoj P, Frimodt-Moller N (1998) Bacteremic Staphylococcus aureus spondylitis. Arch Intern Med 158:509–517
84. Ji B, Lounis N, Maslo C, Truffot-Pernot C, Bonnafous P, Grosset J (1998) In vitro and in vivo activities of moxifloxacin and clinafloxacin against Mycobacterium tuberculosis. Antimicrob Agents Chemother 42:2066–2069
85. Jimenez-Mejias ME, de Dios Colmenero J, Sanchez-Lora FJ, Palomino-Nicas J, Reguera JM, Garcia de la Heras J, Garcia-Ordonez MA, Pachon J (1999) Postoperative spondylodiskitis: etiology, clinical findings, prognosis, and comparison with nonoperative pyogenic spondylodiskitis. Clin Infect Dis 29:339–345
86. Joughin E, McDougall C, Parfitt C, Yong-Hing K, Kirkaldy-Willis WH (1991) Causes and clinical management of vertebral osteomyelitis in Saskatchewan. Spine (Phila Pa 1976) 16:261–264
87. Kemp HB, Jackson JW, Shaw NC (1974) Laminectomy in paraplegia due to infective spondylosis. Br J Surg 61:66–72
88. Kim NH, Lee HM, Suh JS (1994) Magnetic resonance imaging for the diagnosis of tuberculous spondylitis. Spine (Phila Pa 1976) 19:2451–2455
89. Kim SH, Choi SJ, Kim HB, Kim NJ, Oh MD, Choe KW (2007) Diagnostic usefulness of a T-cell based assay for extrapulmonary tuberculosis. Arch Intern Med 167:2255–2259
90. Kim CW, Currier BL, Eismont FJ (2011) Infections of the Spine. In: Herkowitz HN, Garfin SR, Eismont FJ, Bell GR, Balderston RA (eds) Rothman-Simeone the spine, vol 2. Elsevier Saunders, Philadelphia, pp 1513–1570
91. King DM, Mayo KM (1973) Infective lesions of the vertebral column. Clin Orthop Relat Res 96:248–253
92. Koppel BS, Tuchman AJ, Mangiardi JR, Daras M, Weitzner I (1988) Epidural spinal infection in intravenous drug abusers. Arch Neurol 45:1331–1337
93. Korovessis P, Petsinis G, Koureas G, Iliopoulos P, Zacharatos S (2006) Anterior surgery with insertion of titanium mesh cage and posterior instrumented fusion performed sequentially on the same day under one anesthesia for septic spondylitis of thoracolumbar spine: is the use of titanium mesh cages safe? Spine (Phila Pa 1976) 31:1014–1019
94. Korovessis P, Petsinis G, Koureas G, Iliopoulos P, Zacharatos S (2006) One-stage combined surgery with mesh cages for treatment of septic spondylitis. Clin Orthop Relat Res 444:51–59
95. Kowalski TJ, Berbari EF, Huddleston PM, Steckelberg JM, Osmon DR (2006) Do follow-up imaging examinations provide useful prognostic information in patients with spine infection? Clin Infect Dis 43:172–179
96. Krodel A, Kruger A, Lohscheidt K, Pfahler M, Refior HJ (1999) Anterior debridement, fusion, and extrafocal stabilization in the treatment of osteomyelitis of the spine. J Spinal Disord 12:17–26
97. Krogsgaard MR, Wagn P, Bengtsson J (1998) Epidemiology of acute vertebral osteomyelitis in Denmark: 137 cases in Denmark 1978–1982, compared to cases reported to the National Patient Register 1991–1993. Acta Orthop Scand 69:513–517

98. Kuklo TR, Potter BK, Bell RS, Moquin RR, Rosner MK (2006) Single-stage treatment of pyogenic spinal infection with titanium mesh cages. J Spinal Disord Tech 19:376–382
99. Kulowski J (1936) Pyogenic osteomyelitis of the spine: an analysis and discussion of 102 cases. J Bone Joint Surg Am 18:22
100. Lam KS, Webb JK (2004) Discitis. Hosp Med 65:280–286
101. Lazzarini L, Lipsky BA, Mader JT (2005) Antibiotic treatment of osteomyelitis: what have we learned from 30 years of clinical trials? Int J Infect Dis 9:127–138
102. Le Moal G, Roblot F, Paccalin M, Sosner P, Burucoa C, Roblot P, Becq-Giraudon B (2002) Clinical and laboratory characteristics of infective endocarditis when associated with spondylodiscitis. Eur J Clin Microbiol Infect Dis 21:671–675
103. Ledermann HP, Schweitzer ME, Morrison WB, Carrino JA (2003) MR imaging findings in spinal infections: rules or myths? Radiology 228:506–514
104. Legrand E, Flipo RM, Guggenbuhl P, Masson C, Maillefert JF, Soubrier M, Noel E, Saraux A, Di Fazano CS, Sibilia J, Goupille P, Chevalie X, Cantagrel A, Conrozier T, Ravaud P, Liote F (2001) Management of nontuberculous infectious discitis. treatments used in 110 patients admitted to 12 teaching hospitals in France. Joint Bone Spine 68:504–509
105. Lerner RK, Esterhai JL Jr, Polomono RC, Cheatle MC, Heppenstall RB, Brighton CT (1991) Psychosocial, functional, and quality of life assessment of patients with posttraumatic fracture nonunion, chronic refractory osteomyelitis, and lower extremity amputation. Arch Phys Med Rehabil 72:122–126
106. Lew DP, Waldvogel FA (1995) Quinolones and osteomyelitis: state-of-the-art. Drugs 49(Suppl 2):100–111
107. Lew DP, Waldvogel FA (2004) Osteomyelitis. Lancet 364:369–379
108. Light RW, Dunham TR (1974) Vertebral osteomyelitis due to Pseudomonas in the occasional heroin user. JAMA 228:1272
109. Liljenqvist U, Lerner T, Bullmann V, Hackenberg L, Halm H, Winkelmann W (2003) Titanium cages in the surgical treatment of severe vertebral osteomyelitis. Eur Spine J 12:606–612
110. Linhardt O, Matussek J, Refior HJ, Krodel A (2007) Long-term results of ventro-dorsal versus ventral instrumentation fusion in the treatment of spondylitis. Int Orthop 31:113–119
111. Luzzati R, Giacomazzi D, Danzi MC, Tacconi L, Concia E, Vento S (2009) Diagnosis, management and outcome of clinically- suspected spinal infection. J Infect 58:259–265
112. Malincarne L, Ghebregzabher M, Moretti MV, Egidi AM, Canovari B, Tavolieri G, Francisci D, Cerulli G, Baldelli F (2006) Penetration of moxifloxacin into bone in patients undergoing total knee arthroplasty. J Antimicrob Chemother 57:950–954
113. Markus HS (1989) Haematogenous osteomyelitis in the adult: a clinical and epidemiological study. Q J Med 71:521–527
114. Masuda T, Miyamoto K, Hosoe H, Shimizu K (2011) Comparative study on the efficacy of two-staged (posterior followed by anterior) surgical treatment using spinal instrumentation on pyogenic and tuberculotic spondylitis. Arch Orthop Trauma Surg 131:765–772
115. Matsui H, Hirano N, Sakaguchi Y (1998) Vertebral osteomyelitis: an analysis of 38 surgically treated cases. Eur Spine J 7:50–54
116. McHenry MC, Duchesneau PM, Keys TF, Rehm SJ, Boumphrey FR (1988) Vertebral osteomyelitis presenting as spinal compression fracture. Six patients with underlying osteoporosis. Arch Intern Med 148:417–423
117. McHenry MC, Easley KA, Locker GA (2002) Vertebral osteomyelitis: long-term outcome for 253 patients from 7 Cleveland-area hospitals. Clin Infect Dis 34:1342–1350
118. McKinnon PS, Davis SL (2004) Pharmacokinetic and pharmacodynamic issues in the treatment of bacterial infectious diseases. Eur J Clin Microbiol Infect Dis 23:271–288
119. Messer HD, Litvinoff J (1976) Pyogenic cervical osteomyelitis. Chondro-osteomyelitis of the cervical spine frequently associated with parenteral drug use. Arch Neurol 33:571–576
120. Michel SC, Pfirrmann CW, Boos N, Hodler J (2006) CT-guided core biopsy of subchondral bone and intervertebral space in suspected spondylodiskitis. AJR Am J Roentgenol 186:977–980

121. Modic MT, Feiglin DH, Piraino DW, Boumphrey F, Weinstein MA, Duchesneau PM, Rehm S (1985) Vertebral osteomyelitis: assessment using MR. Radiology 157:157–166
122. Mondorf Y, Gaab MR, Oertel JM (2009) PEEK cage cervical ventral fusion in spondylodiscitis. Acta Neurochir (Wien) 151:1537–1541
123. Mylona E, Samarkos M, Kakalou E, Fanourgiakis P, Skoutelis A (2009) Pyogenic vertebral osteomyelitis: a systematic review of clinical characteristics. Semin Arthritis Rheum 39:10–17
124. Nagashima H, Morio Y, Nishi T, Hagino H, Teshima R (2002) Spontaneous fusion of isthmic spondylolisthesis after discitis: a case report. Clin Orthop Relat Res 403:104–107
125. Nagashima H, Yamane K, Nishi T, Nanjo Y, Teshima R (2010) Recent trends in spinal infections: retrospective analysis of patients treated during the past 50 years. Int Orthop 34:395–399
126. Nagashima H, Nanjo Y, Tanida A, Dokai T, Teshima R (2012) Clinical features of spinal infection in individuals older than eighty years. Int Orthop 36:1229–1234
127. Nagashima H, Nanjo Y, Tanida A, Dokai T, Yamane K, Teshima R (2013) Early surgical intervention for spinal infection in patients with malignancy requiring chemotherapy: report of two cases and review of the literature. Eur J Orthop Surg Traumatol 23(Suppl 2):S155–S158
128. Nagel DA, Albright JA, Keggi KJ, Southwick WO (1965) Closer look at spinal lesions. Open biopsy of vertebral lesions. JAMA 191:975–978
129. Nather A, David V, Hee HT, Thambiah J (2005) Pyogenic vertebral osteomyelitis: a review of 14 cases. J Orthop Surg (Hong Kong) 13:240–244
130. Nicolle LE (1994) Urinary tract infection in the elderly. J Antimicrob Chemother 33(Suppl A):99–109
131. Nicolle LE (1994) Prevention and treatment of urinary catheter-related infections in older patients. Drugs Aging 4:379–391
132. Nicolle LE (1997) Asymptomatic bacteriuria in the elderly. Infect Dis Clin North Am 11:647–662
133. Nicolle LE, Mayhew WJ, Bryan L (1987) Prospective randomized comparison of therapy and no therapy for asymptomatic bacteriuria in institutionalized elderly women. Am J Med 83:27–33
134. Nicolle LE, Muir P, Harding GK, Norris M (1988) Localization of urinary tract infection in elderly, institutionalized women with asymptomatic bacteriuria. J Infect Dis 157:65–70
135. Niederman MS, Mandell LA, Anzueto A, Bass JB, Broughton WA, Campbell GD, Dean N, File T, Fine MJ, Gross PA, Martinez F, Marrie TJ, Plouffe JF, Ramirez J, Sarosi GA, Torres A, Wilson R, Yu VL (2001) Guidelines for the management of adults with community-acquired pneumonia. Diagnosis, assessment of severity, antimicrobial therapy, and prevention. Am J Respir Crit Care Med 163:1730–1754
136. Nolla JM, Ariza J, Gomez-Vaquero C, Fiter J, Bermejo J, Valverde J, Escofet DR, Gudiol F (2002) Spontaneous pyogenic vertebral osteomyelitis in nondrug users. Semin Arthritis Rheum 31:271–278
137. O'Daly BJ, Morris SF, O'Rourke SK (2008) Long-term functional outcome in pyogenic spinal infection. Spine (Phila Pa 1976) 33:E246–E253
138. Obana WG, Rosenblum ML (1992) Nonoperative treatment of neurosurgical infections. Neurosurg Clin N Am 3:359–373
139. Oga M, Arizono T, Takasita M, Sugioka Y (1993) Evaluation of the risk of instrumentation as a foreign body in spinal tuberculosis. Clinical and biologic study. Spine (Phila Pa 1976) 18:1890–1894
140. Olk DG, Hamill RJ, Proctor RA (1987) Haemophilus parainfluenzae vertebral osteomyelitis. Am J Med Sci 294:114–116
141. Osenbach RK, Hitchon PW, Menezes AH (1990) Diagnosis and management of pyogenic vertebral osteomyelitis in adults. Surg Neurol 33:266–275
142. Park KH, Chong YP, Kim SH, Lee SO, Choi SH, Lee MS, Jeong JY, Woo JH, Kim YS (2013) Clinical characteristics and therapeutic outcomes of hematogenous vertebral osteomyelitis caused by methicillin-resistant Staphylococcus aureus. J Infect 67:556–564
143. Patzakis MJ, Rao S, Wilkins J, Moore TM, Harvey PJ (1991) Analysis of 61 cases of vertebral osteomyelitis. Clin Orthop Relat Res 264:178–183

144. Pee YH, Park JD, Choi YG, Lee SH (2008) Anterior debridement and fusion followed by posterior pedicle screw fixation in pyogenic spondylodiscitis: autologous iliac bone strut versus cage. J Neurosurg Spine 8:405–412
145. Perronne C, Saba J, Behloul Z, Salmon-Ceron D, Leport C, Vilde JL, Kahn MF (1994) Pyogenic and tuberculous spondylodiskitis (vertebral osteomyelitis) in 80 adult patients. Clin Infect Dis 19:746–750
146. Pigrau C, Almirante B, Flores X, Falco V, Rodriguez D, Gasser I, Villanueva C, Pahissa A (2005) Spontaneous pyogenic vertebral osteomyelitis and endocarditis: incidence, risk factors, and outcome. Am J Med 118:1287
147. Priest DH, Peacock JE Jr (2005) Hematogenous vertebral osteomyelitis due to Staphylococcus aureus in the adult: clinical features and therapeutic outcomes. South Med J 98:854–862
148. Propst-Proctor SL, Dillingham MF, McDougall IR, Goodwin D (1982) The white blood cell scan in orthopedics. Clin Orthop Relat Res 168:157–165
149. Quinn SF, Murray W, Clark RA, Cochran C (1988) MR imaging of chronic osteomyelitis. J Comput Assist Tomogr 12:113–117
150. Rath SA, Neff U, Schneider O, Richter HP (1996) Neurosurgical management of thoracic and lumbar vertebral osteomyelitis and discitis in adults: a review of 43 consecutive surgically treated patients. Neurosurgery 38:926–933
151. Rissing JP (1997) Antimicrobial therapy for chronic osteomyelitis in adults: role of the quinolones. Clin Infect Dis 25:1327–1333
152. Roblot F, Besnier JM, Juhel L, Vidal C, Ragot S, Bastides F, Le Moal G, Godet C, Mulleman D, Azais I, Becq-Giraudon B, Choutet P (2007) Optimal duration of antibiotic therapy in vertebral osteomyelitis. Semin Arthritis Rheum 36:269–277
153. Ross PM, Fleming JL (1976) Vertebral body osteomyelitis: spectrum and natural history. A retrospective analysis of 37 cases. Clin Orthop Relat Res 118:190–198
154. Ruf M, Stoltze D, Merk HR, Ames M, Harms J (2007) Treatment of vertebral osteomyelitis by radical debridement and stabilization using titanium mesh cages. Spine (Phila Pa 1976) 32:E275–E280
155. Salahuddin NI, Madhavan T, Fisher EJ, Cox F, Quinn EL, Eyler WR (1973) Pseudomonas osteomyelitis. Radiologic features. Radiology 109:41–47
156. Sapico FL (1996) Microbiology and antimicrobial therapy of spinal infections. Orthop Clin North Am 27:9–13
157. Sapico FL, Montgomerie JZ (1979) Pyogenic vertebral osteomyelitis: report of nine cases and review of the literature. Rev Infect Dis 1:754–776
158. Sapico FL, Montgomerie JZ (1990) Vertebral osteomyelitis. Infect Dis Clin North Am 4:539–550
159. Schimmer RC, Jeanneret C, Nunley PD, Jeanneret B (2002) Osteomyelitis of the cervical spine: a potentially dramatic disease. J Spinal Disord Tech 15:110–117
160. Schinkel C, Gottwald M, Andress HJ (2003) Surgical treatment of spondylodiscitis. Surg Infect (Larchmt) 4:387–391
161. Schuster JM, Avellino AM, Mann FA, Girouard AA, Grady MS, Newell DW, Winn HR, Chapman JR, Mirza SK (2000) Use of structural allografts in spinal osteomyelitis: a review of 47 cases. J Neurosurg 93:8–14
162. Scuderi GJ, Greenberg SS, Banovac K, Martinez OV, Eismont FJ (1993) Penetration of glycopeptide antibiotics in nucleus pulposus. Spine (Phila Pa 1976) 18:2039–2042
163. Silverthorn KG, Gillespie WJ (1986) Pyogenic spinal osteomyelitis: a review of 61 cases. N Z Med J 99:62–65
164. Smith AS, Blaser SI (1991) Infectious and inflammatory processes of the spine. Radiol Clin North Am 29:809–827
165. Smith AS, Weinstein MA, Mizushima A, Coughlin B, Hayden SP, Lakin MM, Lanzieri CF (1989) MR imaging characteristics of tuberculous spondylitis vs vertebral osteomyelitis. AJR Am J Roentgenol 153:399–405
166. Solis Garcia del Pozo JM, Vives Soto M, Solera J (2007) Vertebral osteomyelitis: long-term disability assessment and prognostic factors. J Infect 54:129–134

167. Song KH, Jeon JH, Park WB, Kim SH, Park KU, Kim NJ, Oh MD, Kim HB, Choe KW (2009) Usefulness of the whole-blood interferon-gamma release assay for diagnosis of extra-pulmonary tuberculosis. Diagn Microbiol Infect Dis 63:182–187
168. Stein GE (1996) Pharmacokinetics and pharmacodynamics of newer fluoroquinolones. Clin Infect Dis 23:S19–S24
169. Stoker DJ, Kissin CM (1985) Percutaneous vertebral biopsy: a review of 135 cases. Clin Radiol 36:569–577
170. Stone DB, Bonfiglio M (1963) Pyogenic vertebral osteomyelitis. A diagnostic pitfall for the internist. Arch Intern Med 112:491–500
171. Sundararaj GD, Babu N, Amritanand R, Venkatesh K, Nithyananth M, Cherian VM, Lee VN (2007) Treatment of haematogenous pyogenic vertebral osteomyelitis by single-stage anterior debridement, grafting of the defect and posterior instrumentation. J Bone Joint Surg Br 89:1201–1205
172. Syvanen J, Peltola V, Pajulo O, Ruuskanen O, Mertsola J, Helenius I (2014) Normal behavior of plasma procalcitonin in adolescents undergoing surgery for scoliosis. Scand J Surg 103:60–65
173. Szypryt EP, Hardy JG, Hinton CE, Worthington BS, Mulholland RC (1988) A comparison between magnetic resonance imaging and scintigraphic bone imaging in the diagnosis of disc space infection in an animal model. Spine (Phila Pa 1976) 13:1042–1048
174. Tali ET, Gultekin S (2005) Spinal infections. Eur Radiol 15:599–607
175. Thompson D, Bannister P, Murphy P (1988) Vertebral osteomyelitis in the elderly. Br Med J (Clin Res Ed) 296:1309–1311
176. Torda AJ, Gottlieb T, Bradbury R (1995) Pyogenic vertebral osteomyelitis: analysis of 20 cases and review. Clin Infect Dis 20:320–328
177. Tsiodras S, Falagas ME (2006) Clinical assessment and medical treatment of spine infections. Clin Orthop Relat Res 444:38–50
178. Visalli MA, Jacobs MR, Appelbaum PC (1996) Activity of CP 99,219 (trovafloxacin) compared with ciprofloxacin, sparfloxacin, clinafloxacin, lomefloxacin and cefuroxime against ten penicillin-susceptible and penicillin-resistant pneumococci by time-kill methodology. J Antimicrob Chemother 37:77–84
179. Waldvogel FA, Papageorgiou PS (1980) Osteomyelitis: the past decade. N Engl J Med 303:360–370
180. Waldvogel FA, Medoff G, Swartz MN (1970) Osteomyelitis: a review of clinical features, therapeutic considerations and unusual aspects. N Engl J Med 282:198–206
181. Waldvogel FA, Medoff G, Swartz MN (1970) Osteomyelitis: a review of clinical features, therapeutic considerations and unusual aspects (second of three parts). N Engl J Med 282:260–266
182. Walter J, Kuhn SA, Reichart R, Kalff R, Ewald C (2010) PEEK cages as a potential alternative in the treatment of cervical spondylodiscitis: a preliminary report on a patient series. Eur Spine J 19:1004–1009
183. Wiesseman GJ, Wood VE, Kroll LL, Linda L (1973) Pseudomonas vertebral osteomyelitis in heroin addicts. Report of five cases. J Bone Joint Surg Am 55:1416–1424
184. Wiley AM, Trueta J (1959) The vascular anatomy of the spine and its relationship to pyogenic vertebral osteomyelitis. J Bone Joint Surg Br 41-b:796–809
185. Wisneski RJ (1991) Infectious disease of the spine. Diagnostic and treatment considerations. Orthop Clin North Am 22:491–501
186. Woertgen C, Rothoerl RD, Englert C, Neumann C (2006) Pyogenic spinal infections and outcome according to the 36-item short form health survey. J Neurosurg Spine 4:441–446
187. Yamane K, Nagashima H, Tanishima S, Teshima R (2010) Severe rotational deformity, quadriparesis and respiratory embarrassment due to osteomyelitis at the occipito-atlantoaxial junction. J Bone Joint Surg Br 92:286–288
188. Yang SC, Fu TS, Chen LH, Chen WJ, Tu YK (2008) Identifying pathogens of spondylodiscitis: percutaneous endoscopy or CT-guided biopsy. Clin Orthop Relat Res 466:3086–3092

189. Yoon SH, Chung SK, Kim KJ, Kim HJ, Jin YJ, Kim HB (2010) Pyogenic vertebral osteomyelitis: identification of microorganism and laboratory markers used to predict clinical outcome. Eur Spine J 19:575–582
190. Yoshimoto M, Takebayashi T, Kawaguchi S, Tsuda H, Ida K, Wada T, Yamashita T (2011) Pyogenic spondylitis in the elderly: a report from Japan with the most aging society. Eur Spine J 20:649–654
191. Zarrouk V, Feydy A, Salles F, Dufour V, Guigui P, Redondo A, Fantin B (2007) Imaging does not predict the clinical outcome of bacterial vertebral osteomyelitis. Rheumatology (Oxford) 46:292–295

Part V

Head Injury

Traumatic Brain Injury in the Elderly

19

Verena Röckelein, Michael Buchfelder,
and Andrea Kleindienst

19.1 Epidemiology and Pathology

19.1.1 Epidemiology

Traumatic brain injury (TBI) is defined as a consequence of force exposure resulting in operational deterioration and/or brain damage as well as an optional contusion or trauma of the callosity, the cranium, the vessels, and/or the dura [1]. As postulated by the World Health Organization (WHO), by the year 2020, TBI might be the main cause of disability and death [2]. As demographic change directs to an increased life expectation, we therefore will also face an increasing number of TBI in the elderly (Fig. 19.1). Furthermore, due to physical changes in context of aging, this subgroup is more likely to sustain TBI. In fact, there is an association between age and TBI-related hospital admissions [3]. Referring to the United States, there are 1.4 million cases of TBI per year, of which 155, 000 patients are 65 years or older [4]. From a geographical point of view, moderate to severe forms of TBI are more common in the agrarian population than in urban environment [5].

A multiplicity of work groups all over the world, consisting of expert physicians and neurosurgeons, has established various more or less country-specific guidelines on the management of TBI [1, 6–11]. Unfortunately, these guidelines currently

V. Röckelein • M. Buchfelder, MD, PhD
Department of Neurosurgery, Friedrich-Alexander-University Erlangen-Nürnberg, Schwabachanlage 6, D-91054 Erlangen, Germany
e-mail: verena.roeckelein@fau.de; Michael.Buchfelder@uk-erlangen.de

A. Kleindienst, MD, PhD (✉)
Department of Neurosurgery, Friedrich-Alexander-University Erlangen-Nürnberg, Schwabachanlage 6, D-91054 Erlangen, Germany

Department of Neurosurgery, Klinikum Amberg, Amberg, Germany
e-mail: Andrea.Kleindienst@uk-erlangen.de

© Springer International Publishing Switzerland 2017

M. Berhouma, P. Krolak-Salmon (eds.), *Brain and Spine Surgery in the Elderly*,
DOI 10.1007/978-3-319-40232-1_19

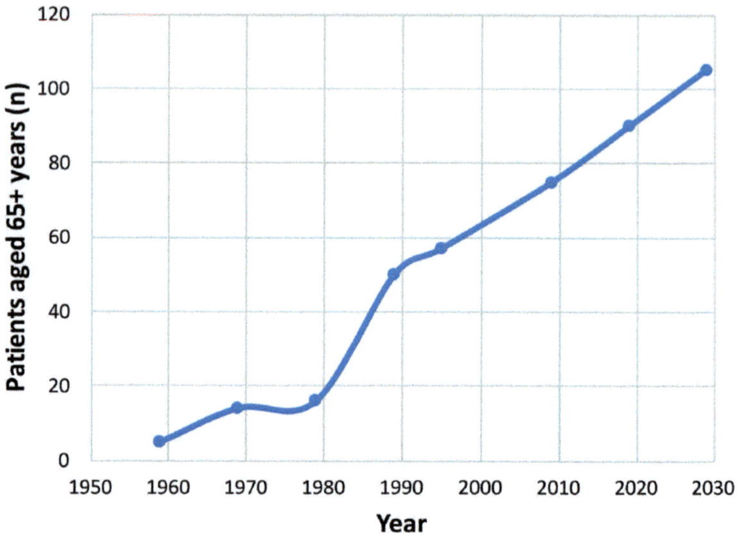

Fig. 19.1 Estimated number of future TBI patients >65 years based on data of a German University Department of Neurosurgery©

available do not provide recommendations that are validated for elderly TBI patients explicitly [1, 6–11].

In the following, the "elderly" patient is defined as being 65 years or older.

19.1.2 Main Causes of Traumatic Brain Injury

A population-based study in New Zealand of 2013 revealed falls to be the most common mechanism for TBI (38 %), followed by mechanical forces (21 %), transport accidents (20 %), and assaults (17 %) [5]. Wee et al. from Singapore declare motor vehicle accidents (48.8 %) to be the main reason for TBI (48.8 %), followed by falls (42.5 %) [12].

Factors that result in fall injuries in patients aged 65 years and older are physical and behavioral conditions (73.4 %), medication (8.4 %), personal (7.6 %), environment (7.1 %), and equipment or facility (3.5 %) [13].

Another risk factor for falls in patients with oral anticoagulation is the existence of at least one comorbidity [14].

In India, 40 % of elderly patients who fell also suffered from head injury, whereas 50 % suffered from a severe head injury (Glasgow Coma Scale, GCS <9) in turn [15].

A study in Taiwan revealed that a main part of falls in the elderly led to injury (71.2 %); among those a major part was mild (56.3 %). Thirty out of 378 patients (7.9 %) even suffered from head injury [13].

As age is correlated to the total number of prescribed drugs, medication is another factor which should be taken into consideration when analyzing the main causes of fall in the elderly population [16]. Anticoagulants, antiplatelets, antihypertensives, and psychotropic drugs go along with a cumulative incidence of TBI. Hospital admission in general is associated with anticoagulants, antiplatelets, narcotics, and analgesics as well [16].

19.1.3 Pathophysiology

The damage of TBI consists of in two parts: a primary, irreversible brain damage caused by the injury itself. Here the physician's treatment aims to minimize the extent of damage.

The secondary brain damage, which lingers from the time of injury and continues for days and weeks afterwards, is caused by a plurality of pathophysiological, cellular, and molecular processes. Homeostasis needs to be restored to protect brain tissue from secondary insults, whereas inflammation in the acute phase seems to deviate from delayed responses after TBI [17].

Following TBI, we can differ two types of brain damage, categorized on the basis of localization: focal damage (including cortical and subcortical contusions, lacerations, and intracranial hemorrhage) caused by direct impingement on the brain, which is often related to severe TBI on one hand, and diffuse injury on the other.

In contrast to focal damage, diffuse injury is also seen in mild forms of TBI and is provoked by strain and tearing of the brain tissue. Direct force effect or skull fractures are not required. The most frequently resulting type of diffuse injury is the diffuse axonal injury (DAI) [18].

19.1.4 Diffuse Axonal Injury

More precisely, the term diffuse axonal injury (DAI) is a misnomer as the damage does not accrue in the whole brain but prevailing in discrete regions such as the brain stem, parasagittal white matter, and gray-white matter junctions of the cerebral cortex and the corpus callosum [19]. Therefore, often the term traumatic axonal injury (TAI) is preferred over DAI [20].

Three grades of DAI can be distinguished: in grade 1, histological correlates of axonal injury are detectable in the white matter of the cerebral hemispheres, the brain stem, the corpus callosum, and in rare cases in the cerebellum. Grade 2 is characterized through focal lesions in the corpus callosum. In grade 3, finally, there are also focal lesions in the dorsolateral quadrant of the rostral brain stem [21]. These focal lesions are often only detectable by microscopic investigation [21].

Damage on cellular level can be linked to various types of cellular injury mechanisms (anoxic or hemorrhagic events, contusion, perfusion-reperfusion damage) or structural correlates (DAI, focal lesion). Having in mind that each injury has its own pattern of receptors and biochemical pathways to regain, recover, it is essential to differentiate these types of injury [19].

Examining axonal damage after dynamic stretching in micro-patterned neuronal cell cultures, an immediate rupture and buckling of the microtubules result in axon undulations. This microtubule disorganization is followed by a delayed elastic response as the microtubule system relaxes back to orientation progressively resulting in recovery of the former straight morphology of the axon [22]. What finally results in axonal damage is the interruption of axonal transport during these undulation processes which procures swelling and degeneration [22].

The examination of the brains from patients deceased from blunt head injury revealed obvious reduction of neurofilament triplet proteins 200 and 68 kDa in the corpus callosum. B-tubulin and tau, though, only display minimally changed concentrations [23]. Compared to healthy individuals, calpain-mediated spectrin breakdown products were significantly increased in head-injured patients. This supports the assumption of axonal damage after TBI resulting in calpain-mediated breakdown of the cytoskeleton [23]. In rats these elevated calpain-specific 145-kDa breakdown products of alpha II-spectrin (SBDP145) can be localized in the neocortex, the subcortical white matter, as well as the thalamus and hippocampus with peaks at 24–48 h after the head injury [24]. As SBDP145 levels in CSF are raised at 24-h post-injury, this breakdown product might serve as a biomarker of diffuse brain injury [24].

Reactive axonal change can be verified by immunocytochemical strategies. It is possible to visualize early axonal damage after trauma by the use of antibodies targeting the neurofilamental subunits. Six hours after the injury, affected axons seem focally swollen but intact. At 12-h post-injury, focal swelling has proceeded, and disconnection has developed. This immunoreactive swelling progresses for 1 week after the injury [25].

Genetic studies on rats disclosed an amount of genes which are upregulated to protect and repair brain tissue after injury, for instance, C1q12, Cbnl, 5dC1 BDNF, MMP9, and CD47 [26]. Several isoforms, though, are only induced in young, but not in elderly animals [27].

19.1.5 Imaging of Traumatic Brain Injury

19.1.5.1 Computed Tomography

Cranial computed tomography (CT) still is the base of imaging in the acute phase of TBI (Fig. 19.2) [20, 28].

However, there is a limitation, as CT is only sensitive enough for moderate to severe forms of TBI [28]. In cases of mild TBI and DAI, where no hemorrhagic mass lesion or punctate lesions exist, only about 10 % of DAI patients show classic structural correlates are detectable by cranial CT scan [19].

In adult patients with minimal, mild, or moderate head injury, who have a GCS score of <15, loss of consciousness, clinical signs of depressed or basal skull fracture, focal neurological deficits or posttraumatic seizures, repeated vomiting, coagulation disorders, anticoagulant therapy, or, in case of elderly patients, antiplatelet medication, a CT scan is indicated [8, 29].

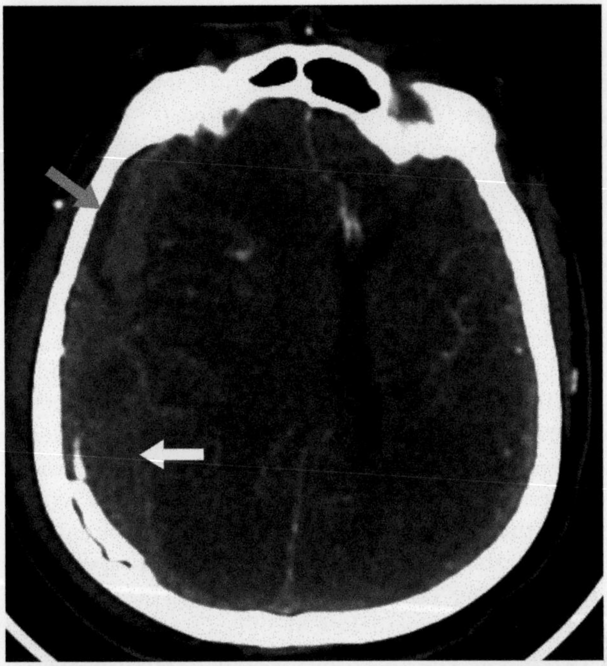

Fig. 19.2 The CT scan of a 75-year-old male patient involved in a car accident as a pedestrian. The initial GCS was 3. He was under oral anticoagulation with rivaroxaban because of a tachyarrhythmia absoluta and an embolic minor stroke. The CT demonstrates an impression fracture, epi- and acute subdural hematoma (*white arrow*), as well as a preexisting chronic subdural hematoma (*gray arrow*)

19.1.5.2 Magnetic Resonance Imaging and Diffusion Tensor Imaging

Compared to cranial CT, magnetic resonance imaging (MRI) scores with its better diagnostic sensitivity for nonhemorrhagic contusions and shear-strain injuries [20].

Diffusion tensor imaging (DTI), an explorative MRI technique, assesses diffusion in at least six (typically 25–30) directions. DTI is based on the intrinsic diffusion properties of neurons and drafts the microstructural characteristics of brain tissue [20].

As DAI causes such changes in neuronal diffusivity, the resulting pathophysiologic correlates can be visualized via DTI. DTI might even be the only tool sensitive enough to detect changes occurring in the acute phase of mild TBI (mTBI) [30].

Recent studies investigating occult white matter integrity and abnormalities in patients suffering from mild TBI confirmed DTI to be more accurate than traditional clinical measures. Consequently, DTI serves as a valuable clinical evaluation tool, also for evaluating the resulting cognitive recovery prospectively [31–33].

Regarding the prediction of the patient's cognitive recovery, DTI might even serve as a noninvasive prognostic marker [33].

Preferentially used DTI-derived measures are the mean diffusivity (MD) and the fractional anisotropy (FA) [30, 33].

Following TBI, changes in MD and FA are measureable [34].

A study including mild TBI patients with negative CT findings showed that mean diffusivity (MD) 24-h post-injury was significantly higher in injured individuals compared to the healthy control group [30].

19.1.6 S100B

S100B is a member of the calcium-binding S100 family [35]. In the molecule's center, the so-called linker region connects the two EF-hand calcium-binding domains [35]. S100B possesses neurotropic and mitogenic activity and operates stimulative on astroglial cell proliferation [36–38]. As highest levels of S100B are existent in the nervous system [39], S100B serves as a marker of brain tissue damage and is measured in the cerebrospinal fluid (CSF) and in serum. CSF performs shock-absorbing to the brain and works as a protective environment. Because of its direct contact to the exterior brain tissue, many cytokines, chemokines, and other proteins released following TBI are also detectable in the CSF [18].

Measurement of S100B level in the CSF of healthy individuals resulted in values of 0.66 ± 0.08 μg/L in CSF and 0.05 ± 0.01 μg/L in serum, which is about 10 % of the concentration detectable in CSF [40].

Following stretch injury to glial-neuronal cell cultures, S100B is released passively and actively secreted [41].

Significant increase of S100B and also of the neuron-specific enolase (NSE) and of cortisol concentrations in serum can be found in boxers being hit on the head during their fight in comparison to those who did not receive direct head blows [42].

Concerning the S100B passage from CSF to serum, Kleindienst et al. established a ratio of S100B serum to CSF. This ratio correlates positively with a better neurological function [40]. Therefore, S100B is a valuable prognostic tool for outcome.

The neuroprotective role of S100B has been demonstrated in cell cultural experiments. Adding S100B to neuronal and glial cultures, which have been subjected to stretch injury before, the resulting neuronal damage at 48 h is significantly reduced [41].

S100B serum levels are not falsified by alcohol intoxication [43].

Regarding the variation of S100B levels in patients 65 years and older, increased serum concentrations are more common in this group. Our own data on 126 TBI patients confirm significantly increased S100B levels in the serum on day 3, 4, and 5 post-injury. However, evaluating the reliability of S100B diagnostics in elderly people, there might be limitations due to poor specificity [43].

19.1.7 Association of TBI and Neurodegenerative Illness

Acute axonal damage due to TBI evokes both degenerative and regenerative tissue responses [18]. Recurrent concussion may be the basis of dementia pugilistica, a long-term neurodegenerative event and a type of chronic traumatic encephalopathy

(CTE) [18]. CTE, a disease characterized through memory disturbances, changes in behavior and personality, parkinsonism, as well as abnormal speech and gait, is possible to arise at a later period of life after repetitive minor blunt head trauma in the past. Pathologic vast tau-immunoreactive neurofibrillary tangles in the brain tissue correlate with the relative deficiency of Aβ deposits [44, 45].

In 30 % of those patients deceased from TBI, Aβ plaques, a pathological correlate of Alzheimer's disease (AD), are existent [46].

Potential markers for Alzheimer's disease in CSF are the tau protein, amyloid beta (Aβ; 42-amino acid forms Aβ (1–42)), as well as apolipoprotein E (APOE) [47].

19.1.7.1 Amyloid Beta

Amyloid beta 42 (Aβ-42) in CSF as well as in serum has a predictive value in estimating mortality. Aβ-42 levels in the CSF are decreased in the acute phase after TBI and even lower in deceased patients compared to survivors [48, 49]. Concentrations of Aβ-42 in serum act conversely: levels are significantly elevated in patients suffering from TBI and lower in the surviving, not the deceased, individuals [48]. Franz et al. found significantly lower concentrations of Ab-42 in TBI patients compared to patients suffering from headache or dementia [49]. Higher levels of Aβ-42 in the CSF are also associated with better neurological outcome, suggesting Aβ-42 as a prognostic marker and monitoring tool for patients with severe TBI [48, 49].

Cutoff levels differ between good (GOS 4 and 5) and poor outcome (GOS 1–3) can be set at an Aβ-42 CSF concentration of 230 pg/mL resulting in a sensitivity of 100 % and a specificity of 82 % [49].

19.1.7.2 Tau

In patients suffering from TBI, tau in CSF is significantly elevated in comparison to control groups [49, 50].

CSF tau increases immediately after TBI resulting in peak values about 2 weeks post-injury [49]. Furthermore, tau in CSF correlates to the extended Glasgow Outcome Scale (GOSe) assessed 1 year after severe brain injury [50].

Total tau levels on day 2–3 serve as a cutoff point. Here, levels above 2126 pg/mL are a predictor for mortality with a sensitivity of 100 % and a specificity of 81 % and levels above 702 pg/mL to differentiate between bad (GOSe 1–4) and good (GOSe 5–8) outcome (sensitivity, 83 %; specificity, 69 %) [50].

All these findings suggest CSF tau as a valuable early biomarker in predicting future outcome [50].

19.1.7.3 Apolipoprotein E ε4

The existence of APOE ε4 comes along with a higher risk of moderate to severe forms of head injury and severe ischemic damage of brain tissue [51]. Thus, APOE ε4 is also associated with unfavorable outcome [51]. As demonstrated in animal experiments, the existence of APOE ε4 delays astroglial repair mechanisms and compromises synaptic remodeling indirectly [52].

In hippocampal slice cultures, higher APO E3 expression led to increased sprouting, whereas the presence of higher APOE ε4 went along with decreased sprouting [53]. This encourages the hypothesis that this deficiency of APO ε4 in supporting neuronal sprouting serves as a gain-of-negative activity and should be taken into consideration in the development of future Alzheimer's disease drugs [53].

In a population-based study, in elderly patients suffered from fall-related TBI, dementia occurred earlier. This was mostly the case if the patient was a carrier of the apolipoprotein E ε4 allele [54].

19.2 Comorbidities, Coagulation Abnormalities, and Intracerebral Hemorrhage

19.2.1 Comorbidities and Coagulation

Referring to the main reasons of fall, one risk factor for falls in elderly patients with oral anticoagulation is the existence of at least one comorbidity [14].

As elderly people are likely to have cardiovascular diseases requiring drugs for anticoagulation, antiplatelet agents, and more, medication is a common cofactor of this population (Fig. 19.3).

The use of anticoagulation (e.g., warfarin) and antiplatelet agents (e.g., aspirin, clopidogrel) is an effective tool of reducing mortality associated with cerebrovascular and cardiovascular diseases. In TBI, though, the influence on coagulation might promote bleeding and be harmful [55]. Involving all types of TBI, elderly patients with intraparenchymal contusions and coagulation abnormalities are more likely to undergo pogressive hemorrhagic injury, which also leds to higher mortality [56]. Recent research supports the hypothesis that the use of warfarin, but not of antiplatelets, increases mortality and a higher degree of demand of neurosurgical treatment [55]. In case the elderly patient's head injury has led to intracranial hemorrhage,

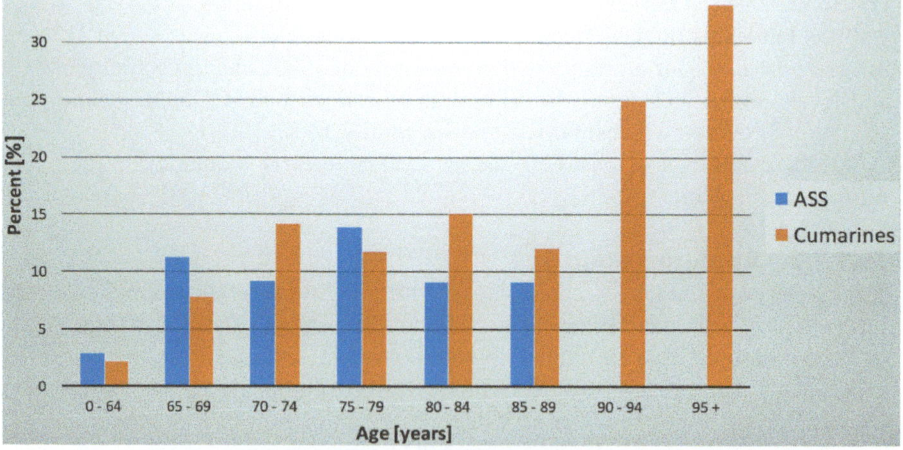

Fig. 19.3 Percentage of elderly TBI patients consuming ASS (*blue column*) or Marcumar (*orange column*) in a German University Hospital within a 5-year period

though, Ohm et al. declare the use of antiplatelet agents as a factor, which increases the risk of mortality [60].

19.2.2 Anticoagulation

In those patients over 65 years that are on oral anticoagulation, the appearance of two and more complications is more likely (288 and 370 %) [14].

In about 20 % of head injured patients aged 65 years and older, who were admitted to an American level I trauma center, were on warfarin [61].

Positive correlation exists between the consumption of warfarin and higher mortality in patients aged 55 years and older [62]. Patients on warfarin suffering from mild TBI are 2.7 times more likely to evolve intracranial hemorrhage (ICH) following TBI. Similarly, a supratherapeutic international normalized ratio (INR) was associated with a traumatic intracerebral hemorrhage (ICH) [63, 64].

Also delayed forms of ICH are more prevalent in elderly TBI patients treated with oral anticoagulation [65]. However, such delayed ICH only occurred in 1 % of the follow-up CT if no ICH was detectable in the initial CT scan [66, 67].

Thus, an INR over 4.0 predicts a higher mortality in TBI patients over 70 years [64]. Initial minor head injuries combined with an average INR of 4.4 result in a mortality of over 80 % [68].

For instance, the 30-day mortality in elderly patients on warfarin is 50 % (mean INR 3.0) compared to a mortality of 20 % in those without warfarin [69]. The INR and initial CT scan should be processed in all TBI patients on warfarin. Repeated cranial CT scan should be performed routinely at 12 to 18 h post-injury respectively when neurological worsening occurs [68].

Scandinavian guidelines on the *initial management of minimal, mild, and moderate head injury* suggest that the combination of older age (75 years and older) and the consumption of antiplatelet medication is an indication for a CT scan, as its coincidence is a risk factor for increased risk of intracranial complications in older patients suffering from mild head injury [8, 29].

19.2.3 Intracranial Hemorrhage

TBI in elderly people results most often in an acute subdural hematoma [70] (see also Chap. 20), analyzing the CT scans of the deceased ones [71].

In many cases traumatic intracranial hemorrhage (ICH) occurs and comes along with scalp hematoma and contrecoup injury [72].

Especially patients with intraparenchymal contusion are more likely to evolve progressive hemorrhagic injury [56].

Both, age and coagulopathy, are associated with a risk of hemorrhagic progression. TBI patients with progressive hemorrhagic injury are older, have fewer hospital-free days, and have higher mortality [56].

In summary, individuals that are most likely to experience progressive hemorrhagic injuries are elderly patients with coagulation abnormalities and IPH [56].

Fig. 19.4 CT findings of elderly patients aged 65 years and older in a German University Hospital within a 5-year period

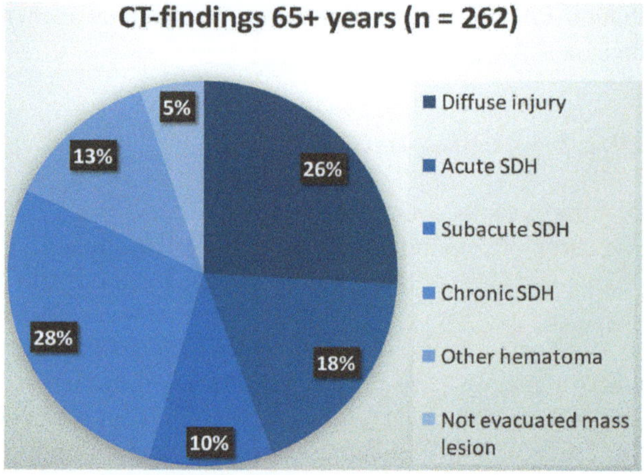

19.2.4 Imaging of Intracerebral Hemorrhage

19.2.4.1 Computed Tomography

Traditionally, CT has been the favored diagnostic imaging modality as it is widespread available and provides the feasibility to assess the patient's initial condition and to exclude ICH [72, 75] (Fig. 19.4).

Computed tomography angiography (CTA) is frequently used in order to detect vascular lesions causing the hemorrhage.

As a more invasive procedure, CTA implicates further risk for the patient and comes along with longer hospital stay and higher rate of intensive care unit (ICU) admission and ICU residence [73]. Apart from that, its results normally do not alter clinical management. Therefore, the existence of clear indications for CTA in TBI patients should be ensured [73].

19.2.4.2 Magnetic Resonance Imaging

The detection of ICH in TBI patients by magnetic resonance imaging (MRI) is at least as sensitive as CT in the acute phase. Furthermore, MRI outweighs CT in cases of subacute and chronic hematoma [72].

The sequences recommended in the hyperacute stage are the gradient echo (GRE) MRI sequences. In detecting intraparenchymal hemorrhage, it is as accurate as CT and therefore superior to traditional T1- and T2-weighted MRI pulse sequences. Furthermore, GRE MRI is even more favorable than CT in chronic hemorrhage [74, 76].

Another advantage of GRE MRI is the possibility to visualize even old, clinically silent cerebral micro hemorrhage (primary intracerebral), that is not detectable by classic CT [72].

In the detection of shearing lesions and diffuse axonal injury after TBI, susceptibility-weighted (SW) magnetic resonance (MR) imaging is favorable, as this high spatial resolution is capable of detecting more small hemorrhagic lesions than GRE MR imaging [77].

19.2.5 Management of Intracerebral Hemorrhage

Optimal clinical management of ICH patients is published within the actual AHA/ASA guidelines [79].

Class I recommendations (evidence for and/or general agreement in usefulness and effectivity of the procedure) are:

- A baseline severity score as well as rapid neuroimaging (CT or MRI) should be included in the initial evaluation of ICH patients [79].
- All clinical management and monitoring should happen in an intensive care unit (ICU) and a stroke unit, respectively, and should be observed by a physician with neuroscience acute care expertise [78, 79].
- Ideal systolic arterial blood pressure (SAP) for patients suffering from ICH is between 150 and 220 mmHg. If no contraindication, SAP may be lowered to 140 mmHg safely in order to enhance functional outcome [78, 79].
- The treatment of hemostasis and coagulopathy includes the substitution of coagulation factors and platelets, respectively.

If vitamin K antagonist has been applied and INR is abnormal, anticoagulation should be paused, vitamin K-dependent factors should be replaced, and vitamin K i.v. should be given [78, 79].

- Glucose levels should be observed and, if necessary, hypoglycemia and hyperglycemia have to be treated [78, 79].
- Antiseizure drugs can be applied to cure seizures [78, 79].
- Patients suffering from cerebellar hemorrhage with neurological deterioration or brainstem compression and/or hydrocephalus due to ventricular obstruction should receive surgical intervention in terms of surgical removal of the hemorrhage as soon as possible [79].
- Before oral intake of medication is initiated, dysphagia should be precluded in all ICH patients to prevent pneumonia [78, 79].
- To prevent recurrence of ICH, blood pressure monitoring is recommended in all patients starting immediately after the hemorrhage [78, 79].
- Multidisciplinary rehabilitation is recommended to all ICH patients [79].

Complications occurring in context of ICH are the expansion of hematoma, perihematomal edema and increased intracranial pressure, seizures, fever, venous thrombotic events, intraventricular extension and hydrocephalus, blood pressure increase, and various infections [80].

Intracranial hematoma above 25 mL predicts a poor outcome [81].

19.3 Prognosis, Outcome, and Rehabilitation

19.3.1 Intensive Care Unit and Treatment

A study including 11, 240 patients assessed in the Western United States illustrates the wide variability in the use of intensive care units (ICU) in minor traumatic ICH (50–97 %). Many of those transferred to the ICU never required critical care intervention (95 %) [82].

However, it is remarkable that senior patients often don't receive a treatment as aggressive as it would be performed in younger patients [83]. A population-based study, which investigated the hospital destination decision directly after trauma, found out that of all TBI cases in 2012, nearly half of them (47.9 %) were treated in a level I or II trauma center directly, whereas another 20.3 % were transferred to a level I or II trauma center subsequently [84]. About half of these 20 %, whose need for trauma center treatment was initially misjudged and who were transferred secondarily, were patients aged 55 or older [84].

19.3.1.1 Oxygenation and Blood Pressure

Hypotension below 90 mmHg systolic as well as hypoxemia below 90 % arterial hemoglobin oxygen saturation (measured with a pulse oximeter) should be avoided in severe TBI as they correlate with an unfavorable outcome [9]. As emphasized in the European guidelines on the *management of bleeding and coagulopathy following major trauma*, in TBI a low volume approach in hypotensive patients is contraindicated [85, 86]. Especially in elderly patients, a reevaluation of permissive hypotension therapy is crucial [86]. Berry et al. recommend to consider patients aged 70 years or older hypotensive, when the systolic blood pressure is below 110 mmHG [85]. If the GCS is below 9 or hypoxemia occurs despite supplemental oxygen, respiratory assurance with endotracheal intubation is indicated [9]. Whenever possible, blood pressure and oxygenation should be observed continuously [9].

19.3.1.2 Surgery

Always reassessed is the benefit of neurosurgical intervention in elderly patients aged 65 years and older. A Japanese study from Shimoda et al. suggests to triage senior TBI patients on the basis of their initial GCS score. In fact, surgical management could not be proven as effective in individuals with a GCS score of 3–5. Neurosurgical intervention, although, was able to improve prognosis in selected elderly TBI patients (GCS score of 6–15) [87, 88]. Suitable case selection and the identification of minor to moderate head injuries are the basis of distinguishing those who benefit from surgical treatment and traumatic hematoma evacuation. This is also valid for relatively younger elderly patients [89].

19.3.1.3 Craniotomy

Following surgical intervention like craniotomy, elderly individuals show good recovery and overall survival in 30–77 % [83, 89, 90–92].

In a cohort study on patients older than 80 years on one hand and 80 years of age and younger on the other, who suffered from single traumatic hematoma and underwent craniotomy, it was remarkable that adequate postoperative therapy enabled not only younger but also elderly patients to return to their preinjury functional conditions [93].

These results are not simply transferable to decompressive craniectomy.

For instance, at 1 year after decompressive craniectomy, 80 % had a poor outcome [94]. Among those who did not survive, the intracranial pressure (ICP) could not be controlled, but no complications due to surgery occurred [94].

19.3.1.4 Intracranial Pressure Monitoring

According to the Brain Trauma Foundation (BTF), one part of supportive therapy in the management of TBI patients is the intracranial pressure (ICP) monitoring. In the *guidelines for the management of severe traumatic brain injury*, the BTF declares ICP in the elderly of being an important topic, but by reason of lack of literature base, consensus could not be found in this issue so far [6]. However, recent studies could not verify a beneficial effect of ICP monitoring on the elderly TBI patients' outcome [87]. Patients who received an ICP monitor were younger in general and their mortality was significantly higher [95, 96]. The indication of ICP monitoring should be reevaluated [96].

19.3.1.5 Hypothermia

Investigations on hypothermia to improve functional outcome by the reduction of intracranial hypertension in TBI patients are inconclusive [97]. Standard care plus therapeutic hypothermia did not improve outcome in patients with an ICP of 20 mmHg and more, compared to standard care alone [97]. Quite the contrary, good outcome (GOSe score from 5 to 8) was achieved in 37 % of the individuals without hypothermia treatment compared to only 26 % in the hypothermia group [97].

19.3.1.6 Medication

In a clinical trial, the medication with progesterone, which was shown to have robust positive effects in animal TBI studies and early single-center trials, revealed no beneficial effects on outcome and mortality compared to placebo on brain-injured patients [98]. On the other hand, the use of statins in elderly TBI patients correlates with a higher probability of good recovery 12 months after the injury and is also associated with lower mortality. This effect might be explained by the immunomodulatory and inflammatory properties of statins [99].

19.3.2 Prognostic Factors

Elderly patients over 65 years have a total mortality of 14–55 %. The main influence coefficient is primarily the initial GCS and secondly the age [58, 100–104].

In the following, we present more detailed factors influencing the outcome of TBI patients and especially those aged 65 years and older.

19.3.2.1 Age

Several studies confirm higher age as an independent predictor of poor outcome [64, 81, 87] and influencing on neurocognitive recovery especially [105].

The Scottish Intercollegiate Guidelines Network even cites an age of over 40 years as a predictor of poor prognosis of mild TBI [10]. Animal studies could demonstrate general worse performance of older mice in comparison to younger animals [106, 107].

This tendency to higher mortality and worse functional outcome contrasts the fact that elderly patients tend to sustain from less severe injuries [4, 89, 102, 103, 108, 109].

Thus, age should not be the sole factor for restricting care in patients with a GCS 6–15 [87].

19.3.2.2 Loss of Consciousness

There is a correlation between the loss of consciousness and poor functional outcome and higher mortality in elderly TBI patients [88, 105].

The duration of coma is associated with the depth of "marker lesions" in CT findings [81].

19.3.2.3 Glasgow Coma Score

The correlation of GCS on admission and the severity of head injury as well as the future outcome have been known for a long time [9, 81, 110]. A large Chinese multicenter study on TBI showed that mild TBI patients (GCS 13–15) survived in 90% of cases. In contrast, among severe TBI victims, only 20% reached a good outcome (GCS 3–8) [104]. Table 19.1 demonstrates data from a German hospital over a 5-year period. The percentage of unfavorable GCS (scores of 3–5) rises with the patient's age.

In the elderly population, even less than one fifth of those suffering from severe TBI resulted in proper outcome, and mortality was higher and reached from 68 to 92.5%.

19.3.2.4 Anticoagulation

In patients that were on oral anticoagulation (e.g., warfarin), significantly elevated mortality was present [64]. This is not valid for consumption of antiplatelet agents [55], but in combination with older age, the use of antiplatelet agents should be considered as a combined risk factor increasing the risks for intracranial complications and indicating a CT scan [8, 29].

19.3.2.5 Pupillary Dilatation

Former guideline recommendations for prehospital management of TBI (2002) declared the data on examination of the pupils on admission as insufficient [9].

Table 19.1 Percentages of elderly TBI patients aged 65 and older ($n=61$) with GCS score of 3–5 within 5 years in a German hospital

Age	65–69	70–74	75–79	80–84	85+
GCS Score 3–5	38%	47%	44%	63%	73%

Recently, a correlation between pupillary dilatation and unfavorable outcome respectively increased mortality could be shown [81, 88]. Moreover, pupillary responsiveness (bilateral unresponsive mydriasis) on admission can serve as a screening tool to detect those TBI patients with risk for brain death in time [111].

19.3.2.6 Stress-Induced Hyperglycemia

In severe forms of TBI in patients not suffering from diabetic hyperglycemia also, stress-induced hyperglycemia is associated with an increased mortality [112].

19.3.2.7 ANP

The atrial natriuretic peptide (ANP) is conductive to body fluid homeostasis, serves as a marker of cardiac dysfunction, and is linked to the development of brain edema following TBI.

Furthermore, as our own data confirm (Fig. 19.5), ANP levels are correlated to the patient's age [113].

In a study of Kleindienst et al., who used of a cutoff of 100 pg/L, ANP was raised in TBI patients on admission and on day 3 (22 %) and on day 7 (31 %). At follow-up investigations, ANP levels had normalized. On one hand, high ANP concentration was positively associated with neuroendocrine stress response (i.e., high cortisol and prolactin levels) and poor outcome (GOS at 6 months post-injury); on the other hand although, ANP levels were not significantly influenced by the severity of injury [113]. One factor that triggers ANP elevation was the injury's volume load [113]. As depicted in Fig. 19.5, there is a positive correlation between the patients' age and ANP levels on day 0, day 3, and day 7 and in context of follow-up investigations.

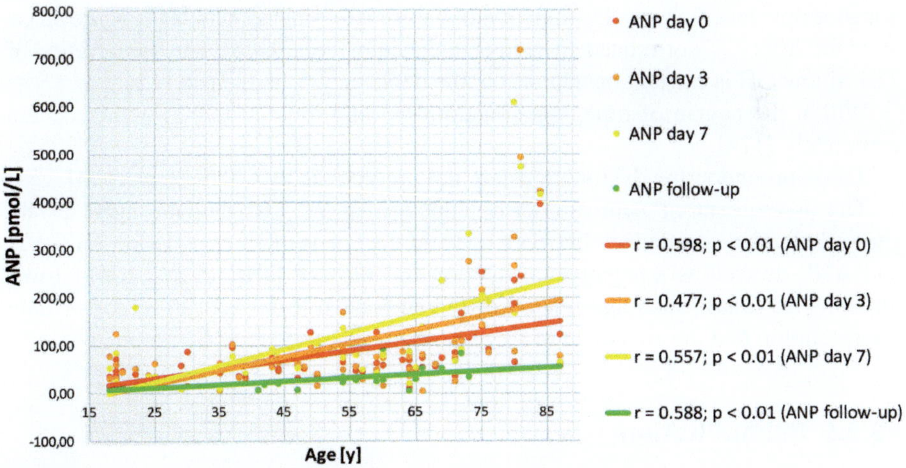

Fig. 19.5 Correlations between the patients' age and ANP levels on day 0 (*red*), day 3 (*orange*), and day 7 (*yellow*) and in context of follow-up investigations (*green*)

19.3.3 Outcome

A study from 1995 found out that in almost 50 % of patients with DAI, residual sequelae like cognitive or focal deficits or post-concussion syndrome were traceable [81].

Regarding future functional but not neurocognitive outcome of elderly patients, loss of consciousness could be proven as a relevant prognostic factor [105]. Long-term cognitive dysfunction is another often arising complication of TBI involving subarachnoid hemorrhage in the elderly [114]. Factors that influence future neurocognitive outcome are the patients' age, gender, and educational level [105].

Latest research suggests a connection between moderate to severe TBI and the development of cognitive degeneration and Alzheimer's disease far afterwards [115–117].

According to a magnetic resonance imaging (MRI)-based study, pathology in the basal ganglia and the frontotemporal lobe might even be a structural correlate of depression resulting from TBI [118].

Depression itself is prevalent in 1.8–8.9 % among community-residing seniors and in 10–25 % of those living in medical and long-term care settings [57, 119].

Thus, TBI might boost the probability of disinhibition in elderly demented patients [120].

19.3.4 Neuroendocrine Dysfunction

Hypopituitarism as an aftereffect of TBI occurs with a prevalence of 30–50 % [121–123]. Neuroendocrine dysfunction after TBI is affected by both the severity of the injury and the treatment with prolonged mechanical ventilation [124].

Patients in a critical condition show significantly increased cortisol concentrations initially and decreased levels afterward in case of ventilation for over 24 h. In ventilated patients also lower values of TSH (day 3), total T3, and free T4 exist as well as gonadotropic insufficiency. Dysfunction of the somatotropic system in the acute phase after the injury is not related to neither mechanical ventilation nor the severity of TBI. If low GH is existent on admission, the deficiency is permanent [124].

Within the course of time, the gonadotropic and thyreotropic system recovers completely [124].

The neuroendocrine dysfunctions are not predictable by CT findings [124].

The assessment of neuroendocrine function in 71 TBI patients aged 18–87 showed positive correlations between age and the levels of cortisol, LH, FSH, AVP, and ANP, as well as a negative correlation for age and DHEAS and IGF-1 (own unpublished data). Such age-related differences have to be kept in mind for data interpretation and improvement of targeted therapy.

19.3.5 Rehabilitation

Elderly TBI patients are sent to inpatient rehabilitation or care facilities for a long period more often, and they are also considered to have poorer outcome. And in fact, death is more likely compared to younger patients [125]. Tendencies of the past two decades show that the number of elderly patients surviving moderate and severe forms of TBI is increasing [59, 108].

Certain deeply comatose elderly TBI patients who benefit from inpatient rehabilitation revealed improved outcome at 6 months after the injury as the modified Barthel Index after rehabilitation gained substantial increase [126].

The risk of repeated critical care intervention is lower in younger adults aged under 65 years with a normal mental status (GCS of 15) who suffer from an isolated brain injury (sensitivity, 98 %; specificity, 50 %) [82].

However, ICU treatment especially in TBI patients aged between 65 and 74 years ("younger elderly") might lower mortality in this subgroup [127].

This cohort even reached a survival rate comparable to those individuals being younger than 65 years, having a GCS of 8 or higher and receiving surgical intervention [127]. By the use of appropriate resources, adequate surgical intervention in time, and the claim of intensive care and neurorehabilitation, also patients of older age have the opportunity to retrieve the same pleasant functional and cognitive outcome as their younger counterparts [89].

Improving targeted therapy for elderly patients should be our future challenge in order to guarantee the best possible treatment for all our patients.

References

1. Firsching R et al (2015) S2e-Leitlinie: Schädelhirntrauma im Erwachsenenalter. [cited 2016 2016/03/21]; Available from: http://www.awmf.org/uploads/tx_szleitlinien/008-001l_S2e_Schaedelhirntrauma_SHT_Erwachsene_2015-12.pdf
2. Hyder AA et al (2007) The impact of traumatic brain injuries: a global perspective. NeuroRehabilitation 22(5):341–353
3. Peschman J, Neideen T, Brasel K (2011) The impact of discharging minimally injured trauma patient: does age play a role in trauma admission? J Trauma 70(6):1331–1336
4. Richmond R et al (2011) Age: is it all in the head? Factors influencing mortality in elderly patients with head injuries. J Trauma 71(1):E8–E11
5. Feigin VL et al (2013) Incidence of traumatic brain injury in New Zealand: a population-based study. Lancet Neurol 12(1):53–64
6. Brain Trauma Foundation, American Association of Neurological Surgeons, Congress of Neurological Surgeons (2007) Guidelines for the management of severe traumatic brain injury. J Neurotrauma 24 Suppl 1:S1–S106
7. Maas AI et al (1997) EBIC-guidelines for management of severe head injury in adults. European Brain Injury Consortium. Acta Neurochir (Wien) 139(4):286–294
8. Undén J, Ingebrigtsen T, Romner B (2013) Scandinavian guidelines for initial management of minimal, mild and moderate head injuries in adults: an evidence and consensus-based update. BMC Med 11(1):1–14
9. Gabriel EJ et al (2002) Guidelines for prehospital management of traumatic brain injury. J Neurotrauma 19(1):111–174
10. Scottish Intercollegiate Guidelines Network (SIGN). Brain injury rehabilitation in adults. Edinburgh: SIGN; 2013. (SIGN publication no. 130). [March 2013].
11. Marshall S et al (2012) Clinical practice guidelines for mild traumatic brain injury and persistent symptoms. Can Fam Physician 58(3):257–267, e128–140

12. Wee JZ, Yang YRJ, Lee QYR, Cao K, Chong CT (2016). Demographic profile and extent of healthcare resource utilisation of patients with severe traumatic brain injury: still a major public health problem. Singapore medical journal 57:491–496
13. Tsai L-Y et al (2014) Fall injuries and related factors of elderly patients at a medical center in Taiwan. Int J Gerontol 8(4):203–208
14. Boltz MM et al (2015) Injuries and outcomes associated with traumatic falls in the elderly population on oral anticoagulant therapy. Injury 46(9):1765–1771
15. Jagnoor J et al (2012) Fall related injuries: a retrospective medical review study in North India. Injury 43(12):1996–2000
16. Montali F et al (2015) Impact of different drug classes on clinical severity of falls in an elderly population: epidemiological survey in a trauma center. J Clin Gerontol Geriatr 6(2):63–67
17. Ziebell JM, Morganti-Kossmann MC (2010) Involvement of pro- and anti-inflammatory cytokines and chemokines in the pathophysiology of traumatic brain injury. Neurotherapeutics 7(1):22–30
18. Blennow K, Hardy J, Zetterberg H (2012) The neuropathology and neurobiology of traumatic brain injury. Neuron 76(5):886–899
19. Meythaler JM et al (2001) Current concepts: diffuse axonal injury–associated traumatic brain injury. Arch Phys Med Rehabil 82(10):1461–1471
20. Kim JJ, Gean AD (2011) Imaging for the diagnosis and management of traumatic brain injury. Neurotherapeutics 8(1):39–53
21. Adams JH et al (1989) Diffuse axonal injury in head injury: definition, diagnosis and grading. Histopathology 15(1):49–59
22. Tang-Schomer MD et al (2010) Mechanical breaking of microtubules in axons during dynamic stretch injury underlies delayed elasticity, microtubule disassembly, and axon degeneration. FASEB J 24(5):1401–1410
23. McCracken E et al (1999) Calpain activation and cytoskeletal protein breakdown in the corpus callosum of head-injured patients. J Neurotrauma 16(9):749–761
24. McGinn MJ et al (2009) Biochemical, structural, and biomarker evidence for calpain-mediated cytoskeletal change after diffuse brain injury uncomplicated by contusion. J Neuropathol Exp Neurol 68(3):241–249
25. Grady MS et al (1993) The use of antibodies targeted against the neurofilament subunits for the detection of diffuse axonal injury in humans. J Neuropathol Exp Neurol 52(2):143–152
26. Colak T et al (2012) Microarray-based gene expression analysis of an animal model for closed head injury. Injury 43(8):1264–1270
27. Mehan ND, Strauss KI (2012) Combined age- and trauma-related proteomic changes in rat neocortex: a basis for brain vulnerability. Neurobiol Aging 33(9):1857–1873
28. Li X-Y, Feng D-F (2009) Diffuse axonal injury: novel insights into detection and treatment. J Clin Neurosci 16(5):614–619
29. Fabbri A et al (2010) Predicting intracranial lesions by antiplatelet agents in subjects with mild head injury. J Neurol Neurosurg Psychiatry 81(11):1275–1279
30. Narayana PA et al (2015) Multi-modal MRI of mild traumatic brain injury. Neuroimage Clin 7:87–97
31. Mayer AR et al (2010) A prospective diffusion tensor imaging study in mild traumatic brain injury. Neurology 74(8):643–650
32. Lipton ML et al (2008) Multifocal white matter ultrastructural abnormalities in mild traumatic brain injury with cognitive disability: a voxel-wise analysis of diffusion tensor imaging. J Neurotrauma 25(11):1335–1342
33. Miles L et al (2008) Short-term DTI predictors of cognitive dysfunction in mild traumatic brain injury. Brain Inj 22(2):115–122
34. Bazarian JJ et al (2012) Subject-specific changes in brain white matter on diffusion tensor imaging after sports-related concussion. Magn Reson Imaging 30(2):171–180
35. Zimmer DB et al (1995) The S100 protein family: history, function, and expression. Brain Res Bull 37(4):417–429

36. Marshak DR (1990) S100 beta as a neurotrophic factor. Prog Brain Res 86:169–181
37. Selinfreund RH et al (1991) Neurotrophic protein S100 beta stimulates glial cell proliferation. Proc Natl Acad Sci U S A 88(9):3554–3558
38. Barger SW, Wolchok SR, Van Eldik LJ (1992) Disulfide-linked S100 beta dimers and signal transduction. Biochim Biophys Acta 1160(1):105–112
39. Zimmer DB, Van Eldik LJ (1987) Tissue distribution of rat S100 alpha and S100 beta and S100-binding proteins. Am J Physiol 252(3 Pt 1):C285–C289
40. Kleindienst A et al (2010) Dynamics of S100B release into serum and cerebrospinal fluid following acute brain injury. Acta Neurochir Suppl 106:247–250
41. Willoughby KA et al (2004) S100B protein is released by in vitro trauma and reduces delayed neuronal injury. J Neurochem 91(6):1284–1291
42. Graham MR et al (2011) Direct hits to the head during amateur boxing is associated with a rise in serum biomarkers for brain injury. Int J Immunopathol Pharmacol 24(1):119–125
43. Calcagnile O et al (2013) S100B levels are affected by older age but not by alcohol intoxication following mild traumatic brain injury. Scand J Trauma Resusc Emerg Med 21:52
44. McKee AC et al (2009) Chronic traumatic encephalopathy in athletes: progressive tauopathy after repetitive head injury. J Neuropathol Exp Neurol 68(7):709–735
45. McKee AC et al (2010) TDP-43 proteinopathy and motor neuron disease in chronic traumatic encephalopathy. J Neuropathol Exp Neurol 69(9):918–929
46. Sivanandam TM, Thakur MK (2012) Traumatic brain injury: a risk factor for Alzheimer's disease. Neurosci Biobehav Rev 36(5):1376–1381
47. Hesse C et al (2000) Cerebrospinal fluid markers for Alzheimer's disease evaluated after acute ischemic stroke. J Alzheimers Dis 2(3–4):199–206
48. Mondello S et al (2014) CSF and plasma amyloid-beta temporal profiles and relationships with neurological status and mortality after severe traumatic brain injury. Sci Rep 4:6446
49. Franz G et al (2003) Amyloid beta 1–42 and tau in cerebrospinal fluid after severe traumatic brain injury. Neurology 60(9):1457–1461
50. Ost M et al (2006) Initial CSF total tau correlates with 1-year outcome in patients with traumatic brain injury. Neurology 67(9):1600–1604
51. Smith C et al (2006) Association of APOE e4 and cerebrovascular pathology in traumatic brain injury. J Neurol Neurosurg Psychiatry 77(3):363–366
52. Blain JF, Sullivan PM, Poirier J (2006) A deficit in astroglial organization causes the impaired reactive sprouting in human apolipoprotein E4 targeted replacement mice. Neurobiol Dis 21(3):505–514
53. Teter B et al (2002) Defective neuronal sprouting by human apolipoprotein E4 is a gain-of-negative function. J Neurosci Res 68(3):331–336
54. Luukinen H et al (2005) Fall-related brain injuries and the risk of dementia in elderly people: a population-based study. Eur J Neurol 12(2):86–92
55. Grandhi R et al (2015) Preinjury warfarin, but not antiplatelet medications, increases mortality in elderly traumatic brain injury patients. J Trauma Acute Care Surg 78(3):614–621
56. Folkerson LE et al (2015) Predicting progressive hemorrhagic injury from isolated traumatic brain injury and coagulation. Surgery 158(3):655–661
57. Menzel JC (2008) Depression in the elderly after traumatic brain injury: a systematic review. Brain Inj 22(5):375–380
58. Flaada JT et al (2007) Relative risk of mortality after traumatic brain injury: a population-based study of the role of age and injury severity. J Neurotrauma 24(3):435–445
59. Fletcher AE, Khalid S, Mallonee S (2007) The epidemiology of severe traumatic brain injury among persons 65 years of age and older in Oklahoma, 1992–2003. Brain Inj 21(7):691–699
60. Ohm C et al (2005) Effects of antiplatelet agents on outcomes for elderly patients with traumatic intracranial hemorrhage. J Trauma 58(3):518–522
61. Pieracci FM et al (2007) Degree of anticoagulation, but not warfarin use itself, predicts adverse outcomes after traumatic brain injury in elderly trauma patients. J Trauma 63(3):525–530

62. Lavoie A et al (2004) Preinjury warfarin use among elderly patients with closed head injuries in a trauma center. J Trauma 56(4):802–807
63. Claudia C et al (2011) Minor head injury in warfarinized patients: indicators of risk for intracranial hemorrhage. J Trauma 70(4):906–909
64. Franko J et al (2006) Advanced age and preinjury warfarin anticoagulation increase the risk of mortality after head trauma. J Trauma 61(1):107–110
65. Itshayek E et al (2006) Delayed posttraumatic acute subdural hematoma in elderly patients on anticoagulation. Neurosurgery 58(5):E851–E856; discussion E851–E856
66. Reynolds FD et al (2003) Time to deterioration of the elderly, anticoagulated, minor head injury patient who presents without evidence of neurologic abnormality. J Trauma 54(3):492–496
67. Peck KA et al (2011) Delayed intracranial hemorrhage after blunt trauma: are patients on preinjury anticoagulants and prescription antiplatelet agents at risk? J Trauma 71(6):1600–1604
68. Cohen DB, Rinker C, Wilberger JE (2006) Traumatic brain injury in anticoagulated patients. J Trauma 60(3):553–557
69. Karni A et al (2001) Traumatic head injury in the anticoagulated elderly patient: a lethal combination. Am Surg 67(11):1098–1100
70. Ushewokunze S et al (2004) Elderly patients with severe head injury in coma from the outset–has anything changed? Br J Neurosurg 18(6):604–607
71. Chisholm KM, Harruff RC (2010) Elderly deaths due to ground-level falls. Am J Forensic Med Pathol 31(4):350–354
72. Kidwell CS, Wintermark M (2008) Imaging of intracranial haemorrhage. Lancet Neurol 7(3):256–267
73. Naraghi L et al (2015) Is CT angiography of the head useful in the management of traumatic brain injury? J Am Coll Surg 220(6):1027–1031
74. Kidwell CS et al (2004) Comparison of MRI and CT for detection of acute intracerebral hemorrhage. JAMA 292(15):1823–1830
75. Fiebach JB et al (2002) CT and diffusion-weighted MR imaging in randomized order: diffusion-weighted imaging results in higher accuracy and lower interrater variability in the diagnosis of hyperacute ischemic stroke. Stroke 33(9):2206–2210
76. Chalela JA et al (2007) Magnetic resonance imaging and computed tomography in emergency assessment of patients with suspected acute stroke: a prospective comparison. Lancet 369(9558):293–298
77. Tong KA et al (2003) Hemorrhagic shearing lesions in children and adolescents with posttraumatic diffuse axonal injury: improved detection and initial results. Radiology 227(2):332–339
78. Badenes R, Bilotta F (2015) Neurocritical care for intracranial haemorrhage: a systematic review of recent studies. Br J Anaesth 115 Suppl 2:ii68–ii74
79. Hemphill JC 3rd et al (2015) Guidelines for the management of spontaneous intracerebral hemorrhage: a guideline for healthcare professionals from the American Heart Association/American Stroke Association. Stroke 46(7):2032–2060
80. Balami JS, Buchan AM (2012) Complications of intracerebral haemorrhage. Lancet Neurol 11(1):101–118
81. Selladurai BM et al (1995) Diffuse axonal injury: a clinical and computerised tomography study of 128 patients. J Clin Neurosci 2(3):216–223
82. Nishijima DK, Haukoos JS, Newgard CD, Staudenmayer K, White N, Slattery D, Maxim PC, Gee CA, Hsia RY, Melnikow JA and Holmes JF (2013). Variability of ICU Use in Adult Patients With Minor Traumatic Intracranial Hemorrhage. Annals of Emergency Medicine 61:509–517.e504
83. Munro PT, Smith RD, Parke TR (2002) Effect of patients' age on management of acute intracranial haematoma: prospective national study. BMJ 325(7371):1001
84. Faul M, Xu L, Sasser SM (2016) Hospitalized Traumatic Brain Injury: Low Trauma Center Utilization and High Interfacility Transfers among Older Adults. Prehospital Emergency Care 20:594–600

85. Berry C et al (2012) Redefining hypotension in traumatic brain injury. Injury 43(11):1833–1837
86. Spahn DR et al (2013) Management of bleeding and coagulopathy following major trauma: an updated European guideline. Crit Care 17(2):R76
87. Shimoda K et al (2014) Outcome and surgical management for geriatric traumatic brain injury: analysis of 888 cases registered in the Japan Neurotrauma Data Bank. World Neurosurg 82(6):1300–1306
88. Herou E, Romner B, Tomasevic G (2015) Acute traumatic brain injury: mortality in the elderly. World Neurosurg 83(6):996–1001
89. Mak CH et al (2012) Traumatic brain injury in the elderly: is it as bad as we think? Curr Transl Geriatr Exp Gerontol Rep 1:171–178
90. Mitra B et al (2008) Management and hospital outcome of the severely head injured elderly patient. ANZ J Surg 78(7):588–592
91. Wong GK et al (2011) Neurological outcomes of neurosurgical operations for multiple trauma elderly patients in Hong Kong. J Emerg Trauma Shock 4(3):346–350
92. Mohindra S et al (2008) Continuation of poor surgical outcome after elderly brain injury. Surg Neurol 69(5):474–477
93. Lau D et al (2012) Postoperative outcomes following closed head injury and craniotomy for evacuation of hematoma in patients older than 80 years. J Neurosurg 116(1):234–245
94. De Bonis P et al (2011) Decompressive craniectomy for elderly patients with traumatic brain injury: it's probably not worth the while. J Neurotrauma 28(10):2043–2048
95. Dang Q et al (2015) More fateful than fruitful? Intracranial pressure monitoring in elderly patients with traumatic brain injury is associated with worse outcomes. J Surg Res 198(2):482–488
96. Tang A et al (2015) Intracranial pressure monitor in patients with traumatic brain injury. J Surg Res 194(2):565–570
97. Andrews PJ et al (2015) Hypothermia for intracranial hypertension after traumatic brain injury. N Engl J Med 373(25):2403–2412
98. Skolnick BE et al (2014) A clinical trial of progesterone for severe traumatic brain injury. N Engl J Med 371(26):2467–2476
99. Schneider EB et al (2011) Premorbid statin use is associated with improved survival and functional outcomes in older head-injured individuals. J Trauma 71(4):815–819
100. Bhullar IS et al (2010) The effect of age on blunt traumatic brain-injured patients. Am Surg 76(9):966–968
101. Gan BK, Lim JH, Ng IH (2004) Outcome of moderate and severe traumatic brain injury amongst the elderly in Singapore. Ann Acad Med Singapore 33(1):63–67
102. Susman M et al (2002) Traumatic brain injury in the elderly: increased mortality and worse functional outcome at discharge despite lower injury severity. J Trauma 53(2):219–223; discussion 223–224
103. Wong GK et al (2009) Traumatic intracerebral haemorrhage: is the CT pattern related to outcome? Br J Neurosurg 23(6):601–605
104. Wu X et al (2008) Epidemiology of traumatic brain injury in eastern China, 2004: a prospective large case study. J Trauma 64(5):1313–1319
105. Jung YJ et al (2014) Prognostic factors of neurocognitive and functional outcomes in junior and senior elderly patients with traumatic brain injury undergoing disability evaluation or appointed disability evaluation. J Korean Neurosurg Soc 55(1):18–25
106. Onyszchuk G et al (2008) Detrimental effects of aging on outcome from traumatic brain injury: a behavioral, magnetic resonance imaging, and histological study in mice. J Neurotrauma 25(2):153–171
107. Onyszchuk G et al (2009) Post-acute pathological changes in the thalamus and internal capsule in aged mice following controlled cortical impact injury: a magnetic resonance imaging, iron histochemical, and glial immunohistochemical study. Neurosci Lett 452(2):204–208
108. Ramanathan DM et al (2012) Epidemiological shifts in elderly traumatic brain injury: 18-year trends in Pennsylvania. J Neurotrauma 29(7):1371–1378

109. Styrke J et al (2007) Traumatic brain injuries in a well-defined population: epidemiological aspects and severity. J Neurotrauma 24(9):1425–1436
110. Jennett B et al (1976) Predicting outcome in individual patients after severe head injury. Lancet 1(7968):1031–1034
111. Egea-Guerrero JJ et al (2013) S100B protein may detect brain death development after severe traumatic brain injury. J Neurotrauma 30(20):1762–1769
112. Bosarge PL et al (2015) Stress-induced hyperglycemia is associated with higher mortality in severe traumatic brain injury. J Trauma Acute Care Surg 79(2):289–294
113. Kleindienst A et al (2012) The atrial natriuretic peptide does not serve osmoregulation but predicts outcome following brain injury. Acta Neurochir Suppl 114:277–281
114. Wong GK, Ngai K, Wong A, Lam SW, Mok VC, Yeung J, Rainer T, Wong R, Poon WS (2012) Long-term cognitive dysfunction in patients with traumatic subarachnoid hemorrhage: prevalence and risk factors. Acta neurochirurgica 154:105–111; discussion 111
115. Plassman BL et al (2000) Documented head injury in early adulthood and risk of Alzheimer's disease and other dementias. Neurology 55(8):1158–1166
116. Goldstein FC, Levin HS (2001) Cognitive outcome after mild and moderate traumatic brain injury in older adults. J Clin Exp Neuropsychol 23(6):739–753
117. Jellinger KA (2004) Traumatic brain injury as a risk factor for Alzheimer's disease. J Neurol Neurosurg Psychiatry 75(3):511–512
118. Rao V et al (2010) Neuroanatomical correlates of depression in post traumatic brain injury: preliminary results of a pilot study. J Neuropsychiatry Clin Neurosci 22(2):231–235
119. Rao V et al (2010) Predictors of new-onset depression after mild traumatic brain injury. J Neuropsychiatry Clin Neurosci 22(1):100–104
120. Rao V et al (2010) Neuropsychiatric symptoms in dementia patients with and without a history of traumatic brain injury. J Neuropsychiatry Clin Neurosci 22(2):166–172
121. Schneider HJ, Stalla GK, Buchfelder M (2006) Expert meeting: hypopituitarism after traumatic brain injury and subarachnoid haemorrhage. Acta Neurochir (Wien) 148(4):449–456
122. Kelly DF et al (2000) Hypopituitarism following traumatic brain injury and aneurysmal subarachnoid hemorrhage: a preliminary report. J Neurosurg 93(5):743–752
123. Lieberman SA et al (2001) Prevalence of neuroendocrine dysfunction in patients recovering from traumatic brain injury. J Clin Endocrinol Metab 86(6):2752–2756
124. Kleindienst A et al (2009) Neuroendocrine function following traumatic brain injury and subsequent intensive care treatment: a prospective longitudinal evaluation. J Neurotrauma 26(9):1435–1446
125. LeBlanc J et al (2006) Comparison of functional outcome following acute care in young, middle-aged and elderly patients with traumatic brain injury. Brain Inj 20(8):779–790
126. Yap SG, Chua KS (2008) Rehabilitation outcomes in elderly patients with traumatic brain injury in Singapore. J Head Trauma Rehabil 23(3):158–163
127. Bouras T et al (2007) Head injury mortality in a geriatric population: differentiating an "edge" age group with better potential for benefit than older poor-prognosis patients. J Neurotrauma 24(8):1355–1361

Chronic Subdural Haematoma in the Elderly

20

Ellie Edlmann, Peter J. Hutchinson, and Angelos G. Kolias

20.1 Introduction

Chronic subdural haematoma (CSDH) is one of the most common conditions a neurosurgeon will come across in the elderly population. The reason for this can be said no better than by Markwalder's words in 1981, "…a disease of older age, in which physiological brain atrophy, frequent head trauma and coagulation disorders...or alcoholic hepatopathy play a cumulative role" [40]. This has become increasingly true, with an aging population and a new generation of anticoagulant drugs being used for wider indications.

A CSDH is essentially a collection of blood and blood breakdown products in the subdural space, between the layers of the arachnoid and dura mater (Fig. 20.1).

Although it is occasionally considered a rather "benign" condition, it shouldn't be forgotten that left untreated, symptomatic CSDHs will lead to a poor outcome in most instances [40]. This is either directly through haematoma enlargement and cerebral decompensation or the inevitable complications such as pneumonia, venous thromboembolism, etc. Ensuring that treatment is efficacious and timely is important in order to minimise the morbidity and mortality associated with this condition. In this chapter, we intend to assess the background pathophysiology, interventions and outcomes that are reported in the literature to date. However, it is important to first recognise that the CSDH literature has some limitations. Although there are meta-analyses, these have a paucity of level 1 evidence, and there are currently only 13 published prospective randomised controlled trials in the field [34]. However, it is an ever-expanding topic area, and now 20 prospective randomised clinical trials

E. Edlmann • P.J. Hutchinson • A.G. Kolias (✉)
Division of Neurosurgery, Department of Clinical Neurosciences, Addenbrooke's Hospital & University of Cambridge, Cambridge, UK
e-mail: angeloskolias@gmail.com

© Springer International Publishing Switzerland 2017

M. Berhouma, P. Krolak-Salmon (eds.), *Brain and Spine Surgery in the Elderly*,
DOI 10.1007/978-3-319-40232-1_20

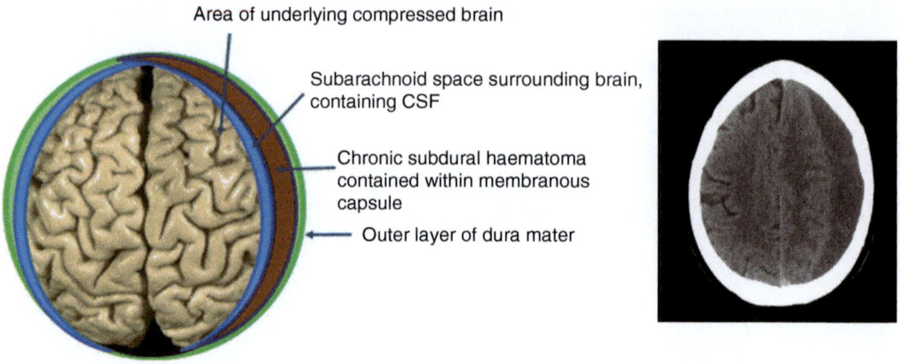

Fig. 20.1 Schematic representation of a CSDH along the left cerebral convexity (*right*) and comparative CT head scan (*left*)

are registered on the WHO-ICTRP website. There is also a problem with the literature using wide-ranging and heterogeneous baseline data and outcomes in CSDH [12, 13]. Core outcome sets have been recommended as a method of increasing congruency of reported outcomes, making published data more comparable and the compilation of systematic reviews easier. This review has therefore tried to use data from meta-analyses, larger studies or those that are well conducted and/or with findings of high relevance/interest.

20.2 Epidemiology

CSDH is well described as being a disease of the elderly and large reviews have reported mean ages from 68.3 to 77.3 years [5, 21, 23, 50, 69]. Therefore, life expectancy of a population has a critical impact on the CSDH incidence seen. In England, the EU and the USA life expectancy is increasing and currently sits between 78 and 81, with 55 % of deaths in England now in those over the age of 80 [18, 48]. What is most interesting is the concurrent and significant rise in life expectancy specifically for the elderly, for example, a man reaching the age of 75 can expect to live a further 12 years and women 13 years [48]. The incidence of CSDH will almost certainly continue to increase with these population statistics.

The incidence of CSDH has been reported as 1.72 per 100,000 per annum in the population of Helsinki, increasing to 7.32 per 100,000 per annum in the peak age group of 70–79 years [19]. This is similar to the incidence of 8.2 per 100,000 per annum reported in over 65-year-olds in North Wales [3].

There is a well-recognised and significant preponderance for CSDHs to affect men, with a ratio of 1.7–2.9:1 of men to women [5, 21, 23, 50, 69]. Many reasons for this have been postulated, such as increased risk of falls and higher use of anti-coagulants or anti-platelets in men [5]. However, no clear reason has been convincingly established.

20.3 Pathophysiology

20.3.1 Trauma

Preceding trauma is often reported in CSDH patients, in the range of 61–80% [5, 21, 50, 60]. However, the trauma may also be too trivial for patients to recollect, or direct head trauma may not have occurred at all. Even indirect acceleration/deceleration forces, such as falling onto buttocks, can be sufficient to result in a subdural haematoma [45]. The time interval from trauma to onset of symptoms can vary widely but on average is around 7–8 weeks after the trauma [21, 40, 41].

20.3.2 Inflammation

Interestingly the role of inflammation in the pathophysiology of CSDH has waxed and waned in popularity over the years. Virchow's original description of CSDH in 1857 identified the inflammatory nature of the condition and referred to it as "pachymeningitis haemorrhagica interna". Since then the theory that bleeding from torn cortical veins is *entirely* responsible for the gradual growth of the subdural collection was considered more likely by some [40, 41, 45]. However, in recent years, a plethora of publications have reported the presence of inflammatory cells and mediators in CSDH, and it is well accepted that this is the main driving force for growth of the collection, despite trauma being the initiator (see Fig. 20.2).

The outer membrane is well recognised as a key factor in CSDH development and is thought to produce areas of recurrent acute bleeding often seen on imaging. The presence of fragile, highly permeable macrocapillaries with large gap junctions and thin or absent basement membrane allows the repeated leakage of blood into the CSDH cavity [53, 73]. Angiogenic markers (Ang-2) have been found to be present in the CSDH membrane and could be the driving force for the development of these vessels, alongside enzymes such as MMP-9, which digest basement membrane

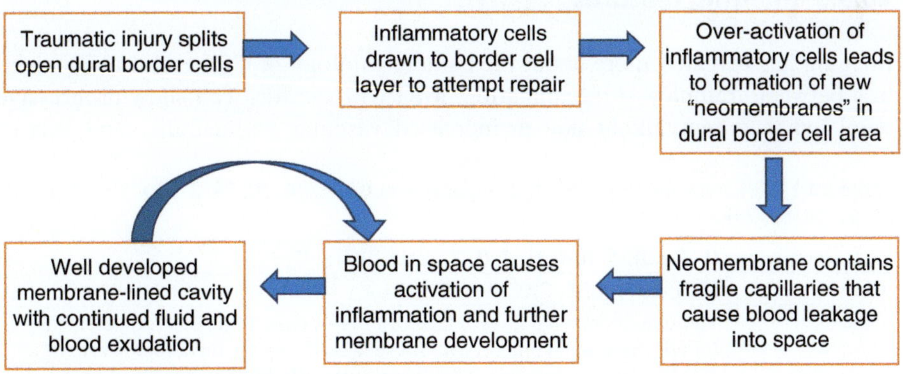

Fig. 20.2 Theory on the process of CSDH formation

causing their friability [26, 43]. There is also evidence of abnormally high concentrations of procollagens which are likely to be involved in aiding development of the CSDH neomembrane [25, 51].

Table 20.1 summarises some of the key mediators found in CSDH fluid or membranes. Concentrations of these markers are significantly higher than in peripheral blood, signifying that inflammatory process is very much a local phenomenon.

Many reports support interleukins as key mediators in the inflammatory process, and high levels of the proinflammatory IL-6 and IL-8 are a common finding. Their levels have also been correlated with risk of recurrence, and therefore, they may be a potential marker for predicting recurrence [20, 27]. Levels of anti-inflammatory cytokines have also been found to be high in some patients and shown to correlate with reduced risk of recurrence; this is also an indirect evidence that the body attempts to regulate the inflammatory response [46, 68].

VEGF is a marker of particular interest due to its key action in angiogenesis and may be produced from inflammatory cells such as neutrophils or macrophages present in the CSDH [26, 54]. Levels of associated markers, such as PGE2, have also been shown to increase with the time interval from trauma; this may represent the escalating inflammatory process occurring over time [24].

Overall it is clear that inflammation in CSDH is multifactorial and as of yet a single key-independent driver has not been identified. It is important to consider the balance of molecules present, both the pro- and anti-inflammatory markers and how their balance changes over time. Not all inflammatory markers are detrimental all of the time, and certain markers which are perceived to be harmful may be required in reparative processes at later time points. One example is VEGF, which has previously been shown to have a role in neurogenesis and aid recovery in TBI [65] and therefore despite contributing to the pathophysiology of CSDH may also be implicated in reparative processes. More work is needed in this area to understand the patterns of markers over time and how they can be targeted by new potential therapies.

20.3.3 Imaging features

Imaging has revealed more about the pathophysiology of CSDH and the correlation between trauma and inflammation. MRI with contrast can show progressive dural enhancement, likely due to increased vascular permeability and loss of

Table 20.1 Key inflammatory mediators implicated in CSDH [6, 20, 24–27, 29, 32, 42, 43, 46, 51, 54, 59, 68, 70]

Cytokines	IL-1ra, IL-5, IL-6, IL-7, IL-8, IL-10, IL-13, IL-17,
Chemokines	MCP-1, CXCL8, CXCL9, CXCL10,
Others	Vascular endothelial growth factor (VEGF), basic fibroblast growth factor (bFGF), prostaglandin E2, cyclooxygenase-2, matrix-metalloproteases (MMP-9 and 2), hypoxia-inducible factor (HIF-1alpha), angiopoietin 2, aquaporin 1, procollagen types 1 and 3

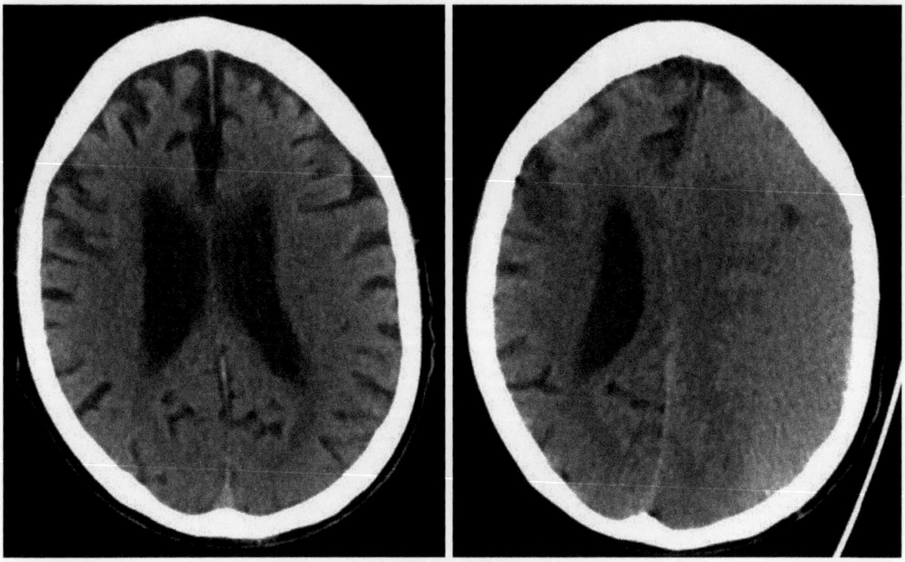

Fig. 20.3 Example of a patient with normal admission CT head following minor head trauma (*left image*) and repeat CT 2 months later (*right image*) with obvious CSDH formation with underlying mass effect on the left side of the brain

capillary integrity in the dura [2, 10]. This process begins before the CSDH collection even appears and supports the theory of an early inflammatory response as the driving force for CSDH collection [2, 58]. This is corroborated by clinical experience, where easy access to CT scanning has allowed CT imaging following even trivial trauma. These early scans can appear entirely normal, but patients may still go on to develop a CSDH as exemplified in Fig. 20.3.

Iso- or hypointense areas on T1 MRI are suggestive of fresh bleeding and found in at least half of CSDHs supporting repeated microhaemorrhage as part of the process in CSDH expansion [33, 66]. However, the fact that approximately half of CSDHs are homogenously hyperintense on T1 MRI, and hence do not show any recent bleeding, supports the theory that it is not just haemorrhage which is important in CSDH [66]. Clearly there is another process which leads to fluid accumulation, and this can be explained by migration of inflammatory cells and fluid exudate into the subdural space. Different distinct patterns in T1 intensity (hypointense versus hyperintense) have been suggested to signify different "stages" of the inflammatory reaction which may correlate with the risk of recurrence [23, 66]. Patients with homogenous hyperintensity on T1 have a much lower risk of recurrence (3.4 % versus 11.6 %) and are considered to represent a more dormant "degenerative" stage of non-haemorrhagic inflammation. Whereas those with hypointensity may reflect the early "proliferative" stage of inflammation where ongoing haemorrhagic occurs (causing T1 hypointensity), and this continued rebleeding makes recurrence more likely [23, 33, 66] (Fig. 20.4).

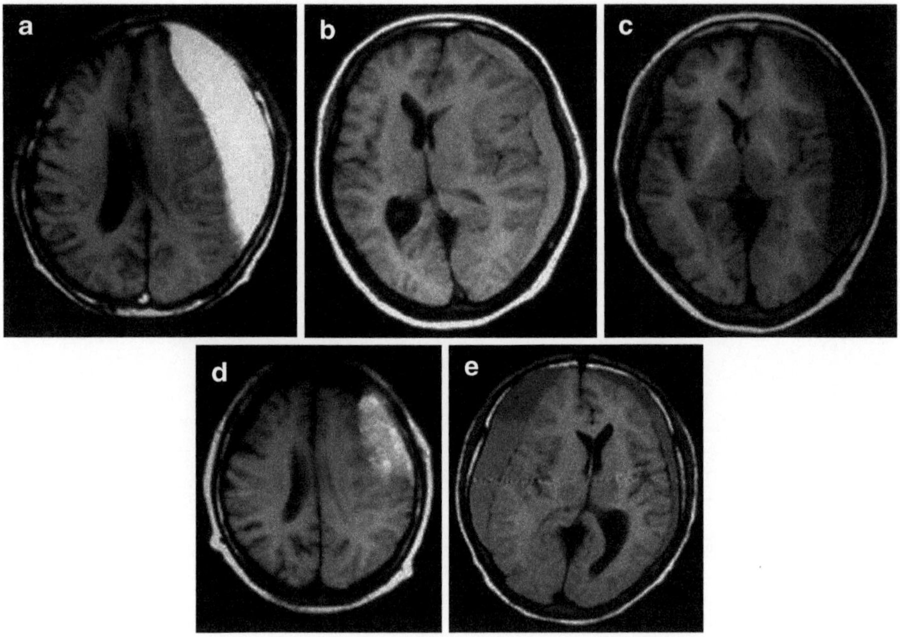

Fig. 20.4 Examples of T1-weighted MRI imaging seen in CSDH with (**a**) hyperintense, (**b**) isointense, (**c**) hypointense, (**d**) mixed high/iso and (**e**) mixed iso/low intensity signal according to Tsutsumi [66]

As well as CSDH forming from a normal scan, there are also those that form from an acute subdural haematoma (ASDH). It is unclear exactly how often CSDHs are the result of a transformed ASDH as the patient may not have been scanned at the time of the acute injury, and not all ASDHs will progress into CSDHs. One series reported that 21 % (8 out of 38) of conservatively managed ASDHs went onto develop CSDH requiring surgery at a mean of 19.4 days after trauma [31]. The operative findings are similar in CSDH's formed from normal scans and those from ASDH's with an outer membrane of granulation tissue, suggesting a similar inflammatory process [31]. The fact that some ASDHs resolve without consequence suggests that this inflammatory reaction is not always activated.

20.4 Clinical Presentation

CSDH can present in many different ways and common presenting symptoms can be found in Table 20.2. Haematoma laterality is likely to impact the type of presentation, and left- and right-sided haematomas are evenly distributed, with approximately 10–20 % occurring bilaterally [21, 34]. Due to the gradual onset of symptoms and age group affected, CSDH can often be mistaken for

Table 20.2 Summary of frequency of presenting symptoms from a review of 205 patients with CSDH [50]

Presenting symptom	Frequency (%)
Gait disturbance	57
Mental deterioration	35
Limb weakness	35
Acute confusion	33
Headache	18
Drowsiness or coma	10
Speech impairment	6
Nonspecific deterioration	3
Collapse	1
Seizures	1
Incontinence	<1
Visual disturbance	<1
Vomiting	<1

other conditions such as dementia and stroke. Transient neurological symptoms can be a feature and explain why transient ischaemic attacks can be suspected [71]; however, in the modern era of CT, early radiological assessment is conclusive.

There is some evidence that younger patients (<70 years) more commonly present with headache, whereas older patients (>70 years) report behavioural disturbance [21]. This may relate to younger patients having less cerebral atrophy and therefore being more sensitive to mass effect as represented with headache. Over 80 % of patients have a GCS of 13 or better at presentation as progression to coma is usually slow and therefore a relatively late feature [50].

Markwalder described a classification system for patients with CSDH, and this is commonly referred to in CSDH research (see Table 20.3). However, in clinical practice, Glasgow Coma Score (GCS) and clinical examination findings are normally sufficient for patient assessment.

20.4.1 Correlating CSDH Pathology with Clinical Signs and Symptoms

One would assume it is purely mass effect which causes neurological deficits in CSDH; however, the process is likely to be much more complex than this. Diffusion tensor imaging (DTI) studies assessing tissue microstructure and the architecture of the white matter tracts have shown a significant correlation between motor weakness and reduced fractional anisotropy (the degree with which white matter fibres run unopposed in one direction) [74]. This does not correlate with haematoma thickness and suggests that not only mass effect but underlying vasogenic oedema is responsible for causing distortion of white matter tracts and hence neurological deficits. The speed at which the CSDH accumulates may be as important

Table 20.3 Markwalder classification [41]

Grade	Symptoms and signs
0	Patient neurologically normal
1	Patient alert and orientated; mild symptoms such as headache; absent or mild neurological deficit such as reflex asymmetry
2	Patient drowsy or disorientated with variable neurological deficit, such as hemiparesis
3	Patient stuporous but responding appropriately to noxious stimuli; severe focal signs such as hemiplegia
4	Patient comatose with absent motor responses to painful stimuli; decerebrate or decorticate posturing

as its volume, as a more rapidly growing CSDH would be likely to cause more underlying oedema.

Further to this, studies on cerebral blood flow (CBF) and perfusion also suggest this may have a causative role in CSDH signs and symptoms. Transcranial Doppler has been used to identify reductions in CBF in relation to presence of CSDH, which improves significantly post-operatively and was not correlated with haematoma volume or midline shift [38]. Inao et al. corroborated this with CT perfusion imaging and showed reductions in CBF in deep regions such as the thalamus was correlated with presence of metal changes such as decreased consciousness and confusion [30]. Perfusion CT also highlights that cerebral perfusion can be impaired throughout *both* cerebral hemispheres despite unilateral CSDH and that this does not appear to correlate with raised intracranial pressure [11, 57, 63]. It has been suggested that there may be a global process of metabolic depression resulting in this widespread reduction in perfusion. Further studies are needed to clarify the true driving force for this phenomenon.

20.5 Imaging

Due to availability and speed, CT is usually the diagnostic imaging modality of choice for CSDH. The characteristic findings are seen in Fig 20.5, with variations in density relating to variations in rebleeding that occur over time [55]. However, on the whole it is very difficult to accurately age a CSDH from imaging alone and the clinical history is essential.

The typical morphology on CT is a crescentic collection along the convexity of the brain surface. It can be homogeneously hypodense or isodense or mixed density. The degree of mass effect and midline shift varies with the volume of the CSDH and the amount of pre-existing cerebral atrophy. In cases of bilateral CSDH (see B, Fig. 20.5), the amount of pressure being exerted on the brain can be underestimated due to lack of midline shift. The loss of normal sulcal patterns should be used instead as a surrogate marker of mass effect.

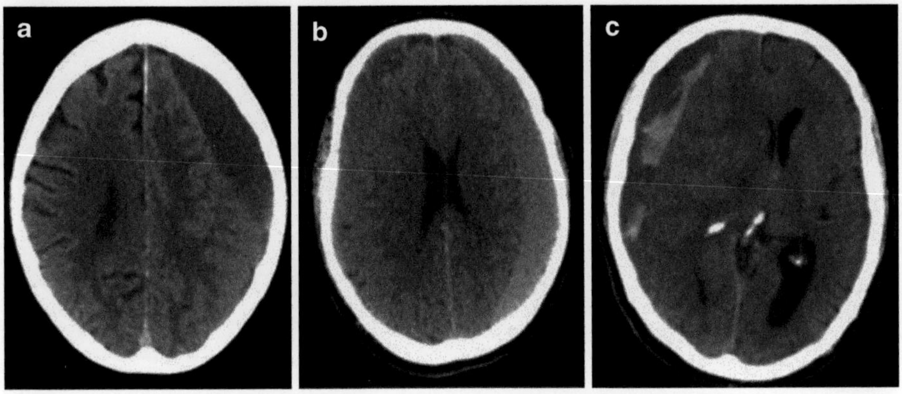

Fig. 20.5 CT examples of (**a**) hypodense, (**b**) isodense (bilateral) and (**c**) mixed density CSDH

20.5.1 Magnetic Resonance Imaging (MRI)

MRI is generally reserved for use in research or if an alternative diagnosis is suspected; however, its clinical use should not be overlooked. MRI does offer superior delineation and localisation of CSDHs, as well as helping distinguishing hygroma from haematoma and identifying the extent of membranes [28, 66, 52]. MRI with diffusion-weighting sequences can also provide more detailed information on the balance of solid and liquid components to aid the surgical planning [31, 36]. High quantities of membranes and multi-layering also confer a higher risk of recurrence, and some authors have suggested that such patients might benefit from a more extensive evacuation with a craniotomy or mini-craniotomy, rather than burr holes [58, 64] (Fig. 20.6).

20.5.2 Post-operative Imaging

Post-operative imaging is not routinely undertaken by all neurosurgeons. However, if undertaken, it should be interpreted in conjunction with clinical evaluation of the patient. Between 43 and 78 % of patients have a residual collection, which is not correlated with recurrence or clinical outcome [23, 40, 41]. These residual collections are likely to occur due to the slow and steady brain re-expansion that occurs post-operatively and is normally resolved by day 40 [40, 41].

20.5.3 Differentials

In rare cases, a collection in the subdural space can appear to be a CSDH but be something entirely different. It is important to be aware of this for patients who do not have typical findings intra-operatively so that histological samples can be taken and alternatives considered. Reported differentials include empyema, lymphoma, dural metastases and sinus histiocytosis [4, 14, 35].

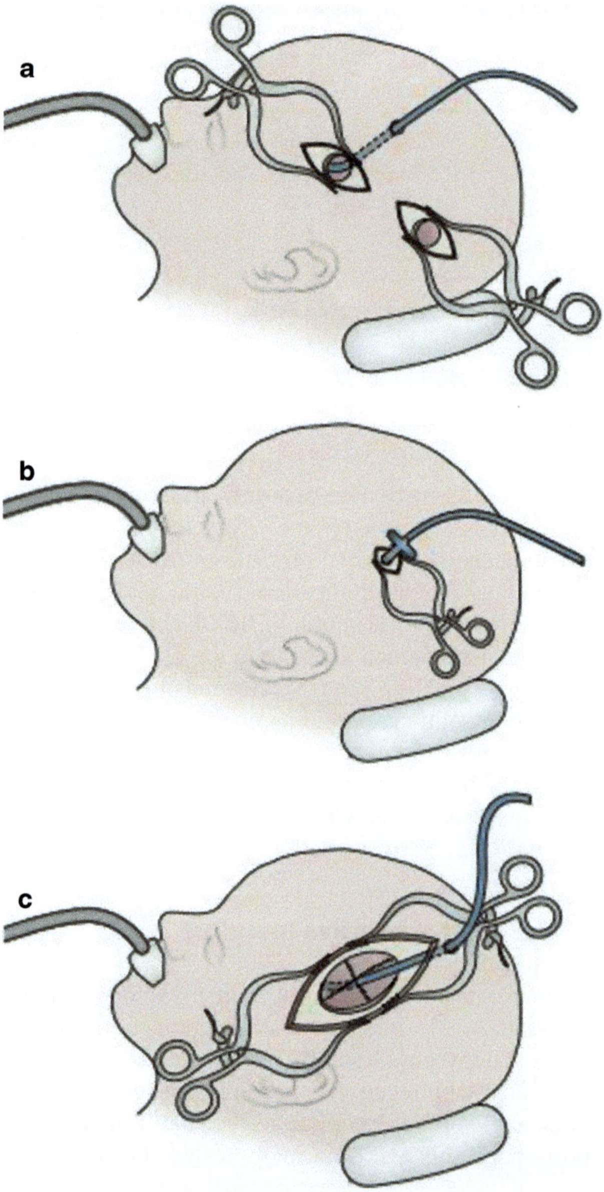

Fig. 20.6 (**a**) Burr-hole craniostomy, (**b**) twist-drill craniostomy with hollow screw, (**c**) mini-craniotomy with subdural drain from Kolias et al. [34]

20.6 Treatment

20.6.1 Surgery

Surgery has long been considered the mainstay of treatment for symptomatic CSDH, with washout of the haematoma leading to resolution of the collection in up to 86.5 % of cases [1, 34]. Trends in practice have changed over time with the more traditional craniotomy being replaced with the less invasive burr-hole craniostomy (BHC). Craniotomy with membranectomy (removal of the internal CSDH membranes, adjacent to the brain surface) used to be considered a key part of evacuating CSDHs. However this has largely fallen out of practice, since the finding that BHC has superior outcomes [62]. There is still debate about whether burr hole craniostomy (BHC), twist-drill craniostomy (TDC) or mini-craniotomy are better (see Fig. 20.6). The proposed benefits of performing a mini-craniotomy include a larger and therefore safer operative approach with easier washout of the haematoma (particularly if mixed density), better identification of membranes allowing their division, easier identification and treatment of the occasional bleeding vessel and the ability to insert a drain under direct vision. However, it is perceived to take longer, requires a general anaesthetic and is considered more invasive than BHC or TDC. Definitive evidence on the superiority of mini-craniotomy is lacking and therefore surgeons preference is usually the main deciding factor [34]. The only excpetion to this is in cases of recurrent CSDH, where there is some evidence to support the superiorty of craniotomy [1].

TDC is the least invasive option and one which can be performed under local anaesthetic in a ward setting. There are mixed views about whether this procedure is sufficient, and it is not practiced as widely as BHC. Lui et al.'s meta-analysis of 19 randomised and quasi-randomised control trials on TCD and BHC found no significant difference in outcome, advocating both as reasonable treatment options. This concurred with Almenawer et al.'s meta-analysis of 250 randomised and observational studies, finding no difference in morbidity, mortality, neurological improvement or recurrence between TCD and BHC. The latter review advocated TDC as first line management given the cost-effective nature of avoiding operating theatres, the safety of avoiding a GA in elderly patients and the non-significant trend towards lower complications with TDC [1]. Support for TCD may continue to increase with the use of an adjunct called subdural exacuating port system (SEPS). This is a device attached to the craniostomy hole which enables continued suction drainage without inserting a catheter into the subdural space. This can still be performed at the bedside, under L.A. and has been shown to be an efficacious way of treating CSDH, although may require repeat drainage [44, 56]. Further studies are needed to assess these interventions and there is currently a randomised trial comparing mini-craniotomy, TDC and BHC ongoing in Brussels, due to complete in 2018 (clinical trials.gov).

20.6.2 Drains

There is substantial support for the use of post-operative drains in reducing recurrence of CSDH, from 20.8 to 8.4 % with an OR of 0.36 [1, 39]. A landmark trial found a significant reduction in 6-month mortality from 18.1 to 8.6 % in conjunction with a reduction in recurrence from 24 to 9.3 % with a drain [50]. This relationship is complex and not fully understood. However, this improved mortality was not seen in the meta-analysis of randomised studies and needs further investigation [39].

There is evidence that drain placement should not remain for longer than 48 h, to minimise risk of complications, and that recurrence risk is maximally reduced with a frontally placed tip [39]. Perhaps surprisingly, neither the use of irrigation *or* the number of burr holes have been shown to be related to outcome following CSDH treatment [1, 39]. However, increased volumes of post-operative fluid drainage (>200 ml) have been correlated with lower recurrence rates [37]. Some authors have suggested that this is due to continuous plasma exudation from the outer membrane diluting anti-clotting and inflammatory factors, reducing recurrence [37]. Large post-operative volumes of fluid could also be signifying good brain re-expansion, displacing whatever remains in the subdural space. Adequate brain re-expansion is anecdotally considered important in preventing recurrence and many techniques have been discussed in the literature to try and improve this. Adequate or hyper-hydration, CO_2 insufflation and post-op bed rest have all been assessed but none have proven significant in affecting outcome [1, 39–41].

20.6.3 Anaesthesia

The use of general anaesthetic (GA) over local anaesthetic (LA) for CSDH surgery varies between individual units throughout the world. Gelabert-Gonzalez (in Spain) reported that 91 % of their patients receive LA with sedation, versus our practice in the UK of more than 90 % of patients receiving a GA [21]. It could be debated that LA is lower risk given the potential complications in relation to GA in an elderly population, however no significant association has been proven and this is an area which warrants further investigation.

20.6.4 Adjuvant Therapies

Evidence first emerged on the use of steroids as a treatment for CSDH in the 1970s. Glover and Labadie used a rat model to show that dexamethasone resulted in smaller, significantly lighter CSDH collections without the presence of a capsule [22]. They correlated this to the fact that dexamethasone inhibited the inflammatory reaction required to develop the CSDH membrane. This membrane contains highly permeable neocapillaries that are responsible for ongoing plasma exudation which drives clot enlargement.

Although steroid treatment has become almost routine practice in some regions [8, 9], there is no level 1 evidence to supports its efficacy in CSDH treatment. However, the results of many observational studies are promising for steroid use as an adjunct to surgery in preventing recurrence, or even as a primary conservative treatment ([7–9, 17, 61] review). Two randomised controlled trials are currently in progress to provide a definitive answer to these questions (DRESH, Dex-CSDH).

There is reason to be cautious about implementing widespread steroid use in this population without good evidence as steroids have previously been shown to cause harm in acute traumatic brain injury patients [49]. Their potential side effects in the

CSDH population have also been highlighted in a recent, trial assessing dexamethasone for conservative management in CSDH [47]. This study highlighted hyperglycaemia, infection, dyspepsia, appetite increase, muscle weakness, fatigue and depression as potential problems. Whilst the risks and side effects of steroids must be taken seriously, it should also be remembered that mortality and morbidity in relation to CSDH are already high and therefore complications are to be expected. There is also a substantial increase in morbidity associated with recurrence, as described in a study of 496 patients where 38.6 % had complications in the recurrent CSDH group compared with only 10.9 % in those with nonrecurrent CSDH [8]. Therefore, any treatment which significantly reduces recurrence may confer benefit despite carrying its own side-effect profile.

The direct application of steroids into the subdural space has also been used and shown to be safe in one small study [72]. There were no recurrences at 12-month follow-up in the 26 patients assessed, but it is difficult to know whether this was a direct effect of the local steroid infiltration due to the small sample size.

Tranexamic acid is another drug therapy being investigated for use in CSDH patients with two randomised trials currently registered (WHO-ICTRP). This drug has received a great deal of interest since the results of the CRASH-2 study showed that it reduced the risk of death in bleeding trauma patients [15]. However, there was a clear indication that the drug had to be given early to allow benefit, and therefore, it will be interesting to see whether it confers any benefit in a chronic condition such as CSDH [16].

20.6.5 Anticoagulants (AC) and Anti-platelet (AP) Agents

Some studies suggest that AC and AP have no influence on risk of CSDH recurrence or imaging characteristics related to more recent haemorrhage (such as T1 hypointensity) [23, 50]. Conversely, Wada et al. reviewed 681 CSDHs with 14 % of patients on AP and found that recurrence was significantly higher in these patients if surgery was performed immediately [69]. If surgery was delayed even by 1 day, then this risk is significantly reduced and their recommendation was to delay surgery 3 days after stopping AP to minimise recurrence risk. This practice is commonly adopted and if urgent surgery is required then platelets are often given to reduce bleeding risk. Alternatively, surgery is delayed for about 7 days for normal platelet function to recover.

It is commonly accepted that patients on AC receive the appropriate reversal, with fresh frozen plasma (FFP), vitamin K and/or prothrombin complex (PCC) before surgical treatment is started. The difficulty arises with novel "direct oral anticoagulants" (DOACs) which are now in common use due to the benefits of not requiring monitoring. However, they also do not have well-recognised mechanisms of reversal, and difficulties have arisen in their management in patients with haemorrhage. There are no neurosurgical studies on patients taking DOACs. Currently activated prothrombin complex (APCC) appears to be the best option for DOAC reversal while clinical trials are ongoing to establish antidotes [67].

20.7 Outcomes

20.7.1 Recurrence and Its Risk Factors

The average time period to recurrence has been reported as 34.9 days in a series of 414 patients and was similar in unilateral and bilateral cases [23]. Rates of recurrence have been reported to range from 6.1 to 22 % ([5, 8, 9, 23, 60], Gelbert). As previously discussed, presence of a subdural drain appears to be the most significant factor in reducing this [1, 39, 50].

Several studies have shown a higher recurrence rate in the more elderly patients (i.e. >70) compared with the younger ones [21, 60]. The cause of this is not well defined but may be related to poorer brain re-expansion in the elderly. Otherwise, a logistic regression analysis showed that neither haematoma laterality, admission GCS, mRS nor neurological deficit was correlated with recurrence [50].

20.7.2 Complications

CSDH can be associated with a high level of complications (up to 38.6 %) [8, 9]. However, it can be difficult to differentiate complications that are a product of the CSDH itself and those which are related to surgical interventions. Medical complications commonly occur, such as pneumonia, and are probably due to a combination of both underlying pathology and general anaesthetic risks; these are considered in Table 20.4 [21].

20.7.3 Mortality

Mortality is difficult to assess in direct relation to CSDH due to the average age of the population and hence deaths occurring from both the CSDH and coincidentally from pre-existing co-morbidities. The reported figures are variable and often dependant on the follow-up period and demographics of patients included. Mortality rates between 0 and 5.3 % at 30 days are common but as high as 18 % at 6 months, depending on surgical treatment strategies [8, 9, 50, 66].

Table 20.4 Complications associated with CSDH and its treatment

Medical	Surgical
Pneumonia	Pneumocephalus
Other systemic infections (e.g. UTI)	Residual/recurrent CSDH
Cardiac complications	Acute subdural haematoma
Seizures	Intracerebral haematoma
	Wound infection
	Subdural empyema

It has been suggested that CSDH is like the "neck of femur fracture" of neurosurgery, and therefore a marker of already declining function rather than necessarily the cause of it. As already discussed, CSDH is often related to trauma, frequently a fall, and recurrent falls are common in frail elderly people at a time of decline. Age and baseline function are clearly important prognostic factors, and the admission mRS score has been shown to be an independent and significant predictor of death at 6 months [50].

Conclusion

CSDH is an interesting and important condition in neurosurgery, and its prevalence is likely to continue to increase with the world-wide aging population. There are still many questions to answer in order to optimise treatment strategies, and randomised clinical trials are crucial in this. Understanding the pathophysiology and hence improving and targeting therapies appropriately could lead to significant improvements in terms of morbidity and mortality, as already seen with the introduction of drains.

References

1. Almenawer SA, Farrokhyar F, Hong C, Alhazzani W, Manoranjan B, Yarascavitch B, Arjmand P, Baronia B, Reddy K, Murty N, Singh S (2014) Chronic subdural haematoma management: a systematic review and meta-analysis of 34,829 patients. Ann Surg 259(3):449–457
2. Atkinson JL, Lane JI, Aksamit AJ (2003) MRI depiction of chronic intradural (subdural) hematoma in evolution. J Magn Reson Imaging 17(4):484–486
3. Asghar M, Adhiyaman V, Greenway MW, Bhowmick BK, Bates A (2002) Chronic subdural haematoma in the elderly–a North Wales experience. J R Soc Med 95(6):290–292
4. Azevedo R, Reis F, Brito AB, Vassallo J, Lima CS (2015) Dural lymphoma mimicking subdural haematoma on computerized tomography. Br J Haematol 169(2):156
5. Baechli H, Nordmann A, Bucher HC, Gratzl O (2004) Demographics and prevalent risk factors of chronic subdural haematoma: results of a large single-center cohort study. Neurosurg Rev 27:263–266
6. Basaldella L, Perin A, Orvieto E, Marton E, Iksvetich D, Dei Tos AP et al (2010) A preliminary study of AQUAPORIN 1 immunolocalization in chronic subdural haematoma membranes. J Clin Neurosci 17(7):905–907
7. Bender MB, Christoff N (1974) Nonsurgical treatment of subdural hematomas. Arch Neurol 31(2):73–79
8. Berghauser Pont LM, Dammers R, Schouten JW, Lingsma HF, Dirven CM (2012) Clinical factors associated with outcome in chronic subdural hematoma: a retrospective cohort study of patients on preoperative corticosteroid therapy. Neurosurgery 70:873–880
9. Berghauser Pont LM, Dirven CM, Dippel DW, Verweij BH, Dammers R (2012) The role of corticosteroids in the management of chronic subdural hematoma: a systematic review. Eur J Neurol 19(11):1397–1403
10. Blitshteyn S et al (2004) Diffuse dural gadolinium MRI enhancement associated with bilateral chronic subdural haematomas. J Clin Imaging 28:90–92
11. Brodersen P, Gjerris F (1975) Regional cerebral blood flow in patients with chronic subdural hematomas. Acta Neurol Scand 51:233–239
12. Chari A, Hocking KC, Broughton E, Turner C, Santarius T, Hutchinson PJ et al (2016) Core Outcomes and Common Data Elements in Chronic Subdural Hematoma: A Systematic Review of the Literature Focusing on Reported Outcomes. J Neurotrauma 33(13):1212–1219

13. Chari, Hocking KC, Edlmann E, Turner C, Santarius T, Hutchinson PJ et al (2016) Core Outcomes and Common Data Elements in Chronic Subdural Hematoma: A Systematic Review of the Literature Focusing on Baseline and peri-operative care data elements. Journal of Neurotrauma 33(17):1569–1575
14. Cheng YK, Wang TC, Yang JT, Lee MH, Su CH (2009) Dural metastasis from prostatic adenocarcinoma mimicking chronic subdural hematoma. J Clin Neurosci 16(8):1084–1086
15. CRASH-2 trial collaborators, Shakur H, Roberts I, Bautista R, Caballero J, Coats T, Dewan Y, El-Sayed H, Gogichaishvili T, Gupta S, Herrera J, Hunt B, Iribhogbe P, Izurieta M, Khamis H, Komolafe E, Marrero MA, Mejía-Mantilla J, Miranda J, Morales C, Olaomi O, Olldashi F, Perel P, Peto R, Ramana PV, Ravi RR, Yutthakasemsunt S (2010) Effects of tranexamic acid on death, vascular occlusive events, and blood transfusion in trauma patients with significant haemorrhage (CRASH-2): a randomised, placebo-controlled trial. Lancet 376(9734):23–32
16. CRASH-2 collaborators, Roberts I, Shakur H, Afolabi A, Brohi K, Coats T, Dewan Y, Gando S, Guyatt G, Hunt BJ, Morales C, Perel P, Prieto-Merino D, Woolley T (2011) The importance of early treatment with tranexamic acid in bleeding trauma patients: an exploratory analysis of the CRASH-2 randomised controlled trial. Lancet 377(9771):1096–1101
17. Delgado-Lopez PD, Martin-Velasco V, Castilla-Diez JM, Rodriguez-Salazar A, Galacho-Harriero AM, Fernandez-Arconada O (2009) Dexamethasone treatment in chronic subdural haematoma. Neurocirugia (Astur) 20(4):346–359
18. Disease control and prevention (DCP). National vital statistics report, 64(2), Feb 2016. U.S. Department of Health and Human Services Centers for Disease Control and Prevention National Center for Health Statistics
19. Foelholm R, Waltimo O (1975) Epidemiology of chronic subdural haematoma. Acta Neurochir (Wien) 32(3–4):247–250
20. Frati A et al (2004) Inflammation markers and risk factors for recurrence in 35 patients with a posttraumatic chronic subdural haematoma: a prospective study. J Neurosurg 100:24–32
21. Gelabert-Gonzalez M, Iglesias-Pais M, Garcia-Allut A, Martinez- Rumbo R (2005) Chronic subdural haematoma: surgical treatment and outcome in 1000 cases. Clin Neurol Neurosurg 107:223–229
22. Glover D, Labadie EL (1976) Physiopathogenesis of subdural hematomas. Part 2: inhibition of growth of experimental hematomas with dexamethasone. J Neurosurg 45:393–397
23. Goto H, Ishikawa O, Nomura M, Tanaka K, Nomura S, Maeda K (2015) Magnetic resonance imaging findings predict the recurrence of chronic subdural hematoma. Neurol Med Chir (Tokyo) 55(2):173–178
24. Hara M, Tamaki M, Aoyagi M, Ohno K (2009) Possible role of cyclooxygenase-2 in developing chronic subdural haematoma. J Med Dent Sci 56(3):101–106
25. Heula AL, Sajanti J, Majamaa K (2009) Procollagen propeptides in chronic subdural hematoma reveal sustained dural collagen synthesis after head injury. J Neurol 256(1):66–71
26. Hohenstein A, Erber R, Schilling L, Weigel R (2005) Increased mRNA Expression of VEGF within the Hematoma and Imbalance of Angiopoietin-1 and -2 mRNA within the Neomembranes of Chronic Subdural Hematoma. J Neurotrauma 22(5):518–528
27. Hong HJ, Kim YJ, Yi HJ, Ko Y, Oh SJ, Kim JM (2009) Role of angiogenic growth factors and inflammatory cytokine on recurrence of chronic subdural hematoma. Surg Neurol 71(2):161–165
28. Hosoda K, Tamaki N, Masumura M, Matsumoto S, Maeda F (1987) Magnetic resonance images of chronic subdural haematomas. J Neurosurg 67(5):677–683
29. Hua C, Zhao G, Feng Y, Yuan H, Song H, Bie L (2016) Role of matrix metalloproteinase-2, matrix metalloproteinase-9, and vascular endothelial growth factor in the development of chronic subdural hematoma. J Neurotrauma 33(1):65–70
30. Inao S, Kawai T, Kabeya R, Sugimoto T, Yamamoto M, Hata N, Isobe T, Yoshida J (2001) Relation between brain displacement and local cerebral blood flow in patients with chronic subdural haematoma. J Neurol Neurosurg Psychiatry 71(6):741–746

31. Izumihara A, Yamashita K, Murakami T (2013) Acute subdural haematoma requiring surgery in the subacute or chronic stage. Neurologia Medico-Chirurgica 53(5):323–328
32. Kalamatianos T, Stavrinou LC, Koutsarnakis C, Psachoulia C, Sakas DE, Stranjalis G (2013) PlGF and sVEGFR-1 in chronic subdural hematoma: implications for hematoma development. J Neurosurg 118(2):353–357
33. Kaminogo M, Moroki J, Ochi A, Ichikura A, Onizuka M, Shibayama A, et al (1999) Characteristics of symptomatic chronic subdural haematomas on high-field MRI. Neuroradiology 41(2):109–116
34. Kolias AG, Chari A, Santarius T, Hutchinson PJ (2014) Chronic subdural haematoma: modern management and emerging therapies. Nat Rev Neurol 10:570–578
35. Kumar KK, Menon G, Nair S, Radhakrishnan VV (2008) Rosai-Dorfman disease mimicking chronic subdural hematoma. J Clin Neurosci 15(11):1293–1295
36. Kuwahara S, Fukuoka M, Koan Y, Miyake H, Ono Y, Moriki A, Mori K, Mokudai T, Uchida Y (2005) Subdural hyperintense band on diffusion-weighted imaging of chronic subdural hematoma indicates bleeding from the outer membrane. Neurol Med Chir (Tokyo) 45(3):125–131
37. Kwon TH, Park YK, Lim DJ, Cho TH, Chung YG, Chung HS, Suh JK (2000) Chronic subdural hematoma: evaluation of the clinical significance of postoperative drainage volume. J Neurosurg 93:796–799
38. Lee EJ, Lee MY, Hung YC (1999) The application of transcranial doppler sonography in patients with chronic subdural haematoma. Acta Neurochir (Wien) 141:835–839
39. Liu W, Bakker NA, Groen RJ (2014) Chronic subdural haematoma: a systematic review and meta-analysis of surgical procedures. J Neurosurg 121(3):665–673
40. Markwalder TM (1981) Chronic subdural haematoma: a review. J Neurosurg 54(5):637–645
41. Markwalder TM, Steinsiepe KF, Rohner M, Reichenbach W, Markwalder H (1981) The course of chronic subdural hematomas after burr-hole craniostomy and closed-system drainage. J Neurosurg 55:390–396
42. Nanko N, Tanikawa M, Mase M, Fujita M, Tateyama H, Miyati T, Yamada K (2009) Involvement of hypoxia-inducible-factor-1a and VEGF in the mechanism and development of chronic subdural haematoma. Neurol Med Chir (Tokyo) 49(9):379–385
43. Nakagawa T, Kodera T, Kubota T (2000) Expression of matrix metalloproteinases in the chronic subdural haematoma membrane. Acta Neurochir (Wien) 142(1):61–66
44. Neal MT, Hsu W, Urban JE, Angelo NM, Sweasey TA, Branch CL Jr (2013) The subdural evacuation port system: outcomes from a single institution experience and predictors of success. Clin Neurol Neurosurg 115(6):658–664
45. Ommaya AK, Yarnell P (1969) Subdural haematoma after whiplash injury. Lancet 2(7614):237–239
46. Pripp AH & Stanisic M (2014) The correlation between pro- and anti-inflammatory cytokines in chronic subdural hematoma patients assessed with factor analysis. PLoS one 9(2):e90149
47. Prud'homme M, Mathieu F, Marcotte N, Cottin S (2016) A Pilot Placebo Controlled Randomized Trial of Dexamethasone for Chronic Subdural Hematoma. Can J Neurol Sci 43(2):284–290
48. PHE – Publie Health England (2016) Recent trends in life expectancy at older ages: update to 2014. PHE publications gateway number:2015661
49. Roberts I, Yates D, Sandercock P, Farrell B, Wasserberg J, Lomas G, Cottingham R, Svoboda P, Brayley N, Mazairac G, Laloë V, Muñoz-Sánchez A, Arango M, Hartzenberg B, Khamis H, Yutthakasemsunt S, Komolafe E, Olldashi F, Yadav Y, Murillo-Cabezas F, Shakur H, Edwards P (2004) CRASH trial collaborators. Effect of intravenous corticosteroids on death within 14 days in 10008 adults with clinically significant head injury (MRC CRASH trial): randomised placebo-controlled trial. Lancet 364(9442):1321–1328
50. Santarius T, Kirkpatrick PJ, Ganesan D, Chia HL, Jalloh I, Smielewski P et al (2009) Use of drains versus no drains after burr-hole evacuation of chronic subdural haematoma: a randomised controlled trial. Lancet 374(9695):1067–1073

51. Sajanti J & Majamaa K (2003) High concentrations of procollagen propeptides in chronic subdural haematoma and effusion. J Neurol Neurosurg Psychiatry 74(4):522–524
52. Senturk S, Guzel A, Bilici A, Takmaz I, Guzel E, Aluclu MU, Ceviz A (2010) CT and MRI imaging of chronic subdural haematomas: a comparative study. Swiss med wkly 140(23–24):335–340
53. Shono T, Inamura T, Morioka T, Matsumoto K, Suzuki SO, Ikezaki K, Iwaki T, Fukui M (2001) Vascular endothelial growth factor in chronic subdural haematomas. J Clin Neurosci 8(5):411–415
54. Shono T, Inamura T, Morioka T, Matsumoto K, Suzuki SO, Ikezaki K, Iwaki T, Fukui M (2001) Vascular endothelial growth factor in chronic subdural haematomas. J Clin Neurosci 8(5):411–415
55. Sieswerda-Hoogendoorn T et al (2014) Age determination of subdural haematoma with CT and MRI: systematic review. Eur J Radiol 83:1257–1268
56. Singla A, Jacobsen WP, Yusupov IR, Carter DA (2013) Subdural evacuating port system (SEPS)–minimally invasive approach to the management of chronic/subacute subdural hematomas. Clin Neurol Neurosurg 115(4):425–431
57. Slotty PJ, Kamp MA, Steiger SH, Cornelius JF, Macht S, Stummer W, Turowski B (2013) Cerebral perfusion changes in chronic subdural haematoma. J Neurotrauma 30(5):347–351
58. Spreer J, Ernestus RI, Lanfermann H, Lackner K (1997) Connective tissue reactions in subdural haematomas; imaging with contrast-enhancement MRI. Acta Neurochir (wein) 139(6):560–565
59. Stanisic M, Aasen AO, Pripp AH, Lindegaard KF, Ramm-Pettersen J, Lyngstadaas SP, et al (2012) Local and systemic pro-inflammatory and anti-inflammatory cytokine patterns in patients with chronic subdural hematoma: a prospective study. Inflamm Res 61(8):845–852
60. Stroobandt G, Fransen P, Thauvoy C, Menard E (1995) Pathogenetic factors in chronic subdural haematoma and causes of recurrence. Acta Neurochir (Wien) 137(1–2):6–14
61. Sun TF, Boet R, Poon WS (2005) Non-surgical primary treatment of chronic subdural haematoma: preliminary results of using dexamethasone. Br J Neurosurg 19(4):327–333
62. Svien HJ, Gelety JE (1964) On the surgical management of encapsulated subdural hematoma. A comparison of the results of membranectomy and simple evacuation. J Neurosurg 21:172–177
63. Tanaka A, Nakayama Y, Yoshinaga S (1997) Cerebral blood flow and intracranial pressure in chronic subdural hematomas. Surg Neurol 47:346–351
64. Tanikawa M, Mase M, Yamada K, Yamashita N, Matsumoto T, Banno T, Miyati T (2001) Surgical treatment of chronic subdural haematoma based on intrahaematomal membrane structure on MRI. Acta Neurochir (Wien) 143(6):613–618
65. Thau-Zuchman O, Shohami E, Alexandrovich AG, Leker RR (2010) Vascular endothelial growth factor increases neurogenesis after traumatic brain injury. J Cereb Blood Flow Metab 30(5):1008–1016
66. Tsutsumi K, Maeda K, Iijima A, Usui M, Okada Y, Kirino T (1997) The relationship of preoperative magnetic resasonance imaging findings and closed system drainage in the recurrence of chronic subdural haematoma. J Neurosurg 87(6):870–875
67. Tummala R, Kavtaradze A, Gupta A, Ghosh RK (2016) Specific antidotes against direct oral anticoagulants: a comprehensive review of clinical trials data. Int J Cardiol 214:292–298
68. Wada M, Kuroda K, Yoshida Y, Ogasawara K, Ogawa A, Endo S (2006) Local elevation of the anti-inflammatory interleukin-10 in the pathogenesis of chronic subdural haematoma. Neurosurg Rev 29(3):242–245
69. Wada M, Yamakami I, Higuchi Y, Tanaka M, Suda S, Ono J, Saeki N (2014) Influence of antiplatelet therapy on postoperative recurrence of chronic subdural hematoma: a multicenter retrospective study in 719 patients. Clin Neurol Neurosurg 120:49–54
70. Weigel R, Schilling L, Schmiedek P (2001) Specific pattern of growth factor distribution in chronic subdural haematoma (CSH): Evidence for an angiogenic disease. Acta Neurochir (Wien) 143(8):811–819

71. Welsh JE, Tyson GW, Winn HR, Jane JA (1979) Chronic subdural hematoma presenting as transient neurologic deficits. Stroke 10(5):564–567
72. Xu XP et al (2015) Local application of corticosteroids combined with surgery for the treatment of chronic subdural haematoma. Turk Neurosurg 25(2):252–255
73. Yamashima T, Yamamoto S, Friede RL (1983) The role of endothelial gap junctions in the enlargement of chronic subdural hematomas. J Neurosurg 59(2):298–303
74. Yokoyama K, Matsuki M, Shimano H, Sumioka S, Ikenaga T, Hanabusa K, et al (2008) Diffusion Tensor Imaging in Chronic Subdural Haematoma: Correlation between clinical signs and Fractional Anisotropy in the Pyramidal tract. Am J Neuroradiol 29(6):1159–1163

Part VI

Neurovascular

21 Subarachnoid Haemorrhage in the Elderly

Mats Ryttlefors and Per Enblad

21.1 Introduction

During the last century, the population structure has changed due to lowered mortality and lowered nativity, altering the shape of the "population pyramid". The elderly now constitute a substantial proportion of the population. The improvement in the general health of the population has not only been evident in the longer life expectancies but also that the elderly are healthier and have more active lifestyles today than before [102]. This has increased the possibilities and the expectations to treat serious and life-threatening diseases in more advanced ages.

Subarachnoid haemorrhage (SAH) is a devastating disease with a high risk of mortality and morbidity [41]. The incidence of SAH increases with age [52, 116], and along with the increasing elderly population, the number of elderly patients with SAH is increasing steadily. Only a few decades ago, elderly SAH patients rarely received active treatment because of the poor outcome results [20, 67, 81]. Today a more active approach in the treatment of SAH is used also in the elderly. However, special considerations must be made in the management of the elderly SAH patients. The frequency of concurrent diseases increases with age [21]. Along with age-related decline in muscle mass and in cardiovascular [13], respiratory [128] and renal function [6], elderly patients are more prone to develop organ dysfunction and are more vulnerable for complications. Furthermore, the elderly are less amenable to rehabilitation efforts after brain injury [28].

In order to meet the imminent challenge of managing the increasing number of elderly SAH patients in the future, it is urgent to increase the knowledge of different aspects of SAH specifically in the elderly.

M. Ryttlefors, MD, PhD (✉) • P. Enblad, MD, PhD
Department of Neuroscience, Neurosurgery, Uppsala University Uppsala University Hospital, 751 85 Uppsala, Sweden
e-mail: mats.ryttlefors@neuro.uu.se

© Springer International Publishing Switzerland 2017

M. Berhouma, P. Krolak-Salmon (eds.), *Brain and Spine Surgery in the Elderly*,
DOI 10.1007/978-3-319-40232-1_21

21.1.1 Limitations of This Chapter

This book chapter is a review of spontaneous aneurysmal SAH in the elderly. In this context elderly was defined as the patient being 65 years or older. All other causes of subarachnoid haemorrhage, other than a ruptured intracranial aneurysm, such as trauma, vasculitis and intracerebral haemorrhage with rupture to the subarachnoid space are not considered in this chapter. Furthermore, the management of elderly patients with unruptured aneurysms is not considered either.

21.2 Aetiology

Approximately 85 % of all spontaneous SAH are caused by the rupture of an intracranial saccular aneurysm located on one of the basal cerebral vessels near the circle of Willis. Around 10 % of spontaneous SAH are non-aneurysmal perimesencephalic haemorrhages with excellent prognosis. The remaining 5 % are caused by a number of more rare conditions [141].

There is no clearly defined theory on the formation of intracranial aneurysms, and their pathogenesis is still debated. It is likely that the pathogenesis is multifactorial, involving haemodynamic stress, structural alterations in cerebral arteries and genetic and environmental factors [22, 51]. It was early thought that intracranial aneurysms were congenital [37] or that congenital defect in the tunica media of the arterial wall was a prerequisite for aneurysm formation [26]. Others emphasized acquired changes to the internal elastic lamina to be the key factor for aneurysm formation [31]. However, the most plausible explanation is that intracranial aneurysms are formed during life due to degenerative changes in the cerebral arterial wall subjected to haemodynamic stress caused by the pulsating bloodstream at the relatively unsupported arterial divisions [22, 130].

The most important modifiable risk factors for SAH consistent in several studies and meta-analyses are cigarette smoking [2, 9, 23, 53, 61, 68, 77, 103, 116], hypertension [2, 9, 23, 53, 68, 77, 116, 135, 139] and excessive alcohol consumption [23, 61, 77].

It is reasonable to believe that the development of an aneurysm is determined by inherent risk factors and the accumulated burden of acquired risk factors, which increases by age. Given the increased prevalence of hypertension in the elderly (65 % for adults 60 years or older) compared to younger adults (32 % in adults aged 40–59 and 7 % in adults aged 18–39 years) [96], it should not be surprising that the prevalence of intracranial aneurysms also is higher in the elderly compared to younger adults. The prevalence of cigarette smoking is lower in the elderly (9 % for men over 65 years, 7 % for women over 65 years) than in younger adults (22 % men 18–44 years, 17 % women 18–44 years) [91]. However, the elderly adults are likely to be former smokers (52 % men, 36 % women) [91].

21.3 Incidence and Prevalence

The incidence of subarachnoid haemorrhage from a ruptured intracranial aneurysm in the general adult population is 9.1 per 100 000 person-years in most regions (but is higher in Japan (22.7) and Finland (15–17)) [17, 95, 109]. The incidence of subarachnoid haemorrhage increases with increasing age [17, 52, 116], reaching 78 per 100 000 person-years in the eighth decade of life [116]. Women have a higher relative risk for SAH than men do overall [17, 69]. The gender difference is age dependent. Before the age of 55, the incidence is higher in men than in women, but in the age group 55–85 years, the incidence is significantly higher in women than in men [17]. Some studies have indicated that the increased incidence of subarachnoid levels off at 60 years in men and at 70 years in women [63, 69]. However, this contradicts other studies [17, 52, 116] that the incidence increases with increasing age and may be due to that elderly patients with SAH were not actively investigated and treated historically.

The estimated prevalence of an intracranial aneurysm in the general population is 2.3 %, but the reported prevalence varies depending on study design from 0.4 to 6 % [109]. The prevalence of intracranial aneurysms has been shown to be higher in elderly patients than in younger adult patients in autopsy studies [49, 54].

21.4 Symptoms and Diagnosis

The presenting sign of SAH is sudden severe headache, typically described as "worst ever" or "explosive", which develops over seconds rather than minutes. The sudden headache is often accompanied by nausea and vomiting. A period of altered consciousness or prolonged unconsciousness occurs in over half of the cases, and focal neurological signs may develop at the time of ictus or shortly thereafter. In the following hours, neck stiffness, neck pain, low-grade fever and photophobia may develop [141]. It has been observed that elderly SAH patients present in a worse neurological condition than younger patients [47, 50, 73, 74].

Computed tomography (CT) of the brain reveals the characteristically hyperdense appearance of extravasated blood in the basal cisterns, Sylvian fissures and/or the sulci over the brain convexities. If the history is strongly suggestive of SAH, but CT scanning does not reveal any subarachnoid blood, lumbar puncture should be undertaken before ruling out SAH. The haemoglobin in the red blood cell is degraded to oxyhaemoglobin and bilirubin, which gives the typical yellow tinge (xanthochromia) to the cerebrospinal fluid (CSF) after centrifugation. On spectrophotometry absorbance is increased at 415 nm (oxyhaemoglobin) and 455 nm (bilirubin). It is essential to wait at least 6 and preferably 12 h after the onset of symptoms before performing the lumbar puncture to allow for sufficient red blood cell lysis and formation of oxyhaemoglobin and bilirubin [141].

The first-hand method for diagnosis of intracranial aneurysms is, nowadays, computed tomography angiography (CTA), which reveals most intracranial aneurysms, but the sensitivity for small aneurysms is limited [144]. If CTA does not disclose an aneurysm but the SAH is highly suggestive of an intracranial aneurysm, a digital subtraction angiography (DSA) should be performed. DSA has a higher sensitivity in detecting an intracranial aneurysm and is considered the gold standard for this purpose but has a higher risk of complications than CTA due to its invasive nature [16, 66].

21.5 Grading Scales

21.5.1 Neurological Grading Scales

The patients' neurological condition at admission is one of the most important predictors for outcome after SAH. Several scales for grading the neurological condition of SAH patients have been used. The most commonly used grading scale overall and particularly in earlier publications is the Hunt and Hess (H&H) scale [44]. It is a five-level ordinal scale that considers not only level of consciousness but also headache, neck stiffness, focal neurological deficits and hemiparesis (Table 21.1).

Due to unclear definitions of the described neurological conditions of the Hunt and Hess scale, it lacked reliability and validity. In more recent years, the neurological grading scale proposed by the World Federation of Neurosurgical Societies (WFNS) has been used more widely [19, 137]. The WFNS scale is essentially based on the patients' score on the Glasgow Coma Scale (GCS) [136] and on the presence of major focal motor deficit, but cranial nerve palsies are not included (Table 21.2).

More recently the Prognosis on Admission of Aneurysmal Subarachnoid Haemorrhage (PAASH) scale, based solely on the patients GCS, has been suggested, but has not been widely used in publications [134].

21.5.2 Radiological Grading Scale

Fisher's classification is a four-level classification, where level 1 represents no visible blood on the CT and level 2 represents a thin layer of subarachnoid blood less than 1 mm on axial slides, corresponding to a low risk of cerebral vasospasm. Level

Table 21.1 Hunt and Hess grading scale [44]

Hunt and Hess	Description
I	Asymptomatic or minimal headache and slight nuchal rigidity
II	Moderate to severe headache, nuchal rigidity, no neurological deficit other than cranial nerve palsy
III	Drowsiness, confusion or mild focal deficit
IV	Stupor, moderate to severe hemiparesis, possibly early decerebrate rigidity and vegetative disturbances
V	Deep coma, decerebrate rigidity, moribund appearance

Table 21.2 World Federation of Neurological Surgeons (WFNS) scale [19, 137]

WFNS	GCS (sum score)	Motor deficit
I	15	–
II	13 or 14	–
III	13 or 14	+
IV	7–12	+/–
V	3–6	+/–

Table 21.3 Fisher's scale for grading of subarachnoid haemorrhage [125]

Fisher grade	CT findings
1	No visible blood
2	Subarachnoid blood <1 mm
3	Subarachnoid blood >1 mm or localized clot
4	Intraventricular haemorrhage, intracerebral haematoma or both

3 represents a layer of subarachnoid blood thicker than 1 mm in vertical cisterns or fissures or a localized clot, which is correlated with a high risk of developing cerebral vasospasm [25]. Level 4 in Fisher's classification represents either the presence of intraventricular haemorrhage or intracerebral haematoma or both (Table 21.3).

21.5.3 Outcome Grading Scales

The optimal timing for functional outcome classification in the elderly is not determined. In different studies, the timing of outcome classification varies from at the time of hospital discharge up to several years after the SAH. Most often follow-up at 3 or 6 months is used. It is well recognized that the aged brain tolerates injury less well than younger and needs longer time to rehabilitate. Therefore, a too short follow-up is most likely misleading in the elderly because of the risk that one classifies the elderly patients in a worse outcome category than the patients have the potential to achieve. However, true long-time follow-up of several years may not be the most accurate outcome measurement either since the risk of other concurrent diseases and advanced age itself would probably influence this outcome much greater than in a population of younger patients.

Two different functional outcome grading scales are often used for assessing the functional outcome after subarachnoid haemorrhage: the Glasgow Outcome Scale [57] and the Rankin Scale [107]. The Glasgow Outcome Scale (GOS) [57] is an ordinal five-point scale (Table 21.4): dead (D), persistent vegetative state (VS), severe disability (SD), moderate disability (MD) and good recovery (GR). This scale is aimed at measuring disability and handicap rather than impairment [138], and it has been tested for reliability, sensitivity and validity [145–147]. To improve the original GOS, the Extended Glasgow Outcome Scale (GOSE) was developed. In GOSE the three categories good recovery, moderate disability and severe disability of the

Table 21.4 Glasgow Outcome Scale (GOS) [57]

GOS category	Summary	Grouping	Grouping
Dead (D)		Poor	Dependent or dead
Vegetative state (VS)	Sleep/awake, non-sentient	Poor	Dependent or dead
Severe disability (SD)	Conscious but dependent	SD	Dependent or dead
Moderate disability (MD)	Disabled but independent	Favourable	Independent
Good recovery (GR)	None or minor symptoms	Favourable	Independent

Description of outcome categories and outline of grouping of outcome used

Table 21.5 Modified Rankin Scale [107]

Description	Rankin	GOS
I have no symptoms at all and cope well with life	0	GR
I have a few symptoms but these do not interfere with my everyday life	1	GR
I have symptoms which have caused some changes in my life but I am still able to look after myself	2	MD
I have symptoms which have significantly changed my life and prevent me from coping fully, and I need some help looking after myself	3	SD
I have quite severe symptoms which mean I need to have help from other people, but I am not so bad as to need attention day and night	4	SD
I have major symptoms which severely handicap me, and I need constant attention day and night	5	VS
Dead	6	D

Description of outcome categories and comparison to the Glasgow Outcome Scale (GOS). Modified Rankin score 0–2 (GOS: GR and MD) denotes independent survival
Modified Rankin score 3–6 (GOS: SD, VS and D) denotes dependency or death

original GOS are split into two categories, "upper" and "lower", creating an eight-point scale for more precise designation of the patient's functional outcome [146].

In several studies modifications of the original Rankin Scale [107] have been made in that the original category 1 is split into two grades – 0 and 1. Deceased patients are then given a Rankin score of 6 (Table 21.5).

21.6 Natural History

The natural course of subarachnoid haemorrhage in patients of all ages is dismal. In a population-based study from Finland, approximately 60 % of persons suffering a subarachnoid haemorrhage were deceased at 6 months after the initial bleeding. The cause most often being the initial bleed or re-haemorrhage from the ruptured aneurysm [76, 101]. Between 12 and 17 % of all SAH patients die before reaching the hospital [75, 119]. Patients over 60 years have been shown to have a higher rate of early mortality from the initial bleed than younger patients [101]. The case fatality rate increases with age, reaching 70 % at 1 year in patients 80 years or older [69].

21.7 Management and Outcome Results Over Time

The management of SAH in the elderly has changed considerably in the last decades. Also the age at which patients were considered elderly has gradually increased, which can be discerned in the literature (see Table 21.6), from 60 years [20, 43, 81] in the 1960s and 1970s to 65 years in the 1980s and 1990s and to 70 years in the 2000s and 2010s. In some studies the age limit 65 years has been used to define an elderly person because 65 years has been considered the retirement age in many societies [58, 59, 115].

21.7.1 Conservative Management

In the 1960s, elderly patients were at a rule treated conservatively on the basis of their advanced age alone and almost inevitably suffered a poor outcome [20]. It was in this era argued that intracranial investigations and surgery were not justifiable in elderly patients, due to poor surgical results compared to conservative treatment in this age group [67, 81]. During this era most authors suggested an upper age limit for surgical aneurysm treatment at 60 or 65 years [20, 67, 81].

21.7.2 Neurosurgical Aneurysm Treatment

Early studies of surgical treatment of subarachnoid haemorrhage included few or none elderly patients [83, 105, 124]. The surgical mortality in elderly patients was 44–51 % [83, 105, 124]. The timing of surgical treatment and the type of surgical treatment, including aneurysm neck clipping, wrapping and carotid ligation, varied widely [83, 105, 124]. Furthermore, only aneurysms in the anterior cerebral circulation were usually considered surgically treatable in the elderly. It was in this era customary to wait several days to weeks after the initial bleed and let the elderly patient recover neurologically from the effects of the SAH. After this time only elderly patients who were deemed suitable for surgery were operated on. Inevitably a large number of elderly patients would during that time period re-bleed or deteriorate due to ischaemic deficits and suffer a poor prognosis. Most reported surgical series are therefore skewed towards good-grade elderly SAH patients who have survived the initial bleed and the first weeks after the bleed without re-bleeding or suffering from ischaemic deficits due to vasospasm and other complications related to the SAH.

On this note, the most robust knowledge on how to manage elderly SAH patients should come from case series reporting total management results from institutions managing patients from a defined community catchment area, population-based studies or randomized clinical trials. Most reported studies in the literature are less well-controlled case series of surgically or in later years endovascularly treated elderly SAH patients. Outcome data are usually presented only for the elderly patients selected for treatment and not for the patients who were deemed to be in too

Table 21.6 Summary of published series of elderly SAH patients over time

First author	Year	Time period	Age Cut-off	No. of Elderly SAH patients	Treatment NS/ EVT/Cons	Main finding/conclusion
Predominately surgical series						
McKissock [83]	1960	1954–1956	60	80	36 Cons 44 NS	Mortality Cons, 67 % Mortality NS, 48 %
Hugosson [43]	1973	1963–1971	60	43	43 NS	9 % mortality, 66 % symptom-free, 13 % minor disability at 1–9 years
Amacher [4]	1977	1952–1975	60	93	93 NS	Surgical results in good-grade patients Favourable outcome 72 % Mortality 17 %
Martindale [81]	1978	1965–1975	60	97	69 Cons 28 NS	Conservative management Independent at 1 year, 16 % Neurosurgical aneurysm treatment Independent at 1 year, 9 % Conclude that 60 is the upper age limit for aneurysm surgery
Sengupta [123]	1978	1971–1977[a]	60	32	32 NS	75 % independent outcome, 25 % poor outcome
Ohmoto [98]	1980	1973–1978	60	148	148 NS	Good-grade patients, 7 % operative mortality the same as for younger patients; should be operated early Grade III patients should be surgically treated with a delay of 2 weeks Poor-grade patients should be conservatively treated
Nukui [94]	1985	Not stated	60	108	108 NS	Good-grade elderly patients should be surgically treated early as for younger patients Poor-grade elderly SAH patients should be managed conservatively

Kassell [64]	1990	1980–1983	60	908	255 Cons 653 NS	Overall outcome (GOS 6 months) Favourable (GR+MD), 50 % Severe disability, 8 % Poor (VS+D), 42 % Surgical outcome (GOS 6 months) Favourable (GR+MD), 64 % Severe disability, 9 % Poor (VS+D), 26 %
Fridriksson [29]	1995	1988–1993	70	76	76 NS	2/3 of patients over 70 can achieve good outcome returning to independent life
Lanzino [74]	1996	1987–1989	60	208	Not stated	Overall outcome (GOS 3 months) Favourable (GR+MD), 50 % Severe disability, 18 % Poor (VS+D), 31 %
Stachniak [129]	1996	1989–1994	65	47	47 NS	Higher mortality and longer stay in NICU for elderly patients compared to younger
Mori [89]	1997	1981–1988	70	24	24 NS	Favourable outcome in 54 % (13/24) elderly patients. Older age, independent predictor of poor outcome
Hamada [38]	1998	1992–1997	80	10	10 NS	8/10 favourable outcome. Advanced age should not preclude surgical aneurysm treatment, but not all aged patients eligible for treatment
Chung [14]	2000	1992–1998	70	89	53 NS 11 EVT 2 NS+EVT 23 Cons	Overall outcome (GOS 6 months) Excellent (GR), 34 % Good (MD), 9 % Fair (SD), 5.6 % Poor (VS), 3.4 % Dead (D), 45 %
Lan [73]	2000	1990–1996	65	38	38 NS	66 % (25/38) favourable outcome (GR+MD) in elderly SAH patients compared to 78 % favourable outcome in patients aged 51–64 and 90 % favourable outcome in patients <50 years

(continued)

Table 21.6 (continued)

First author	Year	Time period	Age Cut-off	No. of Elderly SAH patients	Treatment NS/ EVT/Cons	Main finding/conclusion
Osawa [100]	2001	1988–1998	70	392	392 NS	Surgical outcome at discharge (GOS) Excellent (GR) 27 % Good (MD) 21 % Fair (SD) 16 % Poor (VS) 17 % Dead (D) 19 %
Johansson (Ryttlefors) [58]	2001	1981–1998	65	281	34 Cons 215 NS 32 EVT	Overall outcome (GOS) 1981–1998 Favourable (GR+MD), 57 % Severe disability (SD), 12 % Poor (VS+D), 31 % Increased favourable outcome over time without increasing severe disability, despite elderly patients being older and in more severe clinical grade
Pinsker [104]	2002	1994–2000	70	41	41 NS	Mortality and good outcome at 30 days post-SAH dependent on initial clinical grade 30-day mort, 6 % in Hunt and Hess I–III, 39 % in Hunt and Hess IV–V
Laidlaw [72]	2002	1991–2000	70	74	18 Cons 56 NS	Overall outcome (GOS 3 months) Favourable (GR+MD), 46 % Severe disability (SD), 13 % Poor (VS+D), 41 % Management and surgical outcome in good-grade patients were worse in elderly than in younger patients, but in poor-grade patients, similar as for younger patients

Yano [148]	2003	1996–1999	80	76	45 Cons 31 NS	All patients with Hunt and Hess ≥III had poor outcomes irrespective of treatment. 9/19 H&H I–II patients who underwent surgery had good outcome
Ferch [24]	2003	1990–2000	70	100	100 NS	Surgical outcome (Rankin 6 months) Independent outcome (RDS 1–2), 60 % Mortality (RDS 6), 24 % Predictors of poor outcome in multivariate analysis were worse clinical grade on admission, early hydrocephalus and medical complications
Agazzi [3]	2004	Not stated	70	33	14 Cons 16 NS 3 EVT	Overall outcome (mRS) Independent (mRS 0–2), 27 % Severe disability (mRS 3), 15 % Dependent or dead (mRS 4–6), 58 % Authors suggest that only elderly patients in good clinical grade (WFNS 1–2) and no major co-morbidity should be considered for surgery
Horiuchi [42]	2005	1988–2002	70	538	530 NS 8 EVT	Surgical outcome (GOS discharge) Favourable (GR + MD), 53 % Unfavourable (SD, VS, D), 47 %
Inagawa [48]	2005	1980–1998	70	115	68 Cons 47 NS	Overall outcome (GOS 6 months) Favourable (GR + MD), 28 % Severe disability (SD), 12 % Unfavourable (VS + D), 60 % Surgical results (GOS 6 months) Favourable (GR + MD), 55 % Severe disability (SD), 23 % Unfavourable (VS + D), 22 %
Mino [85]	2006	2002–2003	70	31	31 NS	Surgical results (GOS 3 months) Good outcome (GR + MD), 48 % Poor outcome (SD, VS, D), 52 %

(continued)

Table 21.6 (continued)

First author	Year	Time period	Age Cut-off	No. of Elderly SAH patients	Treatment NS/ EVT/Cons	Main finding/conclusion
Predominately endovascular						
Rowe [112]	1996	1993–1994	70	10	10 EVT	Treatment outcome 6/10 independent outcome
Sawada [118]	2000	1995–1999	70	26	26 EVT	Treatment outcome (GOS 3 months) Favourable outcome (GR+MD), 50 % Severe disability (SD), 19 % Unfavourable outcome (VS+D), 31 %
Birchall [7]	2001	1992–1998	70	14	14 EVT	Treatment outcome (RDS discharge) 12/14 full recovery (RDS 1) 1/14 severe disability (RDS 3) 1/14 dead (RDS 6)
Sedat [122]	2002	1993–1999	65	52	52 EVT	Treatment outcome (GOS 12 months) Favourable (R+MD), 48 % Severe disability (SD), 27 % Poor (VS+D), 25 % Compared to patients under 65 less favourable outcome and higher mortality and a higher rate of thromboembolic complications
Johansson (Ryttlefors) [59]	2004	1996–2000	65	62	62 EVT	Treatment outcome (GOS 6 months) Favourable (GR+MD), 41 % Severe disability (SD), 36 % Poor outcome (VS+D), 22 %

Jain [56]	2004	1996–2002	70	13	13 EVT	All poor-grade patients (H&H IV–V) Treatment outcome (GOS discharge) Favourable outcome (GR+MD), 38 % Severe disability (SD), 15 % Poor outcome (VS+D), 47 %
Lubicz [78]	2004	1996–2002	65	68	68 EVT	Treatment outcome (GOS 6–36 months) Favourable (excellent or good), 59 % Unfavourable (fair, poor, dead), 41 %
Bradac [10]	2005	1994–2004	70	55	55 EVT	Treatment outcome (GOS 8 months–8 years) Favourable outcome (GR+MD), 60 % Severe disability (SD), 7 % Poor outcome (VS+D), 33 %
Cai [11]	2005	1998–2003	70	41	41 EVT	Hunt and Hess I–II Independent (mRS 0–1), 89 % Hunt and Hess III–V Dependent (mRS 4–6), 77 %
Nieuwkamp [92]	2006	1990–2004	75	170	121 Cons 34 NS 13 EVT	Overall outcome (GOS discharge) Independent 15 % Dependent 35 % Dead 50 % Overall outcome (GOS 6 months) Independent 18 % Dependent 12 % Dead 70 %
Lou [79]	2007	1998–2005	70	25	25 EVT	Treatment outcome (GOS 6–36 months) Favourable outcome (GR+MD), 80 % Severe disability (SD), 16 % Poor (VS+D), 4 %

(continued)

Table 21.6 (continued)

First author	Year	Time period	Age Cut-off	No. of Elderly SAH patients	Treatment NS/ EVT/Cons	Main finding/conclusion
Gizewski [30]	2008	1997–2005	65	85	85 EVT	Treatment outcome (GOS 6 months) Favourable (GR+MD), 39 % Severe disability (SD), 34 % Poor outcome (VS+D), 28 %
Ryttlefors [113]	2008	1994–2001	65	278	138 EVT 140 NS	Outcome (mRS 1 year) by randomized treatment Independent survival (mRS 0–2) Endovascular 60 % Neurosurgical 56 % Dependency or death (mRS 3–6) Endovascular 40 % Neurosurgical 44 %
Gu [34]	2012	2003–2010	70	96	96 EVT	Treatment outcome (mRS 6 months) Independent (mRS 0–2), 80 % Dependent (mRS 3–6), 20 % Lower age, better clinical grade and endovascular treatment <24 h were independent predictors of independent outcome
Schöller [121]	2013	1996–2007	60	256	38 Cons 93 EVT 123 NS	Overall outcome (GOS 35 months) Favourable (GR+MD), 41 % Severe disability (SD), 13 % Poor (VS+D), 46 %

NS neurosurgical aneurysm treatment, *EVT* endovascular aneurysm treatment, *Cons* conservative (no) aneurysm treatment, *GOS* Glasgow Outcome Scale, *GR* good recovery, *MD* moderate disability, *SD* severe disability, *VS* vegetative state, *D* dead, *RDS* Rankin Disability Scale, *mRS* modified Rankin Scale

[a]Time period not clearly stated in paper

poor condition to warrant treatment. The reported series of elderly SAH patients are reviewed in the following section.

Hugosson (1973) reported a series of 43 SAH patients aged 60–68 years who were surgically treated at our department. The surgical mortality was 9 % and 66 % were symptom-free, and 13 % had minor disabilities after long-term follow-up 1–9 years after the SAH. He argued that even elderly patients with ruptured intracranial aneurysms could be successfully surgically treated with good results if some contra-indications were observed. These were prolonged initial unconsciousness in association with the SAH, prior clinical signs of arteriosclerosis and angiographically verified arteriosclerosis in the cerebral vessels. Furthermore, the author suggested that it seemed possible to operate elderly SAH patients early after the haemorrhage without increasing the operative risks appreciably [43].

Amacher et al. (1977) demonstrated that surgical outcome results in 93 elderly SAH patients 60 years and older in good neurological grade were similar to that of younger SAH patients if the aneurysm was located in the anterior cerebral circulation. Overall the elderly patients had a favourable outcome in 72 % compared to 82 % of the younger patients. Considering only patients with anterior circulation aneurysms, both the elderly and the younger patients had a favourable outcome in 76 %. In patients with posterior circulation aneurysms, however, the elderly patients fared worse, where the elderly had a favourable outcome in 64 %, while the younger patients had a favourable outcome in 88 % [4].

Sengupta et al. (1978) reported their results on 32 elderly SAH patients between 60 and 65 years old. Twenty-four of 32 patients had a satisfactory outcome returning to an independent life at follow-up at 6 months to 6 years. Of the eight patients who had a poor outcome after surgery, only three were deemed as a result of advanced age [123].

Ohmoto et al. (1980) showed that in good-grade elderly SAH patients (Hunt and Hess I–II), the surgical mortality was approximately the same as for younger patients (7 %). The elderly age limit was considered at 60 years in their series of 494 SAH patients of which 148 were over the age of 60 years. However, the mortality was higher in drowsy (Hunt and Hess III) and poor-grade (Hunt and Hess IV–V) elderly patients than in the younger patients, especially if surgery was conducted early. The authors suggested that good-grade elderly patients should be surgically treated as soon as possible after the SAH, whereas the poor-grade patients should be conservatively treated and that surgery should be postponed 2 weeks after the haemorrhage in Hunt and Hess III patients [98].

Nukui et al. (1985) reported their results of surgical treatment of 108 elderly SAH patients over 60 years of age. Surgical mortality and morbidity were 7 and 3 %, respectively, in the good-grade elderly SAH patients if surgically treated 2 weeks after SAH. In the elderly SAH patients who were operated on early after the SAH, the mortality was dependent on the patient's neurological grade: grade I and II 0 %, grade III 13 %, grade IV 54 % and grade V 100 %. The authors concluded that elderly SAH patients in good neurological grade should be operated on early after SAH, while elderly poor-grade patients should be treated conservatively [94].

Kassell et al. (1990) reported outcome figures for 908 elderly patients 60 years or older who were enrolled in the International Cooperative Study on the Timing of Aneurysm Surgery, which evaluated the results of surgical and medical management of 3521 SAH patients in total. In the elderly patients, overall favourable outcome was achieved in 50 % and severe disability in 9 %, and 42 % were in a vegetative state or dead at 6 months after the SAH. In surgically treated patients, the corresponding figures were 64 %, 9 % and 26 %, respectively. In multivariate analysis, older age was an independent predictor for poor outcome [64].

Fridriksson et al. (1995) showed that approximately two thirds of 76 SAH patients aged 70–74 years treated with neurosurgical clipping had an independent outcome [29].

Lanzino et al. (1996) analysed data from 906 patients who were enrolled to a multicentre randomized trial of nicardipine. Among those, 210 SAH patients were 60 years or older. It was demonstrated that elderly patients were admitted in worse neurological grade; had larger amount of subarachnoid clots, higher incidence of intraventricular haemorrhage and more often hydrocephalus on the admission CT scans; and had higher incidence of associated pre-existing medical conditions and higher re-bleeding rates. Multivariate analysis of overall outcome, adjusted for different prognostic factors, revealed that high age per se was a negative prognostic factor, suggesting that the aging brain has less optimal response to the initial bleeding. The authors conclude however that elderly patients should not be refused active treatment based solely on advanced age [74].

Stachniak et al. (1996) compared treatment results in 219 SAH patients who underwent clipping of the ruptured aneurysm. Forty-seven patients were 65 years or older and 172 were younger than 65 years. The elderly patients had a higher mortality rate (13 % vs. 5 %) and longer stay in the neurointensive care unit [129].

Mori et al. (1997) reported favourable outcome in 54 % (13/24) of elderly patients 70 years or older who were surgically treated for the ruptured aneurysms. Older age was found to be an independent predictor of mortality [89].

Hamada et al. (1999) reported their surgical outcome results after clipping of ruptured anterior circulation aneurysms in ten elderly patients 80–83 years old. All patients were in good neurological grade and with no other prior systemic comorbidities. At discharge 8/10 had a favourable outcome and two had severe disability. Their conclusion was that advanced age alone does not preclude the possibility of successful aneurysm surgery, but the authors also emphasized that aneurysm surgery in aged patients must aim at preserving vitality and not all aged patients with ruptured aneurysms are eligible for operative treatment [38].

Chung et al. (2000) reported on 89 consecutive SAH patients aged 70 years or older. In this series of patients, 60 % were clipped, 12 % were coiled, and 2 % received both treatment modalities, whereas 26 % received no aneurysm treatment due to poor clinical condition or very advanced age. In this study which reflects the total management results, 34 % had an excellent outcome (good recovery), 9 % had a good outcome (moderate disability), 5.6 % had a fair outcome (severe disability), 3.4 % had a poor outcome (vegetative state), and 45 % were dead at 6 months post-SAH [14].

Lan et al. (2000) compared their outcome results of surgically treated SAH patients in different age groups. Of 38 elderly SAH patients aged 65 years or older, 25 (66 %) had a favourable outcome (GOS: GR and MD), compared to 90 % favourable outcome in patients under 50 years and 76 % favourable outcome in patients between 50 and 64 years. The authors suggest that early aneurysm surgery is indicated for aneurysms in elderly patients with good neurological grades, in the absence of organ failure [73].

Osawa et al. (2001) reported surgical management results of 392 elderly SAH patients aged 70 years or older as part of a larger series comprising 2055 SAH patients of all ages. Forty-seven percent (186/392) had a favourable outcome at discharge (able to return to independent lifestyle), 16 % had fair outcome (disability but able to live at home with assistance), and 36 % had poor outcome (severe disability, vegetative state or dead). In their study, age over 60 years increased the risk of poor outcome compared to patients of younger ages [100].

We (Johansson/Ryttlefors et al. 2001) reported total management results of 281 elderly SAH patients 65 years or older managed at our department over an 18-year period, 1981–1998, divided into three 6-year time periods. Over time more elderly patients in more advanced ages and in more severe clinical grades were admitted for neurosurgical treatment. Despite the elderly patients being older and in more severe clinical grades, the proportion of patients with favourable outcome increased over time without increasing the proportion of patients with severe disability. In the later time period 1993–1998 in this study, 85 % of the good-grade elderly patients (H&H I–II) had a favourable outcome at 6 months after the SAH [58].

Pinsker et al. (2001) reported their surgical results on 41 elderly patients 70 years or older and found that the most important factor for favourable outcome was good clinical grade on admission. Thirty-day mortality was 6 % in Hunt and Hess I–III patients and 39 % in Hunt and Hess IV–V patients. They conclude that early surgical clipping and postoperative neurointensive care can attain a favourable outcome in a significant percentage of elderly patients [104].

Laidlaw et al. (2002) reported total management results and surgical results in 56 elderly SAH patients 70 years or older. In this study of the elderly patients in good neurological grade on admission (WFNS 1–3) who were surgically treated, 53 % (19/36) had a favourable outcome (GOS: GR and MD) at the 3-month follow-up. Of the elderly patients in poor neurological grade (WFNS 4–5), 35 % (7/20) had a favourable outcome. The total management results were 53 % (20/38) favourable outcome for good-grade patients and 22 % (8/36) for poor-grade patients. In comparison to younger patients under the age of 70, surgically treated good-grade elderly SAH patients fared worse than the younger patients, but the results did not differ significantly for poor-grade patients. Case fatality rate was 69 % in the elderly poor-grade group. The authors also studied intraoperative difficulties during surgery and did not find any significant difference between elderly and younger patients. The authors advocate ultra-early surgery as part of a coordinated aggressive management strategy, which also includes meticulous fluid management and early mobilization [72].

Yano et al. (2003) studied 76 elderly SAH patients who were 80–89 years old at onset of the SAH. All patients with a Hunt and Hess III or worse on admission had a poor outcome irrespective of treatment. Nineteen of 32 patients with an initial good neurological grade on admission (Hunt and Hess I–II) underwent surgery for the ruptured aneurysms. Nine of these 19 patients had a good outcome at 2 years after the SAH. The authors conclude that also patients aged over 80 years can be considered for surgical clipping of the ruptured aneurysms if the neurological grade on admission is good [148].

Ferch et al. (2003) analysed the complication rate of 100 SAH patients 70 years or older who were surgically treated for the ruptured aneurysm and found that medical complications occurred in 22 %. The clinical grade of haemorrhage, acute hydrocephalus requiring ventriculostomy and medical complication was associated with poor outcome [24].

Agazzi et al. (2004) reported their results of clipping and coiling of ruptured aneurysms in 19 SAH patients 70 years or older. Only patients in good neurological grade (WFNS 1–3) without significant co-morbidity were offered aneurysm treatment. Among those elderly patients, 7/12 of the patients in WFNS 1 had a favourable outcome (mRS 0–2), while all patients in worse clinical grade on admission were dependent or dead at 1–2 years post-SAH. Their recommendation was to offer aneurysm treatment only for those elderly patients that present in a good clinical grade (WFNS 1 or 2) and without major systemic co-morbidities [3].

Horiuchi et al. (2005) reported outcome in 538 SAH patients aged 70 years or older, where all patients underwent neurosurgical clipping except 8 who had endovascular aneurysm treatment. In patients in good preoperative neurological grade (Hunt and Kosnik I–III), 63 % (254/401) had a favourable outcome (GOS: GR and MD) at discharge, whereas 22 % (30/137) of the patients in poor preoperative neurological grade (Hunt and Kosnik IV–V) had a favourable outcome. The authors conclude that advanced age alone should not exclude elderly patients from adequate surgical repair in patients with aneurysmal rupture [42].

Inagawa (2005) reported decreased case fatality rates of elderly SAH patients aged 70 years or older in the latter of two time periods (1980–1989 and 1990–1999) in defined population in Izumo City, Japan. Of 115 elderly SAH patients, 47 were surgically treated for the ruptured aneurysms during both periods. Twenty-six patients (55 %) had a favourable outcome at the 6-month follow-up [48].

Mino et al. (2006) reported favourable outcome in 48 % (15/31) of elderly patients 70 years or older. Most patients were in good neurological grade [85].

Nieuwkamp et al. (2006) reported total management results of a consecutive series of 170 elderly SAH patients 75 years or older admitted to two hospitals over a 14-year period. One hundred twenty-one patients were managed conservatively, 34 were surgically treated, and 13 were treated endovascularly. Overall outcome was poor, 50 % in-hospital death and merely 18 % achieving an independent outcome at 6 months post-SAH. The 6-month outcome for surgically treated patients was independent outcome in 50 %, dependency in 25 % and deceased in 25 %. Corresponding figures for endovascularly treated patients were 25 % independent and 25 % dependency, and 50 % were deceased at 6 months post-SAH. The strongest predictors of poor outcome were the effect of the initial bleed indicated by worse clinical grade on admission, re-bleeding and subdural extension of the haemorrhage [92].

21.7.3 Endovascular Treatment

With the introduction of endovascular aneurysm treatment with detachable coils in the 1990s [35, 36], it was early on suggested that elderly patients in particular would benefit from this less invasive aneurysm treatment approach.

Rowe et al. (1996) presented their early experience with endovascular aneurysm treatment in 13 elderly patients with symptomatic aneurysm of which 10 had ruptured aneurysms. All were in clinical good condition. The procedures were technically successful in 12/13. Procedural complications were seen in 3/12 (25 %), of which none resulted in permanent deficits. At clinical follow-up 2–17 months after the SAH, 6/10 were independent, 1/10 dependent, 1/10 deceased and 1/10 lost to follow-up [112].

Sawada et al. (2000) reported their 3-month outcome results of endovascular coiling of ruptured aneurysms in 26 SAH patients 70 years and older and found that the outcome results much depended on the preoperative neurological grade. Eleven of 13 patients (85 %) in good neurological grade (WFNS 1–3) had a favourable outcome, whereas 11 of 13 patients who presented in a poor neurological grade (WFNS 4–5) had a poor neurological outcome. The periprocedural technical complication rate was 19 % (5/26). The increased technical complication rate was thought to be due to atherosclerotic changes of cerebral arteries in the elderly patients. Their conclusion was that coil embolization is a useful treatment for elderly SAH patients especially for patients presenting in a good neurological grade [118].

Birchall et al. (2001) studied 14 elderly SAH patients 70 years or older who were endovascularly treated. All patients were in good clinical grade (Hunt and Hess I–II). Complete occlusion of the aneurysm was achieved in 47 % and intraprocedural complication occurred in 13 %. Twelve of 14 patients made a full recovery (86 %), one patient was disabled, and one patient died within 2 weeks [7].

Sedat et al. (2002) compared their treatment results in 52 elderly SAH patients 65 years and older with 143 SAH patients younger than 65. The elderly patients had worse clinical grades and more abundant bleeding on CT than the younger patients. In the elderly group, complete occlusion of the aneurysm was achieved in 48 %, and periprocedural complications were observed in 13 %. Clinical outcome 1 year post-SAH was favourable in 48 %, severe disability in 27 % and poor in 25 % in the elderly group, whereas clinical outcome in the younger group was 77 % favourable, 9 % severe disability and 14 % poor. In a logistic regression model, age over 65, worse clinical grade on admission, more severe Fisher grade and previous medical history of hypertension, smoking, cardiovascular disease and brain disease were independent predictors of poor outcome [122].

We (Johansson/Ryttlefors et al.) (2004) studied endovascular aneurysm treatment in 62 elderly SAH patients 65 years or older. In 58 of 62 patients, endovascular treatment was successful. Procedural complications occurred in 11 %, but did not influence outcome negatively. Neck remnant or some residual filling of the aneurysm was observed in 21 % and 11 %, respectively. The conclusions were that endovascular aneurysm treatment can be performed in elderly patients with SAH with a high level of technical success, with acceptable aneurysm occlusion results, with an acceptable rate of procedural complications and with fair outcome results and that middle cerebral artery aneurysms may be less suitable for endovascular coil embolization in elderly patients [59].

Jain et al. (2004) reported their outcome results of 13 poor-grade (Hunt and Hess IV–V) elderly SAH patients who were treated with endovascular coiling of the ruptured aneurysms. Procedural complications occurred in 11 %. Outcome at discharge was good recovery in 15 % (2/13), moderate disability in 23 % (3/13), severe disability in 15 % (2/13) and 47 % (6/13) were deceased. The authors concluded that most elderly patients with a poor clinical grade can now be treated with endovascular aneurysm treatment in the acute phase and that early treatment of the ruptured aneurysms improves overall outcomes by reducing the incidence of re-bleeding and allows for aggressive medical management for prevention and treatment of symptomatic vasospasm [56].

Lubicz et al. (2004) assessed the feasibility and effectiveness of endovascular coiling and clinical outcome in 68 elderly SAH patients 65 years or older. All procedures were technically successful, and complete occlusion was achieved in 69 %. Procedural complications occurred in 12 % of the patients. Clinical outcome at 6–36 months post-SAH was favourable (good or excellent) in 59 % and fair or poor in 21 %, and 21 % were dead [78].

Bradac et al. (2005) studied 55 elderly SAH patients aged 70 years or older who were treated with coiling of the ruptured aneurysms. The coiling results were complete occlusion in 62 % and incomplete occlusion in 27 %, and in five patients the aneurysm could not be endovascularly treated due to vessel tortuosity or unfavourable aneurysm morphology. Overall outcome was good (returning to independent life) in 60 % of the patients. Outcome was primarily related to the initial neurological condition of the patients. Favourable outcome was achieved in 90 % of Hunt and Hess I–II patients, 66 % of Hunt and Hess III patients and 11 % of Hunt and Hess IV–V patients. The authors also compared the results with 260 younger SAH patients, in whom favourable outcome was achieved in 96 % of Hunt and Hess I–II patients, in 87 % of Hunt and Hess III patients and in 43 % of Hunt and Hess IV–V patients. The poor-grade elderly SAH patients had a significantly worse outcome than younger patients. The authors conclude that aneurysm treatment in elderly patients should be considered and that the most relevant factor influencing prognosis in this age group is not the age per se but the clinical grade on admission and that endovascular approach may represent the initial choice of treatment in many cases [10].

Cai et al. (2005) reported their outcome results in 41 elderly SAH patients who were treated with coiling of the ruptured aneurysms. Favourable outcome (mRS 0–1 = independent outcome) was achieved in 89 % (25/28) of the Hunt and Hess I–II patients, while only 20 % (1/5) of Hunt and Hess III and none of the eight Hunt and Hess IV–V patients had a favourable outcome. The authors conclude that elderly patients should be considered for endovascular treatment of both ruptured and symptomatic unruptured intracranial aneurysms, but morbidity and mortality rates remain high in high-grade elderly SAH patients [11].

Luo et al. (2007) reported their experience of endovascular treatment of ruptured aneurysms in 25 elderly SAH patients 70 years or older. All procedures were technically successful, total occlusion rate was 32 % and procedural complications occurred in 16 %. Clinical outcome at 6–36 months was a favourable outcome in 80 % (20/25), severe disability in 16 % (4/25) and death in 4 % (1/25) [79].

Gizewski et al. (2008) analysed the outcome 6 months after the SAH in 85 elderly SAH patients aged 65 years or older. Endovascular treatment was performed within 72 h of SAH onset. Endovascular procedure was technically feasible in 95 %, procedural complications occurred in 13 %, and complete aneurysm occlusion was achieved in 74 %. Overall outcome according to the Glasgow Outcome Scale was good recovery in 24 %, moderate disability in 14 %, severe disability in 34 % and persistent vegetative state in 6 %, and 22 % were deceased at follow-up. All patients who had a good recovery were in good neurological grade on admission, while all patients in poor neurological grade on admission had either severe disability or vegetative state or were dead at follow-up [30].

Gu et al. (2012) reported outcome results in 96 elderly SAH patients who were treated endovascularly for the ruptured aneurysms. Patients treated within 24 h of SAH onset had significantly better outcomes (87 % mRS 0–2) than patients treated after 24 h of SAH onset (70 % mRS 0–2). Eighty-seven percent of the patients in good neurological grade (WFNS 1–3) had an independent outcome (mRS 0–2), and 60 % of the patients in poor neurological grade (WFNS 4–5) had an independent outcome (mRS 0–2). In a multivariate logistic regression model, younger age, lower WFNS grade and ultra-early endovascular treatment were independent predictors of good clinical outcome [34].

Schöller et al. (2013) reported total management outcome results and treatment-related complication rates from 256 elderly SAH patients aged 60 years or older. Among those patients, 123 (48 %) received endovascular aneurysm treatment, 93 (37 %) received neurosurgical clipping, and 38 (15 %) were managed conservatively. Overall management outcome was favourable in 41 %, severe disability in 13 % and poor (GOS: VS or D) in 46 %. Better outcomes were achieved in patients less than 70 years [121].

21.7.4 Neurosurgical Clipping Versus Coil Embolization

Three randomized trials comparing neurosurgical versus endovascular aneurysm treatment including also elderly patients have been published: the Kuopio study [70, 142], the International Subarachnoid Aneurysm Trial (ISAT) [86–88, 113] and the Barrow Ruptured Aneurysm Trial (BRAT) [82, 126, 127].

In the single-centre randomized study in Kuopio, Finland, SAH patients with ruptured aneurysms suitable for both treatments were randomized to either endovascular or neurosurgical treatment. The study included patients of all ages up to 75 years.

There was no statistical difference between the two treatment groups in terms of clinical outcome at 3 months post-SAH [142] or at 1 year post-SAH [70]. However, separate data for the elderly patients were not presented in the publications.

In a subgroup analysis of 278 elderly patients 65 years or older that were included in the ISAT, no significant difference could be demonstrated between the two different treatment allocations in the elderly patient population [113]. Sixty percent of the endovascularly treated patients had an independent outcome compared to 56 % of the patients allocated to neurosurgical aneurysm treatment. Thus, a trend towards better clinical outcome in the endovascular group could be shown in accordance with the findings of the whole ISAT cohort [86–88]. Furthermore, elderly patients allocated to endovascular treatment had a shorter length of stay in the hospital and had less infectious and pulmonary complications and a lower frequency of epilepsy than the elderly patients allocated to neurosurgical treatment. The location of the ruptured aneurysm was found to have a profound influence on the functional outcome depending on the treatment modality. Of the patients with ruptured aneurysms on the internal carotid and posterior communicating artery, 72 % in the endovascular group and 52 % in the neurosurgical group were independent at follow-up. Conversely, for patients with middle cerebral artery aneurysms, 45 % of the patients who received endovascular treatment and 86 % of the patients who were allocated to neurosurgical clipping were independent at follow-up. It was concluded that endovascular coiling should be the treatment of choice for ruptured internal carotid artery and posterior communicating artery aneurysms in the elderly SAH patients, while elderly patients with ruptured middle cerebral artery aneurysms appear to benefit from neurosurgical clipping [113].

The BRAT study was a single-centre prospective, randomized, controlled trial designed to compare the results of surgical clipping to those of endovascular coil therapy for the treatment of ruptured intracranial aneurysms. The study was designed to reflect real-world practicalities of ruptured aneurysm treatment. Adult patients up to the age of 80 years were eligible for enrolment. However, data stratified by age was not presented in the publications. The main finding of this study was that endovascular coiling resulted in a lower rate of poor clinical outcome at the 1-year follow-up [82]. This difference however decreased over time [126, 127].

In a recent meta-analysis of 44 studies reporting outcome results after aneurysm clipping or coil embolization of ruptured aneurysms in elderly patients aged 69 years or older, it was shown that health-related quality of life was higher after coil embolization than after neurosurgical clipping [125].

21.8 Special Considerations in the Clinical Management of Elderly SAH Patients

It is obvious that elderly patients with SAH have a higher risk of an unfavourable clinical outcome than younger patients, although a substantial proportion of elderly may also have favourable outcome [18, 27, 47, 50, 60, 64, 65, 69, 74, 93, 117, 129, 133]. Reasons for worse outcome are thought to be less active management and conservative referral patterns [97, 111], poorer clinical grades on admission [47, 50, 73, 74], higher frequency of co-morbidity [21, 74, 133] and increased incidence of severe complications [74]. In addition, age-related changes in vital organs also contribute to the worse outcome. Therefore, age-related physiological changes in other vital organ systems must also be considered when managing elderly patients with intracranial disease, such as SAH [90, 132]. The total effects of aging on vital extracranial organ systems render the elderly patient more susceptible to dysfunction of several vital organs and more vulnerable for complications.

21.8.1 Age-Related Changes in Vital Organ Systems

With normal aging, the functional metabolism of the brain and its blood supply declines. This accounts for the widespread clinical observations that the elderly tolerate disorders of the brain worse than the young do [84]. The decline in CBF may be secondary to the age-related increase in atherosclerosis, which results in increased cerebrovascular resistance, reduced elasticity and contractility of small arteries and arterioles [15], and the cerebral vasomotor reactivity declines [84].

The effects of aging in the cardiovascular system include a decrease in elasticity and reduced compliance of the vasculature, reduced responsiveness to beta-adrenergic receptor stimulation, decreased reactivity to baro- and chemoreceptors and an increase in circulating catecholamines. This leads to an increased afterload, increased systolic blood pressure and left ventricular hypertrophy [13]. Alpha-adrenergic effects on the vasculature predominate resulting in vasoconstriction, resting cardiac output declines, and cardiovascular performance under stress is reduced.

Age-related changes of the respiratory system include decreased total respiratory system (lung and chest wall) compliance and decline in arterial oxygenation, due to a decreased diffusion capacity caused by increased ventilation/perfusion mismatching and reduced alveolar surface area. Altogether, age-related alterations of the respiratory system cause a reduced pulmonary reserve rendering the elderly patient more susceptible to respiratory complications in situations of positive fluid balance, increased metabolic demands and prolonged bed rest during intensive care. Increased sensitivity to respiratory depressants and muscle weakness in the elderly further increase the risk of respiratory complications. Elderly patients have an increased risk of respiratory failure requiring mechanical ventilation after surgery and a higher risk of long-term ventilator dependency in intensive care [128].

Aging is accompanied by a decline in liver volume, but the clinical significance of this alteration is unclear, and liver function tests have not shown age-related deficits. The rate of liver regeneration after injury decreases, which may increase the rate of progression of hepatic dysfunction in the elderly [120].

The renal mass and the renal blood flow decrease with age. The loss of renal volume is attributed to a reduction in the number of functioning glomeruli accompanied by a reduction in the glomerular filtration rate, limitations in sodium conservation and potassium and acid excretion. Under normal conditions, most elderly individuals can maintain normal fluid and electrolyte homeostasis despite these changes. However, the reserve to withstand disease-related or iatrogenic stress becomes progressively smaller with age and may lead to disturbance in water and electrolyte homeostasis [6].

It is of utmost importance to consider all these age-related infirmities and balance the treatment according to the specific needs of the different vital organ systems in the elderly to achieve the best possible prerequisites for the vulnerable brain. Therefore, it is even more important for the elderly to be managed according to modern neurointensive care (NIC) principles.

21.8.2 Neurointensive Care of Elderly SAH Patients

Due to the seriousness of SAH and its high risk of fatal outcome due to the initial bleed and re-bleeding and subsequent complications, also elderly SAH patients need prompt treatment in NIC units with high level of expertise treating SAH patients [131].

The general goal of NIC is to prevent secondary ischaemic damage to the brain and thereby improve the overall clinical outcome. The aim is to control intracranial dynamics and to maintain normal body physiology. Special attention is paid to prevention, early diagnosis and intensive management of secondary insults contributing to secondary ischaemic brain damage. SAH patients who have survived the initial bleed in good clinical condition with little or no neurological impairment are still at risk for a devastating clinical course and poor outcome due to complications causing secondary brain injury. Parallels can be drawn to patients with traumatic brain injury (TBI) who talk and die [108], in whom potentially avoidable secondary complications were implicated in the development of secondary brain damage, clinical deterioration and death [108, 110]. In SAH the major causes for a "talk and die" scenario are re-bleeding from the ruptured aneurysm and cerebral vasospasm causing secondary cerebral ischaemia.

Elderly SAH patients should be admitted to a unit where continuous surveillance and intensive monitoring by experienced staff are feasible. Intensive monitoring of neurological condition, blood pressure, temperature, fluid and electrolyte balance and blood glucose levels should be undertaken. A ventricular drain should be inserted irrespective of age in all unconscious patients for ICP monitoring and CSF drainage if needed. Normovolaemia, normal electrolyte levels and ICP between 10 and 20 mmHg should be aimed for. Blood glucose levels > 10 mmol/l should be treated, and systolic blood pressure > 180 mmHg and pyrexia should be avoided [131].

21.8.3 Secondary Insults in Elderly SAH Patients

We (Ryttlefors et al. 2010) studied the occurrence of secondary complications during NIC in 99 severe SAH patients with special focus on 29 patients who were elderly over the age of 65. Seventy-six percent (22/29) of the elderly SAH patients were in poor neurological grade (Hunt and Hess IV–V) on admission, and all had massive

Table 21.7 Treatment goals and secondary insult definitions during NIC (Ryttlefors et al. [115])

Variable	Treatment goal	Insult	Severe insult
ICP (mmHg)	<15–20	≥20	≥25
CPP (mmHg)	>60 Individual	≤60 >100	≤55 >110
MAP (mmHg)	Individual Individual	≤80 >120	≤70 >130
BPs (mmHg)	Individual Individual	≤110 >180	≤100 >200
T° (°C)	<38	≥38	≥39
SpO_2 (%)	>95	<95	<90

ICP intracranial pressure, *CPP* cerebral perfusion pressure, *MAP* mean arterial pressure, *BPs* systolic blood pressure, *T°* body temperature, *SpO2* arterial oxygen saturation

subarachnoid clots on the diagnostic CT. Twenty-one patients were endovascularly treated, seven were treated with neurosurgical clipping of the aneurysm, and one patient did not receive any treatment for the ruptured aneurysm. All patients were closely monitored minute by minute for intracranial pressure, cerebral perfusion pressure, mean arterial pressure, systolic blood pressure, oxygen saturation and temperature. Deviations from predefined treatment goals of these parameters were considered a secondary complication (secondary insult) (Table 21.7). In the elderly patients, there was a lower occurrence of ICP insults, and there was a higher occurrence of hypertensive, as well as hypotensive and hypoxaemic insults compared to the younger patients. Functional outcome at 6 months post-SAH was favourable in 24 % of the elderly severe SAH patients and 43 % in the younger age group. The proportion of patients who were severely disabled did not differ substantially between the elderly and the younger age group. Our conclusion was that neurointensive care is justified also in elderly patients with severe SAH and that the occurrence of secondary insults is age dependent. Further studies should focus on providing insights on age-specific secondary insult levels necessary for creating a tailored neurointensive care specific for elderly patients with severe subarachnoid haemorrhage.

Schöller et al. reported rates of intensive care complications in 256 elderly SAH patients 60 years and older. The overall rate of intensive care complications was 38 %. These included cerebral (22 %), respiratory (11 %), renal (13 %), thrombosis (2 %), pulmonary embolism (1 %) and myocardial infarction (2 %). There was no substantial difference in the rate complications between age subgroups grouped by age decade 60–69, 70–79 or ≥80 years, except from a higher rate of myocardial infarction in the eldest age group [121].

21.8.4 Vasospasm in Elderly SAH Patients

The relationship between age and vasospasm after SAH has been an ongoing debate for decades and data is conflicting. In some previous studies, a reduced risk of radiological vasospasm with older age has been shown [5, 40, 45, 55, 62, 80, 99], but in other studies age had no effect on the rate of radiological vasospasm [32, 46]. Likewise the rate of clinical vasospasm or delayed ischaemic neurological deficits (DINDs) or delayed cerebral ischaemia (DCI) has been reported to decrease with age in some studies [12, 106, 121, 140], while in others the rate of DIND in the elderly patients was similar to that of younger patients [40, 46]. The reported lower incidence of vasospasm in older patients may be secondary to the age-related increase in atherosclerosis, which results in impairment of contractility and elasticity of the muscle wall of small arteries and arterioles [15, 84]. This seems to be a reasonable explanation for the lower risk of DIND in the elderly; however, data are conflicting. The definition of vasospasm and the method of proving vasospasm are not uniform in different studies. Also most previous reports are retrospective studies, which make interpretation difficult.

In a retrospective series of Artiola i Fortuny et al., the rate of generalized radiological vasospasm declined in patients ≥60 years [5]. Oka et al. demonstrated 23 % radiological vasospasm in patients ≥65 years compared to 44 % in patients <65 years [99]. In these early series, the effect of age on vasospasm was not controlled for other factors associated with vasospasm, such as clinical grade or severity of the SAH. Inagawa analysed the radiological vasospasm grade in three age groups: <60 years, 61–69 years and ≥70 years in relation to the severity of SAH. The radiological vasospasm grade declined with age, which was consistent in all subgroups [45]. In a later study by Inagawa, the grade of radiological vasospasm was analysed in patients <60 years compared to patients ≥60 years in relation to severity of the SAH and clinical grade. In that study strong correlation of the SAH grades to the radiological vasospasm grade and to the incidence of symptomatic vasospasm was found, but there were no significant differences between older and younger patients [46]. Jabbarli et al. showed that age under 50 was a predictor of severity of cerebral vasospasm both radiologically and on TCD findings [55].

The observed reduced risk of cerebral vasospasm with age in some earlier studies may be explained by imbalances in clinical grade and severity of SAH in the selection of patients in the older and younger age groups. In most series predominately elderly patients in good neurological grade were selected for treatment. The neurological grade is correlated to the amount of subarachnoid blood, which is a well-known predictor of cerebral vasospasm [25]. It is therefore important to control for other known factors predictive of cerebral vasospasm with multivariate analysis, to avoid confounding of the age effect on the risk for vasospasm.

In a retrospective study by Macdonald et al., the degree of radiological vasospasm was analysed using multiple regression with severity of radiological vasospasm as the dependent variable and preoperative angiographical arterial diameter ratio, clinical grade and age as independent variables. Increased age was associated with less radiological vasospasm [80]. In a study by Hoh et al., age over 50 years was negatively related to total vasospasm (combined transcranial Doppler (TCD) abnormalities, radiological vasospasm and symptomatic vasospasm), but not associated with symptomatic vasospasm alone, when other predictors for vasospasm were controlled for in multivariate logistic regression [40]. Rabb et al. analysed admission and treatment variables as to their relation to symptomatic vasospasm using multivariate logistic regression. Clinical grade, amount of SAH and younger age (less than 35 years) were found to be independent predictors of symptomatic vasospasm [106]. In a study by Charpentier et al., age >50 years was an independent factor associated with reduced risk of symptomatic vasospasm, when other predictors for symptomatic vasospasm were controlled for with multivariate logistic regression [12]. Kale et al. reported similar findings. In their retrospective study of 108 SAH patients, age>50 years was an independent factor associated with less risk of any vasospasm when other predictors for vasospasm was controlled for in multiple regression analysis [62]. Torbey et al. demonstrated that the rate of symptomatic vasospasm and TCD-defined vasospasm was significantly lower in patients ≥68 years than in patients <68 years, but no statistically significant difference between the age groups could be detected in the rate of radiological vasospasm [140].

In studies where TCD has been used for detection of vasospasm according to defined criteria [1, 33, 39], elderly patients have a lower rate of cerebral blood flow velocities (CBFV) indicative of vasospasm [8, 140]. The sensitivity of high CBFV for detecting vasospasm in elderly SAH patients was low when using the same criteria as in younger patients [8]. Symptomatic vasospasm occurred at lower CBFV in elderly patients necessitating an age-dependent CBFV limit for detecting vasospasm [140]. Reasons for lower CBFV in older individuals may be explained by the greater prevalence of atherosclerosis but also by age-dependent changes in the anatomical course of the MCA changing the insonation angle when performing the TCD measurements [71].

Thus, even when other predictive factors for vasospasm are controlled for with multivariate analyses, the effect of age on the risk for vasospasm is inconsistent. Differences in the used measure and definition of vasospasm and the used cut-off age for the elderly group in different studies complicate comparison and influence the interpretation.

We (Ryttlefors et al. 2010) investigated the independent effect of age on radiological vasospasm, DIND and TCD abnormalities in the same prospective cohort of patients [114]. Data from CONSCIOUS-1 (Clazosentan to Overcome Neurological Ischemia and Infarct Occurring After Subarachnoid Hemorrhage) study, a dose-finding study of clazosentan, were used. Patient age was considered in three ways: as a continuous variable, dichotomized at age 65 years and categorized by decade. Age was investigated as the main variable, whereas other possible confounding variables were adjusted for in the multiple logistic regression modelling with each of the three dichotomized vasospasm outcome measures, the presence or absence of angiographic vasospasm, DINDs and TCD abnormalities as the dependent variables. The outcome measures, radiological vasospasm, DIND and TCD abnormalities were clearly defined in the protocol, and data was meticulously recorded prospectively. The proportions of patients with angiographic vasospasm, DINDs and TCD abnormalities were 45 %, 19 % and 81 %, respectively. Age, whether considered as a continuous, dichotomous or a categorical variable, was not significantly associated with angiographic vasospasm, DINDs or abnormal TCD measurements [114].

Further well-designed prospective studies with predefined criteria for vasospasm and with a significant number of patients must be conducted in the future to resolve the issue whether elderly patients do in fact have a less risk of symptomatic vasospasm or if this observation is merely a question of patient selection bias.

Regarding prevention and treatment of vasospasm, elderly SAH patients should be managed similar to SAH patients of all ages. The only treatment with proven benefit across several randomized controlled trials is the routine use of orally administered nimodipine [143]. Other treatments, such as triple-H therapy, fasudil, transluminal balloon angioplasty, thrombolytics, endothelin receptor antagonists, magnesium, statins and miscellaneous therapies such as free radical scavengers and antifibrinolytics, require additional study [143]. Hypertension-, hypervolaemia- and haemodilution-therapy (triple-H-therapy) are intended to improve cerebral haemodynamic flow by expanding intravascular volume and decreasing blood viscosity but have inherited risks of complications that may be dismal, including cardiopulmonary failure, renal dysfunction and exacerbation of cerebral oedema. Due to the age-related decline in most extracranial organ functions including cardiac, respiratory, renal function and muscle mass, elderly are at a greater risk of developing complications in these organ systems and have a lesser capacity to tolerate complications than younger patients. Triple-H-therapy should therefore be used judiciously in elderly SAH patients.

21.9 Concluding Remarks and Summary

Subarachnoid haemorrhage in the elderly is a serious life-threatening disease that needs prompt and resolute treatment in centres with high level of expertise treating this condition.

Elderly patients with SAH have a higher risk of an unfavourable clinical outcome than younger patients. Reasons for worse outcome are thought to be caused by less active management and conservative referral patterns, poorer clinical grades on admission, larger amount of subarachnoid clot, higher incidence of intraventricular haemorrhage and hydrocephalus on the admission CT scans, higher frequency of co-morbidity and increased incidence of severe complications. Higher age per se is however also a negative prognostic factor, suggesting that the aging brain has less optimal response to the initial bleeding.

Over time the management outcome for elderly SAH patients has improved, more patients achieving an independent outcome, and case fatality rates have declined.

Elderly SAH patients in good to moderate neurological grade on admission and without serious pre-existing illnesses can be successfully treated for the ruptured aneurysm and vigorously managed in neurointensive care units to detect and avoid complications of the disease, and up to 80 % of these patients have a good functional outcome. Nowadays there seems to be no controversy about treating elderly patients up to the age of 75–80 years if patients are awake and without focal neurological deficits after the initial haemorrhage. Even some selected patients older than 80 years may be treated successfully.

The prognosis is much worse for unconscious elderly SAH patients (Hunt and Hess IV, WFNS IV), but up to one quarter of these patients had a good functional outcome after early aneurysm treatment and intensive care treatment in our study, which can warrant active treatment also in these patients.

Elderly patients in poor neurological grade (Hunt and Hess V, WFNS V) have a very poor prognosis regardless of treatment and should probably receive comfort care only.

The choice of neurosurgical or endovascular aneurysm treatment in elderly SAH patients should be made on case-by-case basis by a neurovascular team with expertise both in endovascular and neurosurgical aneurysm treatment. Factors influencing this decision are the patients' neurological grade, extent of the SAH, the presence of intracerebral haematoma, aneurysm location and aneurysm geometry.

The introduction of endovascular aneurysm treatment has made early aneurysm treatment also for poor-grade elderly SAH patients feasible. This has likely improved the overall treatment outcomes of elderly SAH patients by reducing the incidence of re-bleeding and allowing aggressive neurointensive care management for prevention and treatment of complications of the SAH such as symptomatic vasospasm.

Although still a matter of debate and discrepancy between different studies, there is no compelling evidence that the rate of vasospasm is lower in the elderly SAH patients than in the younger when other factors leading to vasospasm are controlled for.

Elderly SAH patients seem to tolerate neurointensive care well. Therefore, neurointensive care of elderly SAH patients with severe SAH is justified. Elderly SAH patients exhibit age-dependent patterns of treatable secondary insults during neurointensive care. In elderly SAH patients, age-specific adjustments in the treatment goals for physiological parameters are warranted for tailoring neurointensive care specifically for the elderly patients.

References

1. Aaslid R, Huber P, Nornes H (1984) Evaluation of cerebrovascular spasm with transcranial Doppler ultrasound. J Neurosurg 60(1):37–41
2. Adamson J, Humphries SE, Ostergaard JR, Voldby B, Richards P, Powell JT (1994) Are cerebral aneurysms atherosclerotic? Stroke 25(5):963–966
3. Agazzi S, de Tribolet N, Uske A, Regli L (2004) Quality of life after aneurysmal subarachnoid hemorrhage in the elderly. Cerebrovasc Dis 18(2):174–175. doi:10.1159/000079738
4. Amacher AL, Ferguson GG, Drake CG, Girvin JP, Barr HW (1977) How old people tolerate intracranial surgery for aneurysm. Neurosurgery 1(3):242–244
5. Artiola i Fortuny L, Prieto-Valiente L (1981) Long-term prognosis in surgically treated intracranial aneurysms. Part 1: Mortality. J Neurosurg 54(1):26–34
6. Beck LH (1998) Changes in renal function with aging. Clin Geriatr Med 14(2):199–209
7. Birchall D, Khangure M, McAuliffe W, Apsimon H, Knuckey N (2001) Endovascular management of acute subarachnoid haemorrhage in the elderly. Br J Neurosurg 15(1):35–38
8. Boecher-Schwarz HG, Ungersboeck K, Ulrich P, Fries G, Wild A, Perneczky A (1994) Transcranial Doppler diagnosis of cerebral vasospasm following subarachnoid haemorrhage: correlation and analysis of results in relation to the age of patients. Acta Neurochir (Wien) 127(1–2):32–36
9. Bonita R (1986) Cigarette smoking, hypertension and the risk of subarachnoid hemorrhage: a population-based case–control study. Stroke 17(5):831–835
10. Bradac GB, Bergui M, Fontanella M (2005) Endovascular treatment of cerebral aneurysms in elderly patients. Neuroradiology 47(12):938–941

11. Cai Y, Spelle L, Wang H, Piotin M, Mounayer C, Vanzin JR, Moret J (2005) Endovascular treatment of intracranial aneurysms in the elderly: single-center experience in 63 consecutive patients. Neurosurgery 57(6):1096–1102; discussion 1096–1102
12. Charpentier C, Audibert G, Guillemin F, Civit T, Ducrocq X, Bracard S, Hepner H, Picard L, Laxenaire MC (1999) Multivariate analysis of predictors of cerebral vasospasm occurrence after aneurysmal subarachnoid hemorrhage. Stroke 30(7):1402–1408
13. Cheitlin MD (2003) Cardiovascular physiology-changes with aging. Am J Geriatr Cardiol 12(1):9–13
14. Chung RY, Carter BS, Norbash A, Budzik R, Putnam C, Ogilvy CS (2000) Management outcomes for ruptured and unruptured aneurysms in the elderly. Neurosurgery 47(4):827–832; discussion 832–832
15. Claus JJ, Breteler MM, Hasan D, Krenning EP, Bots ML, Grobbee DE, Van Swieten JC, Van Harskamp F, Hofman A (1998) Regional cerebral blood flow and cerebrovascular risk factors in the elderly population. Neurobiol Aging 19(1):57–64
16. Dawkins AA, Evans AL, Wattam J, Romanowski CA, Connolly DJ, Hodgson TJ, Coley SC (2007) Complications of cerebral angiography: a prospective analysis of 2,924 consecutive procedures. Neuroradiology 49:753–759
17. de Rooij NK, Linn FH, van der Plas JA, Algra A, Rinkel GJ (2007) Incidence of subarachnoid haemorrhage: a systematic review with emphasis on region, age, gender and time trends. J Neurol Neurosurg Psychiatry 78:1365–1372
18. Deruty R, Pelissou-Guyotat I, Mottolese C, Amat D, Bognar L (1995) Level of consciousness and age as prognostic factors in aneurysmal SAH. Acta Neurochir (Wien) 132(1–3):1–8
19. Drake C (1988) Report of World Federation of Neurological Surgeons Committee on a universal subarachnoid hemorrhage grading scale. J Neurosurg 68:985–986
20. Ellenbogen BK (1970) Subarachnoid haemorrhage in the elderly. Gerontol Clin (Basel) 12(2):115–120
21. Elliott JP, Le Roux PD (1998) Subarachnoid hemorrhage and cerebral aneurysms in the elderly. Neurosurg Clin N Am 9(3):587–594
22. Etminan N, Buchholz BA, Dreier R, Bruckner P, Torner JC, Steiger HJ, Hanggi D, Macdonald RL (2014) Cerebral aneurysms: formation, progression, and developmental chronology. Transl Stroke Res 5(2):167–173. doi:10.1007/s12975-013-0294-x
23. Feigin VL, Rinkel GJ, Lawes CM, Algra A, Bennett DA, van Gijn J, Anderson CS (2005) Risk factors for subarachnoid hemorrhage: an updated systematic review of epidemiological studies. Stroke 36(12):2773–2780
24. Ferch R, Pasqualin A, Barone G, Pinna G, Bricolo A (2003) Surgical management of ruptured aneurysms in the eighth and ninth decades. Acta Neurochir (Wien) 145(6):439–445. doi:10.1007/s00701-003-0037-y; discussion 445
25. Fisher CM, Kistler JP, Davis JM (1980) Relation of cerebral vasospasm to subarachnoid hemorrhage visualized by computerized tomographic scanning. Neurosurgery 6(1):1–9
26. Forbus WD (1930) On the formation of miliary aneurysms of the superficial cerebral arteries. Bull Johns Hopkins Hosp 47:239–284
27. Fortuny LA, Adams CB, Briggs M (1980) Surgical mortality in an aneurysm population: effects of age, blood pressure and preoperative neurological state. J Neurol Neurosurg Psychiatry 43(10):879–882
28. Frankel JE, Marwitz JH, Cifu DX, Kreutzer JS, Englander J, Rosenthal M (2006) A follow-up study of older adults with traumatic brain injury: taking into account decreasing length of stay. Arch Phys Med Rehabil 87(1):57–62. doi:10.1016/j.apmr.2005.07.309
29. Fridriksson SM, Hillman J, Saveland H, Brandt L (1995) Intracranial aneurysm surgery in the 8th and 9th decades of life: impact on population-based management outcome. Neurosurgery 37(4):627–631; discussion 631–632
30. Gizewski ER, Goricke S, Wolf A, Schoch B, Stolke D, Forsting M, Wanke I (2008) Endovascular treatment of intracranial aneurysms in patients 65 years or older: clinical outcomes. AJNR Am J Neuroradiol 29(8):1575–1580. doi:10.3174/ajnr.A1165

31. Glynn LE (1940) Medial defects in the circle of Willis and their relation to aneurysm formation. J Path Bacteriol 51:213–222
32. Graf CJ, Nibbelink DW (1974) Cooperative study of intracranial aneurysms and subarachnoid hemorrhage. Report on a randomized treatment study. 3. Intracranial surgery. Stroke 5(4):557–601
33. Grolimund P, Seiler RW, Aaslid R, Huber P, Zurbruegg H (1987) Evaluation of cerebrovascular disease by combined extracranial and transcranial Doppler sonography. Experience in 1,039 patients. Stroke 18(6):1018–1024
34. Gu DQ, Zhang X, Luo B, Long XA, Duan CZ (2012) Impact of ultra-early coiling on clinical outcome after aneurysmal subarachnoid hemorrhage in elderly patients. Acad Radiol 19(1):3–7. doi:10.1016/j.acra.2011.09.012
35. Guglielmi G, Vinuela F, Dion J, Duckwiler G (1991) Electrothrombosis of saccular aneurysms via endovascular approach. Part 2: Preliminary clinical experience. J Neurosurg 75(1):8–14
36. Guglielmi G, Vinuela F, Sepetka I, Macellari V (1991) Electrothrombosis of saccular aneurysms via endovascular approach. Part 1: Electrochemical basis, technique, and experimental results. J Neurosurg 75(1):1–7
37. Gull W (1859) Cases of aneurism of the cerebral vessels. Guy's Hosp Rep 5:281–304
38. Hamada J, Hasegawa S, Kai Y, Morioka M, Fujioka S, Ushio Y (1999) Surgery and long-term outcome for ruptured anterior circulation aneurysms in patients in their ninth decade of life. Surg Neurol 52(2):123–126; discussion 126–127
39. Harders AG, Gilsbach JM (1987) Time course of blood velocity changes related to vasospasm in the circle of Willis measured by transcranial Doppler ultrasound. J Neurosurg 66(5):718–728
40. Hoh BL, Topcuoglu MA, Singhal AB, Pryor JC, Rabinov JD, Rordorf GA, Carter BS, Ogilvy CS (2004) Effect of clipping, craniotomy, or intravascular coiling on cerebral vasospasm and patient outcome after aneurysmal subarachnoid hemorrhage. Neurosurgery 55(4):779–786; discussion 786–789
41. Hop JW, Rinkel GJ, Algra A, van Gijn J (1997) Case-fatality rates and functional outcome after subarachnoid hemorrhage: a systematic review. Stroke 28(3):660–664
42. Horiuchi T, Tanaka Y, Hongo K (2005) Surgical treatment for aneurysmal subarachnoid hemorrhage in the 8th and 9th decades of life. Neurosurgery 56(3):469–475; discussion 469–475
43. Hugosson R (1973) Intracranial arterial aneurysms. Considerations on the upper age limit for surgical treatment. Acta Neurochir (Wien) 28(3):157–164
44. Hunt WE, Hess RM (1968) Surgical risk as related to time of intervention in the repair of intracranial aneurysms. J Neurosurg 28(1):14–20
45. Inagawa T (1991) Cerebral vasospasm in elderly patients with ruptured intracranial aneurysms. Surg Neurol 36(2):91–98
46. Inagawa T (1992) Cerebral vasospasm in elderly patients treated by early operation for ruptured intracranial aneurysms. Acta Neurochir (Wien) 115(3–4):79–85
47. Inagawa T (1993) Management outcome in the elderly patient following subarachnoid hemorrhage. J Neurosurg 78(4):554–561
48. Inagawa T (2005) Trends in surgical and management outcomes in patients with aneurysmal subarachnoid hemorrhage in Izumo city, Japan, between 1980–1989 and 1990–1998. Cerebrovasc Dis 19(1):39–48. doi:10.1159/000081910
49. Inagawa T, Hirano A (1990) Autopsy study of unruptured incidental intracranial aneurysms. Surg Neurol 34(6):361–365
50. Inagawa T, Yamamoto M, Kamiya K, Ogasawara H (1988) Management of elderly patients with aneurysmal subarachnoid hemorrhage. J Neurosurg 69(3):332–339
51. Inci S, Spetzler RF (2000) Intracranial aneurysms and arterial hypertension: a review and hypothesis. Surg Neurol 53(6):530–540; discussion 540–542
52. Ingall TJ, Whisnant JP, Wiebers DO, O'Fallon WM (1989) Has there been a decline in subarachnoid hemorrhage mortality? Stroke 20(6):718–724

53. Isaksen J, Egge A, Waterloo K, Romner B, Ingebrigtsen T (2002) Risk factors for aneurysmal subarachnoid haemorrhage: the Tromso study. J Neurol Neurosurg Psychiatry 73(2):185–187
54. Iwamoto H, Kiyohara Y, Fujishima M, Kato I, Nakayama K, Sueishi K, Tsuneyoshi M (1999) Prevalence of intracranial saccular aneurysms in a Japanese community based on a consecutive autopsy series during a 30-year observation period. The Hisayama study. Stroke 30(7):1390–1395
55. Jabbarli R, Glasker S, Weber J, Taschner C, Olschewski M, Van Velthoven V (2013) Predictors of severity of cerebral vasospasm caused by aneurysmal subarachnoid hemorrhage. J Stroke Cerebrovasc Dis 22(8):1332–1339. doi:10.1016/j.jstrokecerebrovasdis.2013.01.006
56. Jain R, Deveikis J, Thompson BG (2004) Endovascular management of poor-grade aneurysmal subarachnoid hemorrhage in the geriatric population. AJNR Am J Neuroradiol 25(4):596–600
57. Jennett B, Bond M (1975) Assessment of outcome after severe brain damage. Lancet 1(7905):480–484
58. Johansson M, Cesarini KG, Contant CF, Persson L, Enblad P (2001) Changes in intervention and outcome in elderly patients with subarachnoid hemorrhage. Stroke 32(12):2845–2849
59. Johansson M, Norback O, Gal G, Cesarini KG, Tovi M, Solander S, Contant CF, Ronne-Engstrom E, Enblad P (2004) Clinical outcome after endovascular coil embolization in elderly patients with subarachnoid hemorrhage. Neuroradiology 46(5):385–391
60. Jomin M, Lesoin F, Lozes G (1984) Prognosis with 500 ruptured and operated intracranial arterial aneurysms. Surg Neurol 21(1):13–18
61. Juvela S, Hillbom M, Numminen H, Koskinen P (1993) Cigarette smoking and alcohol consumption as risk factors for aneurysmal subarachnoid hemorrhage. Stroke 24(5):639–646
62. Kale SP, Edgell RC, Alshekhlee A, Borhani Haghighi A, Sweeny J, Felton J, Kitchener J, Vora N, Bieneman BK, Cruz-Flores S, Abdulrauf S (2013) Age-associated vasospasm in aneurysmal subarachnoid hemorrhage. J Stroke Cerebrovasc Dis 22(1):22–27. doi:10.1016/j.jstrokecerebrovasdis.2011.05.024
63. Kaminogo M, Yonekura M (2002) Trends in subarachnoid haemorrhage in elderly persons from Nagasaki, Japan: analysis of the Nagasaki SAH Data Bank for cerebral aneurysm, 1989–1998. Acta Neurochir (Wien) 144(11):1133–1138; discussion 1138–1139
64. Kassell NF, Torner JC, Haley EC Jr, Jane JA, Adams HP, Kongable GL (1990) The International Cooperative Study on the Timing of Aneurysm Surgery. Part 1: Overall management results. J Neurosurg 73(1):18–36
65. Kassell NF, Torner JC, Jane JA, Haley EC Jr, Adams HP (1990) The International Cooperative Study on the Timing of Aneurysm Surgery. Part 2: Surgical results. J Neurosurg 73(1):37–47
66. Kaufmann TJ, Huston J 3rd, Mandrekar JN, Schleck CD, Thielen KR, Kallmes DF (2007) Complications of diagnostic cerebral angiography: evaluation of 19,826 consecutive patients. Radiology 243(3):812–819
67. Keller AZ (1970) Hypertension, age and residence in the survival with subarachnoid hemorrhage. Am J Epidemiol 91(2):139–147
68. Knekt P, Reunanen A, Aho K, Heliovaara M, Rissanen A, Aromaa A, Impivaara O (1991) Risk factors for subarachnoid hemorrhage in a longitudinal population study. J Clin Epidemiol 44(9):933–939
69. Koffijberg H, Buskens E, Granath F, Adami J, Ekbom A, Rinkel GJ, Blomqvist P (2008) Subarachnoid haemorrhage in Sweden 1987–2002: regional incidence and case fatality rates. J Neurol Neurosurg Psychiatry 79(3):294–299
70. Koivisto T, Vanninen R, Hurskainen H, Saari T, Hernesniemi J, Vapalahti M (2000) Outcomes of early endovascular versus surgical treatment of ruptured cerebral aneurysms. A prospective randomized study. Stroke 31(10):2369–2377
71. Krejza J, Mariak Z, Lewko J (2003) Standardization of flow velocities with respect to age and sex improves the accuracy of transcranial color Doppler sonography of middle cerebral artery spasm. AJR Am J Roentgenol 181(1):245–252

72. Laidlaw JD, Siu KH (2002) Aggressive surgical treatment of elderly patients following subarachnoid haemorrhage: management outcome results. J Clin Neurosci 9(4):404–410
73. Lan Q, Ikeda H, Jimbo H, Izumiyama H, Matsumoto K (2000) Considerations on surgical treatment for elderly patients with intracranial aneurysms. Surg Neurol 53(3):231–238
74. Lanzino G, Kassell NF, Germanson TP, Kongable GL, Truskowski LL, Torner JC, Jane JA (1996) Age and outcome after aneurysmal subarachnoid hemorrhage: why do older patients fare worse? J Neurosurg 85(3):410–418
75. Ljunggren B, Saveland H, Brandt L, Zygmunt S (1985) Early operation and overall outcome in aneurysmal subarachnoid hemorrhage. J Neurosurg 62(4):547–551
76. Locksley HB (1966) Natural history of subarachnoid hemorrhage, intracranial aneurysms and arteriovenous malformations. J Neurosurg 25(3):321–368
77. Longstreth WT Jr, Nelson LM, Koepsell TD, van Belle G (1992) Cigarette smoking, alcohol use, and subarachnoid hemorrhage. Stroke 23(9):1242–1249
78. Lubicz B, Leclerc X, Gauvrit JY, Lejeune JP, Pruvo JP (2004) Endovascular treatment of ruptured intracranial aneurysms in elderly people. AJNR Am J Neuroradiol 25(4):592–595
79. Luo CB, Teng MM, Chang FC, Chang CY (2007) Endovascular embolization of ruptured cerebral aneurysms in patients older than 70 years. J Clin Neurosci 14(2):127–132. doi:10.1016/j.jocn.2006.05.018
80. Macdonald RL, Wallace MC, Coyne TJ (1994) The effect of surgery on the severity of vasospasm. J Neurosurg 80(3):433–439
81. Martindale BV, Garfield J (1978) Subarachnoid haemorrhage above the age of 59: are intracranial investigations justified? Br Med J 1(6111):465–466
82. McDougall CG, Spetzler RF, Zabramski JM, Partovi S, Hills NK, Nakaji P, Albuquerque FC (2012) The Barrow Ruptured Aneurysm Trial. J Neurosurg 116(1):135–144. doi:10.3171/2011.8.JNS101767
83. McKissock W, Paine KWE, Walsh LS (1960) An Analysis of the Results of Treatment of Ruptured Intracranial Aneurysms Report of 772 Consecutive Cases. J Neurosurg 17(4):762–776
84. Meyer JS, Terayama Y, Takashima S (1993) Cerebral circulation in the elderly. Cerebrovasc Brain Metab Rev 5(2):122–146
85. Mino Y, Hirashima Y, Hamada H, Masuoka T, Yamatani K, Takeda S, Masuda R, Nogami K, Endo S (2006) Effect of arachnoid plasty using fibrin glue membrane after clipping of ruptured aneurysm on the occurrence of complications and outcome in the elderly patients. Acta Neurochir (Wien) 148(6):627–631. doi:10.1007/s00701-006-0777-6; discussion 631
86. Molyneux A, Kerr R, Stratton I, Sandercock P, Clarke M, Shrimpton J, Holman R (2002) International Subarachnoid Aneurysm Trial (ISAT) of neurosurgical clipping versus endovascular coiling in 2143 patients with ruptured intracranial aneurysms: a randomised trial. Lancet 360(9342):1267–1274
87. Molyneux AJ, Kerr RS, Birks J, Ramzi N, Yarnold J, Sneade M, Rischmiller J, Collaborators I (2009) Risk of recurrent subarachnoid haemorrhage, death, or dependence and standardised mortality ratios after clipping or coiling of an intracranial aneurysm in the International Subarachnoid Aneurysm Trial (ISAT): long-term follow-up. Lancet Neurol 8(5):427–433. doi:10.1016/S1474-4422(09)70080-8
88. Molyneux AJ, Kerr RS, Yu LM, Clarke M, Sneade M, Yarnold JA, Sandercock P, International Subarachnoid Aneurysm Trial Collaborative G (2005) International subarachnoid aneurysm trial (ISAT) of neurosurgical clipping versus endovascular coiling in 2143 patients with ruptured intracranial aneurysms: a randomised comparison of effects on survival, dependency, seizures, rebleeding, subgroups, and aneurysm occlusion. Lancet 366(9488):809–817. doi:10.1016/S0140-6736(05)67214-5
89. Mori T, Mori K, Kurisaka M, Morimoto M (1997) Survival probability, delayed mortality, and relationship between short-term outcome and long-term survival after aneurysmal subarachnoid hemorrhage. Neurol Med Chir (Tokyo) 37(1):18–24
90. Morioka T, Miyazaki H, Tsuruta K (1980) Problems in neurosurgical operations on elderly patients-from the viewpoint of anesthesiology. Neurol Med Chir (Tokyo) 20(7):713–720

91. Mozaffarian D, Benjamin EJ, Go AS, Arnett DK, Blaha MJ, Cushman M, Das SR, de Ferranti S, Despres JP, Fullerton HJ, Howard VJ, Huffman MD, Isasi CR, Jimenez MC, Judd SE, Kissela BM, Lichtman JH, Lisabeth LD, Liu S, Mackey RH, Magid DJ, McGuire DK, Mohler ER 3rd, Moy CS, Muntner P, Mussolino ME, Nasir K, Neumar RW, Nichol G, Palaniappan L, Pandey DK, Reeves MJ, Rodriguez CJ, Rosamond W, Sorlie PD, Stein J, Towfighi A, Turan TN, Virani SS, Woo D, Yeh RW, Turner MB, American Heart Association Statistics C, Stroke Statistics S (2016) Heart Disease and Stroke Statistics-2016 Update: a report from the american heart association. Circulation 133(4):e38–e360
92. Nieuwkamp DJ, Rinkel GJE, Silva R, Greebe P, Schokking DA, Ferro JM (2006) Subarachnoid haemorrhage in patients>=75 years: clinical course, treatment and outcome. J Neurol Neurosurg Psychiatry 77(8):933–937
93. Niskanen MM, Hernesniemi JA, Vapalahti MP, Kari A (1993) One-year outcome in early aneurysm surgery: prediction of outcome. Acta Neurochir (Wien) 123(1–2):25–32
94. Nukui H, Sasaki H, Kaneko M, Mitsuka S, Shibasaki T, Ohe C, Kohno N, Tsunoda T (1985) Surgical treatment in patients over 60 years of age with ruptured cerebral aneurysms. Neurol Med Chir (Tokyo) 25(4):275–281
95. Numminen H, Kotila M, Waltimo O, Aho K, Kaste M (1996) Declining incidence and mortality rates of stroke in Finland from 1972 to 1991, Results of three population-based stroke registers. Stroke 27(9):1487–1491
96. Nwankwo T, Yoon SS, Burt V, Gu Q (2013) Hypertension among adults in the United States: National Health and Nutrition Examination Survey, 2011–2012. NCHS Data Brief 133:1–8
97. O'Sullivan MG, Dorward N, Whittle IR, Steers AJ, Miller JD (1994) Management and long-term outcome following subarachnoid haemorrhage and intracranial aneurysm surgery in elderly patients: an audit of 199 consecutive cases. Br J Neurosurg 8(1):23–30
98. Ohmoto T, Mino S, Nishimoto A, Higashi T, Miyake S, Doi A (1980) Operative results of ruptured intracranial aneurysms in aged patients. Neurol Med Chir (Tokyo) 20(7):721–728
99. Oka K, Kuromatsu C, Takaki T, Maeyama R, Fukui M, Kitamura K (1987) Therapeutic problems in aged patients with intracranial aneurysms. No Shinkei Geka 15(4):375–379
100. Osawa M, Hongo K, Tanaka Y, Nakamura Y, Kitazawa K, Kobayashi S (2001) Results of direct surgery for aneurysmal subarachnoid haemorrhage: outcome of 2055 patients who underwent direct aneurysm surgery and profile of ruptured intracranial aneurysms. Acta Neurochir (Wien) 143(7):655–663; discussion 663–664
101. Pakarinen S (1967) Incidence, aetiology, and prognosis of primary subarachnoid haemorrhage. A study based on 589 cases diagnosed in a defined urban population during a defined period. Acta Neurol Scand 43(Suppl 29):1–128
102. Persson G, Bostrom G, Allebeck P, Andersson L, Berg S, Johansson L, Thille A (2001) Chapter 5. Elderly people's health--65 and after. Health in Sweden: The National Public Health Report 2001. Scand J Public Health Suppl 58:117–131
103. Petitti DB, Wingerd J (1978) Use of oral contraceptives, cigarette smoking, and risk of subarachnoid haemorrhage. Lancet 2(8083):234–235
104. Pinsker MO, Gerstner W, Wolf S, Trost HA, Lumenta CB (2002) Surgery and outcome for aneurysmal subarachnoid hemorrhage in elderly patients. Acta Neurochir Suppl 82:61–64
105. Pool JL, Potts DG (1965) Aneurysms and arteriovenous anomalies of the brain. Harper and Row Publ, New York
106. Rabb CH, Tang G, Chin LS, Giannotta SL (1994) A statistical analysis of factors related to symptomatic cerebral vasospasm. Acta Neurochir (Wien) 127(1–2):27–31
107. Rankin J (1957) Cerebral vascular accidents in patients over the age of 60. II Prognosis. Scott Med J 2(5):200–215
108. Reilly PL, Graham DI, Adams JH, Jennett B (1975) Patients with head injury who talk and die. Lancet 2(7931):375–377
109. Rinkel GJ, Djibuti M, Algra A, van Gijn J (1998) Prevalence and risk of rupture of intracranial aneurysms: a systematic review. Stroke 29(1):251–256
110. Rose J, Valtonen S, Jennett B (1977) Avoidable factors contributing to death after head injury. Br Med J 2(6087):615–618

111. Rosenorn J, Eskesen V, Schmidt K (1987) Age as a prognostic factor after intracranial aneurysm rupture. Br J Neurosurg 1(3):335–341
112. Rowe JG, Molyneux AJ, Byrne JV, Renowden S, Aziz TZ (1996) Endovascular treatment of intracranial aneurysms: a minimally invasive approach with advantages for elderly patients. Age Ageing 25(5):372–376
113. Ryttlefors M, Enblad P, Kerr RS, Molyneux AJ (2008) International Subarachnoid Aneurysm Trial of Neurosurgical Clipping Versus Endovascular Coiling. Subgroup Analysis of 278 Elderly Patients. Stroke 39:2720–2726
114. Ryttlefors M, Enblad P, Ronne-Engstrom E, Persson L, Ilodigwe D, Macdonald RL (2010) Patient age and vasospasm after subarachnoid hemorrhage. Neurosurgery 67(4):911–917. doi:10.1227/NEU.0b013e3181ed11ab00006123-201010000-00018[pii]
115. Ryttlefors M, Howells T, Ronne-Engstrom E, Nilsson P, Enblad P (2010) Neurointensive care is justified in elderly patients with severe subarachnoid hemorrhage--an outcome and secondary insults study. Acta Neurochir (Wien) 152(2):241–249. doi:10.1007/s00701-009-0496-x; discussion 249
116. Sacco RL, Wolf PA, Bharucha NE, Meeks SL, Kannel WB, Charette LJ, McNamara PM, Palmer EP, D'Agostino R (1984) Subarachnoid and intracerebral hemorrhage: natural history, prognosis, and precursive factors in the Framingham Study. Neurology 34(7): 847–854
117. Sakaki S, Ohta S, Ohue S, Kohno K, Matsuoka K (1989) Outcome in elderly patients with ruptured intracranial aneurysm. Clin Neurol Neurosurg 91(1):21–27
118. Sawada M, Kaku Y, Hayashi K, Ueda T, Yoshimura S, Sakai N (2000) Endovascular Treatment of Ruptured Intracranial Aneurysms using Platinum Coils in Patients over 70 Years of Age. Interv Neuroradiol 6(Suppl 1):85–87
119. Schievink WI, Wijdicks EF, Parisi JE, Piepgras DG, Whisnant JP (1995) Sudden death from aneurysmal subarachnoid hemorrhage. Neurology 45(5):871–874
120. Schmucker DL (2005) Age-related changes in liver structure and function: Implications for disease? Exp Gerontol 40(8–9):650–659
121. Scholler K, Massmann M, Markl G, Kunz M, Fesl G, Bruckmann H, Pfefferkorn T, Tonn JC, Schichor C (2013) Aneurysmal subarachnoid hemorrhage in elderly patients: long-term outcome and prognostic factors in an interdisciplinary treatment approach. J Neurol 260(4):1052–1060. doi:10.1007/s00415-012-6758-1
122. Sedat J, Dib M, Lonjon M, Litrico S, Von Langsdorf D, Fontaine D, Paquis P (2002) Endovascular treatment of ruptured intracranial aneurysms in patients aged 65 years and older: follow-up of 52 patients after 1 year. Stroke 33(11):2620–2625
123. Sengupta RP, Lassman LP, Hankinson J (1978) Scope of surgery for intracranial aneurysm in the elderly: a preliminary report. Br Med J 2(6132):246–247
124. Skultety FM, Nishioka H (1966) Report on the cooperative study of intracranial aneurysms and subarachnoid hemorrhage. Section VII. Part 2. The Results of Intracranial Surgery in the Treatment of Aneurysms. J Neurosurg 25(6):683–704
125. Smith MJ, Sanborn MR, Lewis DJ, Faught RW, Vakhshori V, Stein SC (2015) Elderly patients with intracranial aneurysms have higher quality of life after coil embolization: a decision analysis. J Neurointerv Surg 7(12):898–904. doi:10.1136/neurintsurg-2014-011394
126. Spetzler RF, McDougall CG, Albuquerque FC, Zabramski JM, Hills NK, Partovi S, Nakaji P, Wallace RC (2013) The Barrow Ruptured Aneurysm Trial: 3-year results. J Neurosurg 119(1):146–157. doi:10.3171/2013.3.JNS12683
127. Spetzler RF, McDougall CG, Zabramski JM, Albuquerque FC, Hills NK, Russin JJ, Partovi S, Nakaji P, Wallace RC (2015) The Barrow Ruptured Aneurysm Trial: 6-year results. J Neurosurg 123(3):609–617. doi:10.3171/2014.9.JNS141749
128. Sprung J, Gajic O, Warner DO (2006) Review article: Age related alterations in respiratory function - anesthetic considerations. Can J Anaesth 53(12):1244–1257
129. Stachniak JB, Layon AJ, Day AL, Gallagher TJ (1996) Craniotomy for intracranial aneurysm and subarachnoid hemorrhage. Is course, cost, or outcome affected by age? Stroke 27(2):276–281
130. Stehbens WE (1989) Etiology of intracranial berry aneurysms. J Neurosurg 70(6):823–831

131. Steiner T, Juvela S, Unterberg A, Jung C, Forsting M, Rinkel G, European Stroke O (2013) European Stroke Organization guidelines for the management of intracranial aneurysms and subarachnoid haemorrhage. Cerebrovasc Dis 35(2):93–112. doi:10.1159/000346087
132. Stevens RD, Nyquist PA (2007) The systemic implications of aneurysmal subarachnoid hemorrhage. J Neurol Sci 261(1–2):143–156
133. Suzuki A, Yasui N, Hadeishi H, Mizuno M, Abumiya T, Sampei T, Nakajima S (1990) Early surgery in elderly patients with ruptured intracranial aneurysms--preoperative clinical evaluation and prognosis. Neurol Med Chir (Tokyo) 30(2):95–99
134. Takagi K, Tamura A, Nakagomi T, Nakayama H, Gotoh O, Kawai K, Taneda M, Yasui N, Hadeishi H, Sano K (1999) How should a subarachnoid hemorrhage grading scale be determined? A combinatorial approach based solely on the Glasgow Coma Scale. J Neurosurg 90(4):680–687. doi:10.3171/jns.1999.90.4.0680
135. Taylor CL, Yuan Z, Selman WR, Ratcheson RA, Rimm AA (1995) Cerebral arterial aneurysm formation and rupture in 20,767 elderly patients: hypertension and other risk factors. J Neurosurg 83(5):812–819
136. Teasdale G, Jennett B (1974) Assessment of coma and impaired consciousness. A practical scale. Lancet 2(7872):81–84
137. Teasdale GM, Drake CG, Hunt W, Kassell N, Sano K, Pertuiset B, De Villiers JC (1988) A universal subarachnoid hemorrhage scale: report of a committee of the World Federation of Neurosurgical Societies. J Neurol Neurosurg Psychiatry 51(11):1457
138. Teasdale GM, Pettigrew LE, Wilson JT, Murray G, Jennett B (1998) Analyzing outcome of treatment of severe head injury: a review and update on advancing the use of the Glasgow Outcome Scale. J Neurotrauma 15(8):587–597
139. Toftdahl DB, Torp-Pedersen C, Engel UH, Strandgaard S, Jespersen B (1995) Hypertension and left ventricular hypertrophy in patients with spontaneous subarachnoid hemorrhage. Neurosurgery 37(2):235–239; discussion 239–240
140. Torbey MT, Hauser TK, Bhardwaj A, Williams MA, Ulatowski JA, Mirski MA, Razumovsky AY (2001) Effect of age on cerebral blood flow velocity and incidence of vasospasm after aneurysmal subarachnoid hemorrhage. Stroke 32(9):2005–2011
141. van Gijn J, Rinkel GJ (2001) Subarachnoid haemorrhage: diagnosis, causes and management. Brain 124(Pt 2):249–278
142. Vanninen R, Koivisto T, Saari T, Hernesniemi J, Vapalahti M (1999) Ruptured intracranial aneurysms: acute endovascular treatment with electrolytically detachable coils--a prospective randomized study. Radiology 211(2):325–336
143. Velat GJ, Kimball MM, Mocco JD, Hoh BL (2011) Vasospasm after aneurysmal subarachnoid hemorrhage: review of randomized controlled trials and meta-analyses in the literature. World Neurosurg 76(5):446–454. doi:10.1016/j.wneu.2011.02.030
144. White PM, Teasdale EM, Wardlaw JM, Easton V (2001) Intracranial aneurysms: CT angiography and MR angiography for detection prospective blinded comparison in a large patient cohort. Radiology 219(3):739–749
145. Wilson JT, Edwards P, Fiddes H, Stewart E, Teasdale GM (2002) Reliability of postal questionnaires for the Glasgow Outcome Scale. J Neurotrauma 19(9):999–1005
146. Wilson JT, Pettigrew LE, Teasdale GM (1998) Structured interviews for the Glasgow Outcome Scale and the extended Glasgow Outcome Scale: guidelines for their use. J Neurotrauma 15(8):573–585
147. Wilson JT, Pettigrew LE, Teasdale GM (2000) Emotional and cognitive consequences of head injury in relation to the glasgow outcome scale. J Neurol Neurosurg Psychiatry 69(2):204–209
148. Yano S, Hamada J, Kai Y, Todaka T, Hara T, Mizuno T, Morioka M, Ushio Y (2003) Surgical indications to maintain quality of life in elderly patients with ruptured intracranial aneurysms. Neurosurgery 52(5):1010–1015; discussion 1015–1016

Spontaneous Intracerebral Hemorrhage in the Elderly

22

Moncef Berhouma, Timothée Jacquesson, and Emmanuel Jouanneau

22.1 Introduction

Spontaneous intracerebral hemorrhage (SICH) remains a significant etiology of morbidity and mortality in the general population and particularly the elderly patients. Classically, SICH may be secondary to uncontrolled arterial hypertension, amyloid angiopathy, and iatrogenic coagulopathy. Rarely it reveals a malignant intracerebral tumor, a venous thrombosis, or results from the transformation of an ischemic stroke and vascular malformation rupture as well. The management of SICH remains challenging as it associates the specific treatment of the hemorrhage (medical and/or surgical) but also the associated morbidity inherent to elderly patients such as nosocomial infections particularly urinary and aspiration pneumonia, venous thrombosis, and denutrition.

22.2 Clinical Presentation

The presentation is usually acute or subacute progressing on a few hours associating variably headaches, vomiting, and a decreased level of consciousness, confusion, and motor deficits. Consciousness anomalies are common particularly in large hematomas involving basal ganglia and the brainstem, as well as in cerebellar hematomas compressing the brainstem. Seizures may reveal the hemorrhage especially in cortical and subcortical locations, as well as it can appear during the recovery period (late-onset seizures) in few cases. Cerebellar hematomas are revealed specifically in an acute and sometimes dramatic presentations with headaches, vomiting, vertigo, and ataxia. In several cases of brain hemorrhage in the very

M. Berhouma, MD, MSc, FEBNS (✉) • T. Jacquesson, MD, MSc • E. Jouanneau, MD, PhD
Department of Neurosurgery, University Hospital of Lyon – Hospices Civils de Lyon, Lyon, France
e-mail: berhouma.moncef@gmail.com

© Springer International Publishing Switzerland 2017

M. Berhouma, P. Krolak-Salmon (eds.), *Brain and Spine Surgery in the Elderly*,
DOI 10.1007/978-3-319-40232-1_22

Table 22.1 Correspondence between SICH location and clinical presentation

Location	Possible symptoms and signs
Cortical and subcortical surface	Epilepsy, motor deficits, aphasia, hemianopia, confusion
Brainstem	Ataxia, ophthalmoplegia, hyperthermia, pupillary anomalies, respiratory abnormalities, coma
Thalamus	Aphasia, heminegligence, confusion
Putamen	Hemiparesis, eye deviation
Caudate nucleus	Confusion, stupor, abulia
Cerebellum	Vertigo, vomiting, ataxia
Intraventricular extension	Headaches, coma, hyperthermia

elderly, the hematoma can remain well tolerated despite its large volume because of the brain atrophy and thus the absence of clinically significant brain shift (Table 22.1).

22.3 Age-Related Anatomical and Functional Changes

The structural and functional age-related changes of cerebral microvasculature have been well studied [1]. These include microembolic brain lesions, a decreased vascular density, thickening of the vessel basement membrane, endothelial dysfunction, and blood-brain barrier hyperpermeability. Elsewhere, leukoaraiosis is frequent in elderly patients particularly when a cerebrovascular predisposition is present. This condition associates demyelination, gliosis, spongiosis, and capillary degeneration. Various systemic diseases such as arterial hypertension, diabetes mellitus, atherosclerosis, and atrial fibrillation may also induce pathological modifications encompassing changes in vessel elasticity, blood flow turbulences, and finally endothelial damage promoting thus SICH. Other modifiable risk factors such as smoking and chronic alcohol use may also exacerbate the risk of SICH [2]. Age-related systemic changes explaining the frailty of elderly patients facing SICH comprise the reduction of the physiologic reserve, cardiovascular modifications (consequences of altered response to sympathetic stimulation), kidneys alterations (renal function decline), and respiratory dysfunction [3] (see Chap. 2 for more details).

22.4 Arterial Hypertension

Hypertensive brain hemorrhage usually involves the basal ganglia, the thalamus, or the cerebellum [4–6]. It can also extend to the brainstem, particularly the pons. From a pathological perspective, chronic arterial hypertension is thought to lead to lipohyalinosis and fibrinoid necrosis of very small intraparenchymal arteries particularly in the area of basal ganglia also known as lenticulostriate arterial perforators. The classically described role of Charcot-Bouchard microaneurysms in these basal ganglia hemorrhages in the elderly is still debated. The clinical presentation depends on the location and extent of the hematoma, but also on the association of an intraventricular hemorrhage. The first 24 hours are critical, as several studies have shown that the hematoma may enlarge within this delay. Some features are usually associated to the very elderly patients (>80 years): These had a lower blood pressure profile at admission than the younger patients [7–9], and this should be kept in mind during the intensive care and resuscitation phases. In this same specific subgroup of the very elderly, the thalamic location appears more frequent than in younger patients with SICH [10] as well as a more frequent intraventricular hemorrhage probably due to aging brain plasticity changes [11].

22.5 Cerebral Amyloid Angiopathy

Sporadic cerebral amyloid angiopathy (CAA) is a small vessel disease of the brain characterized by the progressive deposition of amyloid-β (Aβ)-protein in the wall of cortical and pial lobar arteries. Cerebellar, brainstem, or basal ganglia small vessels can be affected very rarely. Sporadic CAA is one of the most frequent etiologies of SICH in the elderly, with an incidence ranging from 5 to 20 % of all SICH [12].

Schematically, CAA causes recurrent cortical and subcortical hemorrhages occurring in non-hypertensive adults after 60 years [13–15], but is also significantly associated to dementia and particularly Alzheimer's disease. CAA is also often concomitant with brain ischemic anomalies including cortical microinfarcts and white matter demyelination and gliosis [16]. Several autopsic studies have revealed a CAA prevalence of 20–40 % in non-demented elderly contrasting with 50–60 % in a demented population [17–21]. The increasing age is actually the only significant risk factor individualized [22], contrary to hypertensive SICH in elderly. Nevertheless, arterial hypertension appears to increase the risk of CAA-related SICH [23–26]. It has been demonstrated that apolipoprotein E (ApoE) alleles are genetic risk factors for sporadic CAA, particularly the ApoE ε4 and ε2 form alleles with a clear relationship with the clinical severity of CAA-related SICH, the younger age at presentation, a greater risk of hematoma expansion in the first hours, and a greater risk of recurrence as well [27–33]. Sporadic CAA affects preferentially posterior cortical areas particularly occipital but also frontal, temporal, and parietal lobes. Typically, the hemorrhage recurrence occurs in the same lobe with an annual risk of 10 % per year in elderly cohorts [34–36]. Characteristically, very distinctive neuroimaging features in CAA-related lobar hemorrhages exist:

- Cerebral microbleeds: These appear clearly on T2* sequences as small well-demarcated hypointensities with a lobar distribution. They reflect the existence of very focal accumulation of macrophages containing hemosiderin located close to small vessels affected by CAA. The parietal lobe seems preferentially involved, and the number of these microbleeds may correlate to the risk of lobar SICH in the elderly [37–39].
- Leukoaraiosis: A radiological term corresponding to white matter anomalies appearing as hyperintensities (T2 and FLAIR) sparing the subcortical U fibers.

Pathologically, leukoaraiosis corresponds to demyelination, gliosis, and axonal loss. It probably results from chronic hypoperfusion of the vulnerable periventricular white matter [40–42].

- Cortical subarachnoid hemorrhage and siderosis: Corresponds to very localized subarachnoid hemorrhage limited to the superficial cortical sulci resulting at term in the accumulation of hemosiderin in the superficial layers of the cerebral cortex better seen on T2* sequences with a gyriform pattern [43, 44].
- Silent acute ischemic lesions: These are associated with the severity of leukoaraiosis and lobar microbleeds and are easily visible on diffusion weighted imaging [45].

In vivo imaging of CAA is actually possible before the onset of consequences. It uses positron emission tomography (PET) with different ligands and mostly [11] C PiB [46]. Apart of autopsic studies and brain biopsies, the diagnosis relies on Boston criteria [47] (Table 22.2). Elsewhere, some CSF markers appear useful such as the assessment of Aβ-levels. In contrast to CSF findings in Alzheimer disease, both

Table 22.2 Boston criteria for CAA diagnosis

Definite CAA
Full postmortem examination showing:
Lobar, cortical, or cortical-subcortical hemorrhage
Severe CAA with vasculopathy
Absence of other diagnostic lesion
Probable CAA with supporting pathology
Clinical data and pathological tissue (evacuated hematoma or cortical biopsy) demonstrating:
Lobar, cortical, or cortical-subcortical hemorrhage
Some degree of CAA in specimen
Absence of other diagnostic lesion
Probable CAA
Clinical data and MRI or CT demonstrating:
Multiple hemorrhages restricted to lobar cortical or cortical-subcortical regions (cerebellar hemorrhage allowed)
Single lobar cortical or cortical-subcortical and focal (3 or fewer sulci) or disseminated (at least 4 sulci) superficial siderosis
Age ≥55 years
Absence of another cause of hemorrhage[a]
Possible CAA
Clinical data and MRI or CT demonstrating:
Single lobar cortical or cortical-subcortical hemorrhage
Or focal or disseminated superficial siderosis
Age ≥55 years
Absence of another cause of hemorrhage[a]

[a]Antecedent of head trauma, hemorrhagic transformation of an ischemic stroke, AVM, hemorrhagic tumor, warfarin therapy with INR > 3, vasculitis

$A\beta_{42}$ and $A\beta_{40}$ are decreased in CAA [48, 49]. Finally, the diagnosis of CAA can be evoked in case of characteristic retinal anomalies including microaneurysms as well as dot and blot hemorrhages [50].

22.6 Iatrogenic Coagulopathy

Over the past decade, there has been a four- to fivefold increase in the incidence of SICH related to anticoagulation and antiplatelets therapy, probably because of the increasing use of oral anticoagulation such as warfarin in the prevention of cardio-embolic stroke in elderly with atrial fibrillation [51, 52]. Anticoagulation is actually responsible for about 15 % of SICH in elderly. Furthermore SICH in an anticoagulated elderly patient can be dramatic in case of underlying CAA [53]. The role of CAA in the pathogenesis of SICH in anticoagulated elderly patients relies on two observations: In the majority of cases, SICH occurs in patients with international normalized ratios within therapeutic range, and elsewhere the ApoE e2 allele is more frequent in warfarin-related SICH than in elderly patients on warfarin without SICH [53]. One should keep in mind that in all patients and particularly the elderly, the risk of SICH can double even when international normalized ratio remains in the therapeutic range between 2 and 3. Elsewhere, the use of new oral anticoagulants (dabigatran etexilate, rivaroxaban, apixaban, and edoxaban) has modified the incidence of SICH. In a meta-analysis, Ruff et al [54] showed that the use of these new oral anticoagulants (NOACs) resulted in a significant reduction of SICH when compared with warfarin (0.48, 0.39–0.59; $p < 0.0001$). Pathogenesis of the decreased risk of SICH with the NOACs is still debated [55–60]. The high concentration of tissue factor (transmembrane receptor for factor VIIa) in the brain may play a pivotal role. It is known that warfarin blocks vitamin K-dependent carboxylation of coagulation factors II, VII, IX, and X. Therefore, NOACs may preserve hemostatic balance in the brain tissue by selectively targeting thrombin without interfering with the arrangement of factor VIIa-tissue factor complex. The role of P-glycoprotein in removing actively NOACs from brain tissue has been questioned [61–63]. Nevertheless, the absence of immediate antidote to NOACs in the acute phase of SICH management still remains pregnant.

22.7 Management and Outcome

The management of SICH in this specific population of patients comprises the limitation of hematoma expansion and mass effect, the reduction of secondary insults to the adjacent brain, and the prevention of decubitus complications (bedsores, pneumopathy, denutrition, urinary infection, depression, etc.). Prevention of SICH in the elderly (control of diabetes mellitus and hypertension, multidisciplinary decision for anticoagulation and antiplatelet therapy, etc.) is of paramount importance as it is now well established that an older age is associated with the initial severity of SICH and poorer outcomes including mortality and disability at 3 months [64]. In addition to the older age, several other factors have been shown to be associated with a worse outcome such as stroke severity as defined by the NIHSS score, the extent of hemorrhage (intraventricular extension and brainstem involvement), diabetes mellitus, comorbid coronary and cardiac diseases, and iatrogenic coagulopathy as well [2, 65]. Particularly in the very old (80 years and more) suffering SICH, a recent study [66] revealed higher hospital mortality comparatively to patients younger than 80 years (35.9 versus 20.0 %) as well as a more frequent unfavorable outcome (modified Rankin Scale>2) (84.9 versus 74.8 %). These authors estimated that by 2050 the number of these very old patients with SICH will be 2.5-fold higher than in 2009 in occidental countries. These data emphasize the challenge when facing the frailty of this particular subgroup and shed the light on the necessity to adapt the management. The surgical evacuation of SICH in elderly but also the resort to external ventricular drainage should be thoroughly discussed within a multidisciplinary board including intensivists, neurologists, neurosurgeons, and geriatricians. The family of the patient should be involved in the decision too. Except for selected cases of cerebellar hematomas without brainstem injury in which surgery can be effective (Fig. 22.1), the surgical treatment of SICH is still debated. The benefice of surgical treatment is mainly questioned in case of deep hematomas particularly when brainstem is involved (Figs. 22.2, 22.3, and 22.4). Lobar and superficial hematomas (Fig. 22.5a, b) are amenable to surgical evacuation, and histopathological examination should be systematic to screen for amyloid angiopathy or underlying neoplasm (particularly metastases from melanomas, kidney, or thyroid cancers) (Table 22.3).

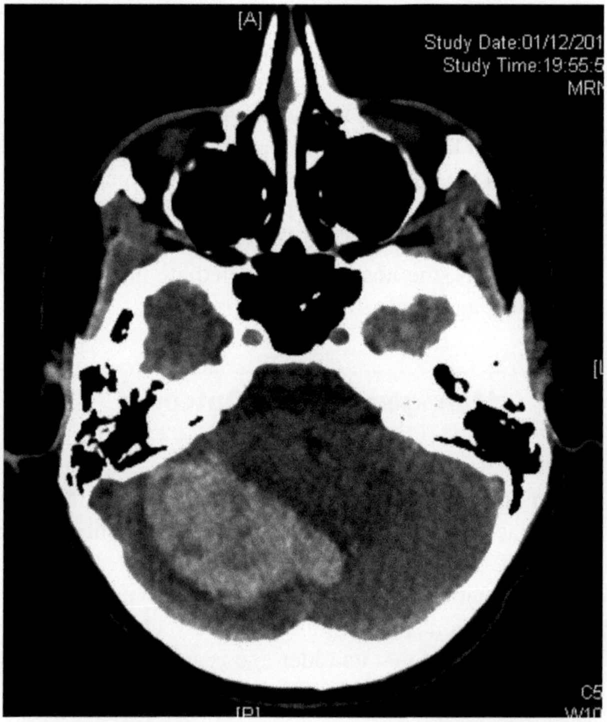

Fig. 22.1 Right cerebellar hematoma superior to 3 cm diameter resulting in fourth ventricle deviation without evident brainstem involvement, amenable to surgical evacuation

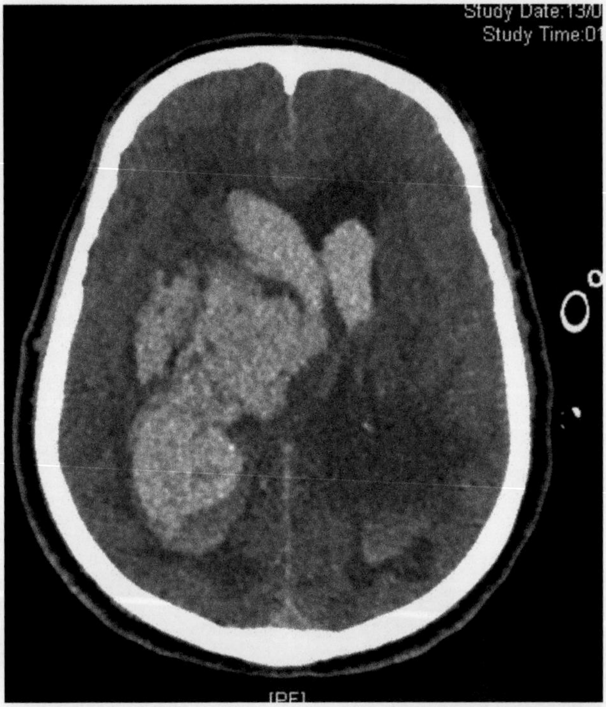

Fig. 22.2 Dramatic extensive and deep right hemorrhage with intraventricular inundation leading to therapeutic limitation and rapid fatal evolution

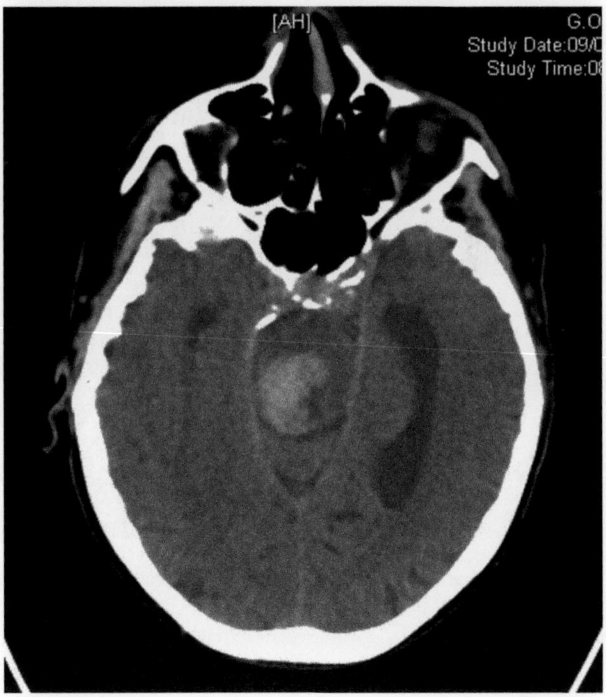

Fig. 22.3 Brainstem hematoma. Indication of conservative management

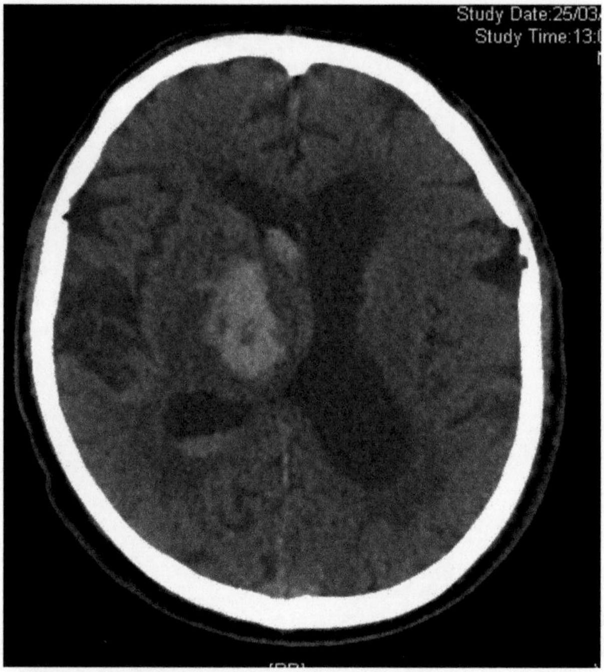

Fig. 22.4 Deep central gray nuclei hemorrhage with intraventricular extension typical of hypertensive hemorrhage

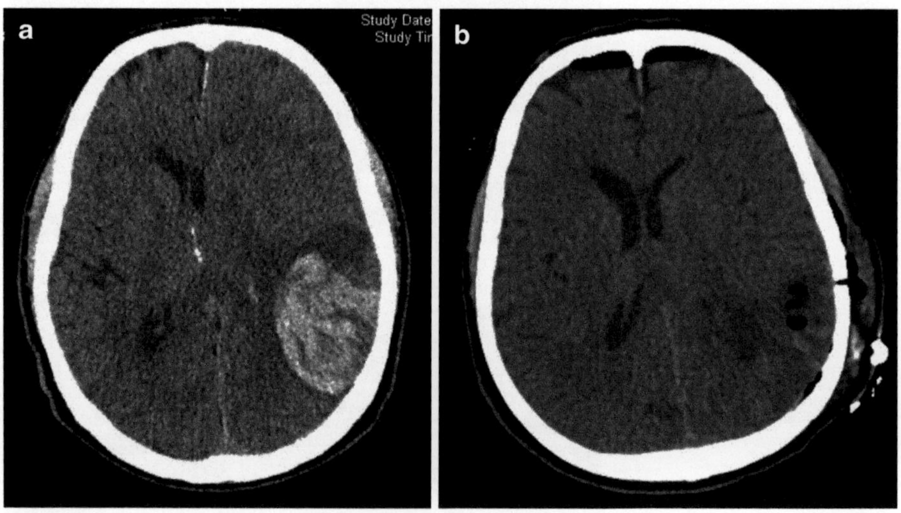

Fig. 22.5 Lobar superficial left parietal hemorrhage (**a**) treated surgically (**b**) with amyloid angiopathy evidence at pathological examination

Table 22.3 Proposal for the management of cerebellar hemorrhage in the elderly

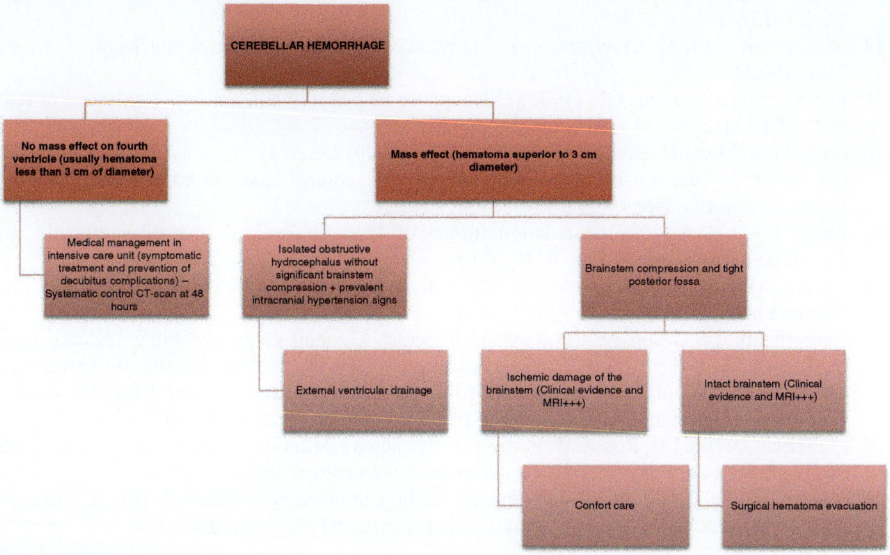

References

1. Brown WR, Thore CR (2011) Review: cerebral microvascular pathology in ageing and neurodegeneration. Neuropathol Appl Neurobiol 37:56–74
2. Ariesen MJ, Claus SP, Rinkel GJE, Algra A (2003) Risk factors for intracerebral hemorrhage in the general population: a systematic review. Stroke 34:2060–2065
3. Pisani MA (2009) Considerations in caring for the critically ill older patient. J Intensive Care Med 24:83–95
4. Aguilar MI, Brott TG (2011) Update in intracerebral hemorrhage. Neurohospitalist 1: 148–159
5. Kreitzer N, Adeoye O (2013) An update on surgical and medical management strategies for intracerebral hemorrhage. Semin Neurol 33:462–467
6. Manno EM (2012) Update on intracerebral hemorrhage. Continuum (Minneap Minn) 18:598–610
7. Thrift AG, McNeil JJ, Forbes A, Donnan GA (1998) Three important subgroups of hypertensive persons at greater risk of intracerebral hemorrhage. Melbourne Risk Factor Study Group. Hypertension 31:1223–1229
8. Sadoshima S, Yoshida F, Ibayashi S, Shiokawa O, Fujishima M (1985) Upper limit of cerebral autoregulation during development of hypertension in spontaneously hypertensive rats – effect of sympathetic denervation. Stroke 16:477–481
9. Salerno JA et al (1995) Brain metabolic function in older men with chronic essential hypertension. J Gerontol A Biol Sci Med Sci 50:M147–M154
10. Chiquete E et al (2007) Hypertensive intracerebral hemorrhage in the very elderly. Cerebrovasc Dis 24:196–201
11. Ruiz-Sandoval JL et al (2006) Hypertensive intracerebral hemorrhage in young people: previously unnoticed age-related clinical differences. Stroke 37:2946–2950
12. Pezzini A et al (2009) Cerebral amyloid angiopathy: a common cause of cerebral hemorrhage. Curr Med Chem 16:2498–2513

13. Itoh Y, Yamada M, Hayakawa M, Otomo E, Miyatake T (1993) Cerebral amyloid angiopathy: a significant cause of cerebellar as well as lobar cerebral hemorrhage in the elderly. J Neurol Sci 116:135–141
14. Jellinger K (1977) Cerebrovascular amyloidosis with cerebral hemorrhage. J Neurol 214:195–206
15. Lee SS, Stemmermann GN (1978) Congophilic angiopathy and cerebral hemorrhage. Arch Pathol Lab Med 102:317–321
16. Cadavid D, Mena H, Koeller K, Frommelt RA (2000) Cerebral beta amyloid angiopathy is a risk factor for cerebral ischemic infarction. A case control study in human brain biopsies. J Neuropathol Exp Neurol 59:768–773
17. Keage HAD et al (2009) Population studies of sporadic cerebral amyloid angiopathy and dementia: a systematic review. BMC Neurol 9:3
18. Love S, Miners JS (2016) Cerebrovascular disease in ageing and Alzheimer's disease. Acta Neuropathol 131:645–658
19. Neuropathology Group (2001) Medical Research Council Cognitive Function and Aging Study. Pathological correlates of late-onset dementia in a multicentre, community-based population in England and Wales. Neuropathology Group of the Medical Research Council Cognitive Function and Ageing Study (MRC CFAS). Lancet 357:169–175
20. Pfeifer LA, White LR, Ross GW, Petrovitch H, Launer LJ (2002) Cerebral amyloid angiopathy and cognitive function: the HAAS autopsy study. Neurology 58:1629–1634
21. Xuereb JH et al (2000) Neuropathological findings in the very old. Results from the first 101 brains of a population-based longitudinal study of dementing disorders. Ann N Y Acad Sci 903:490–496
22. Mastaglia FL, Byrnes ML, Johnsen RD, Kakulas BA (2003) Prevalence of cerebral vascular amyloid-beta deposition and stroke in an aging Australian population: a postmortem study. J Clin Neurosci 10:186–189
23. Arima H et al (2010) Effects of perindopril-based lowering of blood pressure on intracerebral hemorrhage related to amyloid angiopathy: the PROGRESS trial. Stroke 41:394–396
24. Broderick J, Brott T, Tomsick T, Leach A (1993) Lobar hemorrhage in the elderly. The undiminishing importance of hypertension. Stroke 24:49–51
25. Ferreiro JA, Ansbacher LE, Vinters HV (1989) Stroke related to cerebral amyloid angiopathy: the significance of systemic vascular disease. J Neurol 236:267–272
26. Gregoire SM et al (2011) Acute ischaemic brain lesions in intracerebral haemorrhage: multicentre cross-sectional magnetic resonance imaging study. Brain 134:2376–2386
27. Verghese PB, Castellano JM, Holtzman DM (2011) Apolipoprotein E in Alzheimer's disease and other neurological disorders. Lancet Neurol 10:241–252
28. Greenberg SM et al (1996) Apolipoprotein E epsilon 4 is associated with the presence and earlier onset of hemorrhage in cerebral amyloid angiopathy. Stroke 27:1333–1337
29. Premkumar DR, Cohen DL, Hedera P, Friedland RP, Kalaria RN (1996) Apolipoprotein E-epsilon4 alleles in cerebral amyloid angiopathy and cerebrovascular pathology associated with Alzheimer's disease. Am J Pathol 148:2083–2095
30. Biffi A et al (2010) Variants at APOE influence risk of deep and lobar intracerebral hemorrhage. Ann Neurol 68:934–943
31. Nicoll JA et al (1997) High frequency of apolipoprotein E epsilon 2 allele in hemorrhage due to cerebral amyloid angiopathy. Ann Neurol 41:716–721
32. Biffi A et al (2011) APOE genotype and extent of bleeding and outcome in lobar intracerebral haemorrhage: a genetic association study. Lancet Neurol 10:702–709
33. Montaner J (2011) Genetics of intracerebral haemorrhage: a tsunami effect of APOE ε2 genotype on brain bleeding size? Lancet Neurol 10:673–675
34. Vinters HV (1987) Cerebral amyloid angiopathy. A critical review. Stroke 18:311–324
35. Rosand J et al (2005) Spatial clustering of hemorrhages in probable cerebral amyloid angiopathy. Ann Neurol 58:459–462
36. Passero S, Burgalassi L, D'Andrea P, Battistini N (1995) Recurrence of bleeding in patients with primary intracerebral hemorrhage. Stroke 26:1189–1192

37. Poels MMF et al (2010) Prevalence and risk factors of cerebral microbleeds: an update of the Rotterdam scan study. Stroke 41:S103–S106
38. Greenberg SM, Eng JA, Ning M, Smith EE, Rosand J (2004) Hemorrhage burden predicts recurrent intracerebral hemorrhage after lobar hemorrhage. Stroke 35:1415–1420
39. Sveinbjornsdottir S et al (2008) Cerebral microbleeds in the population based AGES-Reykjavik study: prevalence and location. J Neurol Neurosurg Psychiatr 79:1002–1006
40. Debette S, Markus HS (2010) The clinical importance of white matter hyperintensities on brain magnetic resonance imaging: systematic review and meta-analysis. BMJ 341:c3666
41. Smith EE et al (2004) White matter lesions, cognition, and recurrent hemorrhage in lobar intracerebral hemorrhage. Neurology 63:1606–1612
42. Chen YW et al (2006) Progression of white matter lesions and hemorrhages in cerebral amyloid angiopathy. Neurology 67:83–87
43. Linn J et al (2008) Subarachnoid hemosiderosis and superficial cortical hemosiderosis in cerebral amyloid angiopathy. AJNR Am J Neuroradiol 29:184–186
44. Kumar N et al (2006) Superficial siderosis. Neurology 66:1144–1152
45. Kidwell CS, Greenberg SM (2009) Red meets white: do microbleeds link hemorrhagic and ischemic cerebrovascular disease? Neurology 73:1614–1615
46. Nordberg A, Rinne JO, Kadir A, Långström B (2010) The use of PET in Alzheimer disease. Nat Rev Neurol 6:78–87
47. Knudsen KA, Rosand J, Karluk D, Greenberg SM (2001) Clinical diagnosis of cerebral amyloid angiopathy: validation of the Boston criteria. Neurology 56:537–539
48. de Jong D, Kremer BPH, Olde Rikkert MGM, Verbeek MM (2007) Current state and future directions of neurochemical biomarkers for Alzheimer's disease. Clin Chem Lab Med 45:1421–1434
49. Verbeek MM et al (2009) Cerebrospinal fluid amyloid beta(40) is decreased in cerebral amyloid angiopathy. Ann Neurol 66:245–249
50. Lee A et al (2009) Retinal vascular abnormalities in patients with cerebral amyloid angiopathy. Cerebrovasc Dis 28:618–622
51. Flaherty ML et al (2007) The increasing incidence of anticoagulant-associated intracerebral hemorrhage. Neurology 68:116–121
52. Flibotte JJ, Hagan N, O'Donnell J, Greenberg SM, Rosand J (2004) Warfarin, hematoma expansion, and outcome of intracerebral hemorrhage. Neurology 63:1059–1064
53. Rosand J, Hylek EM, O'Donnell HC, Greenberg SM (2000) Warfarin-associated hemorrhage and cerebral amyloid angiopathy: a genetic and pathologic study. Neurology 55:947–951
54. Ruff CT et al (2014) Comparison of the efficacy and safety of new oral anticoagulants with warfarin in patients with atrial fibrillation: a meta-analysis of randomised trials. Lancet 383:955–962
55. Hankey GJ (2014) Intracranial hemorrhage and novel anticoagulants for atrial fibrillation: what have we learned? Curr Cardiol Rep 16:480
56. Mackman N (2009) The role of tissue factor and factor VIIa in hemostasis. Anesth Analg 108:1447–1452
57. Sakata T et al (1995) Suppression of plasma-activated factor VII levels by warfarin therapy. Arterioscler Thromb Vasc Biol 15:241–246
58. Lippi G et al (2006) Influence of warfarin therapy on activated factor VII clotting activity. Blood Coagul Fibrinolysis 17:221–224
59. Deveras RAE, Kessler CM (2002) Reversal of warfarin-induced excessive anticoagulation with recombinant human factor VIIa concentrate. Ann Intern Med 137:884–888
60. Mayer SA et al (2008) Efficacy and safety of recombinant activated factor VII for acute intracerebral hemorrhage. N Engl J Med 358:2127–2137
61. Eyal S, Hsiao P, Unadkat JD (2009) Drug interactions at the blood–brain barrier: fact or fantasy? Pharmacol Ther 123:80–104
62. Stöllberger C, Finsterer J (2015) Relevance of P-glycoprotein in stroke prevention with dabigatran, rivaroxaban, and apixaban. Herz 40(Suppl 2):140–145
63. Wessler JD, Grip LT, Mendell J, Giugliano RP (2013) The P-glycoprotein transport system and cardiovascular drugs. J Am Coll Cardiol 61:2495–2502

64. Rådholm K et al (2015) Older age is a strong predictor for poor outcome in intracerebral haemorrhage: the INTERACT2 study. Age Ageing 44:422–427
65. Chen G et al (2014) Subarachnoid extension of intracerebral hemorrhage and 90-day outcomes in INTERACT2. Stroke 45:258–260
66. Stein M et al (2012) Intracerebral hemorrhage in the very old: future demographic trends of an aging population. Stroke 43:1126–1128

Swollen Middle Cerebral Artery Stroke in the Elderly

23

Desmond A. Brown and Eelco F.M. Wijdicks

23.1 Introduction

Large territorial infarctions of the brain involving virtually an entire hemisphere may swell, cause tissue shift, and become symptomatic. When associated with clinical signs of brain tissue shift, the affix "malignant" has been used but neither all swelling is "malignant" nor clinically recognizable. This term was recently coined to describe the rapidity and relentlessness of neurological deterioration which occurs as a consequence of space-occupying cerebral edema in the context of large middle cerebral artery (MCA) infarctions [1–3] although the syndrome had long been described [4, 5]. Deterioration may occur within the first 24 h or may be more protracted over several days following the initial ischemic insult. The incidence is approximately 10–20 per 100,000 person-years often affecting patients that are approximately decades younger (30–50 years) than the average age of patients presenting with ischemic strokes in general [1].

The outcome following swollen symptomatic large hemispheric ischemic infarcts is universally poor and mortality rates between 41 and 79 % with medical management have been reported [1–3, 6, 7]. Hacke et al. prospectively evaluated 55 patients with complete MCA territory infarction [1]. Patients were between the ages of 18 and 70 experiencing a first ischemic stroke with documented MCA territory involvement on CT without hemorrhagic transformation. The majority of patients required ventilator assistance with intubation occurring between 3 h and 5 days. Need for intubation was a poor prognostic sign as most of the intubated patients died despite maximal medical therapy consisting of hyperventilation and hyperosmolar therapy with occasional barbiturate coma induction. The main cause of death in this and

D.A. Brown, MD, PhD • E.F.M. Wijdicks, MD, PhD (✉)
Department of Neurosurgery (DAB) and Division of Critical Care Neurology (EFMW), Mayo Clinic, 200 First Street SW, Rochester, MN 55905, USA
e-mail: wijde@mayo.edu

© Springer International Publishing Switzerland 2017

M. Berhouma, P. Krolak-Salmon (eds.), *Brain and Spine Surgery in the Elderly*,
DOI 10.1007/978-3-319-40232-1_23

several prior studies was post-ischemic edema brain tissue shift and eventually raised intracranial pressure, and brain death [1, 4, 5, 8–11]. In the early 1980s, decompressive hemicraniectomy was reintroduced as an optional treatment of ischemic brain swelling.

Massive acute cerebral infarction—most certainly in patients with acute carotid artery occlusion extending infarction territory to the anterior circulation—was considered invariably fatal once cerebral edema developed. Antiedema agents were rarely successful and opening of the skull seemed the only option for many patients. Given the role of secondary edema in the ultimate demise of patients with massive MCA infarctions, most neurosurgeons feel that decompressive craniectomy is a viable strategy to prevent further decline and to prevent death.

Currently, only four (4) interventions for acute ischemic stroke are supported by class 1 evidence: (i) care on a stroke unit, (ii) intravenous tissue plasminogen activator within 4.5 h of stroke onset, (iii) aspirin within 48 h of stroke onset, and (iv) decompressive craniectomy for supratentorial malignant hemispheric cerebral infarction. Decompressive craniectomy performed in the setting of severe brain compression occurring as a consequence of malignant MCA infarcts may lower both the morbidity and mortality associated with the typical natural course [12]. In this chapter, we will limit our review to the evidence for decompressive craniectomy for malignant middle cerebral infarctions. Particular attention will be paid to the role of decompressive surgery in the elderly herein defined rather arbitrarily in clinical trials as patients older than 60 years of age and 5 years younger than "retirement age" and the traditional cut off where geriatric medicine begins. This elderly population is excluded from many seminal randomized control trials on the subject, under the assumption that outcomes would be universally poor. We also present a recent case from our institution of an elderly patient (in the parlance of this literature) presenting with a complete left MCA territory infarct. We conclude with some comments on the ethics of this major neurosurgical procedure as a rescue procedure in elderly patients already struck with a disabling stroke with uncertain future prospects.

23.2 Pathophysiology of Ischemia-Related Cerebral Edema

The pathophysiology of cerebral edema following ischemic insult is complex and will not be reviewed in detail here. Suffice it to say, cerebral ischemia triggers a cascade of downstream molecular processes including apoptosis, necrosis, necroptosis, and autophagy with downstream deleterious events. One of the first such deleterious impacts of infarction is microvascular dysfunction resulting in ionic edema with concomitant vasogenic edema. Ischemia-related microvascular dysfunction is mediated at least in part by upregulation of sulfonylurea receptor 1 (SUR1) [13]. SUR1 regulates and opens the NCCa-ATP channel, a nonselective cation channel in ischemic astrocytes in an ATP-dependent manner. Opening of the channel results in cation influx and cytotoxic edema. There is tremendous interest in the use of SUR1 inhibitors (Glibenclamide being the most well studied but a recent trial found despite reduction in swelling no effect on outcome [14]) in curtailing cerebral edema in the aftermath of severe stroke [15]. Cerebral edema leads to local brain compression which may then initiate a catastrophic cycle involving further compression and infarction of adjacent brain tissue with ensuing worsening of edema. Ischemic edema displaces tissue and brainstem and causes a clinical change. The swollen (tumorlike) mass grows and eventually—albeit late in the process—will increase cerebral volume and intracranial pressure. Medical strategies aimed at curtailing ischemia-related edema are drawn from contemporary neurocritical care measures and include interventions to decrease intracranial pressure such as elevation of head of bed, hyperventilation, and prevention of jugular venous congestion, osmolar therapy, and CSF diversion. Additional interventions aimed at preventing further loss of brain tissue include drug-induced comas and hypothermia. Some of these efforts provide only a fleeting decrease in intracranial mass effect and neuroprotection and, in some cases, result in significant morbidity. Decompressive hemicraniectomy provides the potential for immediate reduction in cerebral compression.

23.3 Decompressive Craniectomy for Malignant Middle Cerebral Artery Infarcts

Decompressive craniectomy was first described by Cushing for relief of "cerebral hernia" associated with brain tumors [16]. Rengachary et al. first advocated decompressive surgery for the specific indication of massive cerebral infarction in 1981 in a publication in which they described outcome of only three patients, all of whom had favorable outcomes [17]. Kondziolka and Fazi subsequently reported their small series of five patients with supratentorial cerebral infarction and uncal herniation on whom they performed frontotemporal craniectomy after failure of maximal medical therapy [18]. All five patients survived were ambulatory and two returned to work. Over the next decade, decompressive hemicraniectomy for malignant MCA infarctions gained traction and led to a series of studies to evaluate its efficacy.

Rieke et al. published their open, prospective trial of 32 patients (age 37–68 years; mean 48.8 years) who received decompressive craniectomy and duraplasty compared to 21 patients (age 37 to 69 years; mean 58.4 years) who had nonsurgical management [2]. Surgery was associated with a significant survival advantage with 21 of 32 surgical patients surviving compared to only five survivors in the control group. Surgically treated patients were less likely to be disabled: 5 surgical patients were disabled but independent, 15 were severely disabled but not totally dependent, and 1 was asymptomatic at ICU discharge. In comparison, there were only four survivors in the control group, 4 of whom had global aphasia. There was no statistically significant difference in the ages of survivors versus non-survivors nor was there a difference in the timing of clinical deterioration and outcome. The authors published an update to this open study in which they evaluated outcome following late versus early hemicraniectomy on mortality rate, length of time in the neurocritical care unit, and the mean Barthel index score [19]. Mortality rate was 16 % when performed early, 34.4 % when performed late, and 78 % for nonsurgical controls. ICU stay was 13.3, 7.4, and 12.6 days for late hemicraniectomy, early hemicraniectomy, and natural history controls, respectively. Mean Barthel index was 62.6, 68.8, and 60 for late hemicraniectomy, early hemicraniectomy, and natural history controls, respectively.

The notion that there is a prognostic benefit to earlier craniectomy was explored further by Cho et al. in their 2003 study on ultra-early decompressive craniectomy for malignant middle cerebral artery infarction [20]. The study evaluated 52 patients (age range of 45–80 years) who received ultra-early (<6 h), early (>6 h), or conservative therapy. Survival was 91 %, 63 %, and 20 % in the ultra-early, early, and conservative groups, respectively. Furthermore, the ability to follow commands at 7 days post-onset was 91 %, 55 %, and 0 % for the ultra-early, early, and conservative groups, respectively. The study was not powered to detect subtle differences in outcome within the treatment groups based on age. The results provided further support for a role of craniectomy for malignant infarcts and suggested that the timing of surgery is a critical factor in procuring both survival and good functional outcome. That is, the sooner, the better.

Several additional observational studies suggested efficacy of decompressive hemicraniectomy for malignant strokes [19–24]. A systematic review of 138 cases published by Gupta et al. suggested that the benefits of decompressive hemicraniectomy for malignant middle cerebral artery infarctions were nonuniform with younger patients (<50 years of age) less likely to be dead or severely disabled at 4 months following the procedure (80 % versus 32 %) [25]. This finding was reproduced in a study from our institution in which older age was the sole factor predictive of poor functional outcome in the aftermath of decompressive craniectomy for malignant stroke [26]. Meanwhile, the role of several key traditional techniques for conservative management, including osmolar therapy, hypothermia, and barbiturate coma, was proving to be less efficacious [4, 5, 9, 27, 28]. This combination of a lack of positive evidence regarding decompressive hemicraniectomy and doubts regarding conservative management led to wide variations in practice and underscored the need for high-quality randomized controlled trials to study the effects of decompressive surgery. Furthermore, the findings suggested that trials should be designed to both determine overall efficacy but also specifically, the population most likely to benefit from neurosurgical intervention.

23.4 Randomized Controlled Trials of Decompressive Craniectomy for Malignant Middle Cerebral Artery Infarction

Several randomized controlled trials were undertaken to address the aforementioned gaps in knowledge and to standardize management of patients with hemispheric infarctions. HeADDFIRST was the first randomized control trial aimed at delineating parameters for the design of additional robust trials to evaluate the role of decompressive craniectomy on functional outcome and survival. Three European randomized trials were undertaken in the early 2000s: DECIMAL (France), DESTINY (Germany), and HAMLET (Netherlands). The Hemicraniectomy for Malignant Middle Cerebral Artery Infarction (HeMMI) was a single center randomized controlled clinical trial launched in the Philippines. HeMMI was launched in January 2002 and terminated December 2009 secondary to poor recruitment. It will not be discussed further. A list of studies aimed at exploring the role of decompressive hemicraniectomy for malignant cerebral infarctions is shown in Table 23.1. It should be noted that most of the clinical trials were not completed and most were stopped early and not even half-way. Data from patients less than 60 years old should therefore be subject to critical scrutiny.

23.5 The First Prospective Clinical Trial on Hemicraniectomy: HeADDFIRST

The Hemicraniectomy and Durotomy Upon Deterioration From Infarction-Related Swelling Trial (HeADDFIRST) was actually the first randomized controlled trial aimed at addressing the role of decompressive craniectomy for malignant infarction although the results were not published until 2014 [29]. HeADDFIRST was designed as a pilot clinical trial to provide parameters for the appropriate design of Phase III clinical trials aimed at assessing the benefit of decompressive craniectomy in malignant supratentorial cerebral hemispheric infarction. The study enrolled patients from 20 North American centers (including our own) between March 2000 and September 2002. Of 4909 patients screened, 66 met all inclusion criteria, but after the consenting and randomization procedures, only 25 patients were included, one of whom subsequently withdrew.

The initial inclusion criteria included patients 18–75 years of age presenting with a unilateral middle cerebral artery stroke with National Institutes of Health Stroke Scale (NIHSS) ≥18 who remained responsive to minor stimulation. Neuroimaging criteria were then applied to patients who passed this initial screen. Radiographic inclusion required hypodensity involving ≥50 % of the MCA territory on CT obtained within 5 h of symptom onset, or hypodensity of the entire MCA vascular distribution on CT performed within 48 h of symptom onset. Patients were excluded from the trial if neurological deterioration preceded admission to the participating hospital; or if there was a subdural or confluent parenchymal hematoma or subarachnoid hemorrhage; PTT > 40 s; INR > 1.4; platelet count <100 k/μl prior to correction with blood products; any pre-existing illness limiting life expectancy to less than 6 months; any significant pre-existing disability (mRS > 2); any pre-existing or concurrent brain injury resulting in neurological deficits in addition to that wrought by the stroke; and participation in another clinical trial. These inclusion and exclusion criteria were used to guide the design of subsequent randomized clinical trials including the 3 European trials (see below).

Mortality at 21 days was reduced in the surgically treated patients relative to patients receiving maximal medical therapy (40 % in the surgical groups [90 %

Table 23.1 Clinical trials of decompressive hemicraniectomy for malignant MCA infarctions

Author	Year	Study	Type	*N*	Age (years)	Finding
Rai et al. [50]	2014	Long-term outcome of decompressive hemicraniectomy in patients with MMCAI	Prospective observational	60	20–91	ARR of mortality 45 % at 1 year; ARR of mRS $\geq$4 93.5 %; surgery reduces mortality and functional outcome
Frank et al. [29]	2014	HeADDFIRST	RCT	66	18–75	Early mortality benefit of surgery at 21 days (21 % versus 40 %)
Shao et al. [51]	2013	Comparison between routine and improved decompressive craniectomy on patients with MMCAI without traumatic brain injury	Prospective observational	131	48 $\leq$60; 37 >60 (improved surgical arm)	Improved decompressive craniectomy showed significant functional improvement. Younger achieved better functional outcomes with shorter hospital stay
Geurts et al. [52]	2013	HAMLET 3-year outcomes	RCT	64	18–60	Surgery showed no effect on functional outcome at 3 years (ARR 1 %; 95 % confidence interval, −21 to 22) but improves survival (ARR 37 %; 95 % confidence interval, 14–60)
Hofmeijer et al. [48]	2013	Cost-effectiveness of surgical decompression for space-occupying hemispheric infarction (HAMLET)	RCT	39	18–60	Surgery improves survival and marginal improvement in functional outcome but at a high cost (high estimate of ~€127 000 per QALY gained)
Neugebauer et al. [53]	2013	DEPTH-SOS Trial	RCT		18–60	Ongoing trial
Hernandez-Medrano et al. [54]	2012	Decompressive craniectomy in MMCAI; experience after the implementation of a response protocol	Prospective observational	15	35–69	25 % mortality among those treated within 48 h versus 42.9 % among those treated later; trend toward improved functional outcome in younger patients

Lucas et al. [55]	2012	DCH for MMCAI: reproducing RCTs in daily practice	Prospective observational	31	18–60	mRS ≤4 at 1 year in 22 patients (71.0 %) and ≤3 in 16 (51.6 %); centers without significant experience can produce results congruent with RCTs
Slezins et al. [56]	2012	Preliminary results of randomized controlled study on decompressive craniectomy in treatment of malignant middle cerebral artery stroke	RCT	28	49–81	Surgery increases the probability of survival without increasing the number of severely disabled survivors
Zhao et al. [40]	2012	Decompressive hemicraniectomy in MMCAI: a randomized controlled trial enrolling patients up to 80 years old	RCT	47	29–80	Surgery within 48 h improves survival and functional outcome in patients up to 80 years of age
Juttler et al. [3]	2011	DESTINY II	RCT	≥60		Ongoing trial
Hofmeijer et al. [57]	2009	HAMLET	RCT	64	18–60	Surgical decompression reduces poor outcome (ARR 16 %, −0·1 to 33) and case fatality (ARR 50 %, 34 to 66)
Skoglund et al. [47]	2008	Health status and life satisfaction after decompressive craniectomy for MMCAI	Observational	18	37–66	At 1–6 years, patient remained impaired with good insight and felt life to be still satisfying
Chen et al. [21]	2007	Outcome of and prognostic factors for decompressive hemicraniectomy in MMCAI	Observational	60	19–89	30-day and 1 year mortality of 20 % and 26.6 %, respectively; age ≥60 years of age associated with poor outcome
Pillai et al. [23]	2007	DCH for MMCAI: long-term outcome and factors in patient selection	Observational	26	28–66	1-year postsurgery survival of 73 % a third of whom were independent and over half partially dependent; non-vegetative

(continued)

Table 23.1 (continued)

Author	Year	Study	Type	*N*	Age (years)	Finding
Juttler et al. [58]	2007	DESTINY Trial	RCT	32	29–60	Surgery yields mortality benefit without improvement in functional outcome
Vahedi et al. [11]	2007	DECIMAL	RCT	38	22–55	52.8 % ARR of death in surgically treated patients versus controls without significant difference in functional outcome
Malm et al. [22]	2006	Swedish MMCAI Study	Observational	30	17–67	Decompressive surgery favorable when patients survives acute phase; outcome better in younger patients
Els et al. [43]	2006	DCH +/– mild hypothermia for MMCAI	RCT	25	27–62	Combination of hypothermia with decompressive surgery poses no added risk and may improve functional outcome
Rabinstein et al. [26]	2006	Factors predicting prognosis after DCH for hemispheric infarction	Retrospective	42	15–73	Older age associated with poor functional outcome
Wang et al. [59]	2006	Factors predicting fatality in MMCAI following DCH	Retrospective	62	30–85	Low GCS, coronary artery disease and deterioration during hospitalization predictive of poor outcome; surgery improves survival but may not improve function
Cho et al. [20]	2003	Ultra-early decompressive craniectomy for MMCAI	Observational	52	45–80	Improved survival and functional outcome in patients undergoing surgery with further improvement in survival and function with ultra-early intervention

confidence interval, 15–70 %] versus 21 % in the medically managed group [90 % confidence interval, 6–47 %]). At 6 months, mortality in the surgical group had risen to 36 % without significant change in the medically managed controls. Death was attributed to complications of increased intracranial hypertension with brain stem compression, worsening cerebral infarction, cardiac arrhythmia, and withdrawal of life support. No subgroup analysis was performed to ascertain the impact of age on outcome.

23.6 Other Clinical Trials on Hemicraniectomy and Pooled Analysis of DECIMAL, DESTINY, and HAMLET

DECIMAL, DESTINY, and HAMLET are three multicenter European studies and are the first published randomized trials aimed at assessing the role of decompressive craniectomy for the specific indication of malignant middle cerebral infarctions. The effect of surgical decompression was largely consistent across all three trials in that all three showed a significant mortality benefit in surgically treated patients, with a less stellar improvement in functional outcome. All three studies were terminated prematurely due to a combination of poor recruitment and clear demonstration of statistically significant survival benefit. None attained sufficient power to detect potentially subtle differences in functional outcome—the primary outcome of interest. Thus, Vahedi et al. pooled patients from DECIMAL, DESTINY, and HAMLET to assess the role of early (<48 h after symptom onset) decompressive craniectomy on functional outcome in patients 18–60 years of age presenting with malignant cerebral artery infarction [30].

The pooled analysis included 93 patients from the three trials. The primary endpoint was outcome at 1 year dichotomized as favorable (mRS 0–4) or unfavorable (mRS 5 or death). Results of the pooled analysis supported a role for decompressive surgery in attaining a superior functional result defined as a modified Rankin score (mRS) $\leq$4 in 75 % of surgically treated versus 24 % of conservatively managed patients (absolute risk reduction 51 %; 95 % confidence interval 34–69 %). Similarly, 43 % of surgically treated versus 21 % of conservatively managed patients achieved mRS $\leq$3 (absolute risk reduction 23 %; 95 % confidence interval 5–41 %). Certainly, the most impressive finding remained the overall survival benefit of surgical intervention with 78 % of those undergoing surgery surviving to 1 year compared to 29 % of medically managed patients (absolute risk reduction 50 %; 95 % confidence interval 33–67 %). Based on these findings, the authors reported that only 2 patients would require surgical decompression to obtain survival with mRS $\leq$4 or survival regardless of outcome. When the functional outcome requirement was slightly more stringent (mRS $\leq$3), the number needed to treat was 4. When one considers that the number needed to treat with aspirin to prevent a single heart attack or stroke is 1 in 1667 (an admittedly apples to oranges comparison) [31, 32], decompressive surgery for malignant strokes appear to be a much more palatable intervention. In the subgroup analyses of age, timing of randomization, and presence of aphasia, surgical decompression retained efficacy for the primary outcome of mRS $\leq$4 (P <0.01).

23.7 Decompressive Hemicraniectomy in the Elderly

Germaine to the reader of this text on practices and standards in geriatric neurosurgery is the efficacy of decompressive surgery performed specifically on "elderly" patients particularly when there is a paucity of studies to guide clinical decision making. The European trials all limited the age of patients to ≤60 years based on several previous results from observational studies suggesting poorer outcome and/or survival in older patients [21, 24–26, 33–39]. However, as populations across the world age and present to clinical attention progressively older, clinicians are now forced to reconsider the definition of "elderly" in regard to decompressive hemicraniectomy for malignant middle cerebral infarcts. This has contributed to significant controversy regarding whether decompressive surgery is indicated for patients >60 years of age. Two randomized controlled trials have specifically addressed this question.

The first randomized controlled trial specifically addressing the role of decompressive hemicraniectomy for malignant cerebral artery infarcts was published by Zhao et al. in 2012 [40]. The authors designed the study using protocols derived from the DESTINY and HAMLET trials but included patients age 18–80 years of age. Recruitment began in July 2008 and the study was terminated in May 2010 after recruitment of 47 patients on the advice of the safety monitoring committee. The rationale for termination was that statistical superiority of the primary endpoint had already been determined on interim analysis. The primary end point was functional outcome at 6 months assessed as good (mRS 0–4) or poor (5–6). The secondary outcomes were death rates at 6 months and 1 year as well as functional outcome at 6 months and 1 year dichotomized as 0–3 versus 4–6.

The outcome among all 47 enrolled patients mirrored that obtained in the European trials and will not be described here. In the subgroup analysis of patients >60 years of age, 16 were randomized to surgery and 13 to medical therapy. Among this group, decompressive surgery conferred a clear mortality benefit at 6 months with 12.5 % mortality among the surgical group versus 61.5 % among those elderly patients randomized to medical management (absolute risk reduction 49.0 %; 95 % confidence interval, 18.0–80.1 %; NNT=2; $P=0.016$). The survival benefit remained at 1 year with 18.8 % mortality among surgically treated patients versus 69.2 % among medically treated patients (absolute risk reduction 50.5 %; 95 % confidence interval, 18.9–92.0; NNT=2; $P=0.010$). Similarly, decompressive surgery conferred a benefit on functional outcome among elderly patients. At 6 months, 33.3 % of surgically treated patients versus 82.6 % of conservatively managed patients had mRS >4 (absolute risk reduction 49.3 %; 95 % confidence interval, 24.9–73.7 %; NNT=2; $P=0.001$). The benefit on functional outcome was maintained at 1 year. When the authors analyzed the secondary outcome of mRS > 3 at 6 months and 1 year, there was a trend toward improved functional outcome among surgically treated patients but this did not reach statistical significance. They attributed this to the fact that the study was stopped when the primary endpoint was attained and that with additional recruitment, the secondary functional outcome would likely prove significant. In the absence of clairvoyance, additional studies or pooled analyses (akin to that performed for the European trials) will likely be needed to assess the degree of function attainable among patients >60 years of age undergoing decompressive surgery for malignant strokes.

23.8 DESTINY II

Results of the DESTINY II trial which limits analysis to patients >60 years of age was published in 2014 [41]. The authors randomized 112 patients to hemicraniectomy versus medical management within 48 h of symptom onset following the general protocol used in the original DESTINY trial. The primary endpoint was survival without severe disability (mRS 0–4) 6 months following randomization. The authors determined that surgical intervention statistically improved the primary outcome. Among patients who underwent decompressive surgery, 38 % survived with mRS 0–4 versus 18 % of medically treated controls (odds ratio, 2.91; 95 % confidence interval, 1.06–7.49; $P=0.04$). Complete recovery or recovery with only slight disability (mRS 0–2) was not attained in any patient included in the study. There was a trend toward less severe disability (mRS 3) among patients treated with surgery versus medical management (7 % versus 3 %) but this did not reach statistical significance.

23.9 Therapeutic Hypothermia Combined with Decompressive Craniectomy

A number of studies have demonstrated benefit of therapeutic hypothermia for malignant cerebral infarction with reduction in mortality by almost half [5, 28, 42]. Naturally, it is of interest to learn whether combination of therapeutic hypothermia with decompressive hemicraniectomy would lead to additive benefits in survival and functional outcome and a few prospective studies have evaluated this [43]. Els et al. found no significant difference in survival but did report a trend toward improved functional outcome in patients receiving combination therapy [43]. The Decompressive surgery Plus hypothermia for Space-Occupying Stroke (DEPTH-SOS) is an ongoing multicenter, randomized clinical trial of patients 18–60 to compare surgery versus surgery combined with hypothermia [44].

23.10 Illustrative Case: Malignant Middle Cerebral Artery Infarction

This is a 62-year-old teacher who developed acute right hemiparesis and aphasia while teaching. His relevant past medical history was significant for morbid obesity, obstructive sleep apnea, hypertension, hyperlipidemia, and recent onset of atrial fibrillation for which he was untreated. He was transferred to our facility after presenting to his local emergency department where intravenous tissue plasminogen activator was administered within 3 h of symptom onset. On arrival, he was

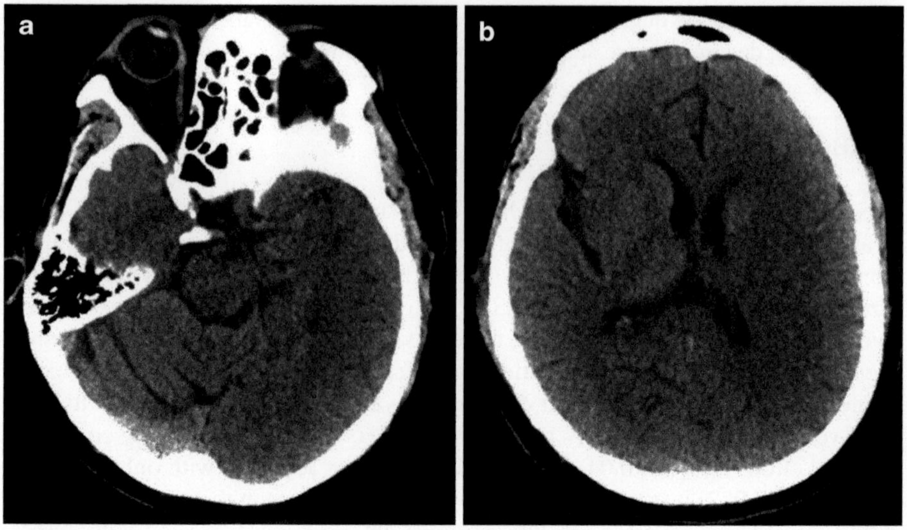

Fig. 23.1 Admission head CT showing a possible hyperdense left MCA sign (**a**) and early infarct characterized by sulcal effacement and loss of gray-white junction (**b**)

markedly hypertensive with systolic blood pressures in excess of 220 mmHg. Initial NIHSS was 26. He was emergently intubated due to severe orolingual edema that developed in the setting of tPA administration. Initial head CT (Fig. 23.1) revealed a hyperdense left MCA with sulcal effacement and loss of distinction of the gray-white junction consistent with early MCA infarction.

Given the lack of symptomatic improvement following IV tPA and the continued presence of a dense MCA, he was taken to angiography for embolectomy. TICI IIa revascularization was attained but was fleeting as he promptly rethrombosed the left M1 segment. He was transferred to the Neurocritical Care service where maximal medical efforts to reduce brain edema were undertaken. Repeat head CT the following morning revealed a large left MCA distribution infarct with a small focus of hemorrhagic transformation and worsening edema without midline shift (Fig. 23.2). Over the course of the day, he became increasingly somnolent and by the following morning (now approximately 44 h from onset), head CT showed worsening edema with new left-to-right midline shift and brain compression (Fig. 23.3). After a thorough discussion with the family including explicit counseling that surgery would likely improve the probability of survival without any significant improvement in his level of disability, the family requested that the surgical team proceed with decompressive hemicraniectomy.

Surgery was performed drawing on principles learned from decompressive craniotomies performed in the setting of battlefield injuries [45]. He was positioned supine with a slight bump under the left shoulder to optimize surgical access. A Mayfield head frame was attached. His head was shaved and the intended Ludwig G. Kempe incision [46] was marked as shown (Fig. 23.4). The incision was opened and carried down to the level of the periosteum, and the temporalis muscle was

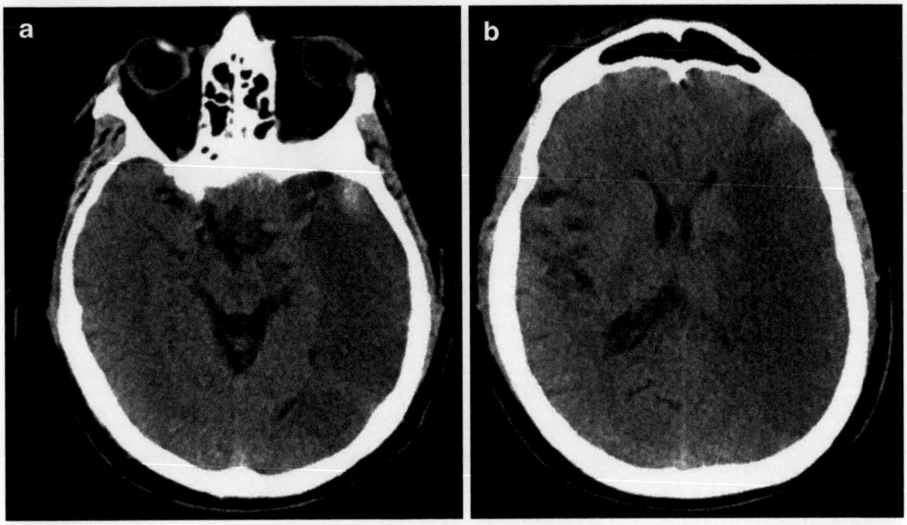

Fig. 23.2 Same areas depicted previously but now showing evolving left MCA hypodensity. Note the increased prominence of the left hyperdense MCA sign (**a**) but no evidence of midline shift (**b**)

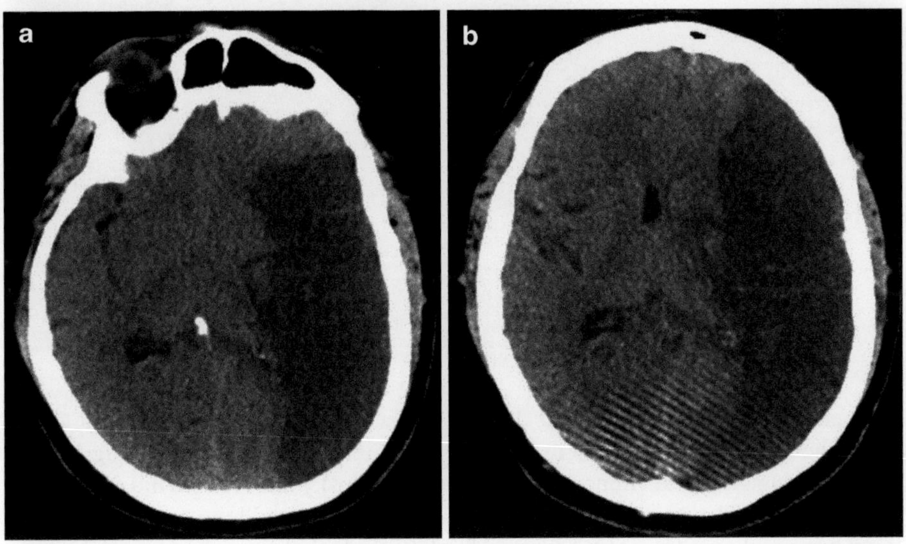

Fig. 23.3 Follow up CT shows (**a**) Brain compression and edema with compression of the third (**a**) and lateral (**b**) ventricles with midline shift of the pineal gland and septum pellucidum

elevated and retracted laterally so that the frontal, parietal, sphenoidal, temporal, and occipital bones were all exposed (Fig. 23.5). Burr holes were made at the pterion, the root of the zygoma, 2 cm above the asterion with an additional 3 burr holes along the midsagittal line approximately 1.5 cm lateral to midline to facilitate

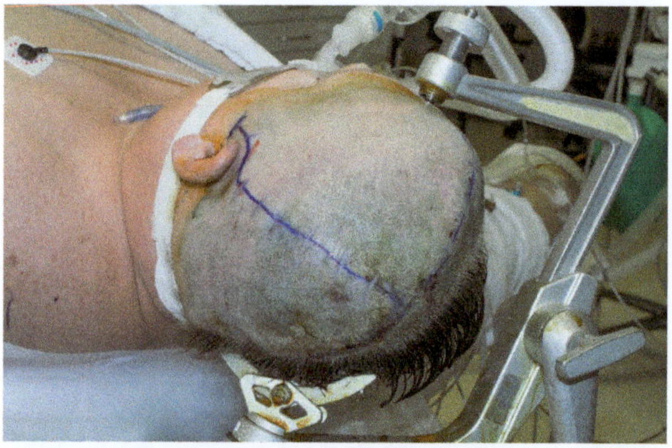

Fig. 23.4 Shows the hemicraniectomy incision with "T-Bar" extension. This is sometimes referred to as a "Tulip" incision

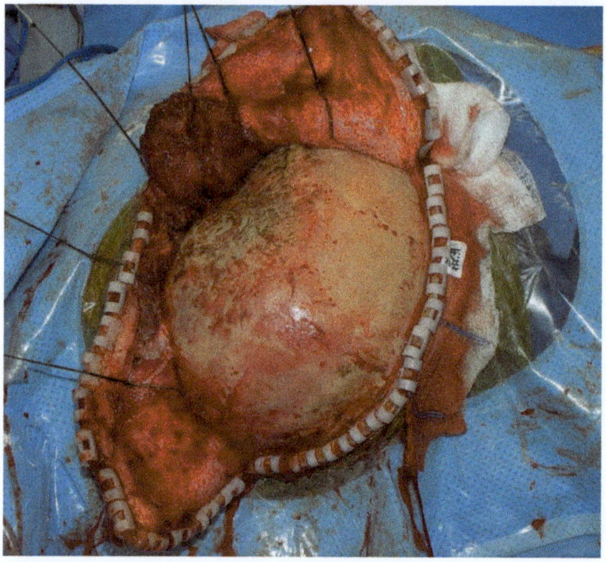

Fig. 23.5 Shows the cranial exposure obtained with this incision. There is exposure of the frontal, parietal, occipital, temporal, and sphenoid bones

safe removal of the bone without damage to the subjacent superior sagittal sinus. The bone flap was removed to expose the entire left hemisphere following stellate dural opening. The brain appeared edematous and dusky and was devoid of pulsatility (Fig. 23.6). The dura was not reapproximated but instead left open. Slabs of gel foam were laid over the brain followed by direct galeal closure. A running, locking stitch was used for skin apposition (Fig. 23.7). Postoperative head CT showed wide decompression with improvement in the mass effect and no further progression of hemorrhagic transformation (Fig. 23.8).

His ICU stay was complicated by hypernatremia in the setting of hyperosmolar therapy and ventilator-associated pneumonia secondary to methicillin-resistant *Staphylococcus aureus* which was diagnosed on postoperative day 8. He was

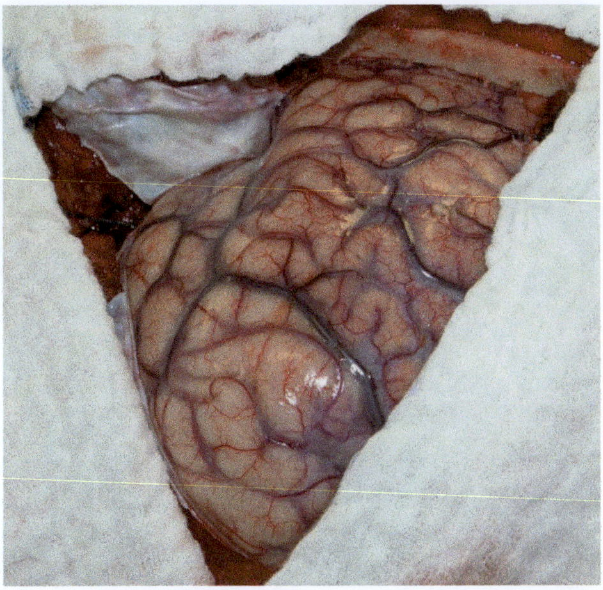

Fig. 23.6 Shows the brain exposure obtained following craniectomy with durotomy

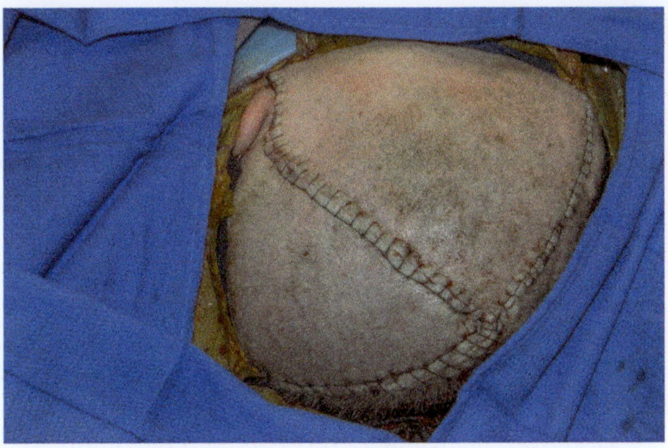

Fig. 23.7 Shows incision closed with running, locking nylon sutures

transferred to the Stroke service for continued cares. His hospital course was further complicated by acalculous cholecystitis requiring percutaneous cholecystostomy. He remained hospitalized for 1 month followed by discharge home with his wife. On discharge, he was globally aphasic but made attempts to communicate with gestures. He had persistent dense right hemiparesis consistent with a modified Rankin Score of 5. Consistent with data found in the literature, his wife and primary care taker believe the appropriate clinical course was undertaken and would make the same decisions again [44, 47].

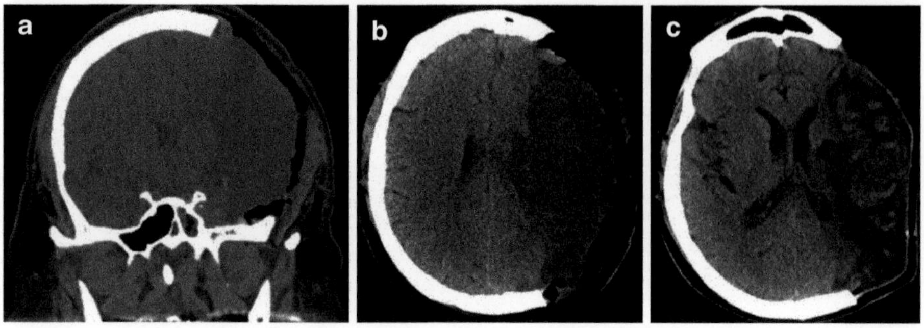

Fig. 23.8 Shows the immediate (**a**, **b**) and 1 month (**c**) postoperative results after decompression. There is bony decompression from the frontal pole to occiput beginning approximately 2–3 cm lateral to midline and extending down to the temporal fossa floor

23.11 Conclusions and Ethical Considerations

Evidence continues to amass in support of decompressive hemicraniectomy to relieve cerebral edema associated with malignant supratentorial infarctions. There is little controversy now about whether this intervention increases survival as all major studies have shown benefit. The question is whether the added survival benefit attained from this procedure represents life deemed by patients and their families as "worth living" a notoriously complex and value laden term. In as much as previous studies have shown a significant survival benefit following decompressive surgery, the data on functional outcome remain far less impressive and survival with significant functional impairment and perhaps lifelong dependence remain the likely outcome. A cost-effectiveness study of decompressive hemicraniectomy for surgical decompression at 3 years post-op reported an improvement of an average of 1 quality-adjusted life year (QALY) at a cost of >€80,000 per QALY [48]! Does survival with significant dependence warrant such herculean efforts and divergence of limited resources? A nation wide sample (2002–2011) showed a major disability with poor outcome (institutional care) in more than 3/4 of patients older than 60 year [49].

Moreover, decisions to proceed with decompressive hemicraniectomy are often made in patients with considerable comorbidity (i.e., congestive heart failure, atrial fibrillation, type 2 diabetes) and in patients with a living will. There is often a reason why patients developed a stroke, and the situation is very different from an unfortunate previously healthy young patient with a spontaneous carotid dissection and subsequent large swollen infarct. Are elderly patients "fit" enough to undergo often intensive neurorehabilitation programs? Is care continued after surgery which may include a tracheostomy and gastrostomy? Are patients eventually going to end up in a nursing home? Is there a support system available to provide long-term care? How do we interpret patient's own wishes if the patient is aphasic and has no means of communication? In our experience, many families of elderly patients opt out, and in patients who underwent decompressive surgery, many were left with the consequences of a devastating stroke. The discussions with family members of an elderly patient struck with a major swollen infarct and the potential for a life saving hemicraniectomy should focus on how the major disability will be dealt with-neurologically, socially, financially and emotionally.

References

1. Hacke W, Schwab S, Horn M, Spranger M, De Georgia M, von Kummer R (1996) 'Malignant' middle cerebral artery territory infarction: clinical course and prognostic signs. Arch Neurol 53(4):309–315
2. Rieke K, Schwab S, Krieger D et al (1995) Decompressive surgery in space-occupying hemispheric infarction: results of an open, prospective trial. Crit Care Med 23(9):1576–1587
3. Juttler E, Bosel J, Amiri H et al (2011) DESTINY II: DEcompressive surgery for the treatment of malignant INfarction of the middle cerebral arterY II. Int J Stroke 6(1):79–86
4. Schwarz S, Schwab S, Bertram M, Aschoff A, Hacke W (1998) Effects of hypertonic saline hydroxyethyl starch solution and mannitol in patients with increased intracranial pressure after stroke. Stroke 29(8):1550–1555
5. Schwab S, Spranger M, Schwarz S, Hacke W (1997) Barbiturate coma in severe hemispheric stroke: useful or obsolete? Neurology 48(6):1608–1613
6. Berrouschot J, Sterker M, Bettin S, Koster J, Schneider D (1998) Mortality of space-occupying ('malignant') middle cerebral artery infarction under conservative intensive care. Intensive Care Med 24(6):620–623
7. Rahme R, Curry R, Kleindorfer D et al (2012) How often are patients with ischemic stroke eligible for decompressive hemicraniectomy? Stroke 43(2):550–552
8. Moulin DE, Lo R, Chiang J, Barnett HJ (1985) Prognosis in middle cerebral artery occlusion. Stroke 16(2):282–284
9. Hofmeijer J, van der Worp HB, Kappelle LJ (2003) Treatment of space-occupying cerebral infarction. Crit Care Med 31(2):617–625
10. Hofmeijer J, van der Worp HB, Amelink GJ, Algra A, van Gijn J, Kappelle LJ (2003) Surgical decompression in space-occupying cerebral infarct; notification of a randomized trial. Ned Tijdschr Geneeskd 147(52):2594–2596
11. Vahedi K, Vicaut E, Mateo J et al (2007) Sequential-design, multicenter, randomized, controlled trial of early decompressive craniectomy in malignant middle cerebral artery infarction (DECIMAL Trial). Stroke 38(9):2506–2517
12. Wartenberg KE (2012) Malignant middle cerebral artery infarction. Curr Opin Crit Care 18(2):152–163
13. Simard JM, Chen M, Tarasov KV et al (2006) Newly expressed SUR1-regulated NC(Ca-ATP) channel mediates cerebral edema after ischemic stroke. Nat Med 12(4):433–440
14. Seth KN, Elm JJ, Molyneaux BJ et al (2016) Safety and efficacy of intravenous glyburide on brain swelling after large hemispheric infarction (GAMES-RP): a randomized, double-blind, placebo-controlled phase 2 trial. Lancet Neurology 15:1160–1169
15. Nakka VP, Gusain A, Mehta SL, Raghubir R (2008) Molecular mechanisms of apoptosis in cerebral ischemia: multiple neuroprotective opportunities. Mol Neurobiol 37(1):7–38
16. Cushing HI (1908) Subtemporal decompressive operations for the intracranial complications associated with bursting fractures of the skull. Ann Surg 47(5):641–644, 641
17. Rengachary SS, Batnitzky S, Morantz RA, Arjunan K, Jeffries B (1981) Hemicraniectomy for acute massive cerebral infarction. Neurosurgery 8(3):321–328
18. Kondziolka D, Bernstein M, Resch L, Tator CH (1988) Brain tumours presenting with tias and strokes. Can Fam Physician 34:283–286
19. Schwab S, Steiner T, Aschoff A et al (1998) Early hemicraniectomy in patients with complete middle cerebral artery infarction. Stroke 29(9):1888–1893

20. Cho DY, Chen TC, Lee HC (2003) Ultra-early decompressive craniectomy for malignant middle cerebral artery infarction. Surg Neurol 60(3):227–232; discussion 232–223
21. Chen CC, Cho DY, Tsai SC (2007) Outcome of and prognostic factors for decompressive hemicraniectomy in malignant middle cerebral artery infarction. J Clin Neurosci 14(4):317–321
22. Malm J, Bergenheim AT, Enblad P et al (2006) The Swedish malignant middle cerebral artery infarction study: long-term results from a prospective study of hemicraniectomy combined with standardized neurointensive care. Acta Neurol Scand 113(1):25–30
23. Pillai A, Menon SK, Kumar S, Rajeev K, Kumar A, Panikar D (2007) Decompressive hemicraniectomy in malignant middle cerebral artery infarction: an analysis of long-term outcome and factors in patient selection. J Neurosurg 106(1):59–65
24. Ziai WC, Port JD, Cowan JA, Garonzik IM, Bhardwaj A, Rigamonti D (2003) Decompressive craniectomy for intractable cerebral edema: experience of a single center. J Neurosurg Anesthesiol 15(1):25–32
25. Gupta R, Connolly ES, Mayer S, Elkind MS (2004) Hemicraniectomy for massive middle cerebral artery territory infarction: a systematic review. Stroke 35(2):539–543
26. Rabinstein AA, Mueller-Kronast N, Maramattom BV et al (2006) Factors predicting prognosis after decompressive hemicraniectomy for hemispheric infarction. Neurology 67(5):891–893
27. Milhaud D, Thouvenot E, Heroum C, Escuret E (2005) Prolonged moderate hypothermia in massive hemispheric infarction: clinical experience. J Neurosurg Anesthesiol 17(1):49–53
28. Schwab S, Schwarz S, Bertram M, Spranger M, Hacke W (1999) Moderate hypothermia for the treatment of malignant middle cerebral artery infarct. Nervenarzt 70(6):539–546
29. Frank JI, Schumm LP, Wroblewski K et al (2014) Hemicraniectomy and durotomy upon deterioration from infarction-related swelling trial: randomized pilot clinical trial. Stroke 45(3):781–787
30. Vahedi K, Hofmeijer J, Juettler E et al (2007) Early decompressive surgery in malignant infarction of the middle cerebral artery: a pooled analysis of three randomised controlled trials. Lancet Neurol 6(3):215–222
31. Baigent C, Blackwell L, Collins R et al (2009) Aspirin in the primary and secondary prevention of vascular disease: collaborative meta-analysis of individual participant data from randomised trials. Lancet 373(9678):1849–1860
32. Group TN. Aspirin to prevent a first heart attack or stroke. 2015; http://www.thennt.com/nnt/aspirin-to-prevent-a-first-heart-attack-or-stroke/
33. Arac A, Blanchard V, Lee M, Steinberg GK (2009) Assessment of outcome following decompressive craniectomy for malignant middle cerebral artery infarction in patients older than 60 years of age. Neurosurg Focus 26(6):E3
34. Holtkamp M, Buchheim K, Unterberg A et al (2001) Hemicraniectomy in elderly patients with space occupying media infarction: improved survival but poor functional outcome. J Neurol Neurosurg Psychiatry 70(2):226–228
35. Leonhardt G, Wilhelm H, Doerfler A et al (2002) Clinical outcome and neuropsychological deficits after right decompressive hemicraniectomy in MCA infarction. J Neurol 249(10):1433–1440
36. Uhl E, Kreth FW, Elias B et al (2004) Outcome and prognostic factors of hemicraniectomy for space occupying cerebral infarction. J Neurol Neurosurg Psychiatry 75(2):270–274
37. Wang DZ, Nair DS, Talkad AV (2011) Acute decompressive hemicraniectomy to control high intracranial pressure in patients with malignant MCA ischemic strokes. Curr Treat Options Cardiovasc Med 13(3):225–232
38. Yang XF, Yao Y, Hu WW et al (2005) Is decompressive craniectomy for malignant middle cerebral artery infarction of any worth? J Zhejiang Univ Sci B 6(7):644–649
39. Yao Y, Liu W, Yang X, Hu W, Li G (2005) Is decompressive craniectomy for malignant middle cerebral artery territory infarction of any benefit for elderly patients? Surg Neurol 64(2):165–169; discussion 169
40. Zhao J, Su YY, Zhang Y et al (2012) Decompressive hemicraniectomy in malignant middle cerebral artery infarct: a randomized controlled trial enrolling patients up to 80 years old. Neurocrit Care 17(2):161–171

41. Juttler E, Unterberg A, Woitzik J et al (2014) Hemicraniectomy in older patients with extensive middle-cerebral-artery stroke. N Engl J Med 370(12):1091–1100
42. Steiner T, Ringleb P, Hacke W (2001) Treatment options for large ischemic stroke. Neurology 57(5 Suppl 2):S61–68
43. Els T, Oehm E, Voigt S, Klisch J, Hetzel A, Kassubek J (2006) Safety and therapeutical benefit of hemicraniectomy combined with mild hypothermia in comparison with hemicraniectomy alone in patients with malignant ischemic stroke. Cerebrovasc Dis 21(1–2):79–85
44. Neugebauer H, Creutzfeldt CJ, Hemphill JC 3rd, Heuschmann PU, Juttler E (2014) DESTINY-S: attitudes of physicians toward disability and treatment in malignant MCA infarction. Neurocrit Care 21(1):27–34
45. Ragel BT, Klimo P Jr, Martin JE, Teff RJ, Bakken HE, Armonda RA (2010) Wartime decompressive craniectomy: technique and lessons learned. Neurosurg Focus 28(5):E2
46. Kempe L (ed) (1968) Hemispherectomy. In: Operative neurosurgery; No. 1 Springer, New York
47. Skoglund TS, Eriksson-Ritzen C, Sorbo A, Jensen C, Rydenhag B (2008) Health status and life satisfaction after decompressive craniectomy for malignant middle cerebral artery infarction. Acta Neurol Scand 117(5):305–310
48. Hofmeijer J, van der Worp HB, Kappelle LJ, Eshuis S, Algra A, Greving JP (2013) Cost-effectiveness of surgical decompression for space-occupying hemispheric infarction. Stroke 44(10):2923–2925
49. Dasenbrock HH, Robertson FC, Aziz-Sultan MA, et al (2016) Patient Age and the Outcomes after Decompressive Hemicraniectomy for Stroke: A Nationwide Inpatient Sample Analysis Neurocritical care (Published Online)
50. Rai VK, Bhatia R, Prasad K et al (2014) Long-term outcome of decompressive hemicraniectomy in patients with malignant middle cerebral artery infarction: a prospective observational study. Neurol India 62(1):26–31
51. Shao A, Guo S, Chen S et al (2013) Comparison between routine and improved decompressive craniectomy on patients with malignant cerebral artery infarction without traumatic brain injury. J Craniofac Surg 24(6):2085–2088
52. Geurts M, van der Worp HB, Kappelle LJ, Amelink GJ, Algra A, Hofmeijer J (2013) Surgical decompression for space-occupying cerebral infarction: outcomes at 3 years in the randomized HAMLET trial. Stroke 44(9):2506–2508
53. Neugebauer H, Kollmar R, Niesen WD et al (2013) DEcompressive surgery plus hypoTHermia for space-occupying stroke (DEPTH-SOS): a protocol of a multicenter randomized controlled clinical trial and a literature review. Int J Stroke 8(5):383–387
54. Hernandez-Medrano I, Matute MC, Abreu F et al (2012) Decompressive craniectomy in malignant middle cerebral artery infarction. Experience after the implementation of a response protocol. Rev Neurol 54(10):593–600
55. Lucas C, Thines L, Dumont F et al (2012) Decompressive surgery for malignant middle cerebral artery infarcts: the results of randomized trials can be reproduced in daily practice. Eur Neurol 68(3):145–149
56. Slezins J, Keris V, Bricis R et al (2012) Preliminary results of randomized controlled study on decompressive craniectomy in treatment of malignant middle cerebral artery stroke. Medicina (Kaunas) 48(10):521–524
57. Hofmeijer J, Kappelle LJ, Algra A, Amelink GJ, van Gijn J, van der Worp HB (2009) Surgical decompression for space-occupying cerebral infarction (the Hemicraniectomy After Middle Cerebral Artery infarction with Life-threatening Edema Trial [HAMLET]): a multicentre, open, randomised trial. Lancet Neurol 8(4):326–333
58. Juttler E, Schwab S, Schmiedek P et al (2007) Decompressive surgery for the treatment of malignant infarction of the middle cerebral artery (DESTINY): a randomized, controlled trial. Stroke 38(9):2518–2525
59. Wang KW, Chang WN, Ho JT et al (2006) Factors predictive of fatality in massive middle cerebral artery territory infarction and clinical experience of decompressive hemicraniectomy. Eur J Neurol 13(7):765–771

Part VII

Miscellaneous

Trigeminal Neuralgia in the Elderly 24

Jonathan Cohen, Hossein Mousavi,
and Raymond F. Sekula Jr.

24.1 Introduction

Trigeminal neuralgia (TN), known as tic douloureux, is a neuropathic pain condition characterized by electric, stabbing, paroxysmal episodes of facial pain in one or more of the sensory distributions of the trigeminal nerve. For those individuals affected by TN, the pain is often characterized as "the worst pain known to man." The existence of this disease has been recognized for centuries, and despite advancement in our current knowledge of TN, management of this disease remains, at times, inadequate. This painful condition incapacitates those affected by it, and its impact on quality of life underscores the need to further enhance both our preclinical and clinical understanding of TN.

The incidence of TN increases with advancing age. The management of TN in elderly patients is considerably nuanced and requires a personalized treatment plan for each patient. The goal of this chapter is to provide an overview of TN treatment in elderly patients and to discuss the composite factors influencing their neurosurgical management.

24.2 Epidemiology

Epidemiological data concerning TN is limited, and the epidemiology of TN in the USA is particularly poor because of a decentralized medical system and inconsistencies in diagnoses. Nevertheless, best available data suggest that the prevalence of

The original version of this chapter was revised.
An erratum to this chapter can be found at DOI 10.1007/978-3-319-40232-1_28

J. Cohen • H. Mousavi • R.F. Sekula Jr. (✉)
University of Pittsburgh, Pittsburgh, PA, USA
e-mail: rsekula@wpahs.org

© Springer International Publishing Switzerland 2017

M. Berhouma, P. Krolak-Salmon (eds.), *Brain and Spine Surgery in the Elderly*,
DOI 10.1007/978-3-319-40232-1_24

TN in the USA is approximately 15,000 cases per year, affecting nearly .01 % of the world's population. No racial differences or geographic tendencies have been found, and a sex-adjusted rate demonstrates that women (5.9 in 100,000) have a higher incidence of TN than men (3.4 in 100,000) [1, 2].

TN disproportionally affects older patients, and the peak onset occurs between the ages of 50 and 70 years. Epidemiological studies have reported that the incidence of TN increases with age from roughly 4.1 per 100,000 persons [1] in the general population to >20 per 100,000 persons over the age of 65 [3].

24.3 Pathogenesis

Because the most effective therapeutic interventions address a disorder's etiopathogenesis, it is imperative, when possible, to properly classify patients with different etiologies of facial pain.

While the exact etiopathogenesis of TN remains unknown, a number of factors have been suggested as potential causes of the disorder. A causal relationship between vascular compression of the trigeminal nerve and facial pain was first suggested by Dandy. Dandy noted, "that in many instances, the nerve is grooved or bent by the artery. This I believe is the cause of tic douloureax" [4]. Clinical evidence of demyelination associated with TN was originally reported by Hilton and colleagues. Staining followed by electron microscopy revealed degraded central myelin at the site of arterial compression in a single patient [5]. This observation was subsequently replicated by Rappaport et al. who published an analysis of biopsy samples obtained from the site of compression in 12 patients with TN undergoing microvascular decompression (MVD). Interestingly, in 11 of 12 patients, both demyelination and axonopathy were noted by biopsy even though only 7 of the 12 patients had intraoperatively confirmed arterial compression of the trigeminal nerve [6]. This data suggests that while demyelination may be present in most patients with TN, vascular compression may not result in demyelination [7]. Furthermore, the authors introduced the concept of the "ignition hypothesis" which holds that damage to the root entry zone of the trigeminal nerve induces parts of the trigeminal ganglion to develop autorhythmicity [8].

Given that TN more often affects patients of advanced age, it is plausible that the aging process predisposes individuals to TN. However, a mechanistic understanding of the age-related changes unique to TN remains to be elucidated. Janetta postulated that the prevalence of TN in elderly patients reflects age-related changes such as cerebral atrophy and atherosclerosis resulting in increased vascular compression. The pathophysiology of TN remains uncertain.

24.4 Medical Treatment of Trigeminal Neuralgia in the Elderly

In an effort to avoid or minimize adverse pharmacologic side effects for patients, medical management of TN requires an understanding of the age-related changes in pharmacological responses in elderly patients. In addition, the presence of multiple comorbidities and the requirement for multiple medications require careful consideration in this population. Poor compliance, reduced homeostatic control, and altered metabolizing ability are some of the factors accounting for the large variability in drug response seen in the elderly population. In effect, elderly patients present with a constrained therapeutic window in the pharmacologic management of TN [9].

Various therapeutic targets for medical management of TN have been identified including glutamate receptors, sodium and calcium channels, monoamines, and neurotropic factors. Antiseizure medications are the standard medical treatment for TN beginning with the use of phenytoin in 1942. Current antiseizure medications including carbamazepine (CBZ) and oxcarbazepine (OXC) are recommended by the American Academy of Neurology (AAN) and European Federation of Neurological Societies (EFNS) as first-line drugs [10]. Only a handful of trials have specifically investigated medical management in the elderly with TN [11].

CBZ and OXC are perhaps the most effective medications currently used to manage the symptoms of TN [12, 13]. Sodium channel activity appears to play an important role in the emergence of pain, and thus inhibition of Na^+ channels by CBZ and OXC can provide effective relief [14]. A series of particularly important randomized control trials demonstrated the efficacy of CBZ with a reduction in both the intensity and frequency of painful paroxysms in 76 % of patients. These trials evaluated the treatment response to CBZ and found the number of patients needed to treat (NNT) to attain meaningful pain relief to be 1.7–1.8. The onset of relief can occur within several hours; however, its efficacy often diminishes after 5 years [12, 15].

CBZ has a narrow therapeutic range with increasingly intolerable effects (e.g. nausea, fatigue, diplopia, memory loss, nystagmus, liver dysfunction, and hemato-suppression) in the elderly. Moreover, CBZ may precipitate skin rash, cardiac defects in patients with preexisting cardiac failure, and symptoms of imbalance, dizziness, and blurred vision, which increase the risk of falling [10, 16, 17]. A series of studies investigating CBZ response in the elderly have demonstrated age-related declines in CBZ metabolism and efficacy. Koyama et al. studied the effects of biological maturation on pharmacological properties of CBZ and found that older patients displayed decreased levels of non-glycated albumin—a major ligand of CBZ—and an accelerated increase in serum CBZ levels, rendering them more sensitive to pharmacological complications and adverse drug interactions [18]. An initial dose of 100 mg/day of CBZ—ranging from 100–2400 mg/day—is recommended for elderly patients, which can then be increased as tolerated [10, 11].

A second treatment of choice, oxcarbazepine (OXC), a keto-derivative of CBZ, is another commonly used antiseizure medication for TN. Despite structural similarities to CBZ, OXC offers several important clinical advantages. OXC, unlike CBZ, bypasses the liver cytochrome system, in doing so avoiding epoxidation and the release of catabolic enzymes that diminish the efficacy of other medications. OXC provides pain relief within 24–72 h [12, 15, 19]. When considering predisposition to comorbidities, one advantage of OXC is its improved safety profile including better tolerability and a reduction in unacceptable side effects. Kuthluay et al. reported that the adverse event profile of OXC in the elderly group was not noticeably different from that in younger adults. In their studies, 81 % of patients in the elderly group experienced at least one OXC-induced adverse event compared to 87 % in the younger group. The four most common adverse events in the elderly group included nausea (17 %), dizziness (17 %), somnolence (15 %), and vomiting (19 %). Interestingly, the reported incidence for dizziness (29 %), nausea (20 %), and somnolence (24 %) was higher in the younger group, although the difference was not statistically significant [20].

Not infrequently, patients are refractory to or develop tolerance to the recommended frontline therapeutics. As suggested by the AAN and EFNS, if a patient is refractory to either CBZ or OXC, second-line medications (including lamotrigine, baclofen, and gabapentin) are recommended [10]. In a small randomized control trial, Fromm et al. provided evidence for the use of baclofen (50–80 mg/day), demonstrating pain relief in 74 % of patients and continued pain relief (>5 years) in 30 % of patients with TN [21]. Moreover, in a crossover randomized control trial, Zakrzewska demonstrated that lamotrigine (200–400 mg/day) in conjunction with CBZ provided superior relief compared to placebo. Consistent with other reports, however, these studies discuss the high incidence of side effects—drowsiness, dizziness, loss of muscle tone, sedation, GI discomfort, and Stevens-Johnson's syndrome—linked to these drugs and thus they are not recommended for the elderly [22].

It is generally recommended that pretreatment assessment and clinical evaluation be performed prior to and during medical treatment including blood work (i.e., measurement of electrolytes, liver enzymes and function, vitamin D levels, and baseline hematology measurements) [11].

24.4.1 Surgical Management of TN

While medical management is often the first-line treatment of TN in all patients, the value of early surgical intervention is increasingly recognized for optimal surgical benefit and avoidance of intolerable side effects [23]. Surgical treatments for TN are either ablative or non-ablative. Techniques aimed at intentional ablation of a component of the trigeminal system include percutaneous glycerol rhizolysis of the Gasserian ganglion (PGZ), percutaneous radiofrequency rhizolysis of the Gasserian ganglion (PRZ), percutaneous balloon compression of the Gasserian ganglion (PBC), and stereotactic radiosurgery rhizolysis of the cisternal segment of trigeminal nerve (SRS). Microvascular decompression (MVD) of the centrally myelinated portion of the trigeminal nerve is the only non-ablative surgical procedure for TN. This section will discuss the various surgical options for TN.

24.5 Microvascular Decompression

Microvascular decompression, wherein a compressive blood vessel is separated from the trigeminal nerve by a prosthesis, is a non-ablative technique for TN [24]. MVD provides the greatest initial efficacy and long-term pain relief with low risk of sensory loss [25–28]. In a series of 1185 patients, Barker et al. reported that 82 % of patients achieved complete pain relief post MVD, 64 % maintained excellent relief 10 years after the procedure, and less than 1 % developed sensory dysfunction [29]. Durable pain relief with infrequent sensory deficits is the hallmark of MVD for TN.

MVD, however, is an invasive procedure that carries with it certain risks not associated with the ablative procedures including cerebellar hematoma, cranial nerve injury, stroke, and death [25, 30]. Historically, the safety of MVD in the elderly has been a concern prompting some neurosurgeons to apply an "age cutoff" when recommending MVD. More recently, however, others have provided data that fitness, rather than age, should be used in the decision to recommend MVD [31–33]. In a prospective study of 36 elderly patients and 53 non-elderly patients having undergone MVD, 86 % of patients realized an excellent outcome following MVD. In most circumstances, MVD is a safe and effective treatment for elderly patients as factors including pain relief, recurrence, complications, and length of stay do not significantly differ between the elderly and non-elderly patients [31, 32, 34–37].

24.5.1 Non-ablative Procedures

Ablative procedures for TN include percutaneous glycerol rhizolysis of the Gasserian ganglion (PGZ), percutaneous radiofrequency rhizolysis of the Gasserian ganglion (PRZ), percutaneous balloon compression of the Gasserian ganglion (PBC), and stereotactic radiosurgery rhizolysis of the cisternal segment of trigeminal nerve (SRS). Despite an increased risk of sensory dysfunction, ablative procedures are more often recommended for the elderly.

The use of percutaneous radiotherapy rhizotomy for TN was made popular by Sweet and Wepsic based on the discovery that thermal lesioning of the trigeminal ganglion blocks nocireceptors on the nerve [38]. Like the other ablative techniques, PRZ offers distinct advantages and disadvantages for patients with TN. Immediate pain relief following PRZ is common, occurring in approximately 98 % of cases. Most suggestive among these was a retrospective study by Tang that included 304 elderly patients (70 years or older) treated with PRZ. Complete pain relief was observed in 100 % of patients at discharge; however, the rate of pain relief dropped to 85 %, 75 %, and 49 % at 1 year, 3 years, and 10 years, respectively [39]. Although PRZ is the most durable ablative procedure (i.e., longest half-life), nearly all patients experience sensory loss following the procedure [38].

Another ablative procedure is percutaneous glycerol rhizolysis of the Gasserian ganglion. The advantages of the glycerol procedure are its rapid action and decreased association with sensory deficits, including dysesthesias, compared to other percutaneous procedures. In a study investigating the efficacy of PGZ for TN, 77 % of patients maintained complete pain relief, and 37 % noted sensory loss at a median follow-up of 7.5 months [40]. Despite this, results from different series have been highly variable, and studies have not addressed the efficacy of PGZ in the elderly specifically.

Stereotactic radiosurgical rhizolysis (SRS) of the cisternal segment of the trigeminal nerve is increasingly used in patients with TN that have demonstrated intolerance or have proven refractory to medical management. SRS, typically performed using the Gamma Knife®, applies radiation to a single 4-mm isocenter positioned at the trigeminal nerve root entry zone. Several studies have reported the efficacy of Gamma Knife treatment for management of TN showing that approximately 41–76.4 % of patients achieve complete pain relief, 22–28 % achieved significant pain relief, while 5–21 % of patients achieved minimal to no pain relief. The onset of pain relief is often delayed (i.e., 30–60 days) and with side effects of facial numbness (9–37 %) and paresthesias (6–13 %) [41, 42]. Because of its delayed effect, SRS is not appropriate for patients with intractable pain. Many studies investigating the outcome of TN patients following surgical interventions are confounded by nonhomogeneous populations due to multiple treatments and differences in TN classification. In a recent report studying outcomes in patients that underwent SRS as their initial surgery, 88 % of patients achieved so-called adequate pain relief (BNI I–IIIa). Moreover, early SRS (within 3 years of symptoms) as the initial surgical procedure for management of refractory TN was associated with faster, better, and longer pain relief when compared to late SRS [23]. Success rates of SRS depend on a number of factors; however, Oh et al. dismissed any causal link between age and outcome following SRS. Consistent with studies in younger patients, favorable outcomes following SRS were observed in 55.6 % of elderly patients with a recurrence rate of 11.1 %. Moreover, the results demonstrated that 5.5 % of patients experienced paresthesia [43]. Karam et al. evaluated the outcomes in patients with TN following GammaKnife RadioSurgery (GKRS) and found a significant correlation between age and pain recurrence with age >70 years predicting a favorable outcome [44].

Percutaneous balloon microcompression (PBC) of the Gasserian ganglion, another ablative procedure, emerged in the field of neurosurgery with the observation that injury to the trigeminal ganglion, via mechanical compression, results in relief of TN. Nearly all patients achieve immediate pain relief however; recurrence rates approximate 6–14 % at 1 year, rising to nearly 20 % and 30 % by 5 and 10 years, respectively. The procedure is not without its risk as incidences of dysesthesia, masseter muscle weakness, hearing loss, anesthesia dolorosa, and subarachnoid hemorrhage can occur [45–48].

While ablative procedures provide immediate or near-immediate pain relief, TN recurrence within a few years is the norm. In our center, because MVD has the best efficacy, durability, and cost-effectiveness in the young and elderly with TN, ablative procedures are reserved for those deemed unfit for MVD, those with a life expectancy of only a few years, or when MVD fails to relieve the pain of trigeminal neuralgia.

24.6 Imaging and TN

Traditionally, identification of candidates for MVD relied on a number of factors such as the patient's clinical history and descriptions of TN-related symptoms. However, several other factors, notably the confirmation of neurovascular contact, have demonstrated significant predication of postoperative outcome. Imaging provides anatomic detail of the trigeminal system, allowing the surgeon to identify abnormal areas of the nerve and particular targets for treatment. Maarbjerg et al. evaluated the prevalence of neurovascular contact in patients with TN using 3.0 T magnetic resonance imaging. Severe neurovascular contact was caused by arteries in 98 % of patients and was more frequently observed on the symptomatic side compared to the asymptomatic side [49].

While a causal link between neurovascular contact and facial pain requires further investigation, we found that the confirmation of neurovascular contact using MRI demonstrated significant discriminatory ability for the prediction of pain-free response to MVD, as 83 % of patients with MRI-based evidence of neurovascular contact maintained pain-free relief at follow-up [24, 50]. The evolution of high-resolution magnetic resonance imaging (MRI) increasingly aids in identifying those patients with characteristic symptoms likely to respond to MVD.

Conclusion

TN remains a challenging disorder to manage, but our understanding of the pathogenesis and options for treatment is improving. In elderly patients, the management of TN is a multidimensional approach that differs from standard medical treatment in its heightened clinical complexity concerning medical, social, and mental factors implicated in advanced age. Due to the increased incidence of TN in elderly patients, management of TN is subject to increasing pressure to improve the delivery of care and the quality of life in this population.

A number of therapeutic options have proved useful in the management of facial pain. Medical management—in particular CBZ and OXC—is considered first-line therapy; however, due to the often unpredictable health status of elderly patients, refractoriness, intolerability, and the emergence of unwanted complications are common in this population. Surgical intervention is performed frequently, with considerable success; however, the fitness of elderly patients and potential complications must be factored into the treatment plan. While MVD provides the best potential for improvement, there is reluctance to perform this technique in older patients due to presumed complications and risks associated with MVD. As such, less invasive methods—including SRS and percutaneous procedures—are preferred for older patients. This view has been questioned more recently by studies demonstrating similar outcomes for elderly and non-elderly patients following MVD. Concerning the appropriate management of elderly patients, several treatments proposed for TN have reported positive results. This leads us to question what factors account for the differences in efficacy among treatments and emphasizes the need for further refinement of the criteria for appropriate management of elderly patients.

References

1. Katusic S, Beard CM, Bergstralh E, Kurland LT (1990) Incidence and clinical features of trigeminal neuralgia, Rochester, Minnesota, 1945–1984. Ann Neurol 27:89–95
2. Manzoni GC, Torelli P (2005) Epidemiology of typical and atypical craniofacial neuralgias. Neurol Sci 26(2):s65–s67
3. Amador N, Gorman D, Pollock BE (2006) Results of repeat posterior fossa exploration for patients with medically intractable trigeminal neuralgia. Neurosurgery 59:471

4. Dandy W (1934) Concerning the cause of trigeminal neuralgia. Am J Surg 24:447–455
5. Hilton DA, Love S, Gradidge T, Coakham HB (1994) Pathological findings associated with trigeminal neuralgia caused by vascular compression. Neurosurgery 5:299–303
6. Rappaport ZH, Govrin-Lippmann R, Devor M (1997) An electron-microscopic analysis of biopsy samples of the trigeminal root taken during microvascular decompressive surgery. Stereotact Funct Neurosurg 68:182–186
7. Sekula RF Jr (2016) Pathogenesis of trigeminal neuralgia. In: Sekula RF Jr (ed) Microvascular decompression surgery. Springer, Dordrecht
8. Devor M, Amir R, Rappaport ZH (2002) Pathophysiology of trigeminal neuralgia: the ignition hypothesis. Clin J Pain 18:4–13
9. Seymour RM, Routledge PA (1998) Important drug–drug interactions in the elderly. Drugs Aging 12(6):485–494
10. Cruccu G et al (2008) AAN-EFNS guidelines on trigeminal neuralgia management. Eur J Neurol 15(10):1013–1028
11. Oomens MA, Forouzanfar T (2015) Pharmaceutical management of trigeminal neuralgia in the elderly. Drugs Aging 32(9):717–726
12. Jorns TP, Zakrzewska JM (2007) Evidence-based approach to the medical management of trigeminal neuralgia. Br J Neurosurg 21(3):253–261
13. Zakrzewska JM (2010) Medical management of trigeminal neuropathic pains. Expert Opin Pharmacother 11(8):1239–1254
14. Ambrósio AF, Soares-Da-Silva P, Carvalho CM, Carvalho AP (2002) Mechanisms of action of carbamazepine and its derivatives, oxcarbazepine, BIA 2-093, and BIA 2-024. Neurochem Res 27:121–130
15. Sindrup SH, Jensen TS (2002) Pharmacotherapy of trigeminal neuralgia. Clin J Pain 18(1):22–27
16. Kramlinger KG, Phillips KA, Post RM (1994) Rash complicating carbamazepine treatment. J Clin Psychopharmacol 14(6):408–413
17. Killian JM, Fromm GH (1968) Carbamazepine in the treatment of neuralgia: use and side effects. Arch Neurol 19(2):129–136
18. Koyama H et al (1999) Age-related alteration of carbamazepine-serum protein binding in man. J Pharm Pharmacol 51(9):1009–1014
19. Gomez-Arguelles JM et al (2008) Oxcarbazepine monotherapy in carbamazepine-unresponsive trigeminal neuralgia. J Clin Neurosci 15(5):516–519
20. Kutluay E et al (2003) Safety and tolerability of oxcarbazepine in elderly patients with epilepsy. Epilepsy Behav 4(2):175–180
21. Fromm GH, Terrence CF, Chattha AS (1984) Baclofen in the treatment of trigeminal neuralgia: double-blind study and long-term follow-up. Ann Neurol 15(3):240–244
22. Zakrzewska JM, Chaudhry Z, Nurmikko TJ, Patton DW, Mullens EL (1997) Lamotrigine (Lamictal) in refractory trigeminal neuralgia: results from a double-blind placebo controlled crossover trial. Pain 73:223–230
23. Mousavi SH, Niranjan A, Huang MJ, Laghari FJ, Shin SS, Mindlin JL, Flickinger JC, Lunsford LD (2015) Early radiosurgery provides superior pain relief for trigeminal neuralgia patients. Neurology 85(24):2159–2165
24. Panczykowski DM et al (2016) Blinded, case-control trial assessing the value of steady state free precession magnetic resonance imaging in the diagnosis of trigeminal neuralgia. World Neurosurg 89:427–433
25. Burchiel KJ et al (1988) Long-term efficacy of microvascular decompression in trigeminal neuralgia. J Neurosurg 69(1):35–38
26. Kalkanis SN, Eskandar E, Carter BS, Barker FG 2nd (2003) Microvascular decompression surgery in the United States, 1996 to 2000: mortality rates, morbidity rates, and the effects of hospital and surgeon volumes. Neurosurgery 52(6):1251–1261
27. Zakrzewska JM, Coakham H (2012) Microvascular decompression for trigeminal neuralgia: update. Curr Opin Neurol 25(3):296–301

28. Zakrzewska JM, Lopez BC, Kim SE, Coakham HB (2005) Patient reports of satisfaction after microvascular decompression and partial sensory rhizotomy for trigeminal neuralgia. Neurosurgery 56(6):1304–1311
29. Barker FG et al (1996) The long-term outcome of microvascular decompression for trigeminal neuralgia. N Engl J Med 334(17):1077–1084
30. McLaughlin MR et al (1999) Microvascular decompression of cranial nerves: lessons learned after 4400 operations. J Neurosurg 90(1):1–8
31. Jödicke A et al (1999) Microvascular decompression as treatment of trigeminal neuralgia in the elderly patient. Minim Invasive Neurosurg 42(02):92–96
32. Sekula RF et al (2008) Microvascular decompression for trigeminal neuralgia in elderly patients. J Neurosurg 108:89–91
33. Ferroli P et al (2010) Advanced age as a contraindication to microvascular decompression for drug-resistant trigeminal neuralgia: evidence of prejudice? Neurol Sci 31:23–28
34. Günther T, Gerganov V, Stieglitz L, Ludemann W, Samii A (2009) Microvascular decompression for trigeminal neuralgia in the elderly: long-term treatment outcome and comparison with younger patients. Neurosurgery 65(3):477–482
35. Javadpour M, Eldridge PR, Varma TR, Miles JB, Nurmikko TJ (2003) Microvascular decompression for trigeminal neuralgia in patients over 70 years of age. Neurology 60(3):520
36. Ryu H et al (1999) Neurovascular decompression for trigeminal neuralgia in elderly patients. Neurol Med Chir 39(3):226–230
37. Ogungbo BI, Kelly P, Kane PJ, Nath FP (2000) Microvascular decompression for trigeminal neuralgia: report of outcome in patients over 65 years of age. Br J Neurosurg 14(5):504
38. Sweet WH, Wepsic JG (1974) Controlled thermocoagulation of trigeminal ganglion and rootlets for differential destruction of pain fibers. J Neurosurg 40(2):143–156
39. Tang YZ, Jin D, Bian JJ, Li XY, Lai GH, Ni JX (2014) Long-term outcome of computed tomography-guided percutaneous radiofrequency thermocoagulation for classic trigeminal neuralgia patients older than 70 years. J Craniofac Surg 25(4):1292–1295
40. Lunsford L (1982) Treatment of tic douloureux by percutaneous retrogasserian glycerol injection. JAMA 248(4):449–453
41. Kondziolka D et al (1998) Gamma knife radiosurgery for trigeminal neuralgia: results and expectations. Arch Neurol 55(12):1524–1529
42. Kondziolka D et al (1996) Stereotactic radiosurgery for trigeminal neuralgia: a multiinstitutional study using the gamma unit. J Neurosurg 84(6):940–945
43. Oh IH et al (2008) The treatment outcome of elderly patients with idiopathic trigeminal neuralgia: micro-vascular decompression versus gamma knife radiosurgery. J Korean Neurosurg Soc 44(4):199–204
44. Karam SD et al (2014) Trigeminal neuralgia treatment outcomes following Gamma knife radiosurgery with a minimum 3-year follow-up. J Radiat Oncol 3(2):125–130
45. Park SS et al (2008) Percutaneous balloon compression of trigeminal ganglion for the treatment of idiopathic trigeminal neuralgia: experience in 50 patients. J Korean Neurosurg Soc 43(4):186–189
46. Brown JA, McDaniel MD, Weaver MT (1993) Percutaneous trigeminal nerve compression for treatment of trigeminal neuralgia: results in 50 patients. Neurosurgery 32:570–573
47. Skirving DJ, Dan NG (2001) A 20-year review of percutaneous balloon compression of the trigeminal ganglion. J Neurosurg 94:913–917
48. Mullan S, Lichtor T (1983) Percutaneous microcompression of the trigeminal ganglion for trigeminal neuralgia. J Neurosurg 59:1007–1012
49. Maarbjerg S et al (2015) Significance of neurovascular contact in classical trigeminal neuralgia. Brain 138(2):311–319
50. Hughes MA et al (2016) MRI of the trigeminal nerve in patients with trigeminal neuralgia secondary to vascular compression. Am J Roentgenol 206(3):595–600

Hydrocephalus in the Elderly: Diagnosis of Idiopathic Normal Pressure Hydrocephalus

25

Albert M. Isaacs, Mark G. Hamilton, and Michael A. Williams

25.1 Background

25.1.1 Introduction

Idiopathic normal pressure hydrocephalus (iNPH) is a neurological disorder of the elderly characterized by gait impairment, urinary urgency or incontinence, and dementia in association with enlargement of the cerebral ventricles secondary to impaired circulation of cerebrospinal fluid (CSF). Hydrocephalus is often classified as either communicating or noncommunicating (or obstructive), based on the presence or absence of an identifiable obstruction in the CSF pathways [42]. The causes of obstruction may be divided into space-occupying lesions, such as brain tumors and aneurysms, or adhesions in the ventricles that are the result of infection, hemorrhage, trauma, or carcinomatosis.

In 1965, Salomón Hakim described normal pressure hydrocephalus (NPH) as an acquired, communicating, slowly progressive form of hydrocephalus, characterized by cognitive dysfunction, gait disturbance, and urinary incontinence in the context of normal cerebrospinal fluid (CSF) pressure [1, 17]. NPH has been

A.M. Isaacs, BSc, MD
Division of Neurosurgery, Department of Clinical Neuroscience, University of Calgary, Calgary, AB, Canada

M.G. Hamilton, MD, CM FRCSC, FAANS (✉)
Division of Neurosurgery, Department of Clinical Neuroscience, University of Calgary, Calgary, AB, Canada

Adult Hydrocephalus Program, Department of Clinical Neuroscience, University of Calgary, Calgary, AB, Canada

M.A. Williams, MD, FAAN
Adult and Transitional Hydrocephalus and CSF Disorders, Departments of Neurology and Neurological Surgery, University of Washington School of Medicine, Seattle, WA, USA
e-mail: maw99@neurosurgery.washington.edu

© Springer International Publishing Switzerland 2017

M. Berhouma, P. Krolak-Salmon (eds.), *Brain and Spine Surgery in the Elderly*,
DOI 10.1007/978-3-319-40232-1_25

subcategorized into idiopathic and secondary [18, 41, 44]. Secondary NPH is typically the result of a neurologic injury such as subarachnoid hemorrhage, infection, or trauma that causes inflammation in the subarachnoid space [18, 41]. Idiopathic NPH, by definition, has no identifiable cause and the patients are typically older (>65 years old).

The only effective treatment of iNPH is CSF diversion with shunt surgery [37, 41]. However, due to reports of high complication rates associated with the shunt surgery for iNPH in the 1960s and 1970s [4, 20], early nihilism developed toward the surgical management of the disease. However, higher treatment success rates and lower complication rates in the last two decades [15, 30] are the result of efforts to improve patient selection, standardize surgical approaches, and improve shunt technology. Therefore, the goal of this chapter is to provide an approach to the diagnosis and management of patients, with particular emphasis around a framework that helps the reader to identify good candidates for surgery.

25.1.2 Epidemiology

The global prevalence of iNPH is unknown. Nevertheless, regional data suggest a rate as high as 1–3 % (1000–3000/100,000) prevalence among community-dwelling elderly patients [2, 21]. The reported prevalence of iNPH is an underestimation, as the syndrome is underdiagnosed [2, 7]. The prevalence of probable iNPH in Norway is approximately 5.5/100,000 [7], while the number of patients with iNPH in Europe and the United States, based on epidemiologic data from Sweden of patients over age 70 [27], has been estimated as 2 million and 700,000, respectively. In addition, the prevalence of iNPH increases with age, with 0.2 % of 70–79-year-olds and 5.9 % of those older than 80 years old [27].

25.1.3 Pathophysiology

Idiopathic NPH is thought to result from an imbalance between the production and absorption of CSF, typically due to impaired resorption [42, 56]. Although iNPH is often described as a disorder of CSF circulation, the reversibility of neurologic symptoms following shunt surgery implies that iNPH causes reversible neuronal or glial dysfunction [54]. Animal models of iNPH have shown diffuse white matter damage, particularly in the periventricular zone, oligodendroglia death, astroglia hyperplasia, and concomitant microglia activation [12, 13]. Human autopsy studies have demonstrated subependymal gliosis [35], leptomeningeal fibrosis, neurofibrillary tangles, senile plaques, and cerebrovascular pathologies including atherosclerosis, arteriosclerosis, and enlarged perivascular spaces [10]. However, these findings lack specificity, as they can be found in other neurocognitive diseases [41]. CSF stasis in the ventricles has been identified in iNPH [29], which could lead to impaired clearance of toxic metabolites such as amyloid beta peptide and tau protein [48]. Vascular compliance is also lower in patients with iNPH when compared with healthy subjects and increases after successful treatment with a shunt [3]. A global reduction in cerebral blood flow in iNPH is evident on single-photon emission computed tomography (SPECT) imaging, especially in the fronto-basal, temporal, and deep nuclei regions [56].

The cognitive dysfunction and gait disturbance associated with iNPH have been attributed to subcortical injury and striatal and corticospinal tract changes, respectively, while the urinary incontinence is potentially secondary to impaired cortical inhibition of the micturition reflex [45]. The pathophysiology of improvement following shunt surgery has been attributed to increased brain perfusion with a simultaneous decrease in brain metabolism and resultant improved neuronal function [52, 54].

25.1.4 Risk Factors

Several case–control studies have implicated hypertension, diabetes, low serum levels of high-density lipoprotein (HDL), cardiovascular disease, and peripheral vascular disease as the major risk factors of iNPH [25, 41]. A large population-based study in Sweden identified hypertension, diabetes mellitus, and moderate to severe white mater lesions in 92 % and a history of stroke or TIA in 57 % of iNPH patients [26]. A positive correlation between the magnitude of arterial hypertension and severity of gait disturbance exists in iNPH [34].

25.1.5 Natural History

Patients may have asymptomatic ventriculomegaly that may be present for decades prior to symptom onset. In an MRI-based epidemiological study, 1 % of elderly population in a Japanese community had asymptomatic ventriculomegaly with features of iNPH. Of those patients, 25 % progressed to symptomatic iNPH after 4–8 years [41]. Studies of untreated iNPH are rare and typically consist of patients who refuse shunt surgery. From the available studies, it is clear that many unshunted iNPH patients may worsen as early as 3 months after diagnosis [43, 47]. A prospective study by Razay et al. showed a 64 and 57 % worsening of gait and cognition, respectively, in 14 unshunted iNPH patients over 3–4 months [43]. Scollato et al. found that over the course of a 2-year follow-up with serial imaging and clinical assessments, nine of nine patients with iNPH had worsening of cognition and urinary symptoms, and eight of nine (89 %) had worsening of gait [47]. A study in Sweden showed that 23 % of 33 patients whose surgery had been delayed for 6–24 months demonstrated decline in gait, balance, and cognition. The improvement of these patients after surgery was not as robust as the improvement of patients who had no delay, which suggests that even though symptom reversal is possible in advanced disease, early intervention is advised [2].

25.2 Approach to Diagnosis

25.2.1 Clinical Presentation

Idiopathic NPH typically affects patients over the age of 65 [33]. The hallmark presentation is an insidious onset, with gradually progressive deterioration of gait, cognition, and bladder function for at least 6 months [2, 55]. Because the three symptoms of iNPH can also be the result of multiple etiologies or comorbidities in the elderly population [36], patients suspected to have iNPH should undergo a careful clinical assessment, including a history, and review of prior medical records. Other disorders should be treated prior to considering iNPH if they are considered severe enough to explain the symptoms [53, 55].

25.2.1.1 Gait Disturbance

The earliest and most common symptom of iNPH is gait disturbance in 94–100 % of patients [39, 41, 53]. A formal gait assessment is important to the diagnosis of iNPH, including assessment of response to tests of CSF removal, as well as assessing the response to shunt surgery [24, 52]. The gait in iNPH is characterized by impaired initiation and transition of movement, foot clearance, turning and stance [55], as well as being slow, unbalanced, broad based, and shuffling [41]. While the iNPH gait may at times appear similar to the gait of Parkinson's disease, the iNPH gait does not improve with verbal or visual cues [41]. Clinically, several assessment tools are employed to quantify gait deficits, including the timed up-and-go test, 10 m straight walk test, Tinetti score, and the Boon scale [5, 41].

25.2.1.2 Cognitive Difficulties

Cognitive impairment is observed in 78–98 % of patients. It is characterized by a gradual decline of psychomotor speed, attention, working memory, and recall memory with preservation of recognition memory [41, 44, 55]. Patients may have frontal–subcortical dysfunction, such as apathy and sleep dysregulation, and they are often unable to perform their instrumental activities of daily living [32, 41, 55]. Cognitive screening tests can be used in the initial evaluation of iNPH patients, including the frontal assessment battery, trail-making tests [41], and the commonly used Montreal Cognitive Assessment (MoCA). Delirium is not a feature of iNPH, and its presence should prompt a search for an alternate cause that should be treated before evaluating the patient for iNPH [53, 55].

25.2.1.3 Bladder Dysfunction

Bladder dysfunction is present in 76–83 % of patients [41] and is characterized by overactive bladder symptoms, such as urinary frequency and urgency with or without incontinence and nighttime urinary frequency [41, 55]. Patients will complain that they cannot inhibit bladder emptying for long enough to get to the toilet. Urodynamic tests have demonstrated a reduced bladder capacity and flow rates, with a concomitant increase in residual volume [41].

25.2.2 Diagnostic Criteria

Two widely accepted guidelines for the diagnosis of iNPH exist, the International [44] and the Japanese [30, 41] guidelines. Both guidelines emphasize the clinical diagnosis of iNPH, as well as the presence of ventricular enlargement, with an Evans ratio >0.3 [23, 39, 41, 55]. Both recommend confirmatory tests to identify patients who have a high likelihood of responding to shunt surgery [24, 52]. Table 25.1 (adapted from Williams et al.) compares the International and Japanese guidelines [55].

25.2.3 Imaging Findings

Most iNPH patients have initial identification of their hydrocephalus on a CT scan of the head. However, MRI is a preferred diagnostic modality, as it better identifies sites of obstruction to CSF flow, such as aqueductal stenosis, and shows additional important diagnostic findings (e.g., cerebral microvascular disease or microhemorrhages) that could contribute to the patient's symptoms [28, 55]. The ventricles should be enlarged, and for screening purposes, the Evans index, which is the ratio of the frontal horn diameter to the widest biparietal diameter on the same cut, can be used. An Evans ratio above 0.3 is considered abnormal (Fig. 25.1b) [23, 39, 55]. In iNPH the typical imaging finding is a communicating, symmetric enlargement of all four ventricles [18, 52]. Ventriculomegaly does not always indicate iNPH, as it may also occur secondary to atrophy, known as "hydrocephalus ex vacuo" [42]. Additional findings include bowing of the corpus callosum seen on sagittal views and an acute callosal angle (<90) [22, 50]. Periventricular white matter hyperintensities (PVH) are common and represent either transependymal flow of CSF [44] or chronic ischemic changes [8, 11, 41].

A subgroup of iNPH patients have enlarged subarachnoid spaces, especially in the Sylvian fissures and over the cerebral convexities, categorized as having disproportionately enlarged subarachnoid spaces hydrocephalus (DESH), which is thought to result from an impairment to CSF flow between the basal cisterns and arachnoid granulations (see Fig. 25.1) [31, 55]. Patients with DESH respond very well to shunt surgery, with as many as 69 % demonstrating improved outcomes at 1 year after shunt insertion [19, 30]; however, the absence of DESH does not exclude the possibility of shunt-responsive iNPH.

25.2.4 Differential Diagnosis

As the primary symptoms of iNPH, gait impairment, urinary urgency and incontinence, and dementia are among the three most common symptoms occurring in the elderly patient. Thus, the principle of differential diagnosis is critical to the evaluation of patients for possible iNPH. Some forms of dementia with motor involvement, such as Lewy body dementia, can mimic iNPH. In addition, iNPH may coexist with

Table 25.1 Comparison between the International and Japanese guidelines for the diagnosis of iNPH

Feature	International guidelines	Japanese guidelines
Essential symptoms	Findings of gait/balance disturbance must be present, plus at least one other area of impairment in cognition, urinary symptoms, or both	More than one of the clinical triad: gait disturbance, cognitive impairment, and urinary incontinence
		Gait disturbance is the most prevalent feature, followed by cognitive impairment and urinary incontinence
Symptom onset	Insidious	Symptoms progress slowly
Symptom duration	Minimum duration of 3–6 months	
Age at onset	After age 40 years	After age 60 years
Etiology	No evidence of an antecedent event such as head trauma, intracerebral hemorrhage, meningitis, or other known causes of secondary hydrocephalus	Preceding diseases possibly causing ventricular dilation are not obvious, including subarachnoid hemorrhage, meningitis, head injury, congenital hydrocephalus, and aqueductal stenosis
Comorbid disorders	No other neurologic, psychiatric, or general medical conditions that are sufficient to explain the presenting symptoms	Clinical symptoms cannot be completely explained by other neurologic or non-neurologic diseases
		Other neurologic diseases, including Parkinson disease, Alzheimer disease, and cerebrovascular diseases, may coexist but should be mild
Gait impairment	At least 2 of the following should be present and not be entirely attributable to other conditions: Decreased step height Decreased step length Decreased cadence (speed of walking) Increased trunk sway during walking Widened standing base Toes turned outward on walking Retropulsion (spontaneous or provoked) En bloc turning (3 or more steps for 180°) Impaired walking balance, as evidenced by 2 or more corrections out of 8 steps on tandem gait testing	Small stride, shuffle, instability during walking, and increase of instability on turning

Table 25.1 (continued)

Feature	International guidelines	Japanese guidelines
Urinary urgency/ incontinence	One of the following should be present: Episodic or persistent urinary incontinence not attributable to primary urologic disorders Urinary and fecal incontinence Or any 2 of the following should be present: Urinary urgency (frequent perception of a pressing need to void) Urinary frequency (more than 6 voiding episodes in an average 12-h period) Nocturia (the need to urinate more than twice a night)	Overactive bladder, mainly manifesting as increased nocturnal urinary frequency, urgency, and urinary incontinence
Cognitive impairment	Documented impairment (adjusted for age and educational attainment) or decrease in performance on a cognitive screening instrument or both	Cognitive impairment is detected on cognitive tests
	Or evidence of at least 2 of the following on examination that is not fully attributable to other conditions: Psychomotor slowing (increased response latency) Decreased fine motor speed Decreased fine motor accuracy Difficulty dividing or maintaining attention Impaired recall, especially for recent events Executive dysfunction Behavioral or personality changes	
Ventricular size	Ventricular enlargement not entirely attributable to cerebral size atrophy or congenital enlargement (Evans index 0.3 or comparable measure)	Ventricular dilation (Evans index 0.3)

(continued)

Table 25.1 (continued)

Feature	International guidelines	Japanese guidelines
Other neuroimaging features	No macroscopic obstruction to CSF flow	Sylvian fissures and basal cistern are usually enlarged
	At least one of the following supportive features: Enlargement of the temporal horns of the lateral ventricles not entirely attributable to hippocampus atrophy Callosal angle of 40° or more Evidence of altered brain water content, including periventricular signal changes on CT and MRI not attributable to microvascular ischemic changes or demyelination An aqueductal or fourth ventricular flow void on MRI	Periventricular changes are not essential
		Narrowing of the sulci and subarachnoid spaces over the high convexity/midline surface (DESH)
CSF Pressure	CSF opening pressure in the range of 5–18 mmHg (or 70–245 mm H_2O), as determined by LP or a comparable procedure; appropriately measured pressures that are significantly higher or lower than this range are not consistent with a probable NPH diagnosis	CSF pressure of #200 mm H_2O and normal CSF content

Reproduced from Williams et al. [55] with permission
Abbreviations: *DESH 5* disproportionately enlarged subarachnoid space hydrocephalus, *LP 5* lumbar puncture

other disorders that contribute to the patient's symptoms. Thus, iNPH has a broad differential diagnosis that needs to be considered before performing tests that are specific for iNPH [55]. Table 25.2 (adapted from Williams et al.) presents a differential diagnosis for an undifferentiated patient with suspected iNPH [55].

25.2.5 Predictive (Confirmatory) Testing

Ancillary tests are helpful for confirming the diagnosis of iNPH and for identifying patients who are likely to benefit from shunt surgery. The most commonly used tests assess the pathophysiology of CSF circulation either by measuring CSF hydrodynamics or by removing CSF to evaluate the clinical response [23, 39, 52].

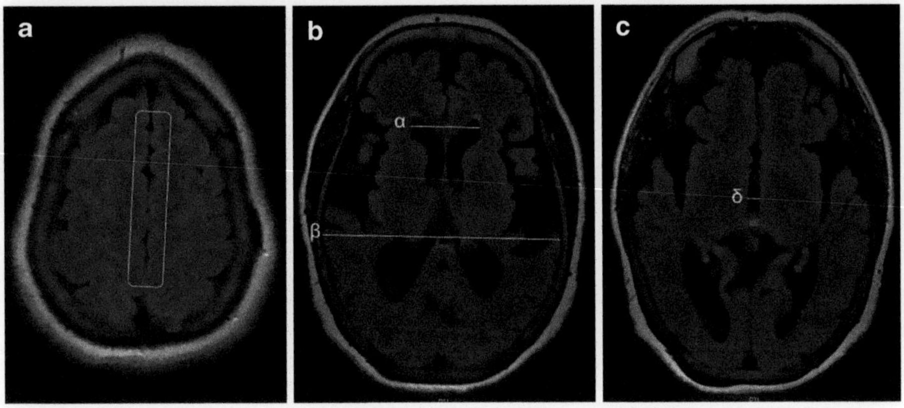

Fig. 25.1 Axial T2-weighted FLAIR MRI images of a 78-year-old male demonstrating lack of sulci at the vertex (**a**) and disproportionately enlarged subarachnoid spaces in the lower sequences (**a, b**) consistent with a DESH pattern hydrocephalus. Abnormal ventriculomegaly is demonstrated by an Evans ratio (α/β) of 0.44 (**b**) and an abnormally enlarged third ventricle (**c**)

25.2.5.1 Cerebrospinal Fluid Tap Test (CSF-TT)

The CSF tap test (CSF-TT) involves removing CSF via a lumbar puncture to observe for clinical improvement. While variation in protocols exists, most centers remove 30–50 ml [24, 51]. Prior to CSF-TT, the gait must be assessed objectively and should be reassessed 2–4 h later [53, 55]. Relying only on the report of the patient or family is unreliable [46]. Gait is the most responsive symptom associated with the CSF-TT [55]. CSF-TT has a positive predictive value of 88–94 % and negative predictive value of 18 % for predicting shunt effectiveness [24, 52].

25.2.5.2 Cerebrospinal Fluid Infusion Test

The cerebrospinal fluid infusion test (CSF-IT) involves infusing artificial CSF into the subarachnoid space either at a constant flow rate and measuring the pressure change or at a variable flow rate to maintain the pressure constant at several different levels, the results of which can be used to calculate the CSF outflow resistance (Rout) [14], which is useful for predicting iNPH shunt responsiveness [6, 49]. In healthy adults, normal Rout has been found to be 5–10 mmHg/ml/min [14]. Infusion testing is in wider use in Europe than in other parts of the world.

25.2.5.3 External Lumbar Drainage

External lumbar CSF drainage (ELD) via a temporary spinal catheter is an alternate method to predict response to CSF drainage [38, 40, 55]. As with the tap test, gait is the most responsive symptom to the ELD test and must be formally assessed before and after the CSF drainage trial. Cognitive improvement is observed in many patients who undergo ELD; thus cognitive assessment testing should be part of the pre- and post-ELD assessment. While some patients do report recovery from their urinary incontinence during the ELD test, the duration of the test is relatively too short to emphasize on the return of continence. A positive ELD response is

Table 25.2 Differential diagnosis of suspected iNPH

	Gait	Dementia	Incontinence
Disorders that may have all 3 symptoms			
iNPH, with or without comorbidities	X	X	X
Parkinsonism	X	X	X
Lewy body dementia	X	X	X
Corticobasal degeneration	X	X	X
Progressive supranuclear palsy	X	X	X
Multiple system atrophy	X	X	X
Vascular dementia	X	X	X
Neurosyphilis	X	X	X
Medication side effects	X	X	X
Multifactorial—any combination of diagnoses, with or without iNPH	X	X	X
Disorders that may have 2 symptoms			
Multifactorial—any combination of diagnoses, with or without iNPH	X	X	X
iNPH, with or without comorbidities	X	X	X
Vitamin B12 deficiency	X	X	
Cervical stenosis and myelopathy	X		X
Lumbosacral stenosis	X		X
Peripheral neuropathy	X		X
Disorders that may have only one symptom			
iNPH	X		
Degenerative arthritis of the hips, knees, ankles	X		
Spinocerebellar degeneration	X		
Peripheral vascular disease (claudication)	X		
Alzheimer dementia		X	
Frontotemporal dementia		X	
Depression		X	
Hypothyroidism		X	
Sleep apnea		X	
Prostatic hypertrophy/obstructive uropathy			X
Pelvic floor abnormalities			X
Interstitial cystitis			X
Disorders that can aggravate other symptoms			
Visual impairment	X	X	
Hearing impairment		X	
Obesity	X		
Cardiovascular disease	X		
Pulmonary disease	X		
Chronic lower back pain	X		
Vestibular disorders	X		

Reproduced with permission from Williams et al. [55]

associated with a 96 % shunt responsiveness [9]. A catheter is inserted into the lumbar subarachnoid space through an 18-gauge Tuohy needle and connected to a drainage system to drain 10 ml/h. The duration of ELD trial varies from 36 to 72 h, depending on the center. ELD is a sensitive test [52], with both high positive and negative predictive values [55]; however, it requires significant resources. The main potential complication is meningitis (1.8–3.6 %), which can be reduced with meticulous attention to sterile technique [16, 37].

References

1. Adams RD, Fisher CM, Hakim S, Ojemann RG, Sweet WH (1965) Symptomatic occult hydrocephalus with “normal” cerebrospinal-fluid pressure. a treatable syndrome. N Engl J Med 273:117–126
2. Andrén K, Wikkelsø C, Tisell M, Hellström P (2014) Natural course of idiopathic normal pressure hydrocephalus. J Neurol Neurosurg Psychiatry 85:806–810
3. Bateman GA (2000) Vascular compliance in normal pressure hydrocephalus. AJNR Am J Neuroradiol 21:1574–1585
4. Bergsneider M, Black PM, Klinge P, Marmarou A, Relkin N (2005) Surgical management of idiopathic normal-pressure hydrocephalus. Neurosurgery 57:S29–S39
5. Boon AJ, Tans JT, Delwel EJ, Egeler-Peerdeman SM, Hanlo PW, Wurzer JA et al (1997) Dutch normal pressure hydrocephalus study: baseline characteristics with emphasis on clinical findings. Eur J Neurol 4:39–47
6. Boon AJW, Tans JTJ, Delwel EJ, Egeler-Peerdeman SM, Hanlo PW, Wurzer HAL et al (2000) The Dutch normal-pressure hydrocephalus study. Surg Neurol 53:201–207
7. Brean A, Eide PK (2008) Prevalence of probable idiopathic normal pressure hydrocephalus in a Norwegian population. Acta Neurol Scand 118:48–53
8. Chang C-C, Asada H, Mimura T, Suzuki S (2009) A prospective study of cerebral blood flow and cerebrovascular reactivity to acetazolamide in 162 patients with idiopathic normal-pressure hydrocephalus. J Neurosurg 111:610–617
9. Chotai S, Medel R, Herial NA, Medhkour A (2014) External lumbar drain: a pragmatic test for prediction of shunt outcomes in idiopathic normal pressure hydrocephalus. Surg Neurol Int 5:12
10. Del Bigio MR, Cardoso ER, Halliday WC (1997) Neuropathological changes in chronic adult hydrocephalus: cortical biopsies and autopsy findings. Can J Neurol Sci 24:121–126
11. Del Bigio MR, Massicotte EM (2001) Protective effect of nimodipine on behavior and white matter of rats with hydrocephalus. J Neurosurg 94:788–794
12. Del Bigio MR, Zhang YW (1998) Cell death, axonal damage, and cell birth in the immature rat brain following induction of hydrocephalus. Exp Neurol 154:157–169
13. Del Bigio MR, Di Curzio DL (2016) Nonsurgical therapy for hydrocephalus: a comprehensive and critical review. Fluids Barriers CNS 13:1–20
14. Eklund A, Smielewski P, Chambers I, Alperin N, Malm J, Czosnyka M et al (2007) Assessment of cerebrospinal fluid outflow resistance. Med Biol Eng Comput 45:719–735
15. Farahmand D, Hilmarsson H, Högfeldt M, Tisell M (2009) Perioperative risk factors for short term shunt revisions in adult hydrocephalus patients. J Neurol Neurosurg Psychiatry 80:1248–1253
16. Greenberg BM, Williams MA (2008) Infectious complications of temporary spinal catheter insertion for diagnosis of adult hydrocephalus and idiopathic intracranial hypertension. Neurosurgery 62:431–436
17. Hakim S, Adams RD (1965) The special clinical problem of symptomatic hydrocephalus with normal cerebrospinal fluid pressure. Observations on cerebrospinal fluid hydrodynamics. J Neurol Sci 2:307–327

18. Halperin JJ, Kurlan R, Schwalb JM, Cusimano MD, Gronseth G, Gloss D (2015) Practice guideline: idiopathic normal pressure hydrocephalus: response to shunting and predictors of response: report of the guideline development, dissemination, and implementation subcommittee of the American Academy of Neurology. Neurology 85:2063–2071
19. Hashimoto M, Ishikawa M, Mori E, Kuwana N (2010) Diagnosis of idiopathic normal pressure hydrocephalus is supported by MRI-based scheme: a prospective cohort study. Cerebrospinal Fluid Res 7:18
20. Hebb AO, Cusimano MD (2001) Idiopathic normal pressure hydrocephalus: a systematic review of diagnosis and outcome. Neurosurgery 49:1166–1186
21. Hiraoka K, Meguro K, Mori E (2008) Prevalence of idiopathic normal-pressure hydrocephalus in the elderly population of a Japanese rural community. Neurol Med Chir (Tokyo) 48:197–200
22. Ishii K, Kanda T, Harada A, Miyamoto N, Kawaguchi T, Shimada K et al (2008) Clinical impact of the callosal angle in the diagnosis of idiopathic normal pressure hydrocephalus. Eur Radiol 18:2678–2683
23. Ishikawa M, Hashimoto M, Kuwana N, Mori E, Miyake H, Wachi A et al (2008) Guidelines for management of idiopathic normal pressure hydrocephalus. Neurol Med Chir (Tokyo) 48(Suppl):S1–S23
24. Ishikawa M, Hashimoto M, Mori E, Kuwana N, Kazui H (2012) The value of the cerebrospinal fluid tap test for predicting shunt effectiveness in idiopathic normal pressure hydrocephalus. Fluids Barriers CNS 9:1
25. Israelsson H, Carlberg B, Wikkelsø C, Laurell K, Kahlon B, Eklund A et al (2015) Cardiovascular risk factors are associated with idiopathic normal pressure hydrocephalus. Fluids Barriers CNS 12:O41
26. Jaraj D, Agerskov S, Rabiei K, Marlow T, Jensen C, Guo X et al (2016) Vascular factors in suspected normal pressure hydrocephalus: a population-based study. Neurology 86:592–599
27. Jaraj D, Rabiei K, Marlow T, Jensen C, Skoog I, Wikkelsø C (2014) Prevalence of idiopathic normal-pressure hydrocephalus. Neurology 82:1449–1454
28. Johansson E, Ambarki K, Birgander R, Bahrami N, Eklund A, Malm J (2016) Cerebral microbleeds in idiopathic normal pressure hydrocephalus. Fluids Barriers CNS 13:4
29. Kawaguchi T, Hirata Y, Bundo M, Kondo T, Owaki H, Ito S et al (2011) Role of computerized tomographic cisternography in idiopathic normal pressure hydrocephalus. Acta Neurochir (Wien) 153:2041–2048
30. Kazui H, Miyajima M, Mori E, Ishikawa M (2015) Lumboperitoneal shunt surgery for idiopathic normal pressure hydrocephalus (SINPHONI-2): an open-label randomised trial. Lancet Neurol 14:585–594
31. Kitagaki H, Mori E, Ishii K, Yamaji S, Hirono N, Imamura T (1998) CSF spaces in idiopathic normal pressure hydrocephalus: morphology and volumetry. AJNR Am J Neuroradiol 19:1277–1284
32. Kizu O, Yamada K, Nishimura T (2001) Proton chemical shift imaging in normal pressure hydrocephalus. AJNR Am J Neuroradiol 22:1659–1664
33. Klinge P, Hellström P, Tans J, Wikkelsø C (2012) European iNPH multicentre study group: One-year outcome in the European multicentre study on iNPH. Acta Neurol Scand 126:145–153
34. Krauss JK, Regel JP, Vach W, Droste DW, Borremans JJ, Mergner T (1996) Vascular risk factors and arteriosclerotic disease in idiopathic normal-pressure hydrocephalus of the elderly. Stroke 27:24–29
35. Leinonen V, Koivisto AM, Savolainen S, Rummukainen J, Sutela A, Vanninen R et al (2012) Post-mortem findings in 10 patients with presumed normal-pressure hydrocephalus and review of the literature. Neuropathol Appl Neurobiol 38:72–86
36. Malm J, Graff-Radford NR, Ishikawa M, Kristensen B, Leinonen V, Mori E et al (2013) Influence of comorbidities in idiopathic normal pressure hydrocephalus - research and clinical care. A report of the ISHCSF task force on comorbidities in INPH. Fluids Barriers CNS 10:22

37. Marmarou A, Black P, Bergsneider M, Klinge P, Relkin N (2005) Guidelines for management of idiopathic normal pressure hydrocephalus: progress to date. Acta Neurochir Suppl 95:237–240
38. Marmarou A, Young HF, Aygok GA, Sawauchi S (2005) Diagnosis and management of idiopathic normal-pressure hydrocephalus: a prospective study in 151 patients. J Neurosurg 102:987–997
39. Marmarou A, Bergsneider M, Relkin N, Klinge P, Black PM (2005) Development of guidelines for idiopathic normal-pressure hydrocephalus: introduction. Neurosurgery 57:S1–S3
40. McGirt MJ, Woodworth G, Coon AL, Thomas G, Williams MA, Rigamonti D (2005) Diagnosis, treatment, and analysis of long-term outcomes in idiopathic normal-pressure hydrocephalus. Neurosurgery 57:699–705
41. Mori E, Ishikawa M, Kato T, Kazui H, Miyake H, Miyajima M et al (2012) Guidelines for management of idiopathic normal pressure hydrocephalus: second edition. Neurol Med Chir (Tokyo) 52:775–809
42. Mori K (1990) Hydrocephalus--revision of its definition and classification with special reference to "intractable infantile hydrocephalus". Childs Nerv Syst 6:198–204
43. Razay G, Vreugdenhil A, Liddell J (2009) A prospective study of ventriculo-peritoneal shunting for idiopathic normal pressure hydrocephalus. J Clin Neurosci 16:1180–1183
44. Relkin N, Marmarou A, Klinge P, Bergsneider M, Black PM (2005) Diagnosing idiopathic normal-pressure hydrocephalus. Neurosurgery 57:S4–S16
45. Sakakibara R, Uchiyama T, Kanda T, Uchida Y, Kishi M, Hattori T (2008) [Urinary dysfunction in idiopathic normal pressure hydrocephalus]. Brain Nerve 60:233–239
46. Schniepp R, Trabold R, Romagna A, Akrami F, Hesselbarth K, Wuehr M et al (2016) Walking assessment after lumbar puncture in normal-pressure hydrocephalus: a delayed improvement over 3 days. J Neurosurg 18:1–10
47. Scollato A, Tenenbaum R, Bahl G, Celerini M, Salani B, Di Lorenzo N (2008) Changes in aqueductal CSF stroke volume and progression of symptoms in patients with unshunted idiopathic normal pressure hydrocephalus. AJNR Am J Neuroradiol 29:192–197
48. Silverberg GD (2004) Normal pressure hydrocephalus (NPH): ischaemia, CSF stagnation or both. Brain 127:947–948
49. Sorteberg A, Eide PK, Fremming AD (2009) A prospective study on the clinical effect of surgical treatment of normal pressure hydrocephalus: the value of hydrodynamic evaluation. Br J Neurosurg 18:149–157
50. Virhammar J, Laurell K, Cesarini KG, Larsson E-M (2014) The callosal angle measured on MRI as a predictor of outcome in idiopathic normal-pressure hydrocephalus. J Neurosurg 120:178–184
51. Wikkelsø C, Andersson H, Blomstrand C, Lindqvist G (1982) The clinical effect of lumbar puncture in normal pressure hydrocephalus. J Neurol Neurosurg Psychiatry 45:64–69
52. Wikkelsø C, Hellström P, Klinge PM, Tans JTJ (2012) The European iNPH Multicentre Study on the predictive values of resistance to CSF outflow and the CSF Tap Test in patients with idiopathic normal pressure hydrocephalus. J Neurol Neurosurg Psychiatr 84:562–568
53. Williams MA, Malm J (2016) Diagnosis and treatment of idiopathic normal pressure hydrocephalus. Continuum (Minneap Minn) 22:579–599
54. Williams MA, McAllister JP, Walker ML, Kranz DA, Bergsneider M, Del Bigio MR et al (2007) Priorities for hydrocephalus research: report from a National Institutes of Health-sponsored workshop. J Neurosurg 107:345–357
55. Williams MA, Relkin NR (2013) Diagnosis and management of idiopathic normal-pressure hydrocephalus. Neurol Clin Pract 3:375–385
56. Wilsson AÅ (2005) On the pathophysiology of idiopathic adult hydrosephalus syndrome: energy metabolism, protein patterns, and intracranial pressure (Doctoral dissertation). Umeå University medical dissertations, ISSN 0346-6612; 955

Hydrocephalus in the Elderly: Surgical Management of Idiopathic Normal Pressure Hydrocephalus

26

Albert M. Isaacs, Michael A. Williams, and Mark G. Hamilton

26.1 Background: History

Idiopathic normal pressure hydrocephalus (iNPH) was first described by Dr. Salomon Hakim in 1964 as a clinical triad of gait disturbance, cognitive difficulties, and urinary incontinence, associated with abnormal ventricular dilatation, despite normal cerebrospinal fluid (CSF) pressures [2, 43]. During his postgraduate studies, Dr. Hakim performed autopsies on patients who had died from neurodegenerative diseases and observed some of the patients had abnormal ventricular dilatation without cortical abnormalities. He subsequently hypothesized his findings were due to what he defined as normal pressure hydrocephalus (NPH). Interestingly, some of the NPH patients had no identifiable etiology for the ventriculomegaly, which prompted a subclassification of those patients as having idiopathic NPH (iNPH) [1, 2, 44]. In the 1960s, Dr. Hakim and his colleagues demonstrated the effectiveness of

A.M. Isaacs, BSc, MD
Division of Neurosurgery, Department of Clinical Neuroscience, University of Calgary, Calgary, AB, Canada
e-mail: akm.isaacs@gmail.com

M.A. Williams, MD, FAAN (✉)
Adult and Transitional Hydrocephalus and CSF Disorders, University of Washington School of Medicine, Seattle, WA, USA
e-mail: maw99@neurosurgery.washington.edu

M.G. Hamilton, MD, CM FRCSC, FAANS
Division of Neurosurgery, Department of Clinical Neuroscience, University of Calgary, Calgary, AB, Canada

Adult Hydrocephalus Program, Department of Clinical Neuroscience, University of Calgary, Calgary, AB, Canada
e-mail: mghamilton.hydro@gmail.com

© Springer International Publishing Switzerland 2017

M. Berhouma, P. Krolak-Salmon (eds.), *Brain and Spine Surgery in the Elderly*,
DOI 10.1007/978-3-319-40232-1_26

CSF diversion surgery (shunting) for patients with iNPH, which to date has remained the only recommended modality of treatment for the disease [2, 44, 57, 92, 102]. However, since the pathophysiology for iNPH remains uncertain, as a consequence, the exact mechanism by which CSF shunting is effective remains somewhat ambiguous.

This chapter will also briefly review the issues associated with the limited role for endoscopic third ventriculostomy (ETV) and pharmacologic agents (drugs) in the treatment of patients with iNPH.

26.2 Surgical Risk Issues in the Elderly and Mitigation of Risks

Idiopathic NPH is a disease of the elderly, a population demographic that has a high prevalence of comorbidities, disability, and frailty. Frailty refers to a lack of physiologic reserve, which may predispose patients to adverse events when subjected to physiological stressors such as surgery. Generally, the physiological stress associated with surgery is not as well tolerated by the elderly, especially when prevalent premorbid conditions reduce physiologic reserve [35, 64]. Frail patients, when compared to non-frail patients, generally have 2.5 times the risk of developing perioperative complications [90, 110]. One should be cautious if using Frailty Index Scales (Table 26.1) [11, 37, 103, 128] to help decide on the surgical candidacy of patients with iNPH, as the invariable gait impairment and functional decline associated with iNPH, which are reversible by the shunt surgery, may overestimate frailty [57, 94, 152, 153].

There is consensus that the risk-benefit ratio of shunting for iNPH is acceptable, and comorbidity-associated perioperative risks of iNPH surgery in the elderly can be kept low [15]. In addition, comorbidities, per se, do not play a major role in predicting shunt responsiveness [45]. Nonetheless, individualized patient assessment must still be carried out prior to iNPH surgery [15], and established guidelines should be used to identify at-risk patients who may benefit from preoperative medical optimization [23]. It is often a useful strategy to consult other medical specialists, such as internists, to assist in the perioperative management of medically complicated patients [35, 64].

26.2.1 Advanced Age

While iNPH afflicts the elderly [94, 152], a patient's age, independent of comorbid factors, is not a risk factor for surgical morbidity and mortality [19, 34, 90], and advanced chronologic age alone should therefore not be a preclusion to surgery [64, 65, 154]. When dealing with properly selected patients undergoing surgery for iNPH, the expected postoperative clinical improvement should typically outweigh the risks of the procedure [15, 39, 113, 138, 152].

Table 26.1 A frailty risk score adapted from the Cardiovascular Health Study Frailty Screening Measure [37] and respective postoperative outcomes of 594 patients who underwent elective surgery [90]

Frailty score	
Characteristic	*Explanation*
Weight loss	A 10 lb weight in the past year or A K value ≥ 0.05: $K = \frac{(\text{Previous year's weight} - \text{Current measured weight})}{\text{Previous year's weight}}$
Exhaustion	Significant self-reported fatigue, tiredness, or weakness in the past month
Low physical activity	Significant decrease in the frequency and duration of physical activity Standardized algorithms may be used to calculate the Kcals of physical activity expended per week: Men with <383 Kcals/week are frail Women with <270 Kcals/week are frail
Walking speed	Time taken to cover a 4 m distance. Generally, $\geq$ 6 or 7 s depending on the patients gender and height may be considered frail
Weakness	Gender and body mass index-based cutoff for grip strength (kg)

Postoperative outcomes

Frailty score	*Category*	*30-day surgical complications (%)*	*Length of stay (days)*	*Discharge to assisted living facility (%)*
0–1	Non-frail	3.9	4.2	2.9
2–3	Intermediate frailty	7.3	6.2	12.2
4–5	Frail	11.4	7.7	42.1

Each frailty criterion is scored with a 0 or 1

26.2.2 Cardiopulmonary Disease and Diabetes Mellitus

The major comorbidities among iNPH surgical candidates include cardiovascular disease, pulmonary disease, and diabetes mellitus [6, 108]. The overall risk of general postoperative cardiovascular complications in the typical iNPH patient age group is approximately 2 %, which may increase up to 5 % in those with a prior history of cardiac disease [27, 41, 81, 84]. Perioperative pulmonary complications such as pneumonia and pulmonary embolism may occur in as many as 7 % and may be a predictor of long-term mortality, especially in patients over 70 years old [142]. Obstructive sleep apnea can also be a significant cardiopulmonary risk factor and is associated with an increased incidence of postoperative acute respiratory failure, myocardial ischemia, and arrhythmias [67, 88, 101, 140]. Diabetes, which affects over 6 % of the world's population, has an even higher incidence in iNPH patients and predisposes them to perioperative complications such as infections, myocardial ischemia, and hypoglycemia [22, 51, 52, 58, 79, 104]. As part of the screening process for potential iNPH surgical candidates, all of these potential perioperative risk issues should be evaluated, and efforts must be undertaken to control or mitigate them.

26.2.3 Anticoagulation in the Elderly

A significant proportion of iNPH patients are being treated with anticoagulant and antiplatelet medication, which can increase the risk of postoperative bleeding complications [3, 36, 46, 126, 143, 155]. However, iNPH surgery is typically performed on a non-emergent basis, which allows ample time to temporarily withdraw anticoagulant or antiplatelet medications before surgery [29, 49]. Information regarding how long before surgery to stop anticoagulant and antiplatelet medications and when they can be restarted is summarized in Table 26.2 [26, 46, 87, 105]. Patients with a high thromboembolic risk, such as those with mechanical heart valves, may require heparin therapy up to a few hours before surgery [60, 109], and some patients may require heparin bridging prior to restarting their regular anticoagulation medication post-op [28]. The risk of temporary interruption of anticoagulation therapy for iNPH surgery is a balance between thrombosis or thromboembolic events and perioperative bleeding and should be determined on an individual patient basis [46].

26.3 Shunts

Shunt surgery, the only recommended treatment for iNPH, involves the diversion of CSF away from the ventricular or subarachnoid space [2, 44, 57, 92, 102] via a mechanical implanted tube device. The present-day three-component shunt system, one valve and two catheters (proximal and distal), is predated by a history that spans over 300 years [9].

26.3.1 History and Overview

LeCat performed the first hydrocephalus shunting procedure in 1744 using a wick. However, Pollock is credited as the first (in 1884) to drain the lateral ventricle using a tube [9, 48]. For over two centuries, CSF shunting only involved direct valveless diversion, and patients experienced a high incidence of mortality secondary to rapid egress of CSF and infection. Materials that were used in those times to limit the rate of CSF drainage included horsehair, silkworm gut, catgut, and rubber tissue. In the 1950s Pudenz and others developed valves, which were incorporated into shunt systems to provide some flow regulation [1, 9, 74, 116, 117]. Over the past 60 years, other valve-regulated shunt systems have been designed, including Dr. Hakim's autoclavable sapphire ball in a stainless steel cone valve, which is the underlying mechanism of many current shunt systems. During the past two decades, there have been major advancements in shunt bioengineering, including siphon-control valves, adjustable valve devices, and flow control valves [9, 114, 115].

Table 26.2 Perioperative management of some of the major oral anticoagulation and antiplatelet interruption [26, 87, 105]

Drug	Half-life (hours)	Duration of interruption prior to surgery (days)	Duration before restarting after surgery (days)[b]	Mechanism of action and comments
Warfarin	36–42	5	5	Inhibition of vitamin K-dependent clotting factors (II, VII, IX, X, protein C and S) Patients with a high risk for venous thromboembolism may require bridging therapy with a heparin or low molecular weight heparin agent
Dabigatran	12–14	4–5[a]	5	Direct thrombin inhibitor. Blocks thrombin from converting fibrinogen to fibrin (factor IIa) Patients can be restarted at the same preoperative dose when hemostasis has been achieved post-op Patients with a high risk for venous thromboembolism may require bridging therapy with a heparin or low molecular weight heparin agent
Rivaroxaban	5–9	4–5[a]	5	Direct factor Xa inhibitor. Blocks factor Xa from converting prothrombin to thrombin Patients can be restarted at the same preoperative dose when hemostasis has been achieved post-op Patients with a high risk for venous thromboembolism may require bridging therapy with a heparin or low molecular weight heparin agent
Apixaban	8–15	4–5[a]	5	
Edoxaban	6–11	4–5[a]	5	
Aspirin		5–7	3–5	Blocks cyclooxygenase and subsequently inhibits the conversion of arachidonic acid into prostaglandin and thromboxane Restart when the perioperative bleeding risk has subsided
Plavix		5–7	5–7	Inhibits adenylyl cyclase and platelet aggregation by blocking the binding of ADP to the platelet receptor, P2Y12 Resume as early as possible post-op. Some patients may require a loading dose post-op

[a]While a 2–3-day presurgical interruption may be adequate for some procedures, we recommend 4–5 days given that iNPH surgery is often elective and the morbidity associated with anticoagulation-related intracranial hemorrhage may be profound. Patients with renal dysfunction may require a longer duration of interruption

[b]Determining the optimal duration to wait before restarting an anticoagulant or antiplatelet agent should be decided with a consideration of the balance of risk associated with withholding the drug with respect to underlying disease for which the agent is used versus the bleeding potential associated with the anticoagulant or antiplatelet drug effect in the postoperative period

26.3.2 Shunt Valves

Most shunt valves operate with a "simple" principle: to promote unidirectional CSF flow. However, in practice, the process is often more complex than the technology allows. The most common valve design used is one that allows flow based on the pressure differential between the proximal and distal ends of the shunt (Fig. 26.1). The manufacturer establishes an "opening pressure" at which the valve permits CSF flow [9, 18], and each valve of this type is preset to a specific fixed differential pressure. There are three common categories of fixed differential pressure valves, "low," "medium," or "high," although the actual pressures (and range of potential opening pressures) for each of these vary between manufacturers.

Other valve types include gravity assisted or flow regulated, and some allow the differential pressure (opening pressure) to be adjusted or modified with an external tool [54, 102]. Gravity-assisted differential pressure valves occlude or permit CSF flow depending on the hydrostatic column created when a patient is recumbent or standing [9]. Flow-regulated valves try to automatically divert CSF according to real-time CSF flow dynamics [9, 74]. At present, all programmable differential pressure systems are magnet-based, and most require evaluation and potential reprogramming when the patient is exposed to a high magnetic field environment such as during a diagnostic MRI scan [102]. Once an opening pressure is set for a programmable differential pressure valve, it functions in the same manner as a fixed differential pressure valve.

CSF overdrainage (also referred to as siphoning) has been a long-standing potential shunting complication [48] that involves excessive CSF flow associated with low resistance in the shunt system. The incorporation of valves into shunt systems during the 1950s was revolutionary, in that these significantly reduced the magnitude of the risks associated with overdrainage [9]. Nonetheless, standard valves and adjustable shunt valves are far from perfect in preventing overdrainage, which may still occur because of the limitations of the basic design of most commonly used shunt systems. The factory determined "opening pressure" for a valve is relevant to a horizontal column of CSF (with the patient supine) and establishes that CSF flow will occur through the valve when the difference between the proximal and distal ends of the shunt exceeds the "opening pressure." When the patient is in the upright position, the pressure differential between the proximal and distal ends of the shunt now includes the length of the peritoneal catheter, and a siphoning effect may occur which can dramatically increase drainage/flow which might not have occurred in the recumbent position.

Antisiphon, siphon-control, or gravity-assisted devices have been developed by different manufacturers to reduce excessive CSF drainage and mitigate the risks of overdrainage. Antisiphon devices are potentially capable of restricting flow or closing the valve when the differential pressure rises precipitously as, for example, in response to the patient standing [9, 80, 96]. Figure 26.2 demonstrates some of the different valve systems currently available for iNPH shunt surgery.

In general, adjustable valves offer versatility for the management of iNPH patients by allowing the opening pressure to be tailored for each patient [15, 91,

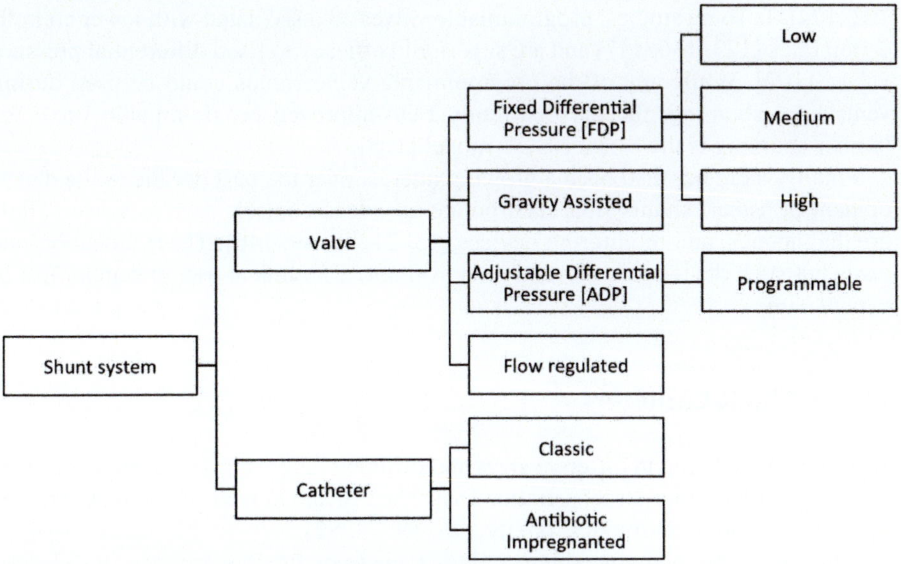

Fig. 26.1 Simplified schematic of the parts and types of shunts

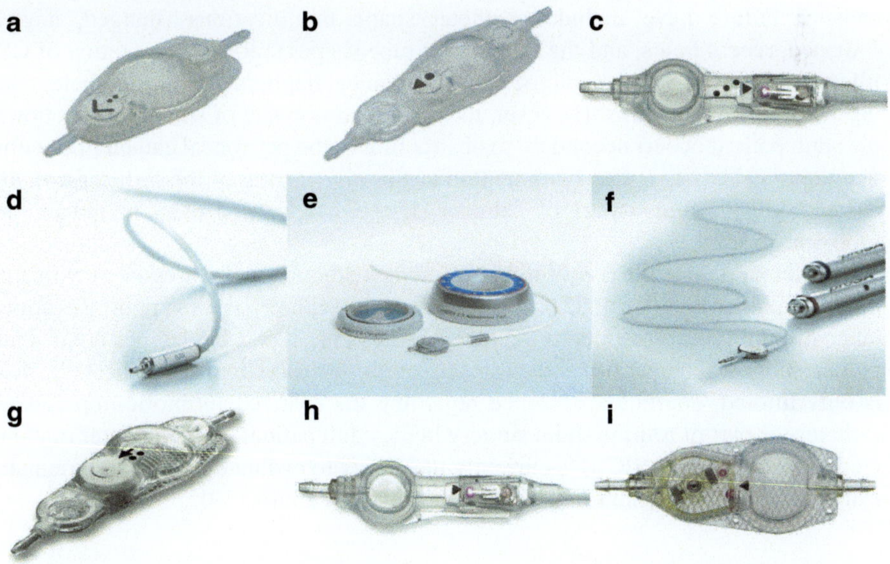

Fig. 26.2 Shunt valve systems. The fixed pressure valves (*top row*) include Medtronic's Flow Contoured Regular (**a**) and Delta (**b**) and Codman Hakim Precision Fixed Pressure In-Line (**c**) valves. The gravity-dependent valves (*middle row*) include Aesculap's GAV (**d**), proGAV (**e**), and proSA (**f**) valves. The adjustable pressure valves (*bottom row*) include Medtronic's Strata (**g**), Codman Hakim Programmable (**h**), and Certas Plus Programmable (**i**) valves (Images **a**, **b** and **g** are courtesy of Medtronic Canada. Images **d**, **e**, and **f** are courtesy of B. Braun Melsungen AG. Images **c**, **h** and **i** are courtesy of CODMAN NEURO. HAKIM is a registered trademark of Hakim USA, LLC and is used under license by Codman & Shurtleff, Inc)

102, 124]. In some studies, programmable valves are associated with lower complication rates [123, 156, 157] and are superior in efficacy to fixed differential pressure valves [102]. While any of the programmable valve shunts could be used during ventricular shunting, the only currently FDA-approved programmable valve for lumbar shunting is the Strata NSC® model [108].

Finally, there has also been a growing interest over the past decade in the development of "smart shunts" that incorporate advanced controls such as sensors, failure diagnostics, and monitoring devices [13, 21, 86, 89, 146]. These are ambitious goals but such devices are currently not available for clinical trial or regular use in patient care.

26.3.3 Shunt Catheters

Shunt catheters come in different sizes and different lengths; may be open or closed at the tip, with or without fenestrations near the tip; and may or may not be impregnated with barium, antibiotics, or silver [9, 59, 74, 82].

Almost all the available shunt tubing is made of flexible silicone [9, 33, 74]. Despite the high efficacy of shunts in treating hydrocephalus, the catheters are prone to relatively high "mechanical" failure rates. Some attempts to reduce proximal catheter failure have included catheter shape modifications (flanged, angled, J-shaped, recess holes, and the Fuji basket tube shapes) [30], incorporation of CSF filters [146], installation of microelectromechanical flappers [16], and catheter coating with debris repellants. However, the most common site of shunt malfunction in the adult patient occurs secondary to obstruction of the peritoneal catheter tip within the peritoneal cavity (often by omentum or fibrous scarring of the catheter tip), and currently no current aspect of catheter design has been proven to reduce this problem.

Finally, to reduce the risk of infection, some catheters are impregnated with antibiotics or silver [9, 59, 74, 82]. While the current evidence does support the importance of quality improvement (QI) care bundles [71, 125, 127, 139] to control and reduce shunt infections (discussed in section "Infection Control Protocols"), there is only limited, conflicted evidence regarding the role for antibiotic-impregnated catheters as part of routine shunt surgery in the adult patient. A multicenter randomized clinical trial (BASICS) is currently underway to evaluate if silver-impregnated catheters can reduce shunt infection in children and adults [59].

26.3.4 Surgical Techniques for Shunt Insertion

CSF diversion can be achieved through a ventricular or lumbar approach [15, 47, 76, 92, 118]. Ventricular shunting involves diverting CSF from the cerebral ventricles to an extracranial compartment such as the peritoneal cavity (ventriculoperitoneal shunt), the right atrium (ventriculoatrial shunt), or the pleural space (ventriculopleural shunt). Lumboperitoneal (LP) shunts on the other hand involve diverting CSF from the lower lumbar subarachnoid space into the intra-abdominal cavity [63, 66, 69, 108]. To date, there are no randomized controlled trials that have identified a significant outcome difference between the ventricular and lumbar shunt methods for the treatment of hydrocephalus [69, 148]. Currently, the majority of surgeons in Europe and North America use ventricular shunts, while lumbar shunts are more commonly used in Japan [47, 76, 93].

26.3.4.1 Ventriculoperitoneal Shunts

Ventriculoperitoneal (VP) shunting, which involves the diversion of CSF from the ventricular system to the intra-abdominal (peritoneal) cavity, is the most common treatment approach for iNPH in Europe and North America [69].

The standard operative approach to VP shunt insertion has been well described [40, 97]. This surgery is typically performed with the patient under general anesthesia. The major steps of the VP shunt insertion include a cranial incision and creation of a 1–1.5 cm burr hole, subcutaneous tunneling of the distal catheter from an abdominal incision to exit at the cranial incision, insertion of the proximal (cranial) catheter into the lateral ventricle via the predetermined entry point and trajectory, connection of the proximal and distal catheters to the valve, and insertion of the distal catheter in the peritoneal cavity after confirming flow of CSF from the end of the distal catheter.

There are three common "standard" entry sites used on the cranium for the creation of a burr hole and insertion of the ventricular catheter. All three sites are based upon external landmarks and "standard measurements": (1) *Kocher's point* (1 cm anterior to the coronal suture and approximately 3 cm lateral to the midline with a trajectory that is perpendicular to the brain with a ventricular catheter insertion length of 3–6 cm depending upon the ventricular size), (2) *Frazier's point* (6–7 cm above the inion and 3–4 cm lateral to the midline with a trajectory aimed at the middle of the forehead and a ventricular insertion length of 4–6 cm depending upon the ventricular size), and (3) *Keen's point* (2.5–3 cm posterior and 2.5–3 cm superior to the pinna with a trajectory that is perpendicular to the brain with a ventricular catheter insertion length of 2–3 cm depending upon the ventricular size) (Fig. 26.3). Frazier's point and Kocher's point represent the two most common sites used for ventricular catheter insertion in the adult patient. Incorrect ventricular catheter insertion is reported to occur 1–10% of the time [106, 135]. However, there is no evidence that either ventricular catheter insertion site results in a decrease in rates of shunt malfunction in adults. A modified approach that includes the use of neuronavigation will be presented when reviewing shunt-related strategies to reduce rates of shunt malfunction (section "Neuronavigation-Assisted Proximal Catheter Insertion").

Insertion of the distal catheter into the peritoneal cavity is commonly done with what is referred to as either the "open technique" or the "trocar technique." The most common locations for insertion are in the area adjacent to the umbilicus. With the open technique (also referred to as minilaparotomy), a 2–3 cm incision is made, and the tissue layers are dissected through until the peritoneal layer is opened after which the catheter is then directed into the peritoneal cavity. With the trocar technique, a 0.5–1 cm incision is made, and the trocar is pushed into the peritoneal

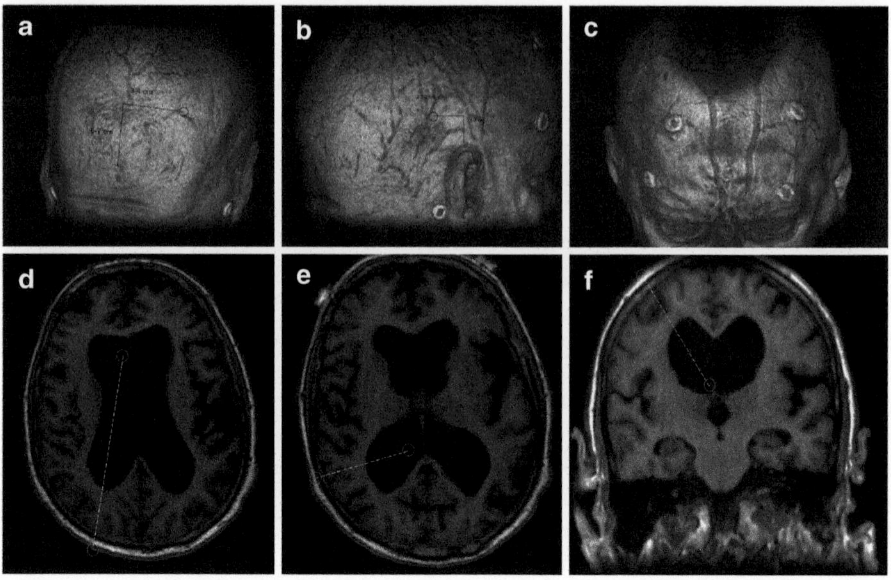

Fig. 26.3 Surface landmark and trajectories for insertion of a VP shunt. A right occipital approach from Frazier's point (**a**) with catheter aimed at the middle of the forehead (**d**) and Keen's point (**b**) with catheter aimed at the antrum of the ventricle (**e**). A right frontal approach can be done from Kocher's point (**c**) with the catheter aimed at the ipsilateral foramen of Monro (**f**)

cavity and used as a conduit for passage of the peritoneal catheter. Trocars are either "peel-away" or open on one side, allowing for easy removal of the trocar after the distal catheter is placed in the peritoneal cavity. Neither of these peritoneal catheter insertion techniques allows for direct visualization of distal catheter placement within the peritoneal cavity. Distal catheter failure rates in the adult patient approach 15–30 % in the first year after shunt surgery [106, 135]. There is no evidence that either of these methods for peritoneal catheter insertion results in a difference in rates of shunt malfunction. A modified approach for peritoneal catheter insertion that includes the use of laparoscopic assistance will be presented when reviewing shunt-related strategies to reduce rates of shunt malfunction (section "Laparoscopic-Guided Distal Catheter Insertion") (Fig. 26.4).

26.3.4.2 Ventriculoatrial Shunts

A ventriculoatrial shunt involves ventricular CSF diversion into the right atrium. While some studies have reported efficacies and complication profiles that are equivalent to VP shunts [95], concerns regarding higher cardiopulmonary complications [78, 98] and the risk of VA shunt infection deter some surgeons from performing VA shunts over VP shunts.

Similar to VP shunts, VA shunts are typically performed under general anesthesia. Following insertion of the proximal (intracranial) catheter in a similar method previously described for a VP shunt, the distal catheter is placed at the tip of the right atrium either via a direct venous cut-down approach or with the Seldinger technique

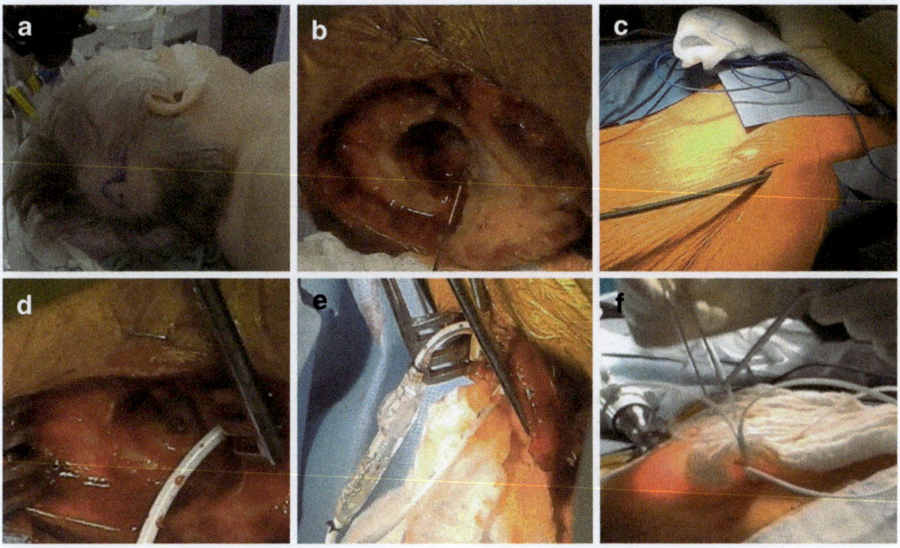

Fig. 26.4 Intraoperative photographs depicting the major steps involved in a VP shunt insertion. The patient is positioned supine and an incision is marked at the right occipital region (**a**). A burr hole is completed after the incision, and a small diameter dura-arachnoid-pia complex coagulated with a fine-tip monopolar cautery (**b**). A tunneler is used to pass (**c**) the distal catheter from the abdomen to the exit at the cranial incision site (**d**). The proximal catheter is inserted and both catheters are attached to the valve (**e**). The abdominal catheter is inserted into the peritoneal cavity (**f**) prior to closure

[50, 136]. The cut-down approach involves a neck incision and dissection to identify the common facial vein, which is cannulated under direct visualization to allow the catheter to be fed directly into the internal jugular vein (IJ). The Seldinger approach, now the preferred technique that is similar to the placement of a central venous catheter, involves cannulation of the IJ, often under ultrasound guidance with a large bore needle. A guidewire is advanced and a sheath dilator is inserted into the IJ over the guidewire. A peel-away sheath is slid over the guidewire and dilator to place the sheath in the IJ. After removal of the wire and dilator, the distal VP shunt catheter is passed into the right atrium through the peel-away sheath. Fluoroscopy is used to confirm correct placement of the catheter tip in the right atrium (at approximately the T6–T8 level). The peel-away sheath is then cracked and removed. The distal catheter is tunneled under the subcutaneous layer from a neck access point to exit at the cranial wound and attached to the distal part of the valve.

26.3.4.3 Lumboperitoneal (LP) Shunts

LP shunts are being used more commonly in Japan [69]. The shift from VP to LP shunting in Japan over the past decade has been attributed to a growing emphasis on the idea of minimally invasive surgery [108]. Although the outcomes of VP and LP shunts for treatment of iNPH appear equal, the practice pattern seems to be driven by regional or cultural differences [15, 69, 108]. A single center retrospective review of LP shunt outcomes compared to previously published VP shunt studies found no statistically significant difference between the respective patient outcomes [108]. Although, no randomized trials comparing LP and VP shunts for iNPH have been performed, the effectiveness of LP shunting has however been clearly shown in several recent studies from Japan [47, 69, 108]. For example, in the non-blinded, randomized LP shunt surgery SINPHONI-2 trial, 65 % of patients who had LP shunt surgery performed better on almost all outcome assessments, compared to 5 % of control patients [69].

While lumboperitoneal shunts may be inserted with local anesthesia, they are most often done with the patient under general anesthesia. The patient is positioned in the lateral decubitus position similar to performing a lumbar puncture procedure, and a Tuohy needle is inserted into the thecal sac at a lower lumbar level (L3–L4 or L4–L5 interspace). The proximal lumbar catheter of the shunt is then guided through the needle bore into the subarachnoid space for about 10–15 cm followed by the removal of the Tuohy needle. Positioning of the incision for the shunt valve is variable but typically located on the flank. The proximal catheter is tunneled from the lumbar to the flank incision and is attached to the proximal hub of the shunt valve device. Another 2–3 cm abdominal incision is made in the periumbilical location to allow for insertion of the distal catheter into the peritoneum. The distal catheter is attached to the valve and tunneled to this incision, and insertion of the distal catheter into the abdomen can be achieved through the open method (minilaparotomy) or trocar method, as previously described. A modified approach for insertion of the peritoneal catheter that includes the usage of laparoscopic assistance will be presented when reviewing shunt-related strategies to reduce rates of shunt malfunction (section "Laparoscopic-Guided Distal Catheter Insertion") (Fig. 26.5).

26.3.5 Surgical Outcomes

Historically, there was a wide variation in the reported outcomes of shunt surgery for iNPH, ranging from 24 to 96 % [14, 120]. However, over the past decade, due to an improved understanding of the iNPH disease process, appropriate patient selection, and standardization of research approaches, contemporary studies have shown less variation and consistently report favorable outcomes ranging between 71 and 90 % [15, 32, 39, 47, 62, 76, 92, 100, 118, 122, 147]. Gait abnormality is the iNPH symptom most dramatically responsive to shunting. It is usually the first improvement seen, the most likely to recover, and may continue to improve even years after the surgery [20, 118, 138]. Shunted patients exhibit improvement in their bladder incontinence, with a reported 30–66 % rate of recovery [56, 73, 77, 94]. Historically, it was thought that shunting did not, or rarely, improve the neurocognitive impairment associated with iNPH [42, 83, 119]. However, contemporary studies and a systematic review of 23 studies have shown cognitive improvement is observed in over 60 % of patients [112, 137].

More specifically, when iNPH patients are selected on the basis of the international or Japanese guidelines [57, 93] (see Sect. 25.2.2 of the previous Chap. 25), outcomes of shunt surgery are generally good. With respect to specific symptoms, (1) Razay reported that 89 % and 78 % of 19 iNPH patients who were shunted

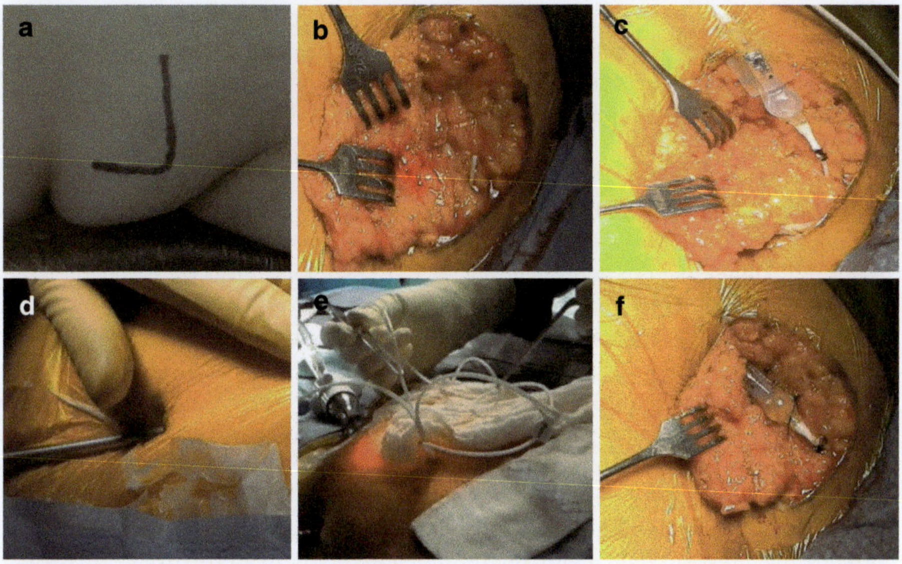

Fig. 26.5 Intraoperative images of insertion of a lumboperitoneal shunt. An infero-costal midaxillary incision is marked (**a**). The proximal lumboperitoneal catheter, which has already been inserted in the subarachnoid space at L4–L5, has been tunneled to exit at the lateral incision site (**b**). The valve is attached (**c**). A tunneler is used to pass the distal catheter to the abdominal insertion site (**d**). The distal catheter is then passed into the peritoneal cavity using a peel-away sheath (**e**). The valve is secured with sutures (**f**) prior to wound closure

showed improvement in gait and global rating, respectively [122]; (2) Williams demonstrated improvement observed in all the triad symptoms of iNPH after shunting, with gait, cognition, and bladder symptoms improving by 87 %, 86 %, and 80 %, respectively [153]; and (3) Kahlon reported that patients who demonstrate positive results on a CSF tap test (CSF-TT) and CSF infusion test (CSF-IT) report up to a 96 % subjective, 83 % gait, and a 46 % memory improvements within 6 months after VP shunting [62]. See also Table 26.3. Furthermore, postoperative improvement is long-lasting and often progressive [118].

Ventricular caliber does not correlate clinical improvement [96] and should not be used as a surrogate for surgical success. Failure to respond to or worsening of symptoms after successful shunt surgery should prompt investigations for possible shunt malfunction. While shunt revision rates are variable [118, 147], over 73 % of patients who undergo revision surgery continue to benefit [118].

26.3.6 Complications and Prevention

26.3.6.1 Shunt Complications

Complications associated with iNPH may be classified as early (perioperative; 15–30 days postoperative) or late (greater than 30 days from the surgery). The reported risk of perioperative mortality associated with VP shunt surgery has historically been reported to be less than 1 %. Patients undergoing a VP shunt should be evaluated for medical comorbidities and surgical risks which should, in consultation with other specialists as needed, be optimized prior to undergoing surgery [15]. Over the past decade, there has been a steady decline in VP shunt surgery-related mortality to 0.2 % [147].

Early (Perioperative) Complications

Cardiopulmonary complications and postoperative thromboembolic disease are the major non-shunt-specific complications of iNPH surgery. Procedure-specific complications include: (1) intracerebral hemorrhage (ICH), subarachnoid hemorrhage (SAH), subdural hemorrhage (SDH), or intraventricular hemorrhage (IVH); (2) inadvertent brain injury; and (3) solid organ or hollow viscous intra-abdominal injury. Asymptomatic mild IVH is not uncommon in VP shunt surgery, which is often identified as a thin layering of blood in the lateral ventricles. However, there is a less than 1 % risk of symptomatic ICH and a 10 % combined rate of SDH, ICH, seizure, and infections in VP shunt surgery [15, 31, 76, 147].

While surgical planning is directed to allow passage of the ventricular catheter through the nondominant hemisphere and non-eloquent brain tissue, there is a potential risk of inadvertent catheter misplacement and subsequent injury to important brain structures. Lung parenchymal or intra-abdominal organ and viscus injury is a possible (but low likelihood) complication that could occur with the passing of the distal catheter of the VP shunt system from the head into the abdominal cavity.

It is important to provide context regarding early surgical hazards and emphasize that while these risks exist, they are generally uncommon, are not typically life threatening (mortality less than 0.2 %), and are more than balanced by the high clinical benefits of shunt treatment in properly selected patients.

Late Complications

The three main late complications of VP shunt surgery are shunt malfunction, overdrainage, and infection [15, 76]. Shunt malfunction could result from a catheter obstruction or breakage or less likely due to valve dysfunction. Obstruction of the peritoneal catheter in the abdomen is the most frequent cause of shunt malfunction in the adult patient [17, 69, 121, 134].

CSF overdrainage is a potential concern in both LP and VP shunts [15, 69, 118] and may cause headache or more significant problems such as subdural effusions or chronic subdural hematoma [7, 15, 108]. These issues have decreased significantly with the use of adjustable shunts and antisiphon devices. LP shunt overdrainage may occur secondary to an inadvertent CSF leak [69], whereas VP shunt overdrainage is often secondary to a valve pressure setting that is too low for the patient [102].

Overall, the infection rates associated with shunt surgery are higher than many routine neurosurgical procedures and can span the spectrum of asymptomatic to cerebritis or meningitis. There is a lack of robust information regarding the risk of shunt infection in the adult patient, and many authors resort to extrapolating information from the pediatric population. Nevertheless, there has been a dramatic

Table 26.3 Shunt outcome studies with improvement in gait, cognition, and bladder

Study	Number of surgically treated patients	Overall improvement	Gait	Cognition	Bladder symptoms
Eide and Sorteberg 2016 [32]	316	90	–	–	–
Klinge et al. 2012 [76]	115	84	77	63	66
Pujari et al. 2008 [118]	55	62	80	76	60

reduction in reported shunt infection rates from 8–17 % in the 1970s to current expectations of less than 4 % [151].

Other shunt-related complications include intra-abdominal CSF pseudocysts or abscess, LP shunt-related radiculopathy, and seizure [7, 15, 108]. Table 26.4 outlines some of the early and delayed complications associated with shunt surgery for iNPH.

26.3.6.2 Strategies for Reduction of Surgical Morbidity and Mortality

Strategies for minimizing the risk of VP shunt-related morbidity and mortality can be classified into shunt-specific and patient-related strategies. Shunt-specific strategies include the modification of operative technique, use of adjunctive technology, and bioengineering of shunt devices. Patient-specific strategies encompass infection control, comorbidity management, and multidisciplinary postoperative follow-up. The rates of revision surgery for all causes of shunt malfunction including infections have reduced from 27 % in the 1990s to 13 % in 2006 [147] and will continue to improve as the following strategies are more broadly utilized.

Shunt-Specific Strategies

Here we present a modified approach for shunt insertion that includes the use of neuronavigation for ventricular catheter insertion and laparoscopic-assisted peritoneal catheter insertion. While it is not yet a “standard of care” for all VP shunt insertions, the available data suggest these techniques lead to lower complication and shunt failure rates when compared to traditional VP shunt insertion approaches [53, 61, 68, 121, 134, 141, 144].

Neuronavigation-Assisted Proximal Catheter Insertion

An ideal shunt catheter placement is one that traverses minimal brain parenchyma (while avoiding any critical structures in its trajectory) and which places the catheter tip away from the choroid plexus. However, due to the variations in human anatomy and at times inadvertent variability in surgical precision, the use of pre-established surface landmarks and trajectories to “blindly” place shunts may lead to nonideal placement. In searching for surgical adjuncts, investigators have

Table 26.4 VP shunt surgery-related complications

Immediate postoperative complications	Early and late complications
Anesthesia related: Cardiopulmonary events	Shunt infection: Localized vs disseminated (bacteremia) Proximal (intracranial) vs distal (intra-abdominal) SIRS→sepsis→shock Meningitis, encephalitis, meningoencephalitis
Hemorrhage Subdural Subarachnoid Intracerebral Intraventricular	Shunt obstruction or breakage: Proximal catheter Valve Distal catheter
Venous thromboembolism	CSF overdrainage: Subdural hematoma Subdural effusion (hygroma) Focal neurologic deficits Seizure
Brain injury	CSF pseudocysts
Traumatic lung injury	
Hollow viscus perforation	
Intra-abdominal solid organ injury	
Seizure	

attempted to use predetermined catheter calculations from skull x-rays [111], x-ray-guided contrast-filled catheters [107, 133], endoscopic approaches [70], and ultrasound-guided [24] and frameless stereotaxy [10, 61]. Of all these, neuronavigation-guided frameless stereotaxic catheter guidance has shown the most promising results in contemporary studies. Azeem et al. observed no proximal catheter failures during a 12-month follow-up of patients whose shunts were placed using frameless stereotaxic techniques, compared to an 18 % failure rate with traditional methods [10]. Jung et al. also showed a relative risk reduction of 20 % among patients whose shunts were placed under neuronavigation guidance, when compared to traditional methods [61]. It is our current practice to insert all ventricular catheters using the Medtronic AxiEM™ Electromagnetic Pinless Navigations System. The AxiEM™ system tracks the tip of the ventricular catheter navigation stylet and allows for precise placement of the ventricular catheter. In our experience, this has required less than 10 min for setup and has added no additional operative time with 100 % accurate ventricular catheter placement over an initial 18-month period.

Laparoscopic-Guided Distal Catheter Insertion

The conventional "blind" approaches for the insertion of the distal catheter of the VP shunt system have been described: open technique (minilaparotomy) or trocar. Approximately 80–90 % of VP shunt failures in the adult patient that require revision surgery are secondary to a distal catheter failure [8, 66, 72, 150]. While some of the distal catheter failures are due to inadvertent supra-peritoneal subcutaneous or submuscular catheter placement, most are secondary to occlusion by the omentum or intra-abdominal fibrous adhesions. As such, obesity and a previous history of intra-abdominal surgery predispose patients to a higher risk of distal catheter failure [72, 129], making recently revised shunts more likely to fail than new shunts. Given the high distal catheter failure rates, some neurosurgeons have sought the collaboration of general surgeons to laparoscopically place the distal catheter for some complex patients [12, 75, 130, 150]. Although the laparoscopic approach may seem to involve more resources than the traditional "standard" approach, it is very cost-effective in the long term as reduced obstruction rates unequivocally lead to reduced costs associated with patient investigations, hospital admissions, and surgical procedures [72, 85, 121, 144, 150].

Most of the laparoscopic approaches described in the literature involve simple direct visualization of the distal catheter insertion within the peritoneal cavity ensuring that the catheter tip has no obvious obstruction. Presently, there are a few centers including that of the author, where the goal of laparoscopic assistance is to "fix" the distal catheter through a small hole created in the falciform ligament which allows the distal catheter to be placed over the dome of the liver and drain into the right paracolic gutter (Fig. 26.6) [144]. This technique provides an "anchor" for the catheter and keeps it free from the omentum, adhesions, or bowel that may obstruct the catheter tip and has been very effective at our center in reducing the rate of distal catheter obstruction for both shunt insertions and shunt revisions.

Patient-Specific Strategies

Infection Control Protocols

At present, there is no accepted/unifying infection control protocol for adult shunt surgery. However, many centers have adopted components of the Hydrocephalus Research Network's (HCRN) pediatric quality improvement (QI) shunt protocol

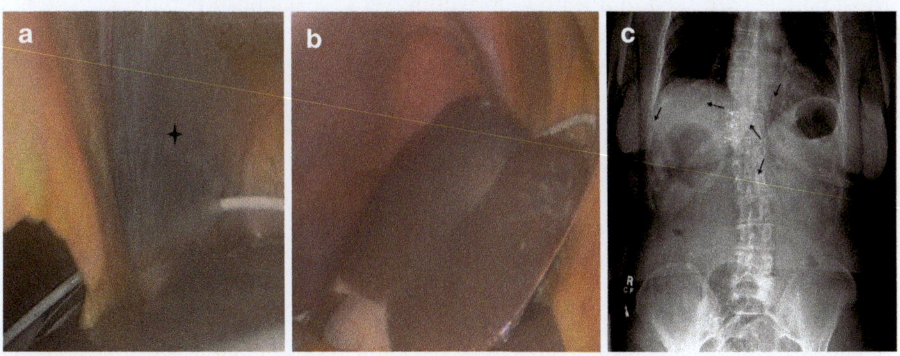

Fig. 26.6 Intraoperative images (**a**, **b**) and a postoperative abdominal x-ray depicting the course of a distal VP shunt catheter, as it traverses the thoracic region to terminate at the paracolic gutter (shown by *successive arrows* on image **c**). The catheter is seen traversing the falciform ligament (**a**, *diamond star*) and placed in the paracolic gutter supero-posterior to the liver (**b**, **c**)

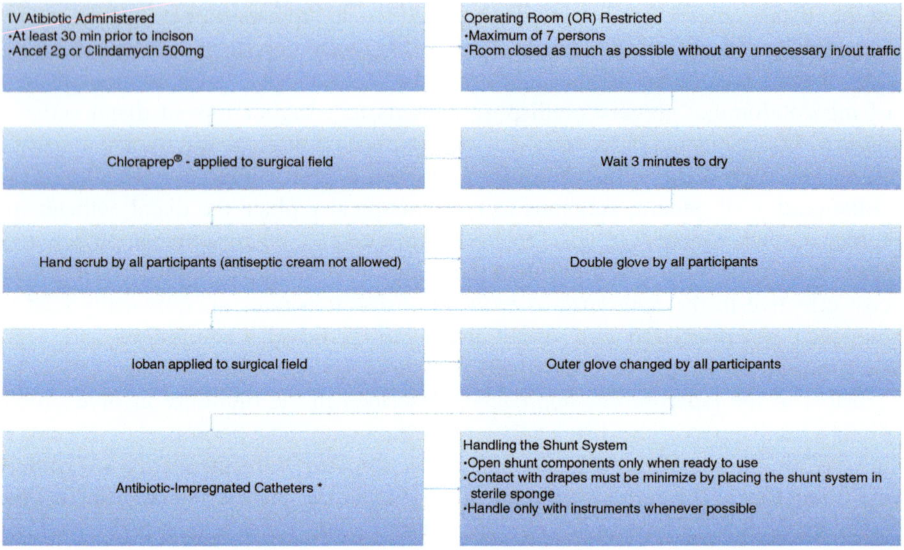

Fig. 26.7 A shunt insertion/revision algorithm modified from Kestle et al.'s HCRN Shunt Protocol [71]. *Antibiotic impregnated catheters are not routinely used at our center

[71]. Preliminary data at the author's institution where a modified version of the protocol has been established (see Fig. 26.7 below) have yielded reduced shunt infection rates (decreased from 6 to 1.7 %).

26.3.7 Postoperative Strategies to Monitor Shunt Function and Complications

Most patients are seen in a follow-up within 6–12 weeks postoperatively. The first clinic visit is geared toward ensuring adequate postoperative wound healing and to assess for interval improvement in gait, cognition, and urinary continence. Gait is typically the first of the triad of iNPH symptoms to improve (usually within the first 6 weeks), followed by cognition and then urinary continence. Therefore, objective gait and cognitive assessments postoperatively are essential not only to appreciate the patient's recovery trajectory but also to identify any delayed complications. It should be noted that substantial improvement in cognition and urinary continence might be delayed up to 6 months post-op.

The duration and frequency of a long-term follow-up is variable among surgeons but should be long term as iNPH is a chronic disease. A plain CT head scan may be obtained during the first post-op visit to ensure there are no subdural effusions or hematoma. However, repeat neuroimaging may not be required unless there is a shunt valve setting change (programmable shunt), lack of clinical improvement, or new symptom suggestive of a complication. The three major potential late complications that should be watched for include: CSF overdrainage, obstruction, and infection.

26.3.8 Overdrainage

There are currently no specific guidelines or preoperative neuroimaging findings that help guide the surgeon in selecting the initial perioperative valve pressure setting. Shunt valve opening pressures that deviate significantly from the patient's ideal may lead to CSF underdrainage or overdrainage. Underdrainage results from a valve pressure that is too high for the patient, which may create inadequate CSF movement through the shunt and lack of clinical improvement after surgery. Overdrainage typically occurs when the set valve opening pressure is too low which can lead to an excessive CSF flow. Patients who suffer from overdrainage often present with insidious symptoms of intracranial hypotension such as headaches (that may be worse with sitting and standing and improve when recumbent), nausea, altered hearing, and on some occasions long tract signs. Characteristically, the symptoms coincide with the presence of subdural effusion(s) or hematoma(s) on neuroimaging (CT or MRI of the head).

Patients treated initially with a programmable valve may often be able to undergo noninvasive elevation of the valve opening pressure. Many of the small (less than 5 mm) or asymptomatic subdural effusions or hematomas can be treated conservatively with valve adjustment, as they tend to regresses over time once the valve pressure has been appropriately adjusted. However, patients with large subdural collections that cause significant clinical impairment may require surgical drainage following pressure adjustment and possibly the addition of an antisiphon device to the valve (if not already present) to restrict CSF outflow.

In order to minimize the dire risks of overdrainage, Mori suggested to start programmable valves at high pressures and titrate down on subsequent clinic visits to achieve the desired clinical effect [102]. Wikkelso reported a study that found reducing shunt valve settings gradually from 200 to 70 mm H_2O over 6 months resulted in better outcomes and equal morbidity (overdrainage problems) as an initial fixed valve setting of 130 H_2O [131]. More research is required to help sort out strategies for different valves in the adult hydrocephalus patient population. It should also be noted that ventricular caliber does not correlate with clinical shunt responsiveness and should not be used alone as a surrogate indicator to initiate "tampering" with the pressure in a programmable shunt valve [96, 102].

If using a fixed pressure valve (rather than a programmable valve), selecting the appropriate type (i.e., opening pressure) is particularly challenging since the occurrence of an underdrainage or overdrainage may require replacement of their valve with one that has a higher opening pressure or removal of the shunt. However, because iNPH is a disease of almost normal pressure, most surgeons who opt for fixed differential valves will frequently select medium or high fixed pressure models.

26.3.9 Shunt Obstruction

CSF flow could be potentially impeded at any point along the course of a shunt: proximal catheter, valve, or distal catheter. However, as previously discussed in contrast to what happens in pediatric hydrocephalus patients, distal catheter (peritoneal) obstructions are the most common cause of shunt obstruction in the adult iNPH population. Distal obstructions are often secondary to wrapping and occlusion of distal catheter ports by omentum or fibrous scar and catheter breakage or disconnection from the valve. In terms of flow dynamics, shunt obstruction may also be classified as (1) *complete*, where there is no CSF flow, or (2) *partial*, which is characterized by reduced or delayed flow. The causes of proximal obstruction include clogging by intraventricular debris, choroid plexus, and catheter breakage at the burr hole site or disconnection from the valve. Strategies to reduce distal catheter failure rates have been previously discussed (section "Laparoscopic-Guided Distal Catheter Insertion").

26.3.10 Infection

The risk of shunt infection in the iNPH population is reported to be 3–10 %. Bacteria or, more rarely, fungi may colonize the proximal or distal portion of a shunt during implantation or later from inoculation by an infected organ or body compartment. Proximal infections often present as headaches, fever, nausea, vomiting, meningismus, and/or focal neurologic deficits. While cerebritis, encephalitis, meningitis, or abscesses due to proximal infections are rare, they carry a high risk of morbidity or mortality to the patient. Patients with isolated distal infection often present with abdominal pain, nausea, vomiting, fevers, chills, tenderness, or peritonitis. Untreated distal infections may track upward to affect the intracranial spaces. Any patient suspected of having a shunt infection must undergo a through clinical exam and laboratory investigations to identify those who may require urgent intervention. A contrast-enhanced CT scan of the head, abdomen, and pelvis may be necessary to identify any infectious collections and for ruling out other pathologies that may mimic a shunt infection. CSF samples should also be obtained by tapping the shunt reservoir and assessed for cell count, glucose, protein, Gram stain, and culture [152].

Any patient with a confirmed infection should have the entire shunt system removed, treated with a full course of appropriate antibiotic or antifungal therapy, and a new system inserted only after CSF samples have become sterile. Most patients with iNPH do not require insertion of a ventricular drain to manage intracranial pressure while their infection is treated with antibiotics. Patients will typically regress with regard to the management of their iNPH symptoms, but the potential risks associated with an external ventricular drain can be avoided for most affected individuals. Intra-abdominal fluid collections (pseudocysts) or abscess may need drainage either with ultrasound or CT guidance or by a general surgeon [151].

26.3.11 Examples of Shunt Complications

The following examples of shunt malfunction or shunt treatment complications are provided to illustrate potential management strategies.

26.3.11.1 Overdrainage Subdural Hematoma Requiring Valve Adjustment

A 77-year-old man with lumbar drainage responsive symptoms compatible with iNPH underwent a right occipital VP shunt insertion with an adjustable differential pressure valve. Three weeks postoperatively, he presented with headaches and muffled hearing. A CT head (Fig. 26.8a) demonstrated a small right subdural hematoma due to shunt overdrainage. His valve was adjusted to a higher pressure and was observed clinically with serial clinic visits. A repeat CT scan of the head 6 weeks later showed complete resolution of the hematoma.

26.3.11.2 Overdrainage Subdural Hematoma Requiring Surgery

An 81-year-old woman with lumbar drainage responsive symptoms compatible with iNPH underwent a right occipital VP shunt insertion with an adjustable differential pressure valve. One month postoperatively, she presented with symptoms (left hemiparesis) secondary to a right subdural hematoma (Fig. 26.9), which had occurred due to shunt overdrainage. Her shunt was removed, and she underwent a successful right-sided frontal burr hole catheter drainage of the hematoma, which improved her left-sided symptoms. Several weeks later, a new VP shunt was inserted through a left occipital approach (Fig. 26.9).

26.3.11.3 Distal Catheter Obstruction

An 85-year-old woman was treated successfully for lumbar drainage responsive symptoms compatible with iNPH. In the ensuing months, her gait and cognition had significantly improved, and her urinary incontinence had completely resolved. However, 15 months later, she presented with a 3-week history of gait and cognitive decline. There was no evidence of any other systemic problems such as infection or medication side effects. Investigations included an unchanged CT scan of the head and a nuclear medicine study, which revealed a distal VP

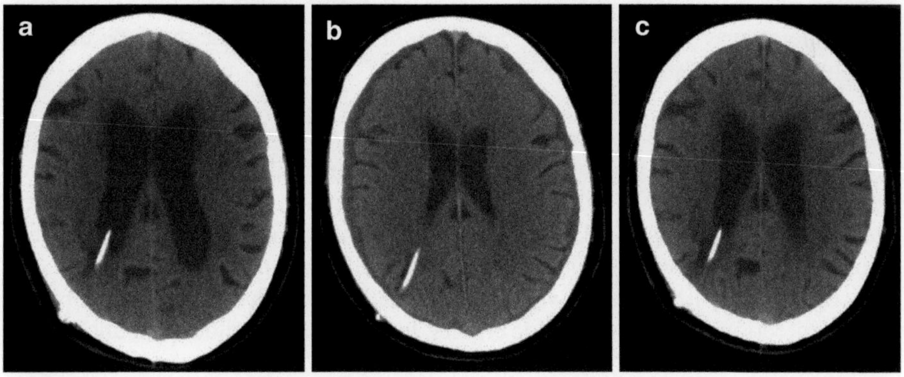

Fig. 26.8 Axial CT head images demonstrating a right lateral ventricle VP shunt via an occipital approach (**a**). Interval development of bilateral subdural hematoma (**b**) and complete resolution after up-adjustment of shunt opening pressure (**c**) can be observed

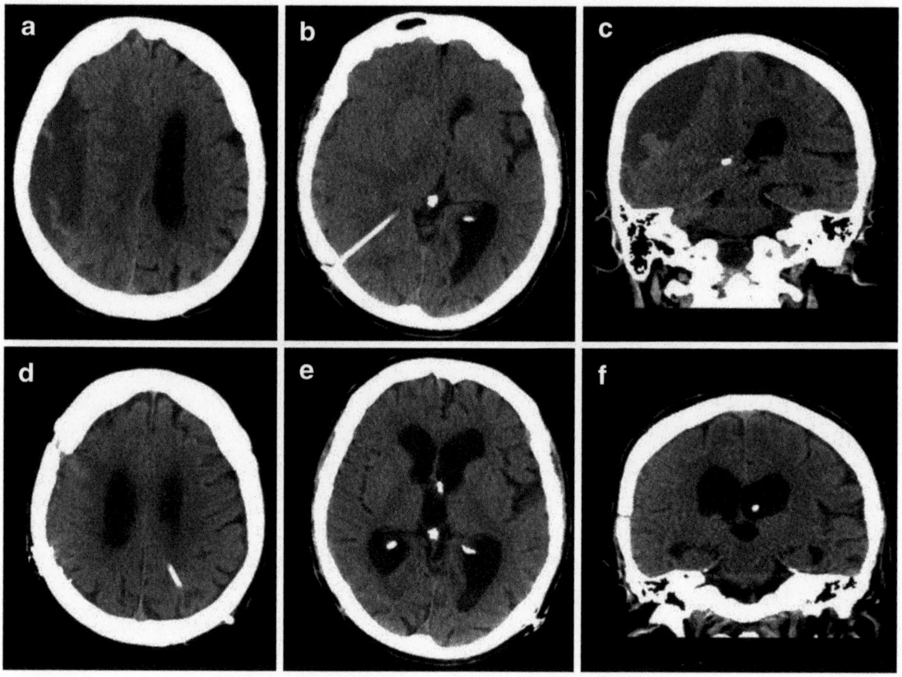

Fig. 26.9 *Top row* images are multiaxial non-contrast CT head images obtained 1 month post-op showing a 3 × 9 cm mixed density subdural hematoma (**a**) with a 1 cm midline shift (**b**), subfalcine herniation, and complete effacement of the right lateral ventricle (**c**). *Bottom row* (**d–f**) images are non-enhanced CT head images demonstrating resolved subdural hematoma following the craniotomy and clot evacuation and interval insertion of a new left occipital VP shunt (**d**)

shunt obstruction (Fig. 26.10). She then underwent a revision of the peritoneal catheter only. Intraoperatively, there was fibrous debris at the distal end of the catheter, which was removed, with restoration of fluid flow from the catheter tip. The catheter was reinserted into the peritoneal cavity using the laparoscopic technique previously described.

26.3.11.4 Proximal Catheter Disconnection

A 75-year-old woman was treated successfully for lumbar drainage responsive symptoms compatible with iNPH. In the ensuing months, her gait and cognition had significantly improved, and her urinary incontinence had completely resolved. However, 36 months later, she presented with an 8-week history of gait and cognitive decline. There was no evidence of any other systemic problems such as infection or medication side effects. Investigations included an unchanged CT scan of the head and a nuclear medicine study, which revealed a proximal VP shunt problem (Fig. 26.11). Intraoperatively, it was determined that the proximal catheter had disconnected from the valve with a broken piece of the valve's

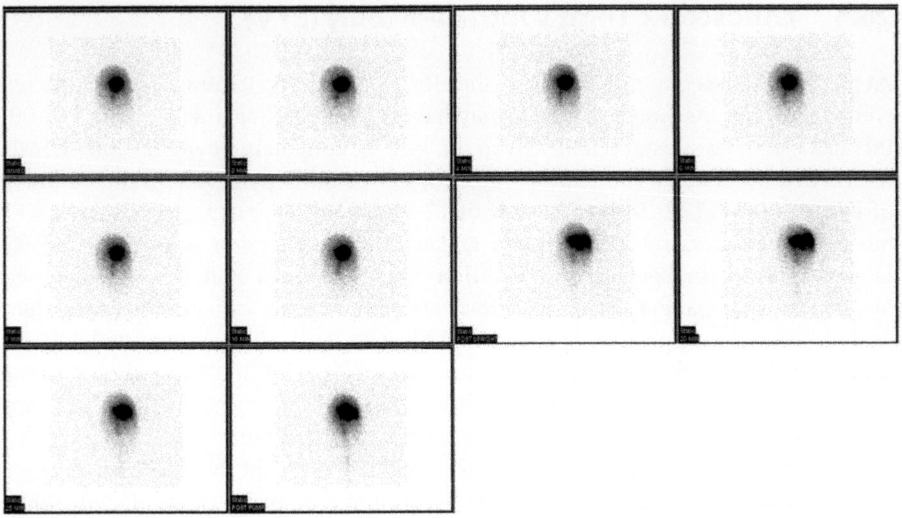

Fig. 26.10 A nuclear medicine (Technetium 99 m) CSF studies showing very delayed flow into the peritoneal cavity

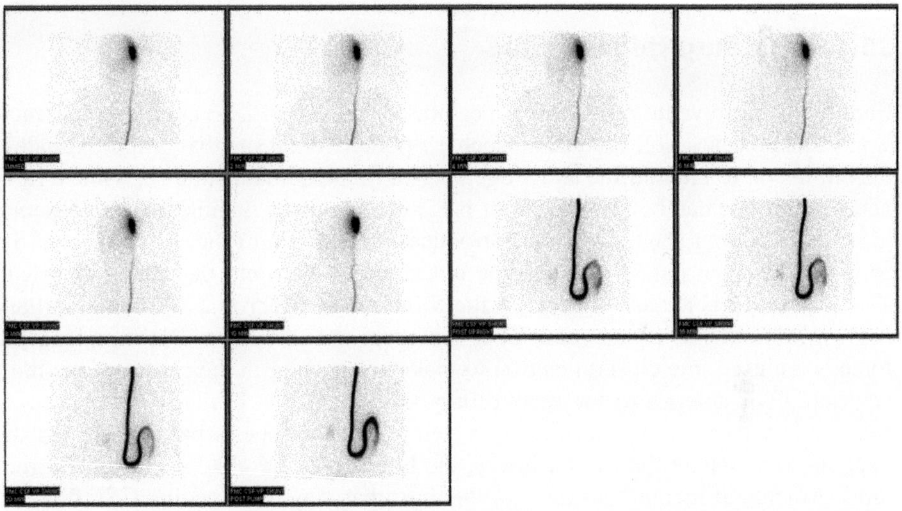

Fig. 26.11 A nuclear medicine (Technetium 99 m) CSF study demonstrating a lack of retrograde migration of contrast material into lateral ventricles. Although some of the contrast opacify the distal tubing, there is no intra-abdominal spill of contrast

proximal connector arm. Thus, the valve was replaced and her symptoms resolved. On further history, it was determined that the patient had sustained a fall 2 months prior to presenting with her recurrent symptoms at which time she impacted (hit) the valve area.

26.4 Endoscopic Third Ventriculostomy (ETV)

At present, there is ongoing debate on the efficacy of ETV in treating iNPH. Although some initial reports suggested ETV may have a role in patients with iNPH [38, 99], this has not been substantiated. Given the lack of convincing evidence, neither the international nor Japanese guidelines advocate for the use of ETV in the treatment of iNPH [57, 94, 132, 149]. A review of 12 studies by Tasiou et al. concluded ETV has a high success rate (50–100 %) and a low complication profile (0–17.9 %). However, all 12 studies were of class III or class IV level of evidence, and there was no uniformity in patient inclusion criteria and significantly variable follow-up duration for the included patients [145]. A Cochrane review by Tudor identified only one randomized trial, which was deemed inconclusive [149]. It has been suggested that the available case series and reports on ETV for iNPH that have shown the most positive results may have represented patients who demonstrated features of secondary rather than idiopathic NPH [102]. Therefore, except in cases where neuroimaging demonstrates complete obstruction of the CSF pathways (e.g., aqueductal stenosis), ETV is not indicated for treatment of hydrocephalus in the elderly population. However, with respect to the occasional situation where ETV is appropriate, a brief description of the operative procedure follows.

26.4.1 ETV Surgical Technique

Endoscopic third ventriculostomy is performed through a 2.5–3 cm transverse incision to create a burr hole located at Kocher's point (frontal site that is approximately 3.5 cm lateral to the midline and 1 cm anterior to the coronal suture). While a rigid neuroendoscope can be used, it is our preference to use a flexible neuroendoscope [55]. A peel-away sheath with an introducer is passed into the ventricle, and the endoscope is then passed through the introducer sheath into the lateral ventricle. The endoscope is advanced through the foramina of Monro, and the mammillary bodies, infundibular recess, and tuber cinereum are identified. Blunt endoscopic forceps are used in a closed position to make an opening in the center of the third ventricle floor anterior to the mammillary bodies and the basilar artery. Once an adequate ventriculostomy has been created, the endoscope is passed through the opening to visualize the basilar artery, the brainstem, the clivus, and other structures. Arachnoid membranes deep to the floor that may be impeding CSF flow are perforated. The ventricular space is copiously irrigated with Ringer's solution during the procedure to clear out any debris or blood products.

26.5 Pharmacologic Management

Presently, there are no pharmacologic agents approved for the treatment of iNPH [5], as none have demonstrated reliable efficacy for the treatment of iNPH [25]. However, the off-label use of some medications has been attempted, including the carbonic anhydrase inhibitor, acetazolamide [4, 5].

References

1. Adams RD (1966) Further observations on normal pressure hydrocephalus. Proc R Soc Med 59:1135–1140
2. Adams RD, Fisher CM, Hakim S, Ojemann RG, Sweet WH (1965) Symptomatic occult hydrocephalus with "normal" cerebrospinal-fluid pressure.a treatable syndrome. N Engl J Med 273:117–126
3. Ageno W, Gallus AS, Wittkowsky A, Crowther M, Hylek EM, Palareti G (2012) Oral anticoagulant therapy: antithrombotic therapy and prevention of thrombosis, 9th ed: American College of Chest Physicians Evidence-Based Clinical Practice Guidelines. Chest 141:e44S–e88S
4. Aimard G, Vighetto A, Gabet JY, Bret P, Henry E (1990) Acetazolamide: an alternative to shunting in normal pressure hydrocephalus? Preliminary results. Rev Neurol (Paris) 146:437–439
5. Alperin N, Oliu CJ, Bagci AM, Lee SH, Kovanlikaya I, Adams D et al (2014) Low-dose acetazolamide reverses periventricular white matter hyperintensities in iNPH. Neurology 82:1347–1351
6. Andrén K, Wikkelsø C, Tisell M, Hellström P (2014) Natural course of idiopathic normal pressure hydrocephalus. J Neurol Neurosurg Psychiatr 85:806–810
7. Aparici-Robles F, Molina-Fabrega R (2008) Abdominal cerebrospinal fluid pseudocyst: a complication of ventriculoperitoneal shunts in adults. J Med Imaging Radiation Oncol 52:40–43
8. Argo JL, Yellumahanthi DK, Ballem N, Harrigan MR, Fisher WS, Wesley MM et al (2009) Laparoscopic versus open approach for implantation of the peritoneal catheter during ventriculoperitoneal shunt placement. Surg Endosc 23:1449–1455
9. Aschoff A, Kremer P, Hashemi B, Kunze S (1999) The scientific history of hydrocephalus and its treatment. Neurosurg Rev 22:67–95
10. Azeem SS, Origitano TC (2007) Ventricular catheter placement with a frameless neuronavigational system. Neurosurgery 60:243–248
11. Bandeen-Roche K, Xue Q-L, Ferrucci L, Walston J, Guralnik JM, Chaves P et al (2006) Phenotype of frailty: characterization in the women's health and aging studies. J Gerontol A Biol Sci Med Sci 61:262–266
12. Bani A, Telker D, Hassler W, Grundlach M (2006) Minimally invasive implantation of the peritoneal catheter in ventriculoperitoneal shunt placement for hydrocephalus: analysis of data in 151 consecutive adult patients. J Neurosurg 105:869–872
13. Basati SS, Harris TJ, Linninger AA (2011) Dynamic brain phantom for intracranial volume measurements. IEEE Trans Biomed Eng 58:1450–1455
14. Benzel EC, Pelletier AL, Levy PG (1990) Communicating hydrocephalus in adults: prediction of outcome after ventricular shunting procedures. Neurosurgery 26:655–660
15. Bergsneider M, Black PM, Klinge P, Marmarou A, Relkin N (2005) Surgical management of idiopathic normal-pressure hydrocephalus. Neurosurgery 57(3 Suppl):S29–S39
16. Bergsneider M, Lee S, Judy JW (2008) Self-Clearing Catheter for Clinical Implantation, Google Patents
17. Bergsneider M, Miller C, Vespa PM, Hu X (2008) Surgical management of adult hydrocephalus. Neurosurgery 62(Suppl 2):643–660
18. Boon AJ, Tans JT, Delwel EJ, Egeler-Peerdeman SM, Hanlo PW, Wurzer HA et al (1998) Dutch Normal-Pressure Hydrocephalus Study: randomized comparison of low- and medium-pressure shunts. J Neurosurg 88:490–495
19. Boyd JB, Bradford B, Watne AL (1980) Operative risk factors of colon resection in the elderly. Ann Surg 192:743–746
20. Bradley WG (2000) Normal pressure hydrocephalus: new concepts on etiology and diagnosis. AJNR Am J Neuroradiol 21(9):1586–1590
21. Bullara, LA (1978) Implantable pressure transducer, Google Patents

22. Casmiro M, D'Alessandro R, Cacciatore FM, Daidone R, Calbucci F, Lugaresi E (1989) Risk factors for the syndrome of ventricular enlargement with gait apraxia (idiopathic normal pressure hydrocephalus): a case–control study. J Neurol Neurosurg Psychiatr 52:847–852
23. Chow WB, Rosenthal RA, Merkow RP, Ko CY, Esnaola NF, American College of Surgeons National Surgical Quality Improvement Program et al (2012) Optimal preoperative assessment of the geriatric surgical patient: a best practices guideline from the American College of Surgeons National Surgical Quality Improvement Program and the American Geriatrics Society. J Am Coll Surg 215:453–466
24. Crowley RW, Dumont AS, Asthagiri AR, Torner JC, Medel R, Jane JA et al (2014) Intraoperative ultrasound guidance for the placement of permanent ventricular cerebrospinal fluid shunt catheters: a single-center historical cohort study. World Neurosurg 81:397–403
25. Del Bigio MR, Di Curzio DL (2016) Nonsurgical therapy for hydrocephalus: a comprehensive and critical review. Fluids Barriers CNS 13:1–20
26. Devereaux PJ, Cohn SL, Eagle KA (2016) Management of cardiac risk for noncardiac surgery. In: Post TW (ed) UpToDate, 5 edn. UpToDate, Waltham, pp 1–14
27. Devereaux PJ, Goldman L, Cook DJ (2005) Perioperative cardiac events in patients undergoing noncardiac surgery: a review of the magnitude of the problem, the pathophysiology of the events and methods to estimate and communicate risk. CMAJ 173(6):627–634
28. Douketis JD (2011) Perioperative management of patients who are receiving warfarin therapy: an evidence-based and practical approach. Blood 117:5044–5049
29. Douketis JD, Spyropoulos AC, Spencer FA, Mayr M, Jaffer AK, Eckman MH et al (2012) Perioperative management of antithrombotic therapy: antithrombotic therapy and prevention of thrombosis, 9th ed: American College of Chest Physicians Evidence-Based Clinical Practice Guidelines. Chest 141:e326S–e350S
30. Drake JM, Sainte-Rose C (1995) The Shunt Book. Wiley-Blackwell, Cambridge
31. Eide PK, Sorteberg W (2010) Diagnostic intracranial pressure monitoring and surgical management in idiopathic normal pressure hydrocephalus: a 6-year review of 214 patients. Neurosurgery 66:80–91
32. Eide PK, Sorteberg W (2016) Outcome of surgery for idiopathic normal pressure hydrocephalus: role of preoperative static and pulsatile intracranial pressure. World Neurosurg 86:186–193.e1
33. Eklund A, Smielewski P, Chambers I, Alperin N, Malm J, Czosnyka M et al (2007) Assessment of cerebrospinal fluid outflow resistance. Med Biol Eng Comput 45:719–735
34. Filsoufi F, Rahmanian PB, Castillo JG, Chikwe J, Silvay G, Adams DH (2008) Excellent early and late outcomes of aortic valve replacement in people aged 80 and older. J Am Geriatr Soc 56:255–261
35. Finlayson E, Fan Z, Birkmeyer JD (2007) Outcomes in octogenarians undergoing high-risk cancer operation: A National Study. J Am Coll Surg 205:729–734
36. Fox BD, Kahn SR, Langleben D, Eisenberg MJ, Shimony A (2012) Efficacy and safety of novel oral anticoagulants for treatment of acute venous thromboembolism: direct and adjusted indirect meta-analysis of randomised controlled trials. BMJ 345:e7498
37. Fried LP, Tangen CM, Walston J, Newman AB, Hirsch C, Gottdiener J et al (2001) Frailty in older adults: evidence for a phenotype. J Gerontol A Biol Sci Med Sci 56:M146–M156
38. Gangemi M, Maiuri F, Buonamassa S, Colella G, de Divitiis E (2004) Endoscopic third ventriculostomy in idiopathic normal pressure hydrocephalus. Neurosurgery 55:129–134
39. Gölz L, Ruppert F-H, Meier U, Lemcke J (2014) Outcome of modern shunt therapy in patients with idiopathic normal pressure hydrocephalus 6 years postoperatively. J Neurosurg 121:771–775
40. Greenberg MS (2010) Handbook of Neurosurgery. Thieme, New York, pp 207–212
41. Group PS (2008) Effects of extended-release metoprolol succinate in patients undergoing non-cardiac surgery (POISE trial): a randomised controlled trial. Lancet 371(9627): 1839–1847
42. Gustafson L, Hagberg B (1978) Recovery in hydrocephalic dementia after shunt operation. J Neurol Neurosurg Psychiatr 41:940–947

43. Hakim S, Adams RD (1965) The special clinical problem of symptomatic hydrocephalus with normal cerebrospinal fluid pressure. Observations on cerebrospinal fluid hydrodynamics. J Neurol Sci 2:307–327
44. Hakim S (1964) Algunas Observaciones Sobre La Presión Del L.C.R. Síndrome Hidrocefálico en El Adulto Con Presión Normal Del L.C.R.: (Presentación De Un Nuevo Síndrome). Javeriana University School of Medicine, Bogotá (Doctoral Thesis)
45. Halperin JJ, Kurlan R, Schwalb JM, Cusimano MD, Gronseth G, Gloss D (2015) Practice guideline: idiopathic normal pressure hydrocephalus: response to shunting and predictors of response: report of the guideline development, dissemination, and implementation subcommittee of the American Academy of Neurology. Neurology 85:2063–2071
46. Hamilton M, Couldwell WT, Golfinos JG (2014) Handbook of bleeding and coagulation for neurosurgery
47. Hashimoto M, Ishikawa M, Mori E, Kuwana N (2010) Diagnosis of idiopathic normal pressure hydrocephalus is supported by MRI-based scheme: a prospective cohort study. Cerebrospinal Fluid Res 7(1):18
48. Haynes IS (1913) I. Congenital internal hydrocephalus: its treatment by drainage of the cisterna magna into the cranial sinuses. Ann Surg 57:449–484
49. Healey JS, Eikelboom J, Douketis J, Wallentin L, Oldgren J, Yang S et al (2012) Periprocedural bleeding and thromboembolic events with dabigatran compared with warfarin: results from the randomized evaluation of long-term anticoagulation therapy (RE-LY) randomized trial. Circulation 126:343–348
50. Higgs Z, Macafee D, Braithwaite BD, Maxwell-Armstrong CA (2005) The Seldinger technique: 50 years on. Lancet 366:1407–1409
51. Hirsch IB, McGill JB, Cryer PE, White PF (1991) Perioperative management of surgical patients with diabetes mellitus. Anesthesiology 74:346–359
52. Hollenberg M, Mangano DT, Browner WS, London MJ, Tubau JF, Tateo IM (1992) Predictors of postoperative myocardial ischemia in patients undergoing noncardiac surgery. The Study of Perioperative Ischemia Research Group. JAMA 268:205–209
53. Huie F, Sayad P, Usal H, Hayek N, Arbit E, Ferzli G (1999) Laparoscopic transabdominal lumboperitoneal shunt. Surg Endosc 13:161–163
54. Hydrocephalus Association (2016) Shunt systems for the management of hydrocephalus. Shunt Systems, from http://www.hydroassoc.org/shunt-systems/
55. Isaacs AM, Bezchlibnyk YB, Yong H, Koshy D, Urbaneja G, Hader W et al (2016) Endoscopic third ventriculostomy for treatment of adult hydrocephalus: long-term follow up of 163 patients. Neurosurg Focus 41(3):E3
56. Ishii K, Hashimoto M, Hayashida K, Hashikawa K, Chang C-C, Nakagawara J et al (2011) A multicenter brain perfusion SPECT study evaluating idiopathic normal-pressure hydrocephalus on neurological improvement. Dement Geriatr Cogn Disord 32:1–10
57. Ishikawa M, Hashimoto M, Kuwana N, Mori E, Miyake H, Wachi A et al (2008) Guidelines for management of idiopathic normal pressure hydrocephalus. Neurol Med Chir (Tokyo) 48 Suppl:S1–S23
58. Jacobs L (1977) Diabetes mellitus in normal pressure hydrocephalus. J Neurol Neurosurg Psychiatr 40:331–335
59. Jenkinson MD, Gamble C, Hartley JC, Hickey H (2014) The British antibiotic and silver-impregnated catheters for ventriculoperitoneal shunts multi-centre randomised controlled trial (the BASICS trial): study protocol. Trials 15:4
60. Joint Task Force on the Management of Valvular Heart Disease of the European Society of Cardiology (ESC), European Association for Cardio-Thoracic Surgery (EACTS), Vahanian A, Alfieri O, Andreotti F, Antunes MJ, et al (2012) Guidelines on the management of valvular heart disease (version 2012). Eur Heart J 33:2451–2496
61. Jung N, Kim D (2013) Effect of electromagnetic navigated ventriculoperitoneal shunt placement on failure rates. J Korean Neurosurg Soc 53:150–155
62. Kahlon B, Sjunnesson J, Rehncrona S (2007) Long–term outcome in patients with suspected normal pressure hydrocephalus. Neurosurgery 60:327

63. Kanemoto H, Kazui H, Suzuki Y, Sato S, Kishima H, Yoshimine T et al (2016) Effect of lumbo-peritoneal shunt surgery on neuropsychiatric symptoms in patients with idiopathic normal pressure hydrocephalus. J Neurol Sci 361:206–212
64. Katlic MR (2010) Consider surgery for elderly patients. CMAJ 182:1403–1404
65. Katlic MR (2013) The holy grail of geriatric surgery. Ann Surg 257:1005–1006
66. Kavic SM, Segan RD, Taylor MD, Roth JS (2007) Laparoscopic management of ventriculo-peritoneal and lumboperitoneal shunt complications. JSLS 11:14–19
67. Kaw R, Chung F, Pasupuleti V, Mehta J, Gay PC, Hernandez AV (2012) Meta-analysis of the association between obstructive sleep apnoea and postoperative outcome. Br J Anaesth 109:897–906
68. Kawahara T, Tokimura H, Higa N, Hirano H, Bohara M (2013) Surgical technique for preventing subcutaneous migration of distal lumboperitoneal shunt catheters. Innovative Neurosurg 1(3–4):169–172
69. Kazui H, Miyajima M, Mori E, Ishikawa M (2015) Lumboperitoneal shunt surgery for idiopathic normal pressure hydrocephalus (SINPHONI-2): an open-label randomised trial. Lancet Neurol 14:585–594
70. Kestle JRW, Drake JM, Cochrane DD, Milner R, Walker ML, Abbott R et al (2003) Lack of benefit of endoscopic ventriculoperitoneal shunt insertion: a multicenter randomized trial. J Neurosurg 98:284–290
71. Kestle JRW, Holubkov R, Douglas Cochrane D, Kulkarni AV, Limbrick DD, Luerssen TG et al (2016) A new hydrocephalus clinical research network protocol to reduce cerebrospinal fluid shunt infection. J Neurosurg Pediatr 17(4):391–396
72. Khosrovi H, Kaufman HH, Hrabovsky E, Bloomfield SM, Prabhu V, el-Kadi HA (1998) Laparoscopic-assisted distal ventriculoperitoneal shunt placement. Surg Neurol 49:127–135
73. Kilic K (2010) Predicting the outcome of shunt surgery in normal pressure hydrocephalus. Neurosurgery 66:E1217; author reply E1217
74. Kim YT, Kim JY (2015) Shunt for the hydrocephalus: the past and the present. Inter Student's J
75. Kirshtein B, Benifla M, Roy-Shapira V, Merkin V, Melamed I, Cohen Z, Cohen A (2004) "Laparoscopically guided distal ventriculoperitoneal shunt placement." Surg Laparosc Endosc Percutan Tech 14(5):276–278
76. Klinge P, Hellström P, Tans J, Wikkelsø C (2012) European iNPH Multicentre Study Group: one-year outcome in the European multicentre study on iNPH. Acta Neurol Scand 126:145–153
77. Klinge P, Marmarou A, Bergsneider M, Relkin N, Black PM (2005) Outcome of shunting in idiopathic normal-pressure hydrocephalus and the value of outcome assessment in shunted patients. Neurosurgery 57:S40–S52
78. Kluge S, Baumann HJ, Regelsberger J, Kehler U, Gliemroth J, Koziej B et al (2010) Pulmonary hypertension after ventriculoatrial shunt implantation. J Neurosurg 113:1279–1283
79. Krauss JK, Regel JP, Vach W, Droste DW, Borremans JJ, Mergner T (1996) Vascular risk factors and arteriosclerotic disease in idiopathic normal-pressure hydrocephalus of the elderly. Stroke 27:24–29
80. Kurtom KH, Magram G (2007) Siphon regulatory devices: their role in the treatment of hydrocephalus. Neurosurg Focus 22:1–8
81. Landesberg G, Beattie WS, Mosseri M, Jaffe AS (2009) Perioperative myocardial infarction. Circulation 119(22):2936–2944
82. Lane JD, Mugamba J, Ssenyonga P, Warf BC (2014) Effectiveness of the bactiseal universal shunt for reducing shunt infection in a sub-Saharan African context: a retrospective cohort study in 160 Ugandan children. J Neurosurg Pediatr 13:140–144
83. Larsson A, Wikkelsø C, Bilting M, Stephensen H (1991) Clinical parameters in 74 consecutive patients shunt operated for normal pressure hydrocephalus. Acta Neurol Scand 84:475–482

84. Lee TH, Marcantonio ER, Mangione CM, Thomas EJ, Polanczyk CA, Cook EF et al (1999) Derivation and prospective validation of a simple index for prediction of cardiac risk of major noncardiac surgery. Circulation 100:1043–1049
85. Li B, Zhang Q, Liu J, Yu H, Hu S (2009) Clinical application of a laparoscope in ventri-peritoneal shunting. Minim Invasive Ther Allied Technol 16:367–369
86. Linninger A, Basati S, Dawe R, Penn R (2009) An impedance sensor to monitor and control cerebral ventricular volume. Med Eng Phys 31:838–845
87. Lip GY, Douketis JD (2016) Perioperative management of patients receiving anticoagulants. In: Post TW, Leung LL, Timaeur JS (eds) UpToDate, 5 edn. UpToDate, Waltham, pp 1–42
88. Lockhart EM, Willingham MD, Abdallah AB, Helsten DL, Bedair BA, Thomas J et al (2013) Obstructive sleep apnea screening and postoperative mortality in a large surgical cohort. Sleep Med 14:407–415
89. Ludin L, Mauge C (2012) Programmable shunt with electromechanical valve actuator, Codman & Shurtleff, Inc
90. Makary MA, Segev DL, Pronovost PJ, Syin D, Bandeen-Roche K, Patel P et al (2010) Frailty as a predictor of surgical outcomes in older patients. J Am Coll Surg 210(6):901–908
91. Marmarou A, Bergsneider M, Klinge P, Relkin N, Black PM (2005) The value of supplemental prognostic tests for the preoperative assessment of idiopathic normal-pressure hydrocephalus. Neurosurgery 57(3 Suppl):S17–S28
92. Marmarou A, Bergsneider M, Relkin N, Klinge P, Black PM (2005) Development of guidelines for idiopathic normal-pressure hydrocephalus: introduction. Neurosurgery 57(3 Suppl):S1–S3
93. Marmarou A, Black P, Bergsneider M, Klinge P, Relkin N (2005) Guidelines for management of idiopathic normal pressure hydrocephalus: progress to date. Acta Neurochir Suppl 95:237–240
94. Marmarou A, Young HF, Aygok GA, Sawauchi S (2005) Diagnosis and management of idiopathic normal-pressure hydrocephalus: a prospective study in 151 patients. J Neurosurg 102(6):987–997
95. McGovern RA, Kelly KM, Chan AK, Morrissey NJ, McKhann GM (2014) Should ventriculoatrial shunting be the procedure of choice for normal-pressure hydrocephalus? J Neurosurg 120:1458–1464
96. Meier U, Mutze S (2004) Correlation between decreased ventricular size and positive clinical outcome following shunt placement in patients with normal-pressure hydrocephalus. J Neurosurg 100:1036–1040. http://dx.doi.org/103171/jns200410061036
97. Meltzer H (2011) Insertion of Ventriculoperitoneal Shunt. In: Jandial R, McCormick P, Black P. Core Techniques in Operative Neurosurgery. Elsevier Saunders. Philadelphia, PA
98. Milton CA, Sanders P, Steele PM (2001) Late cardiopulmonary complication of ventriculoatrial shunt. Lancet 358(9293):1608
99. Mitchell P, Mathew B (1999) Third ventriculostomy in normal pressure hydrocephalus. Br J Neurosurg 13:382–385
100. Miyajima M, Kazui H, Mori E, Ishikawa M (2016) One-year outcome in patients with idiopathic normal-pressure hydrocephalus: comparison of lumboperitoneal shunt to ventriculoperitoneal shunt. J Neurosurg: 1–10
101. Mokhlesi B, Hovda MD, Vekhter B, Arora VM, Chung F, Meltzer DO (2013) Sleep-disordered breathing and postoperative outcomes after elective surgery: analysis of the nationwide inpatient sample. Chest 144:903–914
102. Mori E, Ishikawa M, Kato T, Kazui H, Miyake H, Miyajima M et al (2012) Guidelines for management of idiopathic normal pressure hydrocephalus: second edition. Neurol Med Chir (Tokyo) 52:775–809
103. Morley JE, Vellas B, Van Kan GA, Anker SD, Bauer JM, Bernabei R et al (2013) Frailty consensus: a call to action. J Am Med Dir Assoc 14:392–397
104. Mozaffarian D, Benjamin EJ, Go AS, Arnett DK (2015) Executive summary: heart disease and stroke statistics—2015 update a report from the American Heart Association. Circulation 131(4):e29–e322

105. Muluk V, Macpherson DS, Cohn SL, Whinney C (2016) Perioperative medication management. In: Post TW (ed) UpToDate, 5 edn. UpToDate, Waltham, pp 1–50
106. Naftel RP, Argo JL, Shannon CN, Taylor TH, Tubbs RS, Clements RH et al (2011) Laparoscopic versus open insertion of the peritoneal catheter in ventriculoperitoneal shunt placement: review of 810 consecutive cases. J Neurosurg 115:151–158
107. Nakajima M, Bando K, Miyajima M, Arai H (2009) Lumboperitoneal shunt placement using computed tomography and fluoroscopy in conscious patients. J Neurosurg 111:618–622
108. Nakajima M, Miyajima M, Ogino I, Sugano H, Akiba C, Domon N et al (2015) Use of external lumbar cerebrospinal fluid drainage and lumboperitoneal shunts with Strata NSC valves in idiopathic normal pressure hydrocephalus: a single-center experience. World Neurosurg 83:387–393
109. Nishimura RA, Otto CM, Bonow RO, Carabello BA, Erwin JP, Guyton RA et al (2014) 2014 AHA/ACC guideline for the management of patients with valvular heart disease: a report of the American College of Cardiology/American Heart Association Task Force on Practice Guidelines. J Am Coll Cardiol 63:e57–e185
110. Orandi BJ, Winter JM, Segev DL, Makary MA (2011) Frailty and surgery in the elderly. In: Principles and Practice of Geriatric Surgery. Springer, New York, pp 129–134
111. Pang D, Grabb PA (1994) Accurate placement of coronal ventricular catheter using stereotactic coordinate-guided free-hand passage. J Neurosurg 80:750–755
112. Peterson KA, Housden CR, Killikelly C, DeVito EE, Keong NC, Savulich G et al (2016) Apathy, ventriculomegaly and neurocognitive improvement following shunt surgery in normal pressure hydrocephalus. Br J Neurosurg 30(1):38–42
113. Peterson KA, Savulich G, Jackson D, Killikelly C, Pickard JD, Sahakian BJ (2016) The effect of shunt surgery on neuropsychological performance in normal pressure hydrocephalus: a systematic review and meta-analysis. J Neurol 263(8):1669–1677
114. Pollack IF, Albright AL, Adelson PD (1999) A randomized, controlled study of a programmable shunt valve versus a conventional valve for patients with hydrocephalus. Hakim-Medos Investigator Group. Neurosurgery 45(6):1399–1408
115. Portnoy HD, Schulte RR, Fox JL, Croissant PD, Tripp L (1973) Anti-siphon and reversible occlusion valves for shunting in hydrocephalus and preventing post-shunt subdural hematomas. J Neurosurg 38:729–738
116. Pudenz RH (1957) Experimental and clinical observations on the shunting of cerebrospinal fluid into the circulatory system. Clin Neurosurg 5:98–114; discussion 114–115
117. Pudenz RH, Russell FE, Hurd AH, Shelden CH (1957) Ventriculo-auriculostomy; a technique for shunting cerebrospinal fluid into the right auricle; preliminary report. J Neurosurg 14:171–179
118. Pujari S, Kharkar S, Metellus P, Shuck J, Williams MA, Rigamonti D (2008) Normal pressure hydrocephalus: long-term outcome after shunt surgery. J Neurol Neurosurg Psychiatr 79:1282–1286
119. Raftopoulos C, Deleval J, Chaskis C, Leonard A, Cantraine F, Desmyttere F et al (1994) Cognitive recovery in idiopathic normal pressure hydrocephalus: a prospective study. Neurosurgery 35:397–405
120. Raftopoulos C, Massager N, Balériaux D, Deleval J, Clarysse S, Brotchi J (1996) Prospective analysis by computed tomography and long-term outcome of 23 adult patients with chronic idiopathic hydrocephalus. Neurosurgery 38:51–59
121. Raysi Dehcordi S, De Tommasi C, Ricci A, Marzi S, Ruscitti C, Amicucci G et al (2011) Laparoscopy-assisted ventriculoperitoneal shunt surgery: personal experience and review of the literature. Neurosurg Rev 34:363–371
122. Razay G, Vreugdenhil A, Liddell J (2009) A prospective study of ventriculo-peritoneal shunting for idiopathic normal pressure hydrocephalus. J Clin Neurosci 16:1180–1183
123. Reinprecht A, Czech T, Dietrich W (1995) Clinical experience with a new pressure-adjustable shunt valve. Acta Neurochir (Wien) 134:119–124
124. Relkin N, Marmarou A, Klinge P, Bergsneider M, Black PM (2005) Diagnosing idiopathic normal-pressure hydrocephalus. Neurosurgery 57:S4–S16

125. Riva-Cambrin J, Kestle JRW, Holubkov R, Butler J, Kulkarni AV, Drake J et al (2016) Risk factors for shunt malfunction in pediatric hydrocephalus: a multicenter prospective cohort study. J Neurosurg Pediatr 17(4):382–390
126. Robert-Ebadi H, Le Gal G, Righini M (2009) Use of anticoagulants in elderly patients: practical recommendations. Clin Interv Aging 4:165–177
127. Robinson S (2016) Editorial: reducing the risk of shunt malfunction: beacons of light. J Neurosurg Pediatr 17(4):379–381
128. Rockwood K, Mitnitski A (2007) Frailty in relation to the accumulation of deficits. J Gerontol A Biol Sci Med Sci 62:722–727
129. Roth JS, Park AE, Gewirtz R (2000) Minilaparoscopically assisted placement of ventriculoperitoneal shunts. Surg Endosc 14:461–463
130. Roth J, Sagie B, Szold A, Elran H (2007) Laparoscopic versus non-laparoscopic-assisted ventriculoperitoneal shunt placement in adults. A retrospective analysis. Surg Neurol 68:177–184
131. Sæhle T, Farahmand D, Eide PK, Tisell M, Wikkelsø C (2014) A randomized controlled dual-center trial on shunt complications in idiopathic normal-pressure hydrocephalus treated with gradually reduced or "fixed" pressure valve settings. J Neurosurg 121:1257–1263
132. Sankey EW, Jusué-Torres I, Elder BD, Goodwin CR, Batra S, Hoffberger J et al (2015) Functional gait outcomes for idiopathic normal pressure hydrocephalus after primary endoscopic third ventriculostomy. J Clin Neurosci 22:1303–1308
133. Sato K, Shimizu S, Oka H, Fujii K (2013) Intraoperative fluoroscopy with contrast medium for correct lumbar catheter placement in lumboperitoneal shunts. Kitasato Med J 43:155–158
134. Schubert F, Fijen BP, Krauss JK (2005) Laparoscopically assisted peritoneal shunt insertion in hydrocephalus: a prospective controlled study. Surg Endosc 19:1588–1591
135. Schucht P, Banz V, Trochsler M, Iff S, Krähenbühl AK, Reinert M et al (2015) Laparoscopically assisted ventriculoperitoneal shunt placement: a prospective randomized controlled trial. J Neurosurg 122:1058–1067
136. Seldinger SI (1953) Catheter replacement of the needle in percutaneous arteriography: a new technique. Acta Radiol 39:368–376
137. Shaw R, Everingham E, Mahant N, Jacobson E, Owler B (2016) Clinical outcomes in the surgical treatment of idiopathic normal pressure hydrocephalus. J Clin Neurosci 29:81–86
138. Shaw R, Mahant N, Jacobson E, Owler B (2016) A review of clinical outcomes for gait and other variables in the surgical treatment of idiopathic normal pressure hydrocephalus. Mov Disord Clin Pract. doi:10.1002/mdc3.12335
139. Simon TD, Butler J, Whitlock KB, Browd SR, Holubkov R, Kestle JR, Kulkarni AV, Langley M, Limbrick DD Jr, Mayer-Hamblett N, Tamber M, Wellons JC 3rd, Whitehead WE, Riva-Cambrin J, Hydrocephalus Clinical Research Network (2014) Risk factors for first cerebrospinal fluid shunt infection: findings from a multi-center Prospective Cohort Study. J Pediatr 164:1462–1468.e2
140. Singh M, Liao P, Kobah S, Wijeysundera DN, Shapiro C, Chung F (2013) Proportion of surgical patients with undiagnosed obstructive sleep apnoea. Br J Anaesth 110:629–636
141. Singh K, Raj J, Tiwari DP (2013) Conventional versus neuro-navigation guided shunt surgery. World J Med Res 2:6
142. Smetana GW, Lawrence VA, Cornell JE (2006) Preoperative pulmonary risk stratification for noncardiothoracic surgery: systematic review for the American College of Physicians. Ann Intern Med 144:581–595
143. Spyropoulos DAC, Merli G (2006) Management of venous thromboembolism in the elderly. Drugs Aging 23:651–671
144. Svoboda SM, Park H, Naff N, Dorai Z, Williams MA, Youssef Y (2015) Preventing distal catheter obstruction in laparoscopic ventriculoperitoneal shunt placement in adults: The "Falciform Technique". J Laparoendoscopic Adv Surg Tech 25(8):642–645
145. Tasiou A, Brotis AG, Esposito F, Paterakis KN (2016) Endoscopic third ventriculostomy in the treatment of idiopathic normal pressure hydrocephalus: a review study. Neurosurg Rev 39(4):557–563

146. Thomas GA, Farrow RC, Liu S (2012) No clog shunt using a compact fluid drag path
147. Toma AK, Papadopoulos MC, Stapleton S, Kitchen ND, Watkins LD (2013) Systematic review of the outcome of shunt surgery in idiopathic normal-pressure hydrocephalus. Acta Neurochir (Wien) 155:1977–1980
148. Toma AK, Stapleton S, Papadopoulos MC, Kitchen ND, Watkins LD (2011) Natural history of idiopathic normal-pressure hydrocephalus. Neurosurg Rev 34:433–439
149. Tudor KI, Tudor M, McCleery J, Car J (2015) Endoscopic third ventriculostomy (ETV) for idiopathic normal pressure hydrocephalus (iNPH). Cochrane Database Syst Rev (7):CD010033
150. Turner RD, Rosenblatt SM, Chand B, Luciano MG (2007) Laparoscopic peritoneal catheter placement: results of a new method in 111 patients. Neurosurgery 61:167–174
151. Wells DL, Allen JM (2013) Ventriculoperitoneal shunt infections in adult patients. AACN Adv Crit Care 24:6–12
152. Williams MA, Malm J (2016) Diagnosis and treatment of idiopathic normal pressure hydrocephalus. Continuum Lifelong Learning Neurol 22:577–579
153. Williams MA, Relkin NR (2013) Diagnosis and management of idiopathic normal-pressure hydrocephalus. Neurol Clini Pract 3:375–385
154. Wozniak SE, Coleman J, Katlic MR (2015) Optimal preoperative evaluation and perioperative care of the geriatric patient: a surgeon's perspective. Anesthesiol Clin 33:481–489
155. Zarraga IGE, Kron J (2013) Oral anticoagulation in elderly adults with atrial fibrillation: integrating new options with old concepts. J Am Geriatr Soc 61:143–150
156. Zemack G, Romner B (2000) Seven years of clinical experience with the programmable Codman Hakim valve: a retrospective study of 583 patients. J Neurosurg 92:941–948
157. Zemack G, Romner B (2002) Adjustable valves in normal-pressure hydrocephalus: a retrospective study of 218 patients. Neurosurgery 51:1392–1402

Ethics in Neurosurgery for the Elderly

27

Farshad Nassiri and Mark Bernstein

27.1 Introduction

Physicians today are expected to practice effective medicine that is sensitive to many different factors including academics, technology, philosophy, society, and, most importantly at the center of it all, the patient. Oftentimes, doctors are faced with challenging questions that test their morals. In these cases, the fundamental question remains as to "what is the right thing to do?" Bioethics, the study of ethics in medicine, offers reasoning systems including ethical principles and theories that help guide clinicians when approaching such difficult cases.

With the twentieth century witnessing an unprecedented increase in average human life span and with the baby boomer population approaching the latter centuries of their life, neurosurgeons will be faced with a host of challenges, some of which will be addressed in this chapter. In this chapter, we will summarize the ethical theories that may be useful in guiding clinicians through challenging cases, and we will detail the challenges that neurosurgeons may face in obtaining consent, end-of-life discussions, and research and training with elderly patients. In broad strokes, how is consent to be obtained with elderly neurosurgical patients, how will we deal with difficulties divulging important information to our patients and their families, and how should we approach end-of-life decisions in elderly neurosurgical patients?

F. Nassiri, MD • M. Bernstein, MD (✉)
Division of Neurosurgery, Department of Surgery, University of Toronto,
399 Bathurst Street West, Toronto, ON, Canada, M5T2S8
e-mail: mark.bernstein@uhn.ca

© Springer International Publishing Switzerland 2017

M. Berhouma, P. Krolak-Salmon (eds.), *Brain and Spine Surgery in the Elderly*,
DOI 10.1007/978-3-319-40232-1_27

27.2 Ethical Theories

The answers to the above posed questions may seem simple upon first glance, but if delved into further, it may be evident that there is no clear "right" answer. Through philosophical discourse and theological teaching, we have derived different ethical principles and theories to frame our approaches toward complex ethical scenarios. Principlism is derived from the four common moral principles of ethics in modern medicine: autonomy, beneficence, non-maleficence, and justice [6, 12]. Each principle is in theory, as equal to others; however, specific circumstances may require special attention to any one given principle. When principlism is not sufficient, the main ethical theories of utilitarianism and deontology may provide additional guidance [4]. Below we will briefly introduce each principle and theory and how it may be applied in our population of interest.

27.2.1 Autonomy

The principle of autonomy is the principle of free will. In this regard, patients have the right to choose what they want with regard to their health care. The practice of modern medicine is underpinned by our respect for autonomy and can be seen in how we emphasize autonomy when discussing disclosure of information and obtaining informed consent. In neurosurgery, respect for autonomy is challenging as many of our patients are acutely ill and as such are incapable of making their own medical decisions. In elderly neurosurgical patients, this becomes even more challenging, as those who may not be acutely ill may also not be capable of making decisions [26]. Elderly patients have limited "reserve," and with the added neurological insult, their capacity to make medical decisions for themselves diminishes. Surgeons in general overestimate their patients' abilities to make decisions, and therefore treating surgeons should be mindful of this and advocate for second opinion on capacity assessments when uncertain [26].

27.2.2 Beneficence

Beneficence is the principle of "doing good." In keeping with this, therapeutic strategies offered to patients and families should have a substantial chance of benefiting the health of the patient. Elderly neurosurgical patients often have their judgment clouded by both comorbidities and burden of neurological disease and therefore may not be able to judge which therapies may provide benefit for themselves. Moreover, families of patients may advocate for unorthodox or experimental therapy options in hopes that there may be a slight chance for improvement. There is sometimes conflict between the medical team and family's perception of beneficence compared to maleficence on therapies for patients. Neurosurgeons must use the tenet of serving the patient's best interest and should not offer therapy that will not benefit their patient.

27.2.3 Non-maleficence

The principle of non-maleficence is rooted from the guiding tenets of the Hippocratic oath: "primum non-nocere" [11]. In neurosurgery, this principle guides our decision on whether to offer surgery and which type of operation to offer. There are substantial risks to neurosurgical procedures, and these may be acceptable if the intervention may offer substantial benefit. However, the definition of harm becomes increasingly more difficult as patients age. Is death considered to be the penultimate harm? Would an elderly patient who has lived a full life want to live in a compromised neurological condition? Although there is little data to guide our decision-making in these cases, most neurosurgeons would believe that the answer to both of these questions would be no. However, frequently our decisions are at conflict with families who believe that any life may be worth prolonging – the concept of vitalism. Despite these difficult scenarios, neurosurgeons must ensure that their proposed operation is in keeping with the patient's wishes and that they mitigate any risk to their patient.

27.2.4 Justice

In a resource-constrained system, clinicians have the duty to consider the system as a whole in addition to their patient. Neurosurgeons in particular are challenged with triaging exceptionally ill patients into limited operating room times and beds. How should neurosurgeons triage patients with similar pathology and differing ages? For example, should a 50-year-old with GBM take priority over an 80-year-old with GBM? These questions are at the core of the principle of distributive justice, which raises the question of whether elderly neurosurgical patients might be deprived of expedient access to care because of their age. The literature consistently shows that elderly patients continue to benefit from neurosurgical procedures [2, 3, 18, 23]. Perhaps, similar to pediatric neurosurgery, this suggests that a subspecialty of geriatric neurosurgeons will evolve. It is not advisable that elderly patients be denied neurosurgical procedures solely because of their age.

27.2.5 Utilitarianism

When the tenets of principlism do not help a clinician in reaching a decision, other theories of medical ethics may be of help. In utilitarianism, decisions are made based on the act that produces the best outcome for the largest number of people. Here, the intention of a decision is less important than the consequence of the decision, and in fact, the rights of individuals may be trumped to produce the overall best outcome for society. As an extreme application to the geriatric population in a resource-limited society, this may suggest that barring all else being equal, neurosurgery should be reserved for younger patients as they may benefit from more quality of life years gained after an intervention. Using age as a criterion for specific therapies such as heart transplantation and dialysis has been previously described [29]; however, there has been a general movement away from this as it is found that the elderly can equivalently benefit from these procedures.

27.2.6 Deontology

In contrast to utilitarianism, deontology holds that clinicians have duties to do right for all patients. Using this, the motive and "rightness" behind decisions are more important than outcomes themselves. In neurosurgery, the "right" decision is often not clear, and this becomes more difficult with elderly patients. For example, should an 88-year-old patient with significant vascular risk factors undergo aggressive hemicraniectomy for large traumatic acute subdural hematoma? Should an 85-year-old patient undergo aggressive resection for glioblastoma multiforme? In general, the best interest value for patients can be applied here. For example, maximal safe resection has been shown to be safe and correlated with longer survival times and functional independence for elderly patients with high-grade glioma; therefore, it is not unreasonable to offer elderly patients with GBM aggressive resection [2].

27.3 Informed Consent

The process of informed consent for diagnostic or therapeutic intervention is rooted in our respect for patient autonomy. Physicians and patients engage in shared clinical decision. The concept of consent for a therapeutic procedure and participation in a research study was largely popularized after World War II in the Nuremberg Code. Obtaining informed consent is a delicate process that is more than the acquisition of the patient signature but, rather, a dialogue between the treating surgeon and patient that is built upon the physician-patient relationship. There are five key elements that are critical to obtaining proper informed consent [4]:

1. Competence – the patient must be capable of making decisions regarding their health.
2. Disclosure – surgeons must clearly relay the risks and benefits of their proposed procedure and alternatives to the proposed treatment.
3. Understanding – the patient must understand and appreciate the information disclosed to them.
4. Voluntary – this process must not be coerced.
5. Authorization – the patient must give permission to perform the proposed procedure.

Brain diseases alter the competence of patient's ability to make decisions, and as such these patients are considered to be vulnerable [9, 14]. Elderly neurosurgical patients are at particularly high risk for this. There is currently no known universal tool or guideline for the assessment of capacity in medicine [13].

Validated instruments to assess capacity in Alzheimer's disease have been adapted to be used in neurosurgical population [17]. However, whether these can be reliably adapted for elderly neurosurgical patients is unknown. The treating surgeon should make the determination of capacity. If patients are considered incapable of making specific treatment decisions for themselves and the patient has articulated no known medical directives, the decision at hand is deferred to substitute decision-makers. The hierarchy of substitute decision-makers varies by jurisdiction and is dictated by law; however, generally, substitute decision-makers are family members who may or may not be involved in the patient's life to a significant degree but who feel obligated to help with decision-making. In neurosurgery, patients can be left with debilitating permanent neurological deficits; therefore, it is important for family members to make the best decision for the patient and not for themselves. Lastly, if a patient is considered incapable of providing consent, their involvement in the decision-making should still be encouraged via discussion with, and assent from, the patient, as diminished mental incapacity does not mean the patient's views are irrelevant.

In elderly neurosurgical patients, there is significant risk of perioperative morbidity and mortality, and although not every detail can be relayed, surgeons must remain patient and truthful with patients and their families during the consent process [8]. Unfortunately the rate of recall of disclosed information remains low after the consent process [22], and therefore neurosurgeons should be extra mindful to make additional efforts to ensure that patients understand material risks. It is important to note that understanding does not correlate with delayed recall – in fact, patients may have a good general understanding despite having impaired recall of risks. Simple repeating of one's understanding of disclosed information and consequences of procedures/alternatives may prove to be of sufficient value to determine if patients and/or families understand the risks behind the proposed surgery [25].

For elderly patients, neurosurgeons should ensure that extraneous factors do not contribute to a lack of understanding during consent discussions. For example, if applicable, patients should have their hearing aids inserted and turned on, their dentures in, etc. Surgeons should speak clearly and may need to write down information for their patients. Conversations regarding consent should be held at appropriate hours during the day when patients are less likely to be confused. Moreover, delirium should be managed appropriately prior to commencing discussions regarding consent, if necessary. Lastly, neurosurgeons should ensure that anesthesiologists see their elderly patients in consultation preoperatively, both in urgent but non-emergent scenarios. Elderly neurosurgical patients tend to have significant comorbidities, some of which require optimizing preoperatively and some of which are noteworthy intraoperatively. Moreover, the risks of anesthesia in elderly patients can be a significant part of the risk discussion with patients. Preoperatively anesthesiology consults allow for optimization and planning from an anesthetic induction and intraoperative monitoring perspective [27]. Moreover, it is noteworthy that some awake craniotomies have specific risks that are inherent to the procedure that the patient will need to understand about but may not tolerate [19].

27.4 Confidentiality

Confidentiality is the right of the patient to not have his or her own medical information disclosed to anyone who he/she does not want to have involved in his/her own care. There are few circumstances where doctors are required to breach confidentiality, and these usually involve the law or the greater good of society [20]. Nevertheless, confidentiality is unfortunately breached on a daily basis despite the best intention of the treating neurosurgeon.

For example, with elderly patients, neurosurgeons must speak clearly and sometimes loudly, as some of them suffer from presbycusis. As a result, the patient's neighbors in the room (and their visiting families and friends) are usually well aware of the diagnosis of the patient, their treatment plan, and any neurological deficits. Moreover, these patients are most often not independent at home, and family members and/or friends are heavily involved in their care. As such, neurosurgeons are frequently asked for updates regarding their medical progress. Although family and friends are generally well intended, neurosurgeons must ensure that patients have provided consent for release of information to each particular family member. Although this is practically difficult, it would be inadvisable to release information otherwise. It would be best if neurosurgeons retrieved consent for disclosure of their medical information from patients prior to the start of their medical treatment to ensure confidentiality is respected at all times [4].

27.5 End of Life

By nature of the specialty and disease processes, neurosurgeons are frequently involved in end-of-life care decisions with patients and family members. Elderly patients are frequently burdened by multiple medical comorbidities that complicate their neurosurgical prognosis, thereby making life-sustaining efforts more difficult.

End-of-life discussions with family are always challenging. There are multiple models of end-of-life decision-making, but most western centers utilize a shared decision-making model, whereby the neurosurgical and intensive care staff attempt to learn about the patient's values and goals of care (which may or may not include specific cultural and religious components) and simultaneously share information with patient families to reach a shared understanding and decision [31].

Decisions regarding the goals of care toward the end of life usually end in one of four conclusions [4]:

1. Continuing aggressive care without any limitations
2. Limiting escalation of care (basic medical care only without aggressive interventions such as intubation, cardiopulmonary resuscitation)
3. Not performing interventions on terminally ill patients (palliative comfort measures only)
4. Withdrawal of life-sustaining treatments

One major limitation in discussions of end-of-life care for elderly neurosurgical patients is the uncertainty of prognosis. Physicians rely on a combination of bedside monitoring, clinical examination, imaging, electrophysiology, and biomarkers to determine prognosis. However, among neurosurgeons and intensivist who frequently care for patients with severe traumatic brain injuries, for example, there is significant variation in perceptions of neurological prognosis. Moreover, overall, neurosurgeons are uncomfortable at suggesting withdrawal of life support measures as an initial management plan [21, 28]. The uncertainty and variability in prognostication among elderly neurosurgical patients can lead to confusion among family members regarding end-of-life care decisions. Moreover, these decisions usually depend on degree of functional independence and quality of life, both of which are extremely subjective concepts. Neurosurgeons should keep this in mind during discussion of goals of care with elderly neurosurgical patients and families and should remain truthful and answer questions to the best of their abilities [16]. Unfortunately, sometimes these conversations lead to conflict and disagreement between patients and families and the treating physicians. Usually this leads to physician disengagement from further end-of-life discussions. However, when neurosurgeons have difficulty or are at conflict with family in regard to end-of-life decision-making, an interdisciplinary ethics committee may be helpful in consultation for further guidance [10, 15].

27.6 Training and Research

The care of elderly neurosurgical patients is extremely complex. There are few treatment paradigms that have been shown to be effective specifically for geriatric neurosurgical patients. Given the complexity of this population, it is possible that a subspecialty of geriatric neurosurgeons will develop and evolve. In fact, gaps in geriatric general surgery have been identified, and as such formal geriatric surgical education has been incorporated into the curriculum for general surgical residents [5, 24, 30].

Neurosurgeons who are employed at academic centers have a duty to train residents to become excellent clinicians and surgeons [7]. Trainees on the other hand have the privilege to operate under direct supervision with a graduated level of responsibility. Given that elderly patients generally portend a poorer prognosis compared to a younger cohort of patients, residents and faculty neurosurgeons may have a more nihilistic attitude toward the care of elderly patients and neurosurgical diseases. Although data to support this do not exist, trainees may therefore be given the opportunity to perform procedures that are above or at the edge of their level of surgical training and that they may not otherwise perform on a younger patient. Both faculty and trainees have the duty to provide the patient the best care they can provide, and as such, it is important that both residents and faculty try to remain cognizant of this and refrain from "practicing" on older patients.

Similarly, neurosurgeons are routinely involved in many different types of research, some of which include the involvement of patients. Elderly neurosurgical patients are frequently excluded from neurosurgical trials. However, it has been demonstrated that trials designed specifically for elderly patients have proven efficacy of treatment, and therefore future studies should continue to include elderly neurosurgical patients to expand our indications for treatment of neurosurgical diseases in the elderly and shed more light or their efficacy or lack thereof [1].

27.7 A Case Vignette

It is easy to speak regarding ethical theories and tenets, but it is sometimes difficult to appreciate the nuances in practice. Herein we present a case of an elderly neurosurgical patient with a malignant brain tumor who presented to our institution with a presumed malignant brain tumor. The patient is an 81-year-old female who lives at home with her children. She presented to a peripheral hospital with gradual progressive right-sided hemiparesis and dysphasia for 2 months. She always had a fear of physicians, and as a result, her presentation was delayed. At the time of presentation, she had been non-ambulatory for a few weeks. She was dependent on her children for most of her activities of daily living. MRI showed a left-sided frontotemporal irregular ring-enhancing brain lesion, favored to be glioblastoma (Fig. 27.1). At the time of our initial assessment, the patient requested that the majority of the discussions regarding her care be taken between the medical team and her children and not herself, but she was aware that she had a serious brain tumor. Both aggressive surgical resection and purely palliative options were discussed with the family on the first visit, and the family initially decided to forego surgery and pursue palliation and went home to consider the options. The family discussed options further with the patient, and when reviewed a week after the first visit, the patient herself wanted to pursue aggressive resection as a treatment strategy. The patient underwent an awake left frontal craniotomy and aggressive resection of tumor. In spite of the MRI appearance, the tumor was solid, not cystic. There were no postoperative complications, and almost immediately after the surgery, she was brighter and speaking better, and this improved further over the next few weeks. She was discharged to her home on postoperative day 1. Her pathology came back as glioblastoma with IDH mutation status negative and MGMT methylation negative. The patient was referred to neuro-oncology and was offered adjuvant chemoradiation. She was also referred to the palliative service for home support with physicians and nurses.

In this case we were faced with multiple difficult decisions and ethical dilemmas. Firstly, although the patient had the capacity to consent to procedure, she preferred that the informed consent discussions were held primarily with her family. Although she knew she had a malignant brain tumor and knew that she was to have surgery, she probably did not fully understand the details of the risks and benefits proposed. However, she was deemed capable of making decisions for herself and she deferred the decisions for surgery to her children. Nevertheless, we were careful to ensure

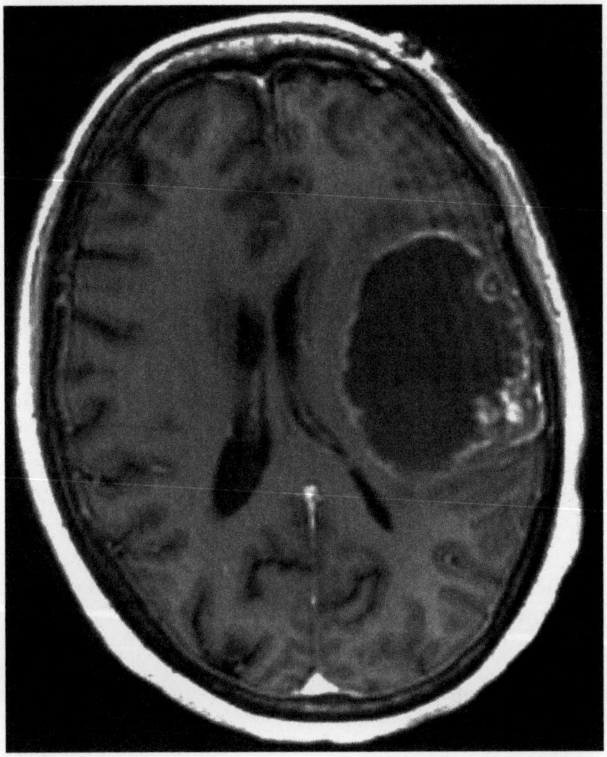

Fig. 27.1 Axial T1-weighted MR images of the brain showing an irregular large left frontal ring-enhancing lesion, compatible with glioblastoma

that we had assent from the patient before continuing with surgery. Moreover, when the patient and her family declined surgery initially, they were offered the opportunity to further consider the options. The patient and her family came to their own decision for surgery on their own terms without coercion. Lastly, the surgery certainly had a large risk of resulting in worsened deficits; however, we felt that with aggressive radiation and treatment, we may have been able to prolong her survival and possibly improve her quality of life. The family understood that her hemiparesis was likely to not improve substantially and in fact may have worsened, and this was a deficit that the patient was willing to accept.

Conclusions

The elderly population represents a growing and especially vulnerable population in neurosurgery. The paucity of available evidence in this cohort leads to many uncertainties in patient care, and therefore neurosurgeons are frequently met with challenging decisions with elderly patients. These patients are burdened by comorbidities and significant intracranial disease that may alter their capacity to make decisions. Neurosurgeons should involve both patients and families in decision-making and use ethical theories and tenets to guide patients through challenging moral decisions.

References

1. Abhinav K, Aquilina K, Gbejuade H, La M, Hopkins K, Iyer V (2013) A pilot study of glioblastoma multiforme in elderly patients: treatments, O-6-methylguanine-DNA methyltransferase (MGMT) methylation status and survival. Clin Neurol Neurosurg 115(8):1375–1378. doi:10.1016/j.clineuro.2012.12.023
2. Almenawer SA, Badhiwala JH, Alhazzani W, Greenspoon J, Farrokhyar F, Yarascavitch B, Algird A, Kachur E, Cenic A, Sharieff W, Klurfan P, Gunnarsson T, Ajani O, Reddy K, Singh SK, Murty NK (2015) Biopsy versus partial versus gross total resection in older patients with high-grade glioma: a systematic review and meta-analysis. Neuro Oncol 17(6):868–881. doi:10.1093/neuonc/nou349
3. Amagasaki K, Watanabe S, Naemura K, Shono N, Nakaguchi H (2016) Safety of microvascular decompression for elderly patients with trigeminal neuralgia. Clin Neurol Neurosurg 141:77–81. doi:10.1016/j.clineuro.2015.12.019
4. Ammar A, Bernstein M (2014) Neurosurgical ethics in practice: value-based medicine. Springer, Heidelberg
5. Barbas AS, Haney JC, Henry BV, Heflin MT, Lagoo SA (2014) Development and implementation of a formalized geriatric surgery curriculum for general surgery residents. Gerontol Geriatr Educ 35(4):380–394. doi:10.1080/02701960.2013.879444
6. Beauchamp TL, Childress JF (2001) Principles of biomedical ethics, 5th edn. Oxford University Press Incorporated, New York
7. Bernstein M (2003) Surgical teaching: how should neurosurgeons handle the conflict of duty to today's patients with the duty to tomorrow's? Br J Neurosurg 17(2):121–123
8. Bernstein M (2005) Fully informed consent is impossible in surgical clinical trials. Can J Surg 48(4):271–272
9. Bernstein M (2014) Neuro-oncology: under-recognized mental incapacity in brain tumour patients. Nat Rev Neurol 10(9):487–488. doi:10.1038/nrneurol.2014.143
10. Bernstein M, Bowman K (2003) Should a medical/surgical specialist with formal training in bioethics provide health care ethics consultation in his/her own area of speciality? HEC Forum 15(3):274–286
11. Brewin T (1994) Primum non nocere? Lancet 344(8935):1487–1488
12. Deigh J (2001) The Cambridge dictionary of philosophy, 2nd edn. Cambridge University Press, Cambridge
13. Etchells E, Sharpe G, Elliott C, Singer PA (1996) Bioethics for clinicians: 3. Capacity. CMAJ 155(6):657–661
14. Ford PJ (2009) Vulnerable brains: research ethics and neurosurgical patients. J Law Med Ethics 37(1):73–82. doi:10.1111/j.1748-720X.2009.00352.x
15. Ford PJ, Kubu CS (2006) Stimulating debate: ethics in a multidisciplinary functional neurosurgery committee. J Med Ethics 32(2):106–109. doi:10.1136/jme.200X.013151
16. Hebert PC, Hoffmaster B, Glass KC, Singer PA (1997) Bioethics for clinicians: 7. Truth telling. CMAJ 156(2):225–228
17. Johnson-Greene D (2010) Informed consent issues in traumatic brain injury research: current status of capacity assessment and recommendations for safeguards. J Head Trauma Rehabil 25(2):145–150. doi:10.1097/HTR.0b013e3181d8287d
18. Jordan JT, Gerstner ER, Batchelor TT, Cahill DP, Plotkin SR (2016) Glioblastoma care in the elderly. Cancer 122(2):189–197. doi:10.1002/cncr.29742
19. Kirsch B, Bernstein M (2012) Ethical challenges with awake craniotomy for tumor. Can J Neurol Sci 39(1):78–82
20. Kleinman I, Baylis F, Rodgers S, Singer P (1997) Bioethics for clinicians: 8. Confidentiality. CMAJ 156(4):521–524
21. Kritek PA, Slutsky AS, Hudson LD (2009) Clinical decisions. Care of an unresponsive patient with a poor prognosis – polling results. N Engl J Med 360(10):e15. doi:10.1056/NEJMclde0900810

22. Krupp W, Spanehl O, Laubach W, Seifert V (2000) Informed consent in neurosurgery: patients' recall of preoperative discussion. Acta Neurochir (Wien) 142(3):233–238; discussion 238–239
23. O'Lynnger TM, Zuckerman SL, Morone PJ, Dewan MC, Vasquez-Castellanos RA, Cheng JS (2015) Trends for spine surgery for the elderly: implications for access to healthcare in North America. Neurosurgery 77(Suppl 4):S136–S141. doi:10.1227/NEU.0000000000000945
24. Petronovich J, Wade TJ, Denson K, Webb TP (2014) Elderly surgical patients: are there gaps in residency education? J Surg Educ 71(6):825–828. doi:10.1016/j.jsurg.2014.04.001
25. Schmitz D, Reinacher PC (2006) Informed consent in neurosurgery – translating ethical theory into action. J Med Ethics 32(9):497–498. doi:10.1136/jme.2005.013144
26. Terranova C, Cardin F, Pietra LD, Zen M, Bruttocao A, Militello C (2013) Ethical and medico-legal implications of capacity of patients in geriatric surgery. Med Sci Law 53(3):166–171. doi:10.1177/0025802412473963
27. Thilen SR, Wijeysundera DN, Treggiari MM (2016) Preoperative consultations. Anesthesiol Clin 34(1):17–33. doi:10.1016/j.anclin.2015.10.003
28. Turgeon AF, Lauzier F, Burns KE, Meade MO, Scales DC, Zarychanski R, Moore L, Zygun DA, McIntyre LA, Kanji S, Hebert PC, Murat V, Pagliarello G, Fergusson DA, Canadian Critical Care Trials Group (2013) Determination of neurologic prognosis and clinical decision making in adult patients with severe traumatic brain injury: a survey of Canadian intensivists, neurosurgeons, and neurologists. Crit Care Med 41(4):1086–1093. doi:10.1097/CCM.0b013e318275d046
29. U.S. Congress OoTA (1987) Life sustaining technologies and the elderly. U.S. Government Printing Office, Washington, DC
30. Webb TP, Duthie E Jr (2008) Geriatrics for surgeons: infusing life into an aging subject. J Surg Educ 65(2):91–94. doi:10.1016/j.jsurg.2007.12.004
31. White DB, Braddock CH 3rd, Bereknyei S, Curtis JR (2007) Toward shared decision making at the end of life in intensive care units: opportunities for improvement. Arch Intern Med 167(5):461–467. doi:10.1001/archinte.167.5.461

Erratum to: Trigeminal Neuralgia in the Elderly

Jonathan Cohen, Hossein Mousavi, and Raymond F. Sekula Jr.

Erratum to:
Chapter 24 in M. Berhouma, P. Krolak-Salmon (eds.), *Brain and Spine Surgery in the Elderly*, DOI 10.1007/978-3-319-40232-1_24

In the chapter titled 'Trigeminal Neuralgia in the Elderly' the affiliation of authors Jonathan Cohen and Hossein Mousavi was incorrect and has been updated in chapter 24 and in the list of contributors.

The correct affiliation is:
J. Cohen • H. Mousavi • R.F. Sekula Jr. (✉)
University of Pittsburgh, Pittsburgh, PA, USA
e-mail: rsekula@wpahs.org

The updated online version of the original chapter can be found under
DOI 10.1007/978-3-319-40232-1_24

J. Cohen • H. Mousavi • R.F. Sekula Jr. (✉)
University of Pittsburgh, Pittsburgh, PA, USA
e-mail: rsekula@wpahs.org

© Springer International Publishing Switzerland 2017

M. Berhouma, P. Krolak-Salmon (eds.), *Brain and Spine Surgery in the Elderly*,
DOI 10.1007/978-3-319-40232-1_28

Appendix: Scores and Scales

1. Muscle Strength Grading Scale
2. Frailty index
3. Karnofsky Performance Scale (KPS)
4. Nurick grading system (cervical myelopathy)
5. Clinical–Radiological Grading System (CRGS) – Meningiomas
6. Modified SKALE (Sex, Karnofsky, ASA, Location, Edema) grading system – Meningiomas
7. The Geriatric Scoring System (GSS) – Meningiomas
8. Markwalder grading (chronic subdural hematoma)

© Springer International Publishing Switzerland 2017

M. Berhouma, P. Krolak-Salmon (eds.), *Brain and Spine Surgery in the Elderly*,
DOI 10.1007/978-3-319-40232-1

Muscle Strength Grading Scale

0/5	No movement
1/5	Barest flicker of movement of the muscle, though not enough to move the structure to which it is attached
2/5	Voluntary movement that is not sufficient to overcome the force of gravity. For example, the patient would be able to slide their hand across a table but not lift it from the surface
3/5	Voluntary movement capable of overcoming gravity, but not any applied resistance. For example, the patient could raise their hand off a table, but not if any additional resistance were applied
4/5	Voluntary movement capable of overcoming "some" resistance
5/5	Normal strength

Frailty index

Deficits counted	Points (max denominator 55)
Cognition	Dementia = 1, mild cog. imp. = 0.5, delirium = 1, agitation = 1, delusions/hallucinations = 1
Emotional state	Anxiety = 1, recent bereavement = 1, depression = 1, fatigue = 1
Sleep	Poor or disrupted = 1, drowsiness = 1
Speech, hearing, vision	Impaired = 1 each
Hemiparesis	Weak arm = 1, weak leg = 1
Grip strength or proximal muscle strength (on non-hemiplegic side)	Weak = 1 each
Weight or weight change	Underweight = 1, obese = 1, slightly overweight = 0, loss = 1, gain = 1
Appetite	Poor = 1, fair = 0.5, normal = 0
Continence	Bowels or bladder incontinent = 1 each
Medical history (scoring 1 point each)	Hypertension, asthma/COPD, stroke/transient ischemic attack, angina/myocardial infarction, heart failure, diabetes, cancer, alcohol excess, pressure sores, hip fracture. osteoarthritis/osteoporosis, Parkinson's
No. of medications in 24 h	0–4 = 0, 5–9 = 1, 10–14 = 2, 15–19 = 3, 20–24 = 4, >25 = 5
Transfers or walking	Dependent = 1, assistance = 0.5
Movements slow	Yes = 1
Sitting balance	Impaired = 1
Falls in the last 6 months	3 or more = 1
Feeding, washing, and dressing (1 each)	Dependent = 1, assistance = 0.5
Manages own medications and finances	Dependent = 1, assistance = 0.5

Karnofsky Performance Scale (KPS)

Condition	%	Description
Able to carry on normal activity and to work. No special care is needed	100	Normal, no complaints, no evidence of disease
	90	Able to carry on normal activity, minor signs or symptoms of disease
	80	Normal activity with effort, some signs or symptoms of disease
Unable to work. Able to live at home, care for most personal needs. A varying degree of assistance is needed	70	Cares for self. Unable to carry on normal activity or to so active work
	60	Requires occasional assistance, but is able to care for most of his needs
	50	Requires considerable assistance and frequent medical care
Unable to care for self. Requires equivalent of institutional or hospital care. Disease may be progressing rapidly	40	Disabled, requires special care and assistance
	30	Severely disabled, hospitalization is indicated although death not imminent
	20	Hospitalization necessary, very sick, active supportive treatment necessary
	10	Hospitalization necessary, very sick, active supportive treatment necessary

Nurick grading system (cervical myelopathy)

Grading	Signs of myelopathy	Gait	Daily activities/working
0	No	Normal	No limitations
1	Yes	Normal	No limitations
2	Yes	Slight disturbance	No limitations
3	Yes	Significant disturbance	Limitations
4	Yes	Only with support	Not possible
5	Yes	Wheel chair/bedridden	Not possible

Clinical–Radiological Grading System (CRGS) – Meningiomas

	Score		
Factor	1	2	3
Size of lesion (cm)	6	4–6	<4
Neurological condition[a]	Unrecoverable	Progressive	No deficits
KPS score	≤50	60–80	90–100
Critical location[b]	Highly	Moderately	Not critical
Peritumoral edema[c]	Severe	Moderate	Absent
Concomitant disease(s)[d]	Decompensated	Compensated	Absent

[a]Unrecoverable deficits: deficits complete and stabilized (e.g., hemiplegia or amaurosis); progressive deficits: deficits incomplete or worsening (e.g., hemiparesis or impairment of visual acuity)
[b]A critical location is present if the tumor is attached to a primary vascular or nervous structure (such as the cranial base or an eloquent area)
[c]Peritumoral edema is classified as moderate (only peritumoral) and severe (with a shift of midline structures)
[d]Concomitant diseases were evaluated as being compensated (controlled by medical therapy) or decompensated (uncontrolled despite medical therapy)

Modified SKALE (Sex, Karnofsky, ASA, Location, Edema) grading system – Meningiomas

	Score		
Factors	0	2	4
Sex	M	F	–
Karnofsky score	≤50	60–70	≥80
ASA class	IV	III	I or II
Location	Highly	Moderately	Not critical
Edema	Severe	Moderate	No edema

The Geriatric Scoring System (GSS) – Meningiomas

Admission parameter	1 point	2 points	3 points
Size	>5 cm	3–5 cm	<3 cm
Neurological deficit	Progressive	Stable severe	None, minor
Karnofsky Performance Scale	<50	60–80	90–100
Tumor location	Falcine, parasagittal Foramen magnum	Tentorial Posterior fossa Jugular foramen	Convexity Intraventricular Sphenoid wing Tuberculum sellae Cavernous sinus Optic nerve
Peritumoral edema	Severe	Mild	None
Diabetes mellitus	Not controlled	Medically controlled	None
Hypertension	Not controlled	Medically controlled	None
Pulmonary disease	Severe	Mild	None

Markwalder grading (chronic subdural hematoma)

Grade	Symptoms and signs
0	Patient neurologically normal
1	Patient alert and orientated; mild symptoms such as headache; absent or mild neurological deficit such as reflex asymmetry
2	Patient drowsy or disorientated with variable neurological deficit, such as hemiparesis
3	Patient stuporous but responding appropriately to noxious stimuli; severe focal signs such as hemiplegia
4	Patient comatose with absent motor responses to painful stimuli; decerebrate or decorticate posturing

Index

© Springer International Publishing Switzerland 2017
M. Berhouma, P. Krolak-Salmon (eds.), *Brain and Spine Surgery in the Elderly*,
DOI 10.1007/978-3-319-40232-1

Q

W

Z

CPI Antony Rowe
Chippenham, UK
2017-09-12 21:37